Sarcopenia

Sarcopenia

Molecular Mechanism and Treatment Strategies

Edited by

Kunihiro Sakuma
Physiologist, Tokyo Institute of Technology, Japan

ELSEVIER

Elsevier
Radarweg 29, PO Box 211, 1000 AE Amsterdam, Netherlands
The Boulevard, Langford Lane, Kidlington, Oxford OX5 1GB, United Kingdom
50 Hampshire Street, 5th Floor, Cambridge, MA 02139, United States

Copyright © 2021 Elsevier Inc. All rights reserved.

No part of this publication may be reproduced or transmitted in any form or by any means, electronic or mechanical, including photocopying, recording, or any information storage and retrieval system, without permission in writing from the publisher. Details on how to seek permission, further information about the Publisher's permissions policies and our arrangements with organizations such as the Copyright Clearance Center and the Copyright Licensing Agency, can be found at our website: www.elsevier.com/permissions.

This book and the individual contributions contained in it are protected under copyright by the Publisher (other than as may be noted herein).

Notices

Knowledge and best practice in this field are constantly changing. As new research and experience broaden our understanding, changes in research methods, professional practices, or medical treatment may become necessary.

Practitioners and researchers must always rely on their own experience and knowledge in evaluating and using any information, methods, compounds, or experiments described herein. In using such information or methods they should be mindful of their own safety and the safety of others, including parties for whom they have a professional responsibility.

To the fullest extent of the law, neither the Publisher nor the authors, contributors, or editors, assume any liability for any injury and/or damage to persons or property as a matter of products liability, negligence or otherwise, or from any use or operation of any methods, products, instructions, or ideas contained in the material herein.

Library of Congress Cataloging-in-Publication Data
A catalog record for this book is available from the Library of Congress

British Library Cataloguing-in-Publication Data
A catalogue record for this book is available from the British Library

ISBN: 978-0-12-822146-4

For information on all Elsevier publications
visit our website at https://www.elsevier.com/books-and-journals

Publisher: Stacy Masucci
Acquisitions Editor: Ana Claudia A. Garcia
Editorial Project Manager: Sam W. Young
Production Project Manager: Niranjan Bhaskaran
Cover Designer: Miles Hitchen

Typeset by SPi Global, India

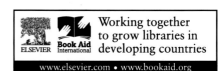

Contents

Contributors xi

Chapter 1: Linking mitochondrial dysfunction to sarcopenia 1
Stephen E. Alway

    Introduction 1
    Sarcopenia and mitochondrial function 2
    Potential sources of mitochondrial dysfunction in aging 3
        Reactive oxygen species-induced damage 3
        Mitochondrial DNA damage and aging 5
        Altered mitochondrial dynamics with aging 5
        Association of reduced activity and mitochondrial dysfunction
            in sarcopenia 7
        Calcium-induced dysregulation of mitochondria in sarcopenia 8
    Mitochondria initiate and mediate cell death signaling in sarcopenia 11
        Mitochondrial-induced nuclear apoptosis in aging muscle 11
        Activation of the mitochondrial permeability transition pore accelerates
            apoptosis in sarcopenia 14
        Mitochondria dysfunction may regulate a fiber type-specific loss
            in sarcopenia 15
    Mitochondrially regulated loss of motor function and mobility in sarcopenia 16
        Motor neurons 16
        Mitochondrial regulation of neural dysfunction in sarcopenia 16
    PGC-1α regulation of mitochondria in sarcopenia 17
        PGC-1α regulation of mitochondria 17
        PGC-1α in mitochondria of aged muscles 17
        PGC-1α regulation of mitochondria in motor neurons 18
    Autophagy/mitophagy and mitochondrial dysfunction in sarcopenia 18
        Removal of dysfunctional mitochondria by mitophagy 18
        Insufficient mitophagy allows unhealthy mitochondria to persist in
            aging muscles 21
    Linking autophagy and apoptosis 22
        BIM and Bcl-2 23
        PGC-1α 23
    Mitochondria, mitophagy, and the ubiquitin-proteasome system 23
        Muscle wasting 23

UPS and sarcopenia 24
UPS and neural dysfunction in aging...26
Mitophagy regulation and the UPS..27
UPS disruption increases dysfunctional mitochondria in muscle and
    neural cells 28
Mitochondrial associated apoptosis, mitophagy, and UPS can be modulated
    by caloric restriction in sarcopenia...28
Conclusions 31
References 32

Chapter 2: The role of the neuromuscular junction in sarcopenia 59
Michael R. Deschenes, Jeongeun Oh, and Hannah Tufts

Introduction 59
Age-related structural adaptations of the NMJ................................61
Age-related functional adaptations of the NMJ...............................66
Preventing and managing the effects of aging on the NMJ 69
Role of NMJ in sarcopenia 70
References 75

Chapter 3: Dietary approaches to maintaining muscle mass 81
Rafael A. Alamilla, Kevin J.M. Paulussen, Andrew T. Askow, and
Nicholas A. Burd

Introduction 81
Dietary protein quality 82
    Defining high-quality protein sources...82
    Plant-based protein sources..84
    Animal-based protein sources..86
    Leucine as a determinant of protein quality................................87
Dietary protein quantity 89
    Protein intake above the RDA 90
    The importance of protein distribution across the day...............91
Dietary considerations for older adults...92
    Dietary protein intake consideration for older adults................93
    Impact of leucine on muscle mass maintenance in older adults 95
Dietary approaches to preserving and gaining muscle mass in those
    with sarcopenia 96
    Dietary protein and amino acid interventions in older adults with
        sarcopenia 97
Conclusions and future work 99
References 100

Chapter 4: Role of muscle stem cells in sarcopenia 109
Ryo Fujita

Introduction 109
Muscle stem cells..111

Support cells that influence the satellite cell activity during regeneration 114
Satellite cell function in aging 116
    Intrinsic changes in muscle stem cells with aging 116
    Extrinsic changes in muscle stem cells with aging 118
Satellite cells and muscle adaptation 120
    Satellite cell in muscle hypertrophy 120
    Satellite cells in muscle atrophy 122
Satellite cells and exercise to combat sarcopenia 126
Concluding remarks 127
Acknowledgment 128
References 129

Chapter 5: Sarcopenia and the inflammatory cytokines 139
Arkadiusz Orzechowski (Bernard)

Histology of skeletal muscle 139
Composition of skeletal muscle 141
Inflammatory response in skeletal muscle 141
Mediators of inflammation 144
Myostatin 145
Interactions between myofibers and adipocytes 145
Proresolving lipid mediators 147
Concluding remarks 151
References 152

Chapter 6: Molecular mechanisms of exercise providing therapeutic rationale to counter sarcopenia 159
Ki-Sun Kwon

Introduction 159
Gene set analysis of exercise that oppose sarcopenia 160
Exercise-induced molecular signaling in skeletal muscle 161
Systemic functions of myokines induced by exercise 162
Exercise mimetics targeting AMPK and PPARβ/δ pathway 163
Anabolic hormones effects on skeletal muscle 163
Roles of autophagy pathway in skeletal muscle 165
Conclusion 166
Acknowledgment 166
References 166

Chapter 7: Myokines: A potential key factor in development, treatment, and biomarker of sarcopenia 171
Wataru Aoi

Introduction 171
The role of myokines in myogenesis 173
The role of myokines in protein anabolism and catabolism 175
MicroRNAs and metabolites as myokines 177

Contents

Perspective 179
References 180

Chapter 8: Defect of autophagy signaling in sarcopenic muscle 187
Kunihiro Sakuma, Akihiko Yamaguchi, and Haruyo Matsuo

Introduction 187
Autophagy-dependent signaling 188
Autophagic adaptation in sarcopenic muscle 190
    Autophagic defect 190
    Possible molecules modulating autophagic defect 192
Factors modulating autophagic defect in sarcopenia 193
    Denervation 193
    Unloading 195
    Cachexia 196
Several therapeutic strategies attenuating sarcopenia due to
    autophagic-activation 197
    Exercise 197
    Calorie restriction 198
    Supplemental approach 199
    Hormonal treatment 200
Concluding remarks 200
Acknowledgments 200
References 200

Chapter 9: Mitophagy in sarcopenic muscle and practical recommendations for exercise training 207
Anthony M.J. Sanchez and Robert Solsona

Introduction 207
Autophagy and mitochondrial dysfunction during aging 209
    Autophagy in skeletal muscle 209
    Mitochondrial dysfunction during aging 212
Parkin pathway in sarcopenia 214
Mul1 and Mdm2 in skeletal muscle mitophagy: Perspectives in
    sarcopenia 216
Exercise modalities and practical recommendations for
    aging people 218
Conclusions and perspectives 220
Acknowledgments 220
Conflict of interest 220
References 221

Chapter 10: Underlying mechanisms of sarcopenic obesity 231
Melanie Rauen, Leo Cornelius Bollheimer, and Mahtab Nourbakhsh

Introduction 231
Diagnostic criteria 232

Obesity 232
　　Sarcopenia 233
　　Sarcopenic obesity 233
　Pathogenesis of sarcopenic obesity 234
　　Metabolism 235
　　Muscle atrophy 239
　　Growth hormones 240
　Intervention strategies in sarcopenic obesity 240
　Conclusion 241
　References 242

Chapter 11: Vascular aging and sarcopenia: Interactions with physiological functions during exercise 249
Naoyuki Hayashi

　Introduction 249
　Role of peripheral blood flow during exercise 250
　Loss of vascular functions relevant to sarcopenia 251
　　Skeletal-muscle vessels 252
　　Cerebral vessels 252
　　Ocular vessels 254
　　Splanchnic vessels 255
　　Skin vessels 256
　　Veins 257
　Other factors resulting in circulatory impairments related
　　to aging 257
　　Central arteries 257
　　Baroreflex 257
　　Blood volume 258
　Possible counteractions to vessel aging 258
　Summary 259
　References 260

Chapter 12: Dysphagia of cachexia and sarcopenia 267
Haruyo Matsuo and Kunihiro Sakuma

　Introduction 267
　Cachexia 268
　　Definition of cachexia 268
　　Condition of cachexia 269
　Sarcopenia 270
　　Definition of sarcopenia 270
　　Condition of sarcopenia 271
　Dysphagia 274
　　Definition of dysphagia 274
　Conclusions 283
　References 283

Contents

Chapter 13: Mechanisms of decline in muscle quality in sarcopenia 295
Takashi Yamada

    Introduction 295
    A decline in muscle quality in sarcopenia 296
    Age-related alterations in intracellular activation-contraction pathway in skeletal muscle fibers 301
    Decreased Ca^{2+} release from the sarcoplasmic reticulum in skeletal muscle fiber from aged subjects 302
    Reduced myofibrillar Ca^{2+} sensitivity in skeletal muscle fiber from aged subjects 303
    Decreased ability of the cross-bridges to generate force in skeletal muscle fiber from aged subjects 304
    Mechanisms behind intrinsic contractile dysfunction in skeletal muscle fiber from aged subjects: Role of disuse 306
    Mechanisms behind intrinsic contractile dysfunction in skeletal muscle fiber from aged subjects: Role of reactive oxygen/nitrogen species (ROS/RNS) 307
        Accelerated reactive oxygen/nitrogen species (ROS/RNS) in skeletal muscle fiber from aged subjects 308
        Increased susceptibility of regulatory proteins to oxidative modification in skeletal muscle fiber 311
    Interventions to counteract the age-related loss of muscle quality 312
    Concluding remarks 313
    References 313

Index 323

Contributors

Rafael A. Alamilla Department of Kinesiology and Community Health, University of Illinois at Urbana-Champaign, Urbana, IL, United States

Stephen E. Alway Laboratory of Muscle Biology and Sarcopenia, Center for Muscle, Metabolism and Neuropathology, Department of Physical Therapy, College of Health Professions; Department of Physiology, College of Medicine, The University of Tennessee Health Science Center, Memphis, TN, United States

Wataru Aoi Laboratory of Nutrition Science, Graduate School of Life and Environmental Sciences, Kyoto Prefectural University, Kyoto, Japan

Andrew T. Askow Department of Kinesiology and Community Health, University of Illinois at Urbana-Champaign, Urbana, IL, United States

Leo Cornelius Bollheimer Geriatric Medicine (Medical Clinic VI), RWTH Aachen University Hospital, Aachen, Germany

Nicholas A. Burd Department of Kinesiology and Community Health; Division of Nutritional Sciences, University of Illinois at Urbana-Champaign, Urbana, IL, United States

Michael R. Deschenes Department of Health Sciences, College of William & Mary, Williamsburg, VA, United States

Ryo Fujita Division of Regenerative Medicine, Transborder Medical Research Center, University of Tsukuba, Tsukuba City, Ibaraki, Japan

Naoyuki Hayashi Faculty of Sport Sciences, Waseda University, Saitama, Japan

Ki-Sun Kwon Aging Research Center, Korea Research Institute of Bioscience and Biotechnology; Aventi Inc., Daejeon, Republic of Korea

Haruyo Matsuo Department of Nursing, Kagoshima Medical Association Hospital, Kagoshima, Japan

Mahtab Nourbakhsh Geriatric Medicine (Medical Clinic VI), RWTH Aachen University Hospital, Aachen, Germany

Jeongeun Oh Department of Health Sciences, College of William & Mary, Williamsburg, VA, United States

Arkadiusz Orzechowski (Bernard) Department of Physiological Sciences, Faculty of Veterinary Medicine, Warsaw University of Life Sciences - SGGW, Warsaw, Poland

Contributors

Kevin J.M. Paulussen Department of Kinesiology and Community Health, University of Illinois at Urbana-Champaign, Urbana, IL, United States

Melanie Rauen Geriatric Medicine (Medical Clinic VI), RWTH Aachen University Hospital, Aachen, Germany

Kunihiro Sakuma Institute for Liberal Arts, Environment and Society, Tokyo Institute of Technology, Tokyo, Japan

Anthony M.J. Sanchez Laboratoire Européen Performance Santé Altitude, EA4604, University of Perpignan Via Domitia, Faculty of Sports Sciences, Font-Romeu, France

Robert Solsona Laboratoire Européen Performance Santé Altitude, EA4604, University of Perpignan Via Domitia, Faculty of Sports Sciences, Font-Romeu, France

Hannah Tufts Department of Health Sciences, College of William & Mary, Williamsburg, VA, United States

Takashi Yamada School of Health Sciences, Sapporo Medical University, Sapporo, Japan

Akihiko Yamaguchi Department of Physical Therapy, Health Sciences University of Hokkaido, Ishikari-Tobetsu, Hokkaido, Japan

CHAPTER 1

Linking mitochondrial dysfunction to sarcopenia

Stephen E. Alway

Laboratory of Muscle Biology and Sarcopenia, Center for Muscle, Metabolism and Neuropathology, Department of Physical Therapy, College of Health Professions, The University of Tennessee Health Science Center, Memphis, TN, United States, Department of Physiology, College of Medicine, The University of Tennessee Health Science Center, Memphis, TN, United States

Abstract
Damaged and dysfunctional mitochondria appear to underlie and mediate much of the signaling that initiates and contributes to molecular signaling pathways in sarcopenia. Dysfunctional mitochondria increase the production of reactive oxygen species and DNA damage. Opening of mitochondrial permeability channels releases their contents to the cytosol, which initiates signaling for apoptosis to eliminate proteins close to dysfunctional muscle mitochondria. Disruption of the ubiquitin-proteasome system along with suppressed mitophagy contributes to the failure to remove dysfunctional mitochondria. This results in an accumulation of dysfunctional mitochondria, which magnifies the apoptotic signaling and muscle cell destruction in both muscle and neural cells sarcopenia. Interventions that remove dysfunctional or damaged mitochondria and improve the quality and quantity of healthy mitochondria in sarcopenic muscles would be expected to reverse or prevent sarcopenia in aging. This chapter summarizes the mitochondria dysfunction and the mitochondrial-associated signaling that contributes to sarcopenia.

Keywords: Mitochondria, Apoptosis, Mitophagy, Reactive oxygen species, Atrophy, Muscle function, Fatigue, Strength

Introduction

Although the average lifespan is generally increasing in nonconflict areas, a complication of living longer is manifested through a general systemic deterioration leading to several geriatric syndromes. An important aging-associated deterioration that negatively impacts mobility in aging is sarcopenia, which encompasses the loss of both muscle mass and muscle function [1–3]. Skeletal muscle comprises approximately 40% of the total body mass of young healthy persons. Aging is associated with a loss of muscle mass, which begins even before middle age. Indeed, sarcopenia occurs after the age of 30 with increasing losses of 2% per year after the age of 60, and muscle loss appears to speed up in older ages [4–8]. Sarcopenia increases the susceptibility for obesity and diabetes [9–13], independently lowers mobility and independence [14–17] and increases mortality [18–22]. It is estimated that 20% of the population of the United States (~ 72,000,000 people) will be 65 years of age or older by 2030 [23]. As there is a rapid increase in the world's older population, sarcopenia is becoming an important global public health concern. Although sarcopenia is primarily a skeletal muscle problem, sarcopenia can also be detrimental to other organs and tissues; therefore, understanding the mechanisms and processes underlying muscle loss is critical to developing strategies to stop or reduce sarcopenia.

Several mediators of sarcopenia have been proposed, but it is difficult to establish which of these is responsible for initiating and regulating muscle loss and which ones are a consequence of the processes involved in muscle atrophy. Examples of changes that might contribute to sarcopenia include an increase in low grade but constant systemic inflammation [24, 25], elevated production or reduced buffering of reactive oxygen species [26–29], altered or impaired innervation [30–36], loss of motor units and alpha motor neurons [37–39], reduced regenerative capability [40–44], and decreased mitochondrial function [45–53]. Low physical activity can exacerbate sarcopenia, whereas exercise can at least partially attenuate some of the aging-associated alterations in mitochondrial function in aging [47, 48, 54–57].

Skeletal muscle has two primary muscle fiber types: type I myosin heavy chain containing fibers and type II myosin heavy chain containing fibers, although there is a continuum of myosin types between these two primary fibers [58]. Type I fibers in human muscles have a mitochondrial volume of approximately 6% of the total cell volume, whereas mitochondria occupy only approximately 3% of the volume of type II fibers [59, 60]. Interestingly, type I fibers appear to be more resistant to sarcopenia, and this raises the possibility that mitochondria could be protective in sarcopenia [61–63]. However, this is a complicated area because there is evidence that shows that dysfunctional mitochondria play an important role in regulating the loss of muscle function that is associated with sarcopenia [37, 49, 50, 64–66]. This is because the optimal mitochondrial function is critical for energy delivery and expenditure, but both mitochondria density is decreased and mitochondria function is impaired in aging [46–48, 67–70].

This chapter will provide evidence that the loss of mitochondrial function and mitochondrial content are central to molecular pathways that mediate muscle and motor neuronal loss and contribute to sarcopenia via activation of signaling. Aberrant mitochondrial signaling includes muscle cell disassembly by apoptosis, autophagy, proteasome, and lysosomal pathways [50, 71].

Sarcopenia and mitochondrial function

Sarcopenia reduces muscle fiber mitochondrial volume, content, and enzyme activity [8, 48, 65, 72–80], suppresses metabolism [81–83], lowers respiration [84–88], and reduces mitochondrial biogenesis [77, 89–91]. Part of the decline in mitochondrial content in aging may be the result of an imbalance between mitochondrial removal and mitochondrial biogenesis. Mitochondrial biogenesis is a complex process consisting of synthesis, assembly, growth by fusion, and division of pre-existing mitochondria by fission dynamics and "recycling" and reusing damaged mitochondria via mitophagy signaling.

The mitochondrial DNA gene encodes for a total of 37 genes, which consists of 13 mRNAs encoding for oxidative phosphorylation enzymes (cytochrome oxidase subunits I, II, III, IV, and V) and 2 ribosomal RNAs (rRNAs) and 22 transfer RNAs (tRNAs) encoding for translational proteins [92–95]. This means that most of the mitochondrial proteins are nuclear-encoded, with mitochondrial proteins synthesized in the cytoplasm and then imported into mitochondria. Since mitochondrial biogenesis can be affected at many different levels including transcriptional regulation by deacetylation and mitochondrial transport [96–101], it is important to be cautious when interpreting mitochondrial markers as outcomes for biogenesis, as they may not fully reflect new mitochondrial assembly. Instead, assessment of mitochondrial protein synthesis provides the best approach for measuring mitochondrial biogenesis [102]. An assessment of the balance between mitochondrial biogenesis and removal of dysfunctional mitochondria via mitophagy are key components for preventing the progression of aging-related diseases, including sarcopenia.

It should be noted that the aging-associated loss of mitochondrial respiration and function has been challenged [103, 104], and reductions in mitochondrial function have been attributed more to the lack of use than aging per se [105–107]. Furthermore, improvements in mitochondrial function in sarcopenic muscle can also be achieved by nutritional intervention or buffering of reactive oxygen species (ROS) without changes in mitochondrial biogenesis [8, 108]. Moreover, it has been suggested that changes (or lack of changes) in mitochondrial respiratory function with age may be influenced by sex [109–111], muscle fiber type, or motor unit recruitment patterns [51, 112–116].

Potential sources of mitochondrial dysfunction in aging

Mitochondrial damage occurs in many different tissues, including sarcopenic muscle. Skeletal muscle, like other tissue types, has a loss of mitochondria, reduced mitochondria function, and increased mitochondria damage. Potential factors contributing to mitochondria dysfunction include a chronic increase in basal levels of ROS, which induces cellular and membrane damage, elevates DNA damage, and alters molecular dynamics with aging in muscle.

Reactive oxygen species-induced damage

There is strong evidence that ROS regulates many functions in skeletal muscle [117, 118], but excessive ROS accumulation under basal conditions, as found in muscles of sarcopenic animals and humans, may underlay much of the mitochondrial dysfunction that accompanies aging muscles. Aging tends to increase ROS production in skeletal muscle, and this is further elevated during reduced muscle activity that is typically closely associated with aging. It is, of course, difficult to separate the impact of aging per se from inactivity, which exacerbates the aging-associated increase in ROS production contributing to the loss of both motor neurons and skeletal muscle in mice [39].

There is a large database specifying that mitochondrial ROS production results in widespread oxidative damage to cells [119–122]. Although the origins of ROS in aging may come from several different sites, generally it has been proposed that high basal levels of ROS occur as a result of an increase in cytokines that occur with aging. Furthermore, myostatin, an anti-hypertrophy gene, has been proposed to generate ROS in muscle cells through tumor necrosis factor-alpha (TNF-alpha) via activation of NF-kappaB (NF-κB) and NADPH oxidase [123, 124]. This is supported by observations that myostatin null mice have lower ROS and sarcopenia [123, 124]. Reducing ROS production would be predicted to attenuate oxidative damage to proteins, lipids, and DNA and reduce mitochondrial damage and dysfunction in aging tissues including skeletal muscle.

The accumulation of ROS is at least as critical of a determinant of the potential for cell damage as the level of ROS production, but clearly, the two are related. ROS accumulation triggers pathways for initiating antioxidant production, which will regulate mitochondrial function for mitochondrial-specific antioxidants and/or the cytosol of a muscle cell to cytosolic-specific antioxidants. Most assessments of oxidative stress likely underestimate the production of total ROS. This is because the muscle has a large antioxidant potential in most of the muscle compartments [125]. The importance of antioxidants in sarcopenia is underscored by data that show that both losses of neural and muscle cytosolic antioxidant CuZn-superoxide dismutase (CuZnSOD) appear to recapitulate sarcopenia [126]. Furthermore, recent studies [39,127] demonstrate that mice lacking Cu/Zn-superoxide dismutase (SOD1) in their muscles had high levels of oxidative stress/damage and had a 30% decrease in lifespan, whereas SOD1 overexpression in neurons prevented mitochondrial damage in muscle. SOD1 loss appears to accelerate and exacerbate sarcopenia [39]. Furthermore, increased oxidative stress, such as that measured in sarcopenia, results in a loss of muscle levels of SOD1, further permitting the elevation of ROS accumulation. It is, however, noteworthy that the loss of CuZnSOD in only neural or muscle cells did not manifest full sarcopenic muscle loss [126], but this, nevertheless, emphasizes the point that tissue cross-talk likely occurs between neurons and muscle in aging. Nevertheless, as muscles and neurons in sarcopenic aged models are associated with an increased ROS accumulation and a reduction of many antioxidant enzyme mRNAs and proteins [71,120,128–135], aging likely increases the potential for greater ROS-induced damage to mitochondrial components in motor neurons and muscle cells [127].

The interactions between low activity levels and aging with ROS production, along with lower antioxidant levels [48,71,133,134,136–141], increase the likelihood for mitochondrial damage in aged muscles as compared to young skeletal muscle cells. It has been proposed that ROS production might be secondary to denervation that occurs in aged muscles [29,142], again emphasizing the potential cross talk between neural and muscle cells in sarcopenia. Whatever the initial source(s) of ROS production, it is clear that accumulation of excessive ROS leads to damaged mitochondria in muscle and neural cells, which in turn can result in more dysfunctional mitochondria.

Mitochondrial DNA damage and aging

Mitochondrial DNA (mtDNA) mutations or deletions have been proposed to contribute to mitochondrial dysfunction that leads to aging-related muscle fiber loss and atrophy and result in sarcopenia [143–148]. Indeed, there is evidence that sarcopenia is associated with increased mtDNA mutations in areas of muscle oxidative damage [149–152]. Similarly, in neurons, DNA damage precedes neuronal apoptosis [153–160]. On the other hand, forced repair of DNA damage rescues neurons from elimination by apoptosis [159–161]. Although not all increases in ROS production are the result of mitochondrial DNA deletions or lead to mtDNA mutations [152,162–165], it is clear that such deletions represent important contributors to mitochondrial ROS production in sarcopenic muscles and neurons [152,166–168]. Furthermore, aging-induced mitochondrial DNA deletions are linked closely to the loss of mitochondrial function in motor neurons [161,169–171] and neuronal malfunction in neural diseases such as Parkinson's disease [172,173] and Alzheimer's disease [174,175] and in sarcopenia [150,152,166]. Together, these observations highlight the important role of mitochondria in maintaining neural and muscle function in aging.

Altered mitochondrial dynamics with aging

Mitochondria are very dynamic organelles. They can form individual units or can generate an extensive reticulum. Mitochondria can be located in the subsarcolemmal or intermyofibrillar regions of muscle cells although both mitochondria subtypes appear to communicate [176–180]. Mitochondrial morphology can be more fragmented or large and complex through its regulation by interactions between fusion and fission regulatory proteins. Fusion proteins such as Mitofusins 1 and 2 (Mfn1 and 2) and Optic atrophy 1 (Opa1) can join mitochondrial membranes together to form larger mitochondria or increase the size of the mitochondrial reticular network [69,181–184]. Fission proteins such as dynamin-related protein 1 (Drp1) and fission protein 1 (Fis1) promote mitochondrial fission, which can result in smaller, individual, or fragmented mitochondria [161,181–186].

These processes of fission and fusion are important to maintain the proper balance to establish healthy mitochondria because they allow for the exchange of the matrix proteins between mitochondria [187–191]. Abnormal mitochondrial fission and turnover will negatively influence mitochondrial quality and health. For example, the protein abundance of fusion and fission proteins along with their mRNA transcripts has been reported to be lower in sarcopenic skeletal muscle as compared to young adult skeletal muscle [192,193]. This presents the potential that mitochondria from aged muscle may be unable to respond adequately to environmental changes as compared to mitochondria from young muscle. Indeed, this appears to be the case, because biochemical analyses and electron microscopic evaluations have shown very different mitochondrial profiles in the sarcopenic muscle [74]. Small, more fragmented mitochondria have been found in sarcopenic muscles as compared with mitochondria from younger muscles [194,195]. However, this is not a universal finding because very large mitochondria have also been observed in sarcopenic muscles of old animals [69,181,196].

There is some evidence to suggest that muscles of aged rodents and humans have a greater overall rate of fission [192,193,197] and lower levels of the fusion proteins such as Opa1 [197] as compared with younger muscles. Fragmented mitochondria tend to have a lower respiratory capacity and are less efficient, including increased production of ROS, which increases the susceptibility of mitochondria to damage and greater propensity to open the mitochondrial permeability pore and release the mitochondria contents and enzymes to the cytosol. This mitochondrial leakage would activate the apoptotic pathways to initiate cell death. Thus, it is not surprising that sarcopenia and muscle disuse, which have excessively fragmented mitochondria, are also accompanied by muscle loss [198], at least in part by activation of apoptotic signaling [50,199–202]. It is interesting that a knockout of Mfn1/2 in skeletal muscle, which prevents mitochondrial fusion, increases the accumulation of mtDNA defects and results in muscle atrophy [203]. Together, these observations are consistent with the hypothesis that muscle mitochondria are important regulators of muscle size in sarcopenia [50]. However, to provide a balanced perspective, it is important to point out that other studies have found higher fusion profiles in muscles of humans [204], prematurely aged mice [205], and larger mitochondria in sarcopenic muscles of aged mice [181,196]. Nevertheless, it is interesting that even in studies reporting a higher fusion index in aged muscles, as shown by ratios of Mfn1/Mfn2 [114] or Mfn2/Drp1 [69,181,196], the protein contents of Mfn1, Mfn2, Opa1, or Drp1 did not change. This means that even when higher fusion indices are found, the mitochondria could be still more fragmented and smaller in sarcopenic muscles with aging [45,194,196,206].

The impact of age-associated changes in mitochondrial dynamics in motor neurons and their potential role in sarcopenia have not been studied in detail. Nevertheless, dysregulation of mitochondrial fission and fusion and lysosomal dysfunction has been reported as an early event in amyotrophic lateral sclerosis (ALS) [207–211], a profound motor neuron disease. Furthermore, increased mitochondrial fragmentation has been found to precede glutamate-induced death of motor neurons [208,212]. Thus, similar to mitochondrial dynamic changes in sarcopenia, motor neuron dysfunction and death may converge upon mitochondria, and mitochondrial dynamics may play an important role in the regulation of neuronal dysfunction and contribute to accelerated sarcopenia.

The changes in fission and fusion protein-mediated functions to regulate mitochondria may be related to mitochondrial damage that occurs with aging, including an accumulation of mtDNA defects, increased production of ROS, excessive uptake of cytosolic calcium, and/or inappropriate import or assembly of electron transport proteins. Generally, exercise is thought to regulate and reduce at least part of the mitochondrial deficits [45,46,48,51,213–216].

However, high-intensity exercise induces mitochondrial damage and dysregulation of mitochondrial fusion and fission proteins, thereby altering the mitochondrial structure [217]. Such damage, largely as a result of excessive ROS production and/or accumulation, can lead to increased mitochondrial permeability (producing leaky mitochondria) and the release of mitochondria-specific proteins, including apoptosis-inducing factor (AIF) and cytochrome c, into the cytosol through the mitochondrial permeability transition pore (mPTP), which triggers death-signaling pathways including apoptosis. Mitochondrial DNA (mtDNA) deletions or DNA mutations have been proposed to contribute to sarcopenia and muscle wasting [146,152,218–221]. Indeed, there is evidence that mtDNA mutations increase in areas of muscle oxidative damage [145,148,149,152,220,222]. Although not all increases in ROS production are the result of mitochondrial DNA deletions, nor does an increase in ROS necessarily lead to mtDNA mutations [163], it is clear that mtDNA deletions and damage provide strong contributions to mitochondrial ROS in aging muscles [164,166,223–227]. Furthermore, mitochondrial DNA deletions are linked closely to muscle loss with aging [165,168], again emphasizing the important role that mitochondrial damage plays in maintaining muscle mass, which underpins sarcopenia in aging [50, 65]. Improving mitochondrial structure and increasing mitochondrial biogenesis by supplementing old mice with growth differentiation factor 11 [228] or caloric restriction [167,168,196,229,230] further supports the idea that healthy mitochondria with proper mitochondria turnover play a critical role in maintaining muscle mass and function to suppress/delay/prevent sarcopenia. Furthermore, early alterations of mitochondrial quality control and autophagic removal and recycling of damaged mitochondria flux occur before the onset of sarcopenia [231], but it will eventually contribute to cell destruction and sarcopenia [50].

Association of reduced activity and mitochondrial dysfunction in sarcopenia

Sarcopenia appears to promote a decrease in mitochondrial quality and quantity [74,232,233]. The loss of mitochondria volume per muscle fiber volume is apparent with aging [74,234]. It has been argued that the loss of mitochondria is the result of lower mobility and activity [234]. Certainly, reduced activity decreases mitochondrial enzyme levels and metabolism and increases ROS [118,235], but mitochondrial content per fiber volume is not markedly different for sedentary young adults than more active people [59, 60]. Thus, while inactivity may decrease the mitochondrial volume in aged muscles, the aging process must increase the susceptibility to reduced mitochondrial volume per fiber volume. This does not rule out the potential that lack of activity might not increase the susceptibility of the mPTP to open or contribute to another ROS-associated mitochondrial dysfunction. Nevertheless, it is important to note that at least some of this mitochondria volume can be regained through elevations of exercise, and this may offset or delay aging comorbidities and reduced function [234]. However, while mitochondrial volume density (mitochondrial volume per muscle fiber volume) may increase with exercise, training appears limited to improve overall muscle size.

That means that the total number of mitochondria in a given muscle of an older person must be lower than for a young healthy adult, even if the normalized mitochondrial volume density is similar in young and older muscles. Thus, a key factor to muscle metabolism, mobility and health, and resistance to sarcopenia including increases in muscle mass and function, may be related more to the total number and total volume of mitochondria [234], which can support greater protein synthesis and metabolic pathways to reverse or offset sarcopenia. However, we cannot discount other effects of exercise that have the potential to improve mitochondria function through reduced levels of ROS [48,236], and more exercise-induced mitochondria (or mitochondrial volume per fiber volume) could also improve calcium buffering in aged muscles [237,238].

Calcium-induced dysregulation of mitochondria in sarcopenia

The sarcoplasmic reticulum (SR) is the known calcium storing and releasing unit for skeletal muscle. In human beings, there is a difference in the sarcoplasmic reticulum volume per fiber volume, with type I fibers having about 6% of the type II fiber as SR and sarcoplasmic reticulum volume, occupying about 3% of the volume of type I fibers [49,60,239,240]. Ca^{2+} release from the ryanodine receptor of the SR initiates cross-bridge interactions and generation of force. However, Ca^+ must be returned to the SR to remove the "on" signal for contraction and induce muscle relaxation. Mitochondria are essential to supply ATP for not only the myosin/actin cross-bridge cycle and but for the reuptake of Ca^{2+} by the sarcoendoplasmic reticulum ATPases (SERCA) [241]. In addition, mitochondria provide an important Ca^{2+} buffering function by assisting the SR in removing cytosolic Ca^{2+} between contractions to allow muscle relaxation [241]. In contrast, the mitochondrial volume in type I fibers is ~ 6% and type II fibers ~ 3% of the fiber volume [49,60,239,240]. This differential is important because the SR ryanodine receptors become "leaky" with increased age [242,243], and so, calcium buffering becomes very important. As mitochondria are very good calcium buffering organs, type I fibers have a much larger ability to buffer calcium and have less total calcium to buffer than type II fibers. Indeed, entry of Ca^{2+} into mitochondria occurs without an apparent threshold that is needed through the mitochondrial calcium uniporter (MCU) [244].

The uptake of calcium by mitochondria occurs as a result of a hydrogen ion gradient across the inner mitochondrial membrane that is produced by mitochondrial respiration [245,246]. In addition, mitochondria and SR are positioned closely together, which facilities an increase of local Ca^{2+} entry to the SR via voltage-dependent Ca^{2+} channels (Fig. 1A). Ca^{2+} first moves across the outer mitochondrial membrane (OMM). Initially, the OMM was considered to be permeable to Ca^{2+} mostly via the voltage-dependent anion channel (VDAC). After passing through the OMM, Ca^{2+} moves into the inner mitochondria membrane (IMM) through a single transport mechanism mediated by a Ca^{2+}-selective channel, the mitochondria calcium

Young healthy muscle

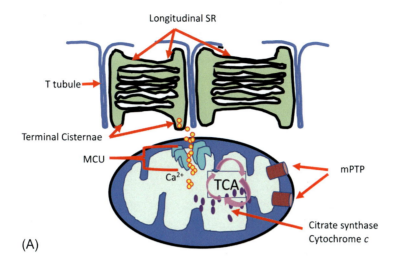

Sarcopenic muscle

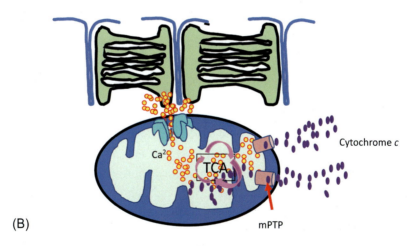

Fig. 1

Regulation of Ca^{2+} signaling between the sarcoplasmic reticulum and mitochondria. Ca^{2+} is released by the terminal cisternae via the ryanodine receptor of the sarcoplasmic reticulum as part of excitation–contraction coupling and muscle cross-bridge regulation for force production. Ca^{2+} is returned to the lateral cisternae at the termination of the action potential by SERCA pumps. Calcium is also taken into the mitochondria via the mitochondria calcium uniporter (MCU) to help buffer and lower cytosolic calcium levels. (A) In young muscle, the sarcoplasmic reticulum efficiently returns Ca^{2+} to maintain the ion gradient. Ca^{2+} that increases in mitochondria can modulate mitochondria function, including increasing activity of the TCA cycle for generating ATP and substrate utilization.
(B) In sarcopenic muscle, the sarcoplasmic reticulum is "leaky," SERCA pumps less efficient at returning Ca^{2+} and cytosolic Ca^{2+} and mitochondria levels are elevated. Mitochondria permeability pore opening is more sensitive to elevated Ca^{2+} levels, and when this occurs, the mitochondrial contents escape the mitochondria and can activate apoptotic pathways. Thus, MCU import of Ca^{2+} appears to be elevated in sarcopenic muscle so mitochondria dysfunction occurs as a result of elevated Ca^{2+}. Other contributors (e.g., ROS) can contribute to increased mitochondria permeability pore opening.

uniporter (MCU) [247–249]. This MCU uptake of Ca^{2+} is important for many mitochondrial functions, including substrate utilization, and may regulate the TCA cycle [250]. However, excessive calcium import can induce mitochondrial permeability pore opening and cell death [251–255]. Thus, there is a threshold where cytosolic Ca^{2+} is available for muscle contraction but does not remain high between contractions, because excessive cytosolic calcium will activate protease, and therefore, it is important that cytosolic calcium remains low in resting states (Fig. 1). It is important to note that the Ca^{2+} content of mitochondria from muscles of young animals is lower than that of old animals, and this difference is observed before the onset of sarcopenia [74]. Thus, this suggests that mitochondria from old animals may have a lower reserve capacity to buffer calcium, and high levels of calcium would be expected to cause mitochondria damage. Although speculative, if mitochondria were to be oversaturated with calcium as a result of aging-associated leaky SR resulting in high basal levels of Ca^{2+} (Fig. 1B), mitochondria will not be able to quickly buffer Ca^{2+} and restore low levels of this ion quickly. This would prolong muscle contraction and muscle time to relax but would increase the risk for elevated Ca^{2+} in muscle proteolysis and increase the permeability of the mitochondria to release mitochondria contents such as cytochrome c to the cytosol. This would activate caspase-initiated death signaling and apoptosis.

Aging muscle has a higher resting calcium level than young adult muscle [256]. Is it possible but unproven that much of the sarcopenic preservation of type I fibers vs type II fibers in aging is related to the greater ability to buffer calcium in the slow contracting fibers? This seems possible becuase type I fibers have lower SR and calcium released in response to an action potential, but a higher volume of mitochondria for buffering Ca^{2+} as compared to type II fibers. Given that sarcopenia is generally not worse in women and maybe lower, and in general, women have a longer life span, it is interesting to note that recent data suggest that mitochondria calcium uptake is higher in type II muscle fibers from female mice as compared to male mice, in part, because there was a greater intermyofibrillar mitochondrial content in the muscles from female mice [257]. Alternatively, would improving mitochondria calcium uptake in either fiber type offset sarcopenia from pathways that could stimulate anabolic muscle growth? This speculation is supported by data that suggest that MCU-dependent mitochondrial Ca^{2+} uptake has a marked anabolic effect that does not depend on mitochondria metabolism per se. Rather, the anabolic effect of mitochondria-calcium appears to activate both skeletal muscle PGC-1α and IGF1-Akt/PKB pathways, which protect muscle loss and stimulate muscle growth [258,259]. In addition, MCU overexpression protects from denervation-associated muscle wasting [246,259]. However, this is not a simple pathway because other data suggest that skeletal muscle-specific deletion of the MCU in mice did not impair myofiber intracellular Ca^{2+} handling, but it did inhibit acute mitochondrial Ca^{2+} influx and mitochondrial respiration that was activated by Ca^{2+} [260]. Nevertheless, this was not evaluated in muscles from old mice. Indeed, exercise in aging human beings was shown to improve MCU function [238]. Together these data suggest that Ca^{2+}-dependent organelle-to-nucleus signaling and regulation of cytoplasmic levels of Ca^{2+} may be important functions, which are reduced in sarcopenic muscle but can be increased by exercise. An interesting question to pose is if muscle mitochondria can remain healthy, perhaps through increased exercise and activity [261], mitochondrial number and MCU number or activity can be increased to sufficiently buffer Ca^{2+} fluxes appropriately, would we see a reduction in muscle proteolysis and atrophy and suppress sarcopenia in aging?

Mitochondria initiate and mediate cell death signaling in sarcopenia

Three independent pathways are involved in regulating signaling for cell death, but two of them involve mitochondria. These include the intrinsic mitochondrial pathway, the TNF-α inflammatory pathway, which connects to mitochondria signaling, and the ER-stress pathway. Nuclear apoptosis [50,69,134,166,176,200,201,213,216,223,262–276] and autophagy [52,81,277–281] pathways are activated in response to dysfunctional or damaged mitochondria in aging. While the proper balance between these signaling pathways is important for optimizing the health of the muscle fiber, altered signaling and dysregulation of one or both pathways are common in sarcopenia [50,201,268,280–284].

Low levels of physical activity, immobilization, or muscle disuse can exacerbate sarcopenia, whereas exercise can at least partially attenuate some of the aging-associated alterations, including improvements of mitochondrial function in aging [48,81,285,286]. Healthy mitochondria provide optimal cellular metabolism, low excessive levels of generating ROS, and high production of ATP. In contrast, excessively high levels of ROS result in dysfunctional or damaged mitochondria that can initiate intrinsic (mitochondrial) death pathways that result in the removal of nuclei via nuclear apoptosis [50,201,268,287–289]. Although autophagy can be acutely upregulated during periods of muscle wasting, the overall pattern to disassemble dysfunctional mitochondria by autophagy (mitophagy) provides a strategy to eliminate the source of the death (apoptotic) signaling. Ultimately removing dysfunctional mitochondria will save the muscle cell from complete removal by the apoptotic death pathway [290–293]. Although a proper balance between removing "sick" and "leaky" mitochondria and ramping up biogenesis by making new healthy mitochondria optimize muscle health, it also minimizes internal signals that are active in generating muscle loss for sarcopenia [50,264,284,292,294–296].

Mitochondrial-induced nuclear apoptosis in aging muscle

The decline of mitochondrial function with aging appears to precede sarcopenia, and increasing mitochondria dysfunction increases sarcopenia once it begins [74]. Losses of mitochondrial function may limit the synthesis of sufficient levels of adenosine triphosphate (ATP) that is needed for contracting muscle, regulating calcium SERCA pumps, biosynthesis of proteins, and general homeostasis. Thus, attenuated ATP levels could contribute to loss of cellular integrity and apoptosis signaling [297].

Although there are similarities in signaling that regulate death in single cells that contain only one nucleus and the multinucleated skeletal muscle cells, there are also some important differences. The similarities include the same mitochondrial-dependent and independent pathways, and the result of DNA fragmentation and elimination of a nucleus. A key difference is that loss of a single nucleus (e.g., via apoptosis) does not result in complete cell death in multinucleated muscle cells, whereas the single nucleated cell will die once its only nucleus is eliminated. In skeletal muscle, targeting one nucleus in a muscle region but not another suggests that signaling for cell death is not controlled systemically but rather is controlled by local targeted signaling networks.

There are three primary pathways for apoptosis, but the intrinsically mediated mitochondrial signaling pathway is attractive for explaining much of the apoptotic signaling associated with sarcopenia. Nuclear apoptosis is characterized by increases in DNA fragmentation and proapoptotic proteins such as Bax, caspase-3, apoptosis protease activating factor-1 (Apaf-1), and AIF [202,296,298–304]. There is a large body of data from our laboratory and other research laboratories that shows that nuclear apoptosis has an important role in regulating muscle mass losses in sarcopenia [270,272,275,305–309]. Furthermore, there is evidence that increasing apoptotic signaling and the abundance of apoptotic proteins can accelerate the loss of muscle mass and function in aging. In addition, apoptosis is a major initiator of muscle loss that is associated with denervation [142,293,294,310–317], and sarcopenia is also associated with denervation and loss of neuromuscular junction function. In addition, an upregulation of apoptotic signaling has been identified in premature aging models that exhibit accelerated sarcopenia [318–320]. Increased levels of caspase-3 and DNA fragmentation have also been reported in sarcopenic muscles of rats and other mammals including human beings [49,321,322].

Fig. 2 summarizes the primary features of mitochondrial-associated (intrinsic) apoptotic signaling, which contributes to nuclear apoptosis in aging-induced sarcopenia. Increased mitochondria permeability results in the escape of mitochondrially-housed proteins into the cytosol of the cell, and this provides the initiation of intrinsic apoptosis signaling in sarcopenia. This permeability is initiated by Bax:Bax (or Bax:Bak) dimerization, which creates a pore in the OMM. Alternatively, mitochondrial permeability can occur via a greater sensitization and opening of the muscle mitochondrial permeability pore (mPTP) by excessive ROS or calcium, both of which are increased in sarcopenia. When these channels open, they allow for the release of mitochondrially-housed proteins such as cytochrome *c* to the cytosol in sarcopenic muscles [323,324]. In the cytoplasm, cytochrome *c* acts as a proapoptotic protein by binding dATP and apoptosis protease activating factor-1 (Apaf-1), forming an apoptosome that cleaves and activates caspase-9 (Fig. 2). An aging-associated increase in the proapoptotic Apaf-1 protein and increases in the abundance of the proapoptotic cleaved caspase-9 protein, along with increased DNA fragmentation, have been found in the gastrocnemius muscles of aged rats. Cleaved caspase-9 will cleave and activate caspase-3, the final effector caspase in the mitochondria apoptotic pathway. Mitochondrial-associated caspase signaling is important in sarcopenia, but it is not the only

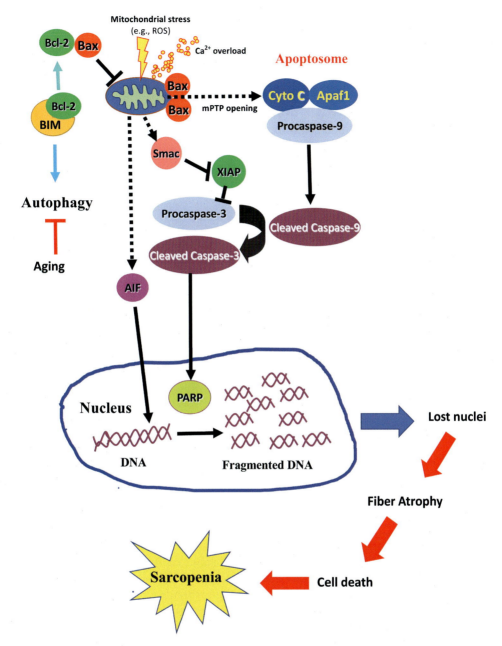

Fig. 2
Mitochondrial initiated nuclear apoptosis leading to apoptosis. Dysfunctional mitochondria can occur by a variety of factors including mitochondrial stress, such as ROS accumulation (*lightning bolt*), DNA damage, and/or elevations in cytosolic Ca^{2+} (*yellow circles*). Mitochondrial stress results in dissociation of the antiapoptotic B-cell lymphoma (Bcl)-2 protein and the proapoptotic Bcl-2-associated X protein (Bax). A Bax:Bax pore is formed in the outer membrane, and a mitochondrial permeability transition pore (mPTP) is formed (not shown) in the inner mitochondrial membrane. The mPTP and Bax:Bax pore allows mitochondrial-housed contents (e.g., cytochrome c) to leak into the cytosol, forming an apoptosome, which activates and cleaves caspase-9 and subsequently activates and cleaves the effector caspase-3 protein. Cleaved caspase-3 enters a nucleus,
(Continued)

source of mitochondrial-associated apoptotic signaling. Caspase-independent signaling can also be initiated as a result of mitochondrial dysfunction and permeability and has been shown to occur in aging-associated muscle loss. The release of endonuclease G (EndoG), AIF, the second mitochondrial-derived activator of caspase/direct inhibitor of apoptosis-binding protein with low pI (Smac/DIABLO), and X-linked inhibitor of apoptosis protein (XIAP), from the mitochondria to the cytosol can initiate mitochondrial apoptotic signaling without the need for activating the caspase-dependent signaling. Thus, it is clear that mitochondria are critically intertwined as part of the initiation of the apoptotic signaling cascades in sarcopenia. However, it is interesting that nuclear apoptosis in skeletal muscle involves cell signaling that is so precise that specific individual myonuclei can be targeted for elimination in multinucleated skeletal myofiber without targeting other nuclei. While apoptosis signaling can provide a general approach to activate the removal of a single-nucleated nonmuscle cell, full cell death will not occur by elimination of a single nucleus in the multinucleated skeletal muscle cell. This type of targeting requires a rather precise focus for eliminating one nucleus without targeting another nucleus in skeletal muscle. One model that has been proposed is that the local signaling from individual dysfunctional mitochondria will provide a localized signal that targets only nuclei within its vicinity [50].

Activation of the mitochondrial permeability transition pore accelerates apoptosis in sarcopenia

It has been well established that apoptosis occurs in sarcopenia [50,69,115,134,142,166,176, 199–202,213,216,223,266,270–272,275,296,303,304,307,323,325–340] including human muscles [183,269,341,342]. Much of the greater susceptibility of sarcopenic muscle to apoptosis is related to the elevated mitochondrial sensitivity to open

---

Fig. 2, cont'd
which is in close proximity to the dysfunctional mitochondria. The enzyme poly-ADP ribose polymerase (PARP) is activated, which cleaves nuclear DNA. Non-caspase-dependent DNA fragmentation can be caused by direct activation of mitochondrial housed components, such as apoptosis-inducing factor (AIF), which leak from porous mitochondria and enter an adjacent nucleus to cause DNA fragmentation. Mitochondrial-housed second mitochondria-derived activator of caspase/direct inhibitor of apoptosis-binding protein with low pI (Smac/DIABLO) can promote caspase-9 cleavage and activation via inhibition of the antiapoptotic X-linked inhibitor of apoptosis protein (XIAP). Although not all DNA damage that occurs in this fashion will result in nuclear removal, sufficient damage will result in the elimination of the nucleus that is targeted by apoptosis. Aging is associated with a blunting of mitophagy that would normally be in place to remove dysfunctional nuclei and in doing so would remove the signaling mechanism for apoptosis. However, blunted mitophagy results in an accumulation of dysfunctional and leaky mitochondria, which elevate the death signaling pathways for apoptosis, eventually resulting in the loss of nuclei and cell death, which reduces muscle mass and function and leads to sarcopenia. The intersections of extrinsic and endoplasmic reticulum pathways that exist for inducing apoptosis are not shown.

the mPTP [269], thereby releasing the contents from mitochondria to the cytosol to initiate apoptotic signaling [176,307,308,340,343].

It could be argued that inactivity that typically accompanies aging, perhaps through inactivity-induced ROS production, might explain some of the increased mPTP susceptibility for opening. However, mPTP opening in aging cannot be solely the function of inactivity, because increased mitochondrial susceptibility to permeability transition opening has also been observed in muscles from active human beings [269]. Exercise as a stimulus to improve mitochondria number and function can, at least, partially reverse aging-associated apoptosis, as exercise training has been reported to decrease catabolic and apoptotic signaling in muscles of aged rodents [344,345]. It is also important to note that the susceptibility for mPTP opening is exacerbated by an imbalance of Ca^{2+} homeostasis that likely results from leaky ryanodine receptors that occur in aged skeletal muscles [242,243], as illustrated in Fig. 1. Sensitization of the mPTP in aging skeletal muscle may be an important contributor to the initiation of mitochondrial initiating apoptosis and muscle loss leading to sarcopenia. Aging-associated muscle denervation contributes to increased mPTP that, in turn, induces muscle apoptosis and muscle loss [142,232,269,346–348].

Mitochondria dysfunction may regulate a fiber type-specific loss in sarcopenia

Type II fibers have few mitochondria as compared to type I fibers, and therefore, it is not unreasonable to think that the signal for mitochondrial-apoptosis should then be low in type II fibers. Yet, type II fibers are lost most frequently in sarcopenia than type I fibers [349] in muscles from aged human beings. In addition, the loss of fiber size and function in sarcopenic rodents is generally most prominent in type II myosin-containing fibers [350–354].

If mPTP opening is a critical component of initiating apoptotic signaling from dysfunctional mitochondria as we think it is, it is perhaps curious as to why the glycolytic type II fibers, which contain less than 3% of the fiber volume as mitochondria [59, 60] also are eliminated in aging. Although it is true that type II fibers contain a lower mitochondrial volume density as compared to type I fibers, type II fibers have a greater susceptibility to ROS damage than type I fibers [355]. This means that although there are fewer mitochondria in type II fibers, the greater mitochondrial damage quickly leads to mPTP opening [356], further mitochondrial DNA damage [357], and mitochondrial-associated apoptotic signaling [50,66,71,176,262,358–360] as compared to type I fibers. Although mitophagy is presumed to be important for the removal of dysfunctional mitochondria in both type I and type II fibers, it is not clear if there are fiber-type differences of mitophagy signaling in sarcopenic muscles.

Irrespective of fiber types, the levels of death signaling in apoptosis are intimately linked to the health or quality of mitochondria in skeletal muscles [166,277–279,285,360–364]. It will be important in future studies to determine if mitophagy is suppressed more in type II than in type I fibers in aging and if the phenotypic switch from type II to type I fibers are protective against sarcopenia.

Mitochondrially regulated loss of motor function and mobility in sarcopenia

Motor neurons

The impact of age-associated changes in mitochondrial dynamics in motor neurons and their potential role in sarcopenia has not been studied. However, mitochondrial dynamic dysfunction has been reported as an early event in ALS [208,365–368], which is a common motor neuron disease. Furthermore, increased mitochondrial fragmentation has been found to precede glutamate-induced death of motor neurons [369,370]. Thus, similar to mitochondrial dynamic changes in muscle with aging, motor neuron dysfunction and death may converge upon mitochondria, and mitochondrial dynamics may play an important role in the regulation of neuronal function that contributes to accelerated sarcopenia.

The general pathways that are initiated by signaling from dysfunctional mitochondria have been summarized in Fig. 1. These pathways assume that stress to mitochondria in aged cells results in irreparably damaged mitochondria, but aging attenuates the removal of these damaged mitochondria. The accumulation of dysfunctional mitochondria initiates the apoptotic death signaling pathway in muscle cells and motor neurons, and communication between these cell types accelerates muscle wasting and denervation and leads to sarcopenia. Evidence for the components of this pathway is given below.

Mitochondrial regulation of neural dysfunction in sarcopenia

Loss of motor function in sarcopenia is partially dependent upon the reduction of muscle cross-sectional area, and partly related to reduced neuronal function, denervation and disruption, and fragmentation of the neuromuscular junction. Neural conduction and resetting membrane potentials after each action potential is an energy-consuming event, so that mitochondrial health would be expected to be important for optimizing function in motor neurons. Indeed, decreases in motor neuron mitochondrial enzyme content [371] and the loss of mitochondrial content [371] may precede neuronal death in aging. Given the importance of mitochondrial in the motor neuron, it is not surprising that mitochondria have been implicated in the decline of neuron function and number in aging [371]. Nevertheless, although the role of mitochondria in aging has been well characterized in muscle cells, their importance in regulating motor neuron aging deficits or motor neuron death is not well understood.

Mitochondria morphological abnormalities and reduced respiratory activity of several enzymes occur in motor neuron degeneration models such as the wobbler mouse [372], but it is less clear if this is a common aging-associated phenomenon that is independent of disease. Thus, we have a good reason to think that mitochondrial dysfunction occurs in motor neurons with aging. Furthermore, with an aging-induced increase in ROS production and perhaps a reduced antioxidant activity, ROS accumulation could impair neural mitochondria in a similar mechanism as proposed for skeletal muscle mitochondria. Denervation has also been suggested to be an important regulator of mitochondrial dysfunction in neural tissue [127,142], but it is less clear if denervation is the initiator or the contributor to mitochondrial dysfunction.

PGC-1α regulation of mitochondria in sarcopenia
PGC-1α regulation of mitochondria

Peroxisome proliferator-activated receptor γ coactivator 1α (PGC-1α) is thought to be a master regulator of mitochondrial biogenesis and it has a role in regulating antioxidant proteins. Aging decreases PGC-1α levels along with muscle mass [46,75,176,359,373]. In contrast, transgenic mice that had a muscle-specific overexpression of PGC-1α had elevated mitochondrial biogenesis, oxidative capacity, greater resistance to muscle fatigue, and improved aerobic performance [74,374–376]. PGC-1α also plays a key role in preventing deterioration of mitochondrial function in response to immobilization [75,377] and conserves mitochondria [378] and skeletal muscle mass in response to catabolic stimuli [379,380]. Overexpression of PGC-1α can block the expression of atrophy-associated genes (atrogenes) and minimize muscle loss that is induced by TNF-like weak inducer of apoptosis (TWEAK)-Fn14 [381,382]. The culmination of these data supports the idea that PGC-1α regulated mitochondrial biogenesis is important for maintaining muscle mass and function and in reducing sarcopenia. However, increasing mitochondrial biogenesis without removing dysfunctional mitochondria would also provide a muscle milieu with a mixture of healthy and unhealthy mitochondria. Thus, not only is the abundance of mitochondria important, but the health of the mitochondria is equally important for maintaining muscle mass. Furthermore, even newly generated healthy mitochondria would be subjected to damaging signaling if the dysfunctional mitochondria are permitted to remain.

PGC-1α in mitochondria of aged muscles

There is also evidence to support an important role for PGC-1α to regulate antioxidant proteins in the aging muscle [383,384]. Reduced mRNA levels CuZnSOD, MnSOD, and/or GPX1 [383–385] have been reported in PGC-1α knockout mice as compared to age-matched wildtype mice. Furthermore, mice that overexpress PGC-1α have greater MnSOD in skeletal muscle, which is primarily housed in the mitochondria [386,387]. Indeed, the effect of PGC-1α overexpression is profound because it has been shown to reduce sarcopenia, by inhibiting mitochondria-associated apoptosis, autophagy, and proteasome protein degradation. In addition, a PGC-1α mediated increase in antioxidant production with a corresponding reduction of inflammation has been reported in skeletal muscles of aged mice [386–388]. Thus, an important component of mitochondrial health and mitochondria muscle volume for maintaining muscle mass and function in aging is highlighted by the dramatic regulation of mitochondria by PGC-1α to offset or eliminate sarcopenia.

PGC-1α regulation of mitochondria in motor neurons

It is likely that there is cross-talk between neural and muscle compartments. This is shown in a study where muscle-specific expression of PGC-1α in mice resulted in a remodeling of the postsynaptic and presynaptic components of the neuromuscular junction in the absence of greater physical activity [389–392]. Furthermore, PGC-1α overexpression increased mitochondrial enzymes, improved motor neuron function, and reduced cell death in a mouse model of ALS [393–395]. Although we do not know if the same result would be found in aged motor neurons, it is reasonable to speculate that a motor neuronal overexpression of PGC-1α would be expected to have a protective effect against age-associated mitochondrial dysfunction and motor neuronal death.

Autophagy/mitophagy and mitochondrial dysfunction in sarcopenia

Autophagy is a network of cellular recycling that involves identifying and tagging damaged organelles, capturing and surrounding them with doubled wall membrane vesicles known as autophagosomes, and degrading the organelle within the lysosome (Fig. 2). Accelerated and extensive autophagy has been identified in many diseases and excessive autophagy in muscle can contribute to muscle wasting [396,397]. However, more modest and appropriately controlled autophagy signaling, particularly autophagic removal of dysfunctional mitochondria (mitophagy), is an important suppressor of the overall apoptotic death-signaling program [81,233,398]. Thus, dismantling and removal of dysfunctional mitochondria by mitophagy removes the source for apoptotic death signaling, thereby promoting cell survival.

Removal of dysfunctional mitochondria by mitophagy

Failure to remove dysfunctional mitochondria by mitophagy results in an accumulation of damaged mitochondria, which together magnify the death-signaling pathway and accelerate sarcopenia. Thus, the progression of the steps leading to sarcopenia hinges upon whether dysfunctional mitochondria can be removed or if they are being permitted to continue with their apoptotic death signaling cascade.

In young cells, signaling for mitochondrial disassembly via fusion and autophagy occurs when ROS damage is high or when the mitochondrial membrane potential ($\Delta \psi m$) is reduced. Mitophagy is the selective removal of dysfunctional mitochondria by autophagic processes

[399,400]. Mitophagy requires tagging of dysfunctional mitochondria so that they can be recognized for disassembly. The selectivity of mitophagy is controlled by the loss of $\Delta \psi m$ and by several important proteins, including function mutations of phosphatase and tensin homolog-induced putative kinase 1 (Pink1), Parkin, B-cell lymphoma (Bcl)-2 and 19 kDa interacting protein-3 (Bnip3), and Bnip3L/Nix [193,398,401–403]. After identification, dysfunctional mitochondria are engulfed in the double-membrane autophagosome. The autophagosome fuses with a lysosome, and the proteolytic contents of the lysosome are emptied into the autophagosome, which then digests the dysfunctional mitochondria [399,404,405].

An overview of some of the elements that are part of the mitophagy signaling pathway is shown in Fig. 3; however, this description is not meant to be exhaustive. Pink1 acts as a primary regulator to target mitophagy in dysfunctional mitochondria. Recent work indicates that under basal physiological conditions in healthy mitochondria, Pink1 is imported to the mitochondria. After it is imported, Pink1 becomes localized to the inner mitochondrial membrane and the intermembrane space and matrix [406]. In healthy mitochondria from young hosts, Pink1 is quickly degraded and therefore does not induce mitophagy. However, Pink1 is activated as a result of a loss of $\Delta \psi m$, which occurs as a result of mitochondrial damage [403,407], depolarization [406], or an increase in mitochondrial pH [408] that can occur in aging and disease. Depolarized mitochondria prevent the import of Pink1 inside the mitochondria [406], which results in an accumulation of Pink1 on the OMM. In addition, Pink1 that is inside the mitochondria is not degraded but translocates to the OMM of a depolarized mitochondria [406]. At the surface of dysfunctional mitochondria, Pink1 recruits the cytosolic ubiquitin ligase Parkin to the outer mitochondria membrane. Pink1 then activates Parkin [406,409–411] and phosphorylates ubiquitin [410,411] to initiate the formation of ubiquitin chains on mitochondria [46,412–414]. The phosphorylated form of Parkin accelerates the formation of ubiquitin links on the OMM, which then further feeds Pink1 as a substrate. Furthermore, Pink1 activates Drp1 [399,415]. The fission property of Drp1 has a role in the degradation of mitochondria as part of the mitophagy process [399,400,415]. The autophagy adaptor protein p62 binds to the ubiquitin tags on the mitochondria membrane and links to the activated form of microtubule-associated protein 1 light chain 3 (LC3). In addition, Bnip3 and Nix translocate to the mitochondria where they act as other autophagy receptors to connect the mitochondria to the autophagosome. Elongation of the double-layered membrane is controlled through linkage of autophagy-related (ATG) proteins 12-ATG5-ATG16L and the conjugation of microtubule-associated protein 1 light chain 3 (LC3)-I with phosphatidylethanolamine (PE) to form the activated lipidated LC3-II-PE, which forms a vital membrane component of the autophagosome and binding partner for autophagy receptors. Elongation of the lipid membrane circles and engulfs the dysfunctional mitochondria (Fig. 3). After forming the mature autophagosome, it fuses with the lysosome to degrade the isolated mitochondria by proteolytic enzymes that are contained in the lysosome [401,402].

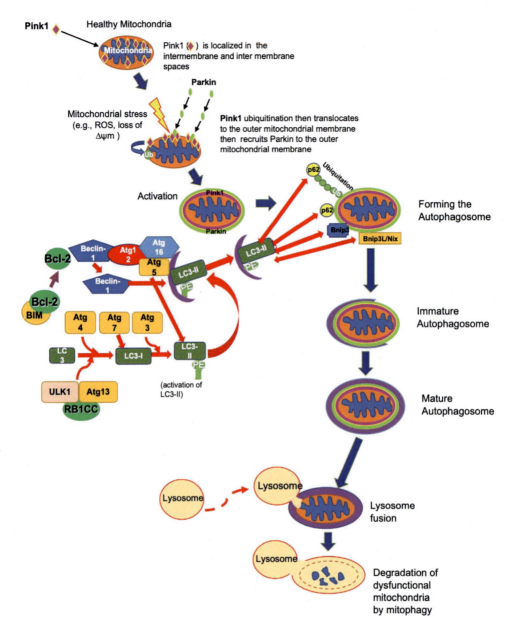

Fig. 3
Removal of dysfunctional mitochondria by mitophagy. With aging, there is an accumulation of ROS, mitochondrial Ca^+ levels, mtDNA damage, and/or other stresses that cause a further reduction in the mitochondrial membrane potential. Pink1 moves to dysfunctional mitochondria (probably as a result of reduced mitochondrial membrane potential) where it is inserted into the intermembrane and intermembrane spaces. Pink1 can be degraded in healthy mitochondria from young nonsarcopenic muscles. However, in sarcopenia where mitochondrial depolarization is presented, Pink1 is recruited to the outer mitochondrial membrane, and transport of Pink1 to the inside of the mitochondria is prevented, resulting in an accumulation of Pink along the outer mitochondrial membrane (depicted by the pink rink around the outer mitochondrial membrane). The E3 ligase Parkin (*green*) is recruited to the outer mitochondrial membrane where it is inserted there. Parkin ubiquitinates the outer mitochondrial membrane proteins

Mitophagy is not a simple process in aging, because it has been both reported to increase [416,417] or decrease [183,203,279,418–422] in sarcopenic muscle. Although there is evidence for increasing the migration of Parkin and p62 to the mitochondria with aging, suggestive of increased mitophagy, there is also a paradoxical accumulation of lipofuscin granules, which suggests an impairment in lysosomal function in aging [416]. These data implicate a failure for the lysosome to remove dysfunctional mitochondrial as this would account for the increase in lipofuscin granules. Indeed, lipofuscin deposits have been previously reported in many tissues including muscles of aged rodents or other mammals [423]. Improved removal of dysfunctional mitochondria perhaps via increased activation of lysosomal activity [52,277,424,425] may include exercise interventions, although the responses might be regulated, at least in part, in a fiber–type-specific fashion [81,426]. Further work is needed to determine if failure of mitophagy progression in sarcopenia may encompass, at least in part, with lysosomal dysfunction [427,428], or if improper signaling upstream of the lysosome is more important in regulating lysosome function.

Insufficient mitophagy allows unhealthy mitochondria to persist in aging muscles

Failure to regulate proper mitophagy and proteasome removal of mitochondria are both upstream of sarcopenic muscle fiber loss. There is strong evidence for an aging-suppression of mitophagy in skeletal muscle and motor neurons [114,295,419,429]. Not only does Mfn2 have a role in mitochondrial fusion, but Mfn2 also has an important role in acting as a receptor for Pink1 and Parkin-targeted mitophagy [430]. Mfn2 abundance declines in muscle

Fig. 3, cont'd
(shown by a green ring around the mitochondria), resulting in the recruitment of ubiquitin-binding autophagy receptors, such as p62, Bnip3, and Bnip3L/Nix to the mitochondria. B-cell lymphoma (Bcl)-2 prevents the induction of autophagy by binding to Beclin-1, which is an important initiator of mitophagy. Displacement of Bcl-2 from Beclin-1 leads to activation of the phagophore nucleation. Elongation of the membrane requires 2 ubiquitin-like conjugation systems: autophagy proteins (ATG) and activation of microtubule-associated protein 1 light chain 3 from its inactive form LC3-I to the active form of LC3-II. After activation, LC3-II is conjugated to phosphatidylethanolamine (PE) to form lipidated (activated) LC3-II (LC3-II-PE). LC3-II-PE can bind autophagy receptors and localize to the outer mitochondrial membrane. The p62 receptor contains a ubiquitin-binding domain, which localizes it to Parkin-ubiquitinated mitochondria. This creates a targeting motif for the identification of mitochondria that are to be removed. LC3-II-PE also participates in autophagosomal membrane elongation (shown in *light purple*). Bnip3 and its homolog Bnip3L/Nix are also mitophagy receptors that, when expressed, localize to the outer mitochondria membrane. Some data suggest that p62 can also bind to ubiquitinated chains (Ub) that are attached to the mitochondria. LC3-II-PE binds to the autophagy receptors (e.g., p62, Bnip3, Bnip3L/Nix, and others) (as depicted by the *red double arrows*), which then links the developing membrane of the autophagosome to the outer mitochondrial membrane. LC3-II-PE complex participates in the elongation of the double-layered membrane that surrounds the damaged mitochondria. After the mature form of the autophagosome is generated, it fuses with a lysosome. The lysosome then injects its contents into the mitochondria to degrade it to complete the mitophagy removal of the dysfunctional mitochondria.

with aging and loss of Mfn2 produces an aging-like phenotype, including age-associated mitochondrial dysfunction, higher ROS accumulation, and muscle fiber atrophy [431,432]. Thus, it is tempting to attribute the aging-associated deficiency in Mfn2 as a potential link between impaired mitophagy and sarcopenic muscle loss [431,432]. However, it should be pointed out that other data have not found changes in Mfn2 and rather, an increase in the Mfn2 to Drp1 ratio that was associated with muscle atrophy in aged mice [69]. Thus, it is clear that while mitophagy is suppressed with aging, the mechanisms that account for this have not been fully identified. Further work is needed to determine the mechanism for loss of mitophagy and to determine if the failure of mitophagy progression in sarcopenia may lie, at least in part, with lysosomal dysfunction [427], or if improper signaling upstream of the lysosome, and particularly the loss of Mfn2 or some other protein involved in mitochondrial dynamics that in turn leads to loss of mitophagy to induce pathways leading to sarcopenia.

Similar to sarcopenic muscles, dysfunctional mitochondria and Mfn2 have been implicated in the reduction of mitophagy in motor neurons. For example, a loss in inhibition of the E3 ligase Omi/HtrA2 in the mitochondria of neuronal cells has been shown to contribute to a decrease in Mfn2 leading to reduced mitophagy Mfn2 [90,231,403,433,434]. Furthermore, it is well known that defective mitophagy is an underlying process that contributes to the progression of motor neuron death in ALS [435]. Furthermore, lithium-induced induction of mitophagy [435–437] and mitochondrial biogenesis [436,437] improve mitochondrial morphology in motor neurons of a G93A SOD-1 ALS mouse model. Other autophagy proteins have also been implicated in the loss of mitophagy in aging-associated neuron diseases, including Parkinsoń's disease. For example, the cleavage product of mitochondrial autophagy proteins, Pink1, Pink152, can exit the mitochondria in neuron cells and cleave Parkin, which then suppresses its translocation to the mitochondria and autophagic signaling, to prevent the elimination of the dysfunctional mitochondria by mitophagy [438]. Thus, reduced mitophagy appears to be a common mechanism in both muscle and neurons that can potentially be permissive for apoptosis and therefore result in cell death and hence contribute to loss of muscle mass and function.

Linking autophagy and apoptosis

Mitochondria are central to signaling for both providing ATP for protein synthesis and inducing signaling for degradation through apoptosis and mitophagy-associated redox-sensitive pathways. This includes pathways involving the communication of signaling proteins from apoptosis and autophagy pathways, dysregulation of PGC-1α, mitochondrial fusion and fission proteins, mitophagy, and sirtuins, which can be activated via nutritional or caloric restriction interventions. A decrease of mitochondrial inner membrane potential and increase of mitochondrial fission can trigger cascades of mitophagy, leading to the loss of mitochondrial homeostasis, inflammation, and apoptosis. The outcomes of dysregulation of apoptosis and mitophagy result in loss of muscle function and fiber atrophy.

BIM and Bcl-2

The proapoptotic BH3 only protein BIM (BCL2L11) is an important link between autophagy and apoptotic signaling pathways (Fig. 2). BIM is a member of the Bcl-2 apoptotic protein family that can interact with the antiapoptotic proteins B-cell lymphoma-2 (Bcl-2) and B-cell lymphoma-2 extra-large (Bcl-xL) [401,402]. However, BIM can also function independently through the regulation of the autophagy protein Beclin-1 [366,439]. This occurs when BIM is removed from its interaction with dynein light chain 1 (LC8), which can induce apoptosis by inactivating Bcl-2. In turn, this activates Bax-Bcl-2 antagonist/killer (Bak) or Bax-Bax homodimerization to induce mPTP pore opening in the outer mitochondria membrane. The resulting permeabilized mitochondria empty their contents to the cytosol to initiate apoptotic-signaling cascades. Thus, BIM appears to have roles in both inhibiting autophagy and promoting apoptosis [366,439].

Bcl-2 is also an important protein in both autophagy and apoptotic pathways, which highlights the crosstalk between these two death-signaling pathways. It is likely that there is required coordination between autophagy and apoptosis to maintain a healthy overall tissue environment. Although it is possible that disruption of the coordination between autophagy and apoptosis, perhaps by BIM or other proteins, permits dysfunctional mitochondria from being removed by mitophagy, the permeabilized mitochondria will perpetuate the apoptotic death signal.

PGC-1α

PGC-1α is normally considered to be a master regulator of mitochondrial biogenesis, but it has recently been shown to increase levels of autophagic proteins in skeletal muscle [362,363,440]. Indeed overexpression of PGC-1α in denervated mouse muscle leads to increased lysosomal capacity, reduced localization of the autophagy protein p62, and reduced lipidation of LC3-II and subsequent binding to mitochondria [362,363,440]. While PGC-1α overexpression did not reduce the Bax/Bcl-2 ratio and caspase-3 activity in immobilized mouse muscles [378], it is not known if other apoptotic proteins in the mitochondrial pathway might have been suppressed in this model.

Together, the data support the idea that some mitochondrial proteins such as PGC-1α, Bcl-2, and BIM, and perhaps other mitochondrial-associated proteins, may have multiple roles in regulating both the autophagy and the apoptotic death signaling pathways. These mitophagy-apoptosis signaling connections are critically linked through their mitochondrial targets.

Mitochondria, mitophagy, and the ubiquitin-proteasome system
Muscle wasting

Although it is clear that mitochondrial-centered signaling pathways are important for initiating cellular destruction, another major factor believed to complement mitochondrial signaling to contribute to sarcopenia is an acceleration of protein turnover. Enhanced protein loss without a concomitant increase in protein synthesis results in a net loss of protein, which leads to muscle wasting.

The forkhead box class O proteins (FOXO) transcription factor family regulates two main proteolytic systems: the ubiquitin-proteasome system (UPS) and the autophagy-lysosome system. The primary elements of the UPS for degradation of mitochondria and contractile elements that were begun through dysfunctional mitochondria-initiated signaling are shown in Fig. 4. FOXOs regulate the mammalian target of rapamycin complex 1 (mTORC1) signaling, which is associated with muscle hypertrophy [441–444] and inhibition of mitochondrial autophagy (mitophagy) in skeletal muscle [445–447]. FOXO proteins are thought to regulate the UPS, which is a tightly controlled system responsible for intracellular protein turnover, including regulation of normal protein turnover and elimination of misfolded and dysfunctional protein [448–453].

Damaged proteins are targeted by the conjugation of a polyubiquitin chain for stepwise proteasomal degradation into individual peptides and then, eventually, into individual amino acids (Fig. 4). Ubiquitinated proteins are recognized by the 26S proteasome, which consists of a 20S core and two 19S regulatory subunits [453–457]. The 19S subunits recognize and bind the ubiquitinated proteins and begin their adenosine triphosphate (ATP)-dependent disassembly and removal [458,459]. In skeletal muscles, polyubiquitination-targeting of proteins for degradation and disassembly by the 26S proteasome [460] occurs through Muscle RING Finger 1 (MuRF1) and muscle atrophy F-box (MAFbx/Atrogin-1) [455], which are muscle-specific E3 ubiquitin ligases [460]. Studies have shown that the inhibition of MAFbx/Atrogin-1 complex reduces muscle wasting [461,462]. Recent reports also indicate that a loss of MuRF1, which reduced skeletal muscle protein degradation in aging [453], was linked to inhibition of m-TOR signaling in muscles of older individuals or animals [463]. These findings indicate that the UPS may be an important element in the disassembly of skeletal muscle proteins under many atrophic conditions, as one of the systems underlying sarcopenia.

However, FOXO regulation is not simple, because mTORC1 is upregulated in denervation-induced muscle atrophy [444], which occurs in aging muscles. Interestingly, inhibition of mTORC1 reduces muscle atrophy via inhibition of MuRF1 and MAFbx/Atrogin-1 in response to denervation [444]. These data suggest that regulation of protein turnover pathways is tightly controlled because mTORC1, which is generally considered important in pathways of anabolism, is also a critical component of muscle atrophy and protein catabolism. It will be important in future studies to understand if failure to regulate FOXO control of mTORC1 properly by additional proteins, might contribute to increased degradation of muscle proteins in sarcopenia.

UPS and sarcopenia

There are conflicting studies that have examined the role of the UPS in sarcopenia and the role of mitochondria in the UPS. For example, increased levels of ubiquitin [464], 26S proteasomes, and polyubiquitinated proteins [465–467] along with increased MuRF1

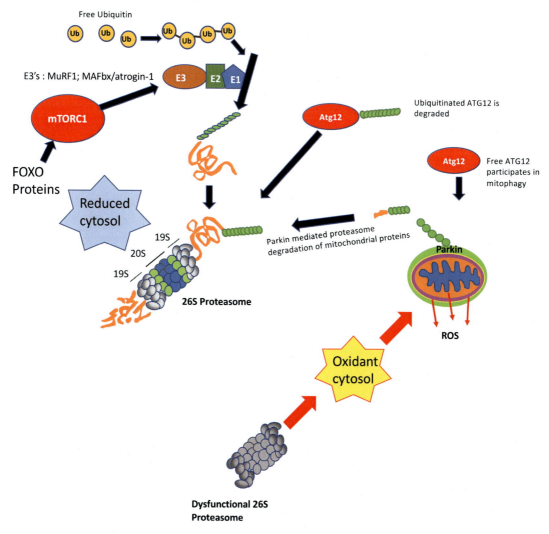

Fig. 4

UPS regulation of sarcopenia. Free ubiquitin conjugates form a polyubiquitin chain and targets damaged proteins in skeletal muscle. Targeting damaged proteins for proteolysis by the 26S proteasome occurs through muscle RING finger 1 (MuRF1) and MAFbx/Atrogin, which are muscle-specific E3 ubiquitin ligases. The 19S subunits recognize and bind the ubiquitinated proteins and begin their adenosine triphosphate (ATP)-dependent disassembly and removal in the 26S proteasome. Proteasome degradation results in small peptides that are further digested into amino acids, while lysosomal degradation directly produces single amino acids. Protein degradation from healthy proteasomes results in a reduced cytosolic environment, but dysfunctional proteasomes induce a highly oxidant cytosolic environment, which, in turn, damages mitochondrial membranes and causes increased ROS production from the damaged mitochondria. Independent from mitophagy, Parkin ubiquitinates outer mitochondrial membrane components for degradation by the proteasome in depolarized mitochondria. While ATG12 participates in mitophagy, when ubiquitinated, it is degraded in the proteasome to prevent mitophagy functions, and therefore, the proteasome has direct and indirect effects on mitochondria turnover.

and MAFbx/Atrogin-1 expression were reported to be elevated in hindlimb muscles of sarcopenic aged rats [465–468], where the mitochondrial function is known to be diminished. Furthermore, ubiquitin was found to be greater in quadriceps muscles of 70–79-year-old human subjects as compared to 20–29-year-old young adults [464]. In contrast, MuRF1 and MAFBx/Atrogin-1 expression have been reported to be lower in muscles of aged rats than young adult rats [223,469,470] and not changed with aging in the vastus lateralis muscle of human beings [342]. The discrepancy between these studies might be due to variability introduced by a low number of subjects in each study, and perhaps by some differences in the age and sex of the older subjects that were studied. It is also possible that MuRF1 and MAFbx/Atrogin-1 regulation were up or downregulated in aged muscles as a result of lifestyle factors, such as activity, nutritional history, health, and smoking habits in these studies. Finally, atrogen signaling could also be based on mitochondrial health because buffering of oxidative stress in mitochondria reduced the UPS activation, showing that mitochondrial oxidative stress is a primary trigger initiating the quality control systems of the UPS [471]. A proper balance of some UPS activation in basal conditions appears to be important to maintain mitochondrial import and health [472]. However, aging can lead to excessive UPS activation, a reduced mitochondrial biogenesis, an increased contractile protein degradation, and a lower net protein balance that together contribute to sarcopenia [473].

Muscles from older hosts have been reported to have a lower proteasome activity than muscles from younger animals or human beings in some [474–476] but not all studies [467,477,478]. Hwee and colleagues [453] reported that the 20S and 26S proteasome subunit activities were reduced with aging in muscles of old mice but maintained in muscles from MuRF1 null mice. This suggested that deletion of MuRF1 maintains skeletal muscle protein and muscle mass while oxidative stress in aged muscles. FOXO regulation of the UPS autophagy pathway in skeletal muscle is also thought to occur through mTORC1-mediated phosphorylation of ULK1 at Ser757 and the subsequent activation of the ULK1-ATG13-RP6KB/ribosomal protein p70S6 kinase (RB1CC1). Inhibition of mTORC1 in muscles of TSC knockout mice reduced autophagy and caused a loss of muscle mass and a reduction in the ability to generate muscle force [445,446,479]. Thus, the FOXO mediated UPS appears to be an important regulator of muscle mass in aging.

UPS and neural dysfunction in aging

While proper control of the UPS is important to maintain optimal cellular function and muscle mass in aging [473,480] reduced proteasome function, and the subsequent accumulation of ubiquitin-tagged proteins have been implicated in aging-associated neurodegenerative diseases [481–484]. An aging-associated reduction of UbcM2, a ubiquitin-conjugating enzyme, has been linked to lower UPS activity and neural degeneration [485]. Furthermore, decreased proteasome activity has been documented in the spinal cord of old rats, and this was accompanied by evidence for increased ROS damage in spinal neurons [486–489]. Loss of proteasome activity may be associated with an age-associated loss of the chaperone heat-shock protein 70 (HSP70) because restoration of HSP70 was shown to reduce autophagy-associated lipofuscin and increase proteasome activity in neurons [490,491]. This is similar to muscle cells, in that proteasome activity via the UPS is suppressed in aging neuronal cells [492–495].

Mitophagy regulation and the UPS

It is clear that autophagy and proteasome-mediated degradation are interconnected so that perturbation of one pathway can affect the function of the other. Thus, it is possible that in studies where the UPS was increased with aging, autophagy signaling was concurrently elevated, but this was not measured. However, it is clear that mitochondrial signaling impacts protein degradation in sarcopenia through the UPS.

The autophagy proteins ATG12–ATG5 are required for LC3-II conjugation to phosphatidylethanolamine (PE) that drives autophagosome membrane expansion. Besides its essential role in autophagy, the ATG12 also carries out various autophagy-independent roles. These include the promotion of mitochondrial fusion and activation of mitochondrial apoptosis [496,497]. ATG12 conjugation to ATG3 supports mitochondrial fusion, whereas free ATG12 directly regulates mitochondrial apoptosis in a similar manner to proapoptotic BH3-only proteins [498]. However, ATG12 is also a ubiquitin-like protein, which is directly ubiquitinated. Once ubiquitinated ATG12 promotes its proteasomal degradation via the UPS, whereas accumulation of free ATG12 contributes to proteasome inhibitor-mediated apoptosis [498,499].

Another important mitochondrial mitophagy protein, Parkin, mediates proteasome-dependent degradation of DRP1 [405,500,501] and OMM proteins, such as Tom20, Tom40, Tom70, and Omp25, when mitochondria become depolarized [401,402]. This is a unique nonautophagy function for Parkin because proteasome-dependent degradation of outer membrane proteins and outer membrane rupture is not required for mitophagy [401,402]. The loss of ATG7 or Parkin in denervated muscle induces dysfunctional mitochondrial mitophagy but also an accumulation of polyubiquitinated proteins. Furthermore, the accumulation of damaged and dysfunctional mitochondria attenuates the transcriptional activity of nuclear factor erythroid-derived 2-related factors (Nrf2), which have been reported to regulate the transcription of proteasome subunits [502–504]. Together, these findings suggest that the mitochondrially targeted mitophagy Parkin protein is also essential for the progression of the UPS degradation in muscle. Further connections between mitophagy and UPS pathways have been shown, including a report that a deficiency of MuRF1 increased the expression of MAFbx/Atrogin-1 and simultaneously reduced Beclin-1 expression in skeletal muscle after denervation [293,455]. This observation suggests that inhibition of UPS signaling via MuRF1 may decrease autophagic signaling, at least during denervation. Thus, proper mitophagy signaling to remove dysfunctional mitochondria appear to be important for not only regulating mitochondrial quality but for fine-tuning other proteolytic pathways.

UPS disruption increases dysfunctional mitochondria in muscle and neural cells

Age-associated conditions, such as Parkinson's and Alzheimer's disease, are associated with high ROS levels in neural cells. Reduced Pink1 and Parkin-regulated ubiquitination of the OMM of damaged mitochondria in aged neurons [505–510] can result in a greater accumulation of ROS, which, in turn, can damage more mitochondria and potentially elevate ROS levels even higher. A dysfunctional proteasome system results in a high oxidant environment [46,449,511,512] that damages the mitochondria and increases ROS production from mitochondria in muscle and neurons [46,507,513]. It is therefore likely that proteasome dysfunction contributes to the higher potential for ROS to be generated in muscle and neuron cells of older human beings or animals. Although more work is needed, it is likely that higher ROS accumulation increases the oxidant inducing potential to further damage mitochondria and initiate apoptotic death-signaling cascades and activates UPS signaling, leading toward loss of muscle and motor neurons, thereby contributing to sarcopenia.

UPS and mitochondria are also linked by a splice variant of mitochondrial regulator PGC-1α. PGC-1α2, PGC-1α3, and PGC-1α4 have been shown to stimulate protein synthesis and suppress UPS activity in cultured myotubes and mouse skeletal muscle [397,452,514,515]. Furthermore, PGC-1α reduces muscle protein degradation by the UPS via blocking NF-κB and FOXO3 activity [380,516,517]. Future studies are needed to determine if one or more of the splice variants of PGC-1α are critical regulators of mitochondrial-mediated UPS function in aging muscles and motor neurons.

Mitochondrial associated apoptosis, mitophagy, and UPS can be modulated by caloric restriction in sarcopenia

Given the impact of oxidative stress on reducing mitochondria function, it is not surprising that excessive nutrition (e.g., obesity), disuse, and aging, all of which greatly increase oxidative stress and reduce mitochondrial function, have been associated with exacerbation of sarcopenia [20,77,518–521]. Reduction of nutritional intake via caloric restriction has been proposed as an intervention to improve a host of deleterious events associated with aging and sarcopenia, including lowering oxidative stress and improving mitochondria function and mitophagy [196,522–525].

Although not strictly an antioxidant, histone deacetylases (HDACs) play a critical role in skeletal muscle that include antioxidant roles. The class II HDACs regulate muscle formation and repair through the transcription factor myocyte enhancer factor-2 [526]. As neural disruption and elimination occur in aging, the HDAC4 is relevant to sarcopenia because it is involved in innervation-regulated gene transcription [527]. Pharmacological inhibition of HDACs by butyrate has been shown to reduce muscle loss in aged mice via lowering of both oxidative stress and oxidative damage markers, including catalase and SOD1, and lower carbonylated proteins and markers of apoptosis, including DNA fragmentation and X-linked inhibitor of apoptosis protein (XIAP) [528,529].

A 30%–40% reduction in calorie consumption from ad libitum feeding without malnutrition attenuates age-associated muscular atrophy and reduces the loss of fibers and muscle stem cells in aging rodents and nonhuman primates [120,167,196,229,350,525,530]. Caloric restriction also attenuates the age-induced decrease in muscle force production per cross-sectional area in rodents [525,531–533]. Moreover, caloric restriction improved mitochondrial oxidative capacity [534,535] and reduced apoptosis signaling in aged muscles [522,536–540]. Part of the improvement in muscle function has been attributed to decreased ROS production and oxidative damage in aging [541–547], increased antioxidant production (to reduce oxidative damage), and attenuated acceleration of the UPS (reviewed in Ref. [548]). A combination of caloric restriction and aerobic exercise has been shown to reduce body fat without losing lean body mass in obese older women with a starting BMI $\geq 30\,\text{kg/m}^2$ and a fat mass > 40% [549].

Several groups have investigated the effects of caloric restriction on mitochondrial health. Long-term 30% caloric restriction has been investigated in middle-aged men and women (aged 52) [550,551]. Data from muscle biopsies showed an increase in autophagy markers, Beclin-1 and LC3, and an elevation in antioxidant enzymes MnSOD in muscles from calorically restricted human subjects [550,551] (Table 1).

Alternations in mitochondrial membrane integrity during caloric restriction may also be an important deterrent to apoptosis [536–539,551,555–559] by decreasing long-chain n-3 polyunsaturated fatty acid (PUFA) content and increasing the degree of membrane saturation [560–562]. This change is hypothesized to affect aging beneficially by protecting membranes against lipid peroxidation and preventing oxidative damage [541,545,560,563–566]. Mitochondrial dynamics, which are closely associated with autophagy signaling, appear to be altered by caloric restriction. In rodents, caloric restriction increased mitochondrial biogenesis and attenuates the decrease in PGC-1α gene expression in skeletal muscles of old rodents [534,535]. The relatively greater level of PGC-1α may be, at least, partially responsible for maintaining the oxidative capacity in muscles of old calorically restricted animals [534,535]. In young human beings (36.2 years), caloric restriction has been shown to increase muscle transcripts from several genes involved in mitochondrial biogenesis, including PGC-1α, transcription factor A, mitochondrial (TFAM), and SIRT1 [567,568]. However, it is not known if similar changes would be found in sarcopenic muscles of aged persons undergo nutritionally balanced caloric restriction. The caloric restriction appears to work, at least in part, via the mitochondrial metabolic regulator AMPK, because when AMPK is knocked out in mice muscles, the anticipated increase in autophagy proteins Beclin-1, ATG5, and LC3II/LC3I was all blunted [433,569,570]. Caloric restriction has also been reported to attenuate apoptosis susceptibility by reducing AIF, APAF-1, DNA fragmentation, and several caspases and also reduce mPTP opening, which results in a reduced migration of cytochrome c release from the mitochondria to the muscle cell cytosol [223,275,303,304,306,331,338,522,558,571–577]. These findings are particularly important because they suggest that reducing calorie intake while maintaining adequate nutritional homeostasis can act as a mediator to reduce mitochondrial dysfunction and apoptosis and improve mitophagy in sarcopenia (Table 1).

Table 1: Regulation of cellular signaling by caloric restriction in sarcopenia.

Nutritional compound	Model	Tissue	Muscle responses	Markers of oxidative stress	Regulators of apoptosis	Regulators of autophagy	Apoptosis markers	Autophagy Markers	UPS signaling	Reference
20% CR	27 months Fisher Brown Norway rats	WG	Mitochondrial respiration →	SIRT1 → PCG-1α ↑	SIRT1 →					[331]
8% lifelong CR (10 weeks to 24 months)	24 months F344 rats	Plantaris					Endo G-nucleosome ↓ AIF ↓ HSP 27 ↑ HSP70 →			[550]
8% lifelong CR (10 weeks to 24 months)	24 months F344 rats	Plantaris	Fiber CSA ↑ Connective tissue space in muscle ↓				Endo G-nucleosome ↓ AIF ↓ HSP 27 ↑ HSP70 →			[552]
30% CR, 3–15 years	Women and Men aged 52 years	Vastus lateralis	Serum cortisol ↑	MnSOD ↑				ULK1 ↑ LC3 ↑ Beclin-1 ↑		[551]
12.5% CR	Men and women aged 36.8 year	Vastus lateralis		TFAM ↑	Sirt1 ↑ PCG1-α ↑					[553]
25% CR-40% CR	26 months F344 rats	GAS	Muscle mass ↓				Procaspase-3 ↓ Cleaved caspase 3 ↓ Procaspase-9 → Cleaved procaspase-9 → Procaspase-12 ↓ Cleaved caspase-12 ↓ XIAP ↓ DNA fragmentation → Mitochondria ARC ↓ APAF-1 ↓ AIF ↓			[82]
40% CR for 14 days	8-, 16-month-old Sprague Dawley rats		S6K ↓ AKT ↓ mTOR ↓						FOXO3a ↓ atrogin ↓ MuRF1 ↓ proteasome subunits alpha 7 and beta 5 ↓ Ubiquitinated proteins ↓	[554]
40% CR	10-week-old C57BL/6 mice				Mfn1 ↑			Beclin 1 ↑ p62 ↑ Pink1 ↑ Parkin ↑		[522]

It would be particularly interesting to investigate the effects of caloric restriction that is combined with nutritional supplements, such as HMB, EGCg, resveratrol, or GTE, to determine if the benefits of caloric restriction and the nutritional interventions work in the same or different pathways to reduce sarcopenia. It has been intriguing, though, to note that there are some suggestions that the effects of caloric restriction attenuate aging-related changes in mitochondrial dynamics in type II glycolytic muscle fibers, but the apparent antiaging effects on mitochondrial morphology are largely restricted to type I oxidative fibers, which are relatively rich in mitochondria [196]. Caloric restriction-induced reduction of content and/or phosphorylation levels of key proteins in mTOR signaling and the UPS has been shown to occur in muscles of middle-aged and sarcopenic animals, but not in muscles of young animals [554]. This suggests that the benefits of caloric restriction on mitochondrial-induced signaling are important for reducing sarcopenia, but this is an age-specific response.

In conditions of starvation, which is not the same as caloric restriction, BIM is phosphorylated by MAPK8/JNK, which removes the BIM-LC8 interaction, allowing dissociation of BIM and Beclin-1. Bcl-2 sequesters Beclin-1 to reduce its availability for initiating autophagy [366,578]. Thus, starvation is a negative regulator of autophagy, whereas caloric restriction is a positive moderator of autophagy, although starvation has also been reported to upregulate autophagy [579].

Conclusions

Mitochondrial associated apoptosis, mitophagy, and UPS can be modulated by caloric restriction in sarcopenia. The data suggest that mitochondria health regulates a variety of pathways beyond energy metabolism and generation of ATP. This can include catabolic and anabolic signaling. Mitochondrial dysfunction arises with increasing age in the skeletal muscle, similar to other tissue types. The loss of muscle mass and function with increasing age defines sarcopenia and this loss appears to be intimately related to mitochondria health and abundance. Aging increases ROS production and accumulation, mtDNA damage, and is associated with higher levels of cytosolic calcium as a result of leaky ryanodine receptors, perhaps due to oxidative damage to the SR calcium channel. Mitochondrial import of calcium to attempt to maintain low basal Ca^{2+} levels through the MCU, modulates mitochondrial function, but excessive Ca^{2+} import into mitochondria will also increase the susceptibility of opening the mtPTP. The increase in mitochondrial permeability permits the mitochondrial contents to leak into the cytosol and initiate caspase-dependent and -independent apoptotic signaling. With aging, there is a suppression of mitophagy signaling and UPS function, so there is an accumulation of dysfunctional mitochondria in sarcopenic muscle. The dysfunctional mitochondria contribute to a large apoptotic signaling cascade, upregulation of the UPS, and the elimination of nuclei and can also lead to necrosis. This type of signaling for dismantling muscle fibers also occurs in neurons that have aging-induced dysfunctional mitochondria and apoptotic death of motor neurons. Death of muscle fibers, neurons, and dysregulation and fragmentation of the neuromuscular junction all contribute to a loss of muscle force and function. Strategies that are designed to reduce mitochondrial damage (e.g., reduce ROS production and ROS-induced damage), increase mitophagy to remove damaged and dysfunctional mitochondria (e.g., caloric restriction, exercise), increase the number of healthy mitochondria (e.g. PGC-1-induced biogenesis), increase mitochondria-UPS mediated regulation, improve Ca^{2+} buffering, and reduce the susceptibility of the remaining mitochondria to permeability, and therefore apoptotic signaling are all important to evaluate as a means to improve mitochondrial health in aging muscle. Returning mitochondrial health to the sarcopenic muscle appears to be one strategy to reduce the deleterious signaling associated with loss of muscle mass and function in aging.

References

[1] Evans WJ. What is sarcopenia? J Gerontol A Biol Sci Med Sci 1995;50. Spec No 5–8.
[2] Bauer J, Morley JE, Schols A, Ferrucci L, Cruz-Jentoft AJ, Dent E, et al. Sarcopenia: a time for action. An SCWD position paper. J Cachexia Sarcopenia Muscle 2019;10(5):956–61.
[3] Carmeli E. Frailty and primary sarcopenia: a review. Adv Exp Med Biol 2017;1020:53–68.
[4] Lexell J. Human aging, muscle mass, and fiber type composition. J Gerontol A Biol Sci Med Sci 1995;50. Spec No: 11–6.
[5] Jochum SB, Kistner M, Wood EH, Hoscheit M, Nowak L, Poirier J, et al. Is sarcopenia a better predictor of complications than body mass index? Sarcopenia and surgical outcomes in patients with rectal cancer. Colorectal Dis 2019;21(12):1372–8. https://doi.org/10.1111/codi.14751.
[6] Marques A, Queiros C. Frailty, sarcopenia and falls. In: Hertz K, Santy-Tomlinson J, editors. Fragility fracture nursing: holistic care and management of the orthogeriatric patient, Chapter 2. Cham, China: Springer; 2018. p. 15–26. https://doi.org/10.1007/978-3-319-76681-2_2.
[7] Schaap LA, van Schoor NM, Lips P, Visser M. Associations of sarcopenia definitions, and their components, with the incidence of recurrent falling and fractures: the longitudinal aging study Amsterdam. J Gerontol A Biol Sci Med Sci 2018;73(9):1199–204.
[8] Aversa Z, Zhang X, Fielding RA, Lanza I, LeBrasseur NK. The clinical impact and biological mechanisms of skeletal muscle aging. Bone 2019;127:26–36.
[9] Kim TN, Park MS, Yang SJ, Yoo HJ, Kang HJ, Song W, et al. Prevalence and determinant factors of sarcopenia in patients with type 2 diabetes: the Korean Sarcopenic Obesity Study (KSOS). Diabetes Care 2010;33(7):1497–9.
[10] Tamosauskaite J, Atkins JL, Pilling LC, Kuo CL, Kuchel GA, Ferrucci L, et al. Hereditary hemochromatosis associations with frailty, sarcopenia and chronic pain: evidence from 200,975 older UK biobank participants. J Gerontol A Biol Sci Med Sci 2019;74(3):337–42.
[11] Khadra D, Itani L, Tannir H, Kreidieh D, El Masri D, El Ghoch M. Association between sarcopenic obesity and higher risk of type 2 diabetes in adults: a systematic review and meta-analysis. World J Diabetes 2019;10(5):311–23.
[12] Stangl MK, Bocker W, Chubanov V, Ferrari U, Fischereder M, Gudermann T, et al. Sarcopenia—endocrinological and neurological aspects. Exp Clin Endocrinol Diabetes 2019;127(1):8–22.
[13] Mesinovic J, Zengin A, De Courten B, Ebeling PR, Scott D. Sarcopenia and type 2 diabetes mellitus: a bidirectional relationship. Diabetes Metab Syndr Obes 2019;12:1057–72.
[14] Murphy RA, Ip EH, Zhang Q, Boudreau RM, Cawthon PM, Newman AB, et al. Transition to sarcopenia and determinants of transitions in older adults: a population-based study. J Gerontol A Biol Sci Med Sci 2014;69(6):751–8.

[15] Larsson L, Degens H, Li M, Salviati L, Lee YI, Thompson W, et al. Sarcopenia: aging-related loss of muscle mass and function. Physiol Rev 2019;99(1):427–511.
[16] Ebeling PR, Cicuttini F, Scott D, Jones G. Promoting mobility and healthy aging in men: a narrative review. Osteoporos Int 2019;30(10):1911–22.
[17] Grosicki GJ, Englund DA, Price L, Iwai M, Kashiwa M, Reid KF, et al. Lower-extremity torque capacity and physical function in mobility-limited older adults. J Nutr Health Aging 2019;23(8):703–9.
[18] Metter EJ, Talbot LA, Schrager M, Conwit R. Skeletal muscle strength as a predictor of all-cause mortality in healthy men. J Gerontol A Biol Sci Med Sci 2002;57(10):B359–65.
[19] Vatic M, von Haehling S, Ebner N. Inflammatory biomarkers of frailty. Exp Gerontol 2020;133:110858.
[20] Atmis V, Yalcin A, Silay K, Ulutas S, Bahsi R, Turgut T, et al. The relationship between all-cause mortality sarcopenia and sarcopenic obesity among hospitalized older people. Aging Clin Exp Res 2019;31(11):1563–72. https://doi.org/10.1007/s40520-019-01277-5.
[21] Gilligan LA, Towbin AJ, Dillman JR, Somasundaram E, Trout AT. Quantification of skeletal muscle mass: sarcopenia as a marker of overall health in children and adults. Pediatr Radiol 2019;50(4):455–64. https://doi.org/10.1007/s00247-019-04562-7.
[22] Hajibandeh S, Hajibandeh S, Jarvis R, Bhogal T, Dalmia S. Meta-analysis of the effect of sarcopenia in predicting postoperative mortality in emergency and elective abdominal surgery. Surgeon 2019;17(6):370–80.
[23] Centers for Disease Control and Prevention. The state of aging and health in America 2013. Atlanta, GA: Centers for Disease Control and Prevention; 2013. www.cdc.gov/aging.
[24] Ferrucci L, Fabbri E. Inflammageing: chronic inflammation in ageing, cardiovascular disease, and frailty. Nat Rev Cardiol 2018;15(9):505–22.
[25] Tran JR, Chen H, Zheng X, Zheng Y. Lamin in inflammation and aging. Curr Opin Cell Biol 2016;40:124–30.
[26] Jackson MJ, Vasilaki A, McArdle A. Cellular mechanisms underlying oxidative stress in human exercise. Free Radic Biol Med 2016;98:13–7.
[27] Jackson MJ, McArdle A. Role of reactive oxygen species in age-related neuromuscular deficits. J Physiol 2016;594(8):1979–88.
[28] Ji LL, Kang C, Zhang Y. Exercise-induced hormesis and skeletal muscle health. Free Radic Biol Med 2016;98:113–22.
[29] Pollock N, Staunton CA, Vasilaki A, McArdle A, Jackson MJ. Denervated muscle fibers induce mitochondrial peroxide generation in neighboring innervated fibers: role in muscle aging. Free Radic Biol Med 2017;112:84–92.
[30] Hepple RT, Rice CL. Innervation and neuromuscular control in ageing skeletal muscle. J Physiol 2016;594(8):1965–78.
[31] Larsson L. Motor units: remodeling in aged animals. J Gerontol A Biol Sci Med Sci 1995;50. Spec No: 91–5.
[32] Pannerec A, Springer M, Migliavacca E, Ireland A, Piasecki M, Karaz S, et al. A robust neuromuscular system protects rat and human skeletal muscle from sarcopenia. Aging (Albany NY) 2016;8(4):712–29.
[33] Rudolf R, Khan MM, Labeit S, Deschenes MR. Degeneration of neuromuscular junction in age and dystrophy. Front Aging Neurosci 2014;6:99.
[34] Rudolf R, Deschenes MR, Sandri M. Neuromuscular junction degeneration in muscle wasting. Curr Opin Clin Nutr Metab Care 2016;19(3):177–81.
[35] Scalabrin M, Pollock N, Staunton CA, Brooks SV, McArdle A, Jackson MJ, et al. Redox responses in skeletal muscle following denervation. Redox Biol 2019;26:101294.
[36] Vasilaki A, Richardson A, Van Remmen H, Brooks SV, Larkin L, McArdle A, et al. Role of nerve-muscle interactions and reactive oxygen species in regulation of muscle proteostasis with ageing. J Physiol 2017;595(20):6409–15.
[37] Migliavacca E, Tay SKH, Patel HP, Sonntag T, Civiletto G, McFarlane C, et al. Mitochondrial oxidative capacity and NAD(+) biosynthesis are reduced in human sarcopenia across ethnicities. Nat Commun 2019;10(1):5808.

[38] Tomlinson BE, Irving D. The numbers of limb motor neurons in the human lumbosacral cord throughout life. J Neurol Sci 1977;34(2):213–9.
[39] Deepa SS, Van Remmen H, Brooks SV, Faulkner JA, Larkin L, McArdle A, et al. Accelerated sarcopenia in cu/Zn superoxide dismutase knockout mice. Free Radic Biol Med 2019;132:19–23.
[40] Rajasekaran NS, Shelar SB, Jones DP, Hoidal JR. Reductive stress impairs myogenic differentiation. Redox Biol 2020;34:101492.
[41] Ungvari Z, Tarantini S, Nyul-Toth A, Kiss T, Yabluchanskiy A, Csipo T, et al. Nrf2 dysfunction and impaired cellular resilience to oxidative stressors in the aged vasculature: from increased cellular senescence to the pathogenesis of age-related vascular diseases. GeroScience 2019.
[42] Sousa-Victor P, Gutarra S, Garcia-Prat L, Rodriguez-Ubreva J, Ortet L, Ruiz-Bonilla V, et al. Geriatric muscle stem cells switch reversible quiescence into senescence. Nature 2014;506(7488):316–21.
[43] Garcia-Prat L, Sousa-Victor P, Munoz-Canoves P. Functional dysregulation of stem cells during aging: a focus on skeletal muscle stem cells. FEBS J 2013;280(17):4051–62.
[44] Sousa-Victor P, Garcia-Prat L, Munoz-Canoves P. New mechanisms driving muscle stem cell regenerative decline with aging. Int J Dev Biol 2018;62(6–7–8):583–90.
[45] Tanaka T, Nishimura A, Nishiyama K, Goto T, Numaga-Tomita T, Nishida M. Mitochondrial dynamics in exercise physiology. Pflugers Arch 2020;472(2):137–53.
[46] Kadoguchi T, Shimada K, Miyazaki T, Kitamura K, Kunimoto M, Aikawa T, et al. Promotion of oxidative stress is associated with mitochondrial dysfunction and muscle atrophy in aging mice. Geriatr Gerontol Int 2020;20(1):78–84.
[47] Hood DA, Memme JM, Oliveira AN, Triolo M. Maintenance of skeletal muscle mitochondria in health, exercise, and aging. Annu Rev Physiol 2019;81:19–41.
[48] Rezus E, Burlui A, Cardoneanu A, Rezus C, Codreanu C, Parvu M, et al. Inactivity and skeletal muscle metabolism: a vicious cycle in old age. Int J Mol Sci 2020;21(2).
[49] Alway SE, Morissette MR, Siu PM. Aging and apoptosis in muscle. In: Masoro EJ, Austad S, editors. Handbook of the biology of aging. 7th. New York: Elsevier; 2011. p. 63–118.
[50] Alway SE, Mohamed JS, Myers MJ. Mitochondria Initiate and Regulate Sarcopenia. Exerc Sport Sci Rev 2017;45(2):58–69.
[51] Anagnostou ME, Hepple RT. Mitochondrial mechanisms of neuromuscular junction degeneration with aging. Cells 2020;9(1):197.
[52] Carter HN, Kim Y, Erlich AT, Zarrin-Khat D, Hood DA. Autophagy and mitophagy flux in young and aged skeletal muscle following chronic contractile activity. J Physiol 2018;596(16):3567–84.
[53] Chabi B, Ljubicic V, Menzies KJ, Huang JH, Saleem A, Hood DA. Mitochondrial function and apoptotic susceptibility in aging skeletal muscle. Aging Cell 2008;7(1):2–12.
[54] Adelnia F, Cameron D, Bergeron CM, Fishbein KW, Spencer RG, Reiter DA, et al. The role of muscle perfusion in the age-associated decline of mitochondrial function in healthy individuals. Front Physiol 2019;10:427.
[55] No MH, Heo JW, Yoo SZ, Kim CJ, Park DH, Kang JH, et al. Effects of aging and exercise training on mitochondrial function and apoptosis in the rat heart. Pflugers Arch 2020;472(2):179–93.
[56] Koo JH, Kang EB, Cho JY. Resistance exercise improves mitochondrial quality control in a rat model of sporadic inclusion body myositis. Gerontology 2019;65(3):240–52.
[57] Ji LL, Yeo D. Mitochondrial dysregulation and muscle disuse atrophy. F1000Res 2019;8.
[58] Moreillon M, Conde Alonso S, Broskey NT, Greggio C, Besson C, Rousson V, et al. Hybrid fiber alterations in exercising seniors suggest contribution to fast-to-slow muscle fiber shift. J Cachexia Sarcopenia Muscle 2019;10(3):687–95.
[59] Alway SE. Is fiber mitochondrial volume density a good indicator of muscle fatigability to isometric exercise? J Appl Physiol (1985) 1991;70(5):2111–9.
[60] Alway SE, MacDougall JD, Sale DG, Sutton JR, McComas AJ. Functional and structural adaptations in skeletal muscle of trained athletes. J Appl Physiol (1985) 1988;64(3):1114–20.
[61] Deschenes MR. Effects of aging on muscle fibre type and size. Sports Med 2004;34(12):809–24.
[62] Frontera WR, Suh D, Krivickas LS, Hughes VA, Goldstein R, Roubenoff R. Skeletal muscle fiber quality in older men and women. Am J Physiol Cell Physiol 2000;279(3):C611–8.

[63] Rogers MA, Evans WJ. Changes in skeletal muscle with aging: effects of exercise training. Exerc Sport Sci Rev 1993;21:65–102.
[64] Alway SE, Siu PM. Nuclear apoptosis contributes to sarcopenia. Exerc Sport Sci Rev 2008;36(2):51–7.
[65] Alway SE. Mitochondrial dysfunction: linking type 1 diabetes and sarcopenia. Exerc Sport Sci Rev 2019;47(2):63.
[66] Alway SE, McCrory JL, Kearcher K, Vickers A, Frear B, Gilleland DL, et al. Resveratrol enhances exercise-induced cellular and functional adaptations of skeletal muscle in older men and women. J Gerontol A Biol Sci Med Sci 2017;72(12):1595–606.
[67] Akbari M, Kirkwood TBL, Bohr VA. Mitochondria in the signaling pathways that control longevity and health span. Ageing Res Rev 2019;54:100940.
[68] Habiballa L, Salmonowicz H, Passos JF. Mitochondria and cellular senescence: implications for musculoskeletal ageing. Free Radic Biol Med 2019;132:3–10.
[69] Leduc-Gaudet JP, Reynaud O, Hussain SN, Gouspillou G. Parkin overexpression protects from ageing-related loss of muscle mass and strength. J Physiol 2019;597(7):1975–91.
[70] Memme JM, Erlich AT, Hood DA, Phukan G. Exercise and mitochondrial health. J Physiol 2021;599(3):803–17. https://doi.org/10.1113/JP278853.
[71] Jackson JR, Ryan MJ, Alway SE. Long-term supplementation with resveratrol alleviates oxidative stress but does not attenuate sarcopenia in aged mice. J Gerontol A Biol Sci Med Sci 2011;66(7):751–64.
[72] Nagarajan P, Agudelo Garcia PA, Iyer CC, Popova LV, Arnold WD, Parthun MR. Early-onset aging and mitochondrial defects associated with loss of histone acetyltransferase 1 (Hat1). Aging Cell 2019;18(5):e12992.
[73] Muller-Hocker J. Mitochondria and ageing. Brain Pathol 1992;2(2):149–58.
[74] Del Campo A, Contreras-Hernandez I, Castro-Sepulveda M, Campos CA, Figueroa R, Tevy MF, et al. Muscle function decline and mitochondria changes in middle age precede sarcopenia in mice. Aging (Albany NY) 2018;10(1):34–55.
[75] Kang S, Fernandes-Alnemri T, Alnemri ES. A novel role for the mitochondrial HTRA2/OMI protease in aging. Autophagy 2013;9(3):420–1.
[76] Kang C, Chung E, Diffee G, Ji LL. Exercise training attenuates aging-associated mitochondrial dysfunction in rat skeletal muscle: role of PGC-1alpha. Exp Gerontol 2013;48(11):1343–50.
[77] Kim C, Hwang JK. The 5,7-dimethoxyflavone suppresses sarcopenia by regulating protein turnover and mitochondria biogenesis-related pathways. Nutrients 2020;12(4).
[78] Melouane A, Yoshioka M, St-Amand J. Extracellular matrix/mitochondria pathway: a novel potential target for sarcopenia. Mitochondrion 2020;50:63–70.
[79] Ljubicic V, Menzies KJ, Hood DA. Mitochondrial dysfunction is associated with a pro-apoptotic cellular environment in senescent cardiac muscle. Mech Ageing Dev 2010;131(2):79–88.
[80] Ljubicic V, Joseph AM, Saleem A, Uguccioni G, Collu-Marchese M, Lai RY, et al. Transcriptional and post-transcriptional regulation of mitochondrial biogenesis in skeletal muscle: effects of exercise and aging. Biochim Biophys Acta 2010;1800(3):223–34.
[81] Picca A, Calvani R, Leeuwenburgh C, Coelho-Junior HJ, Bernabei R, Landi F, et al. Targeting mitochondrial quality control for treating sarcopenia: lessons from physical exercise. Expert Opin Ther Targets 2019;23(2):153–60.
[82] Dirks AJ, Leeuwenburgh C. Aging and lifelong calorie restriction result in adaptations of skeletal muscle apoptosis repressor, apoptosis-inducing factor, X-linked inhibitor of apoptosis, caspase-3, and caspase-12. Free Radic Biol Med 2004;36(1):27–39.
[83] Johannsen DL, Ravussin E. The role of mitochondria in health and disease. Curr Opin Pharmacol 2009;9(6):780–6.
[84] Al-Menhali AS, Banu S, Angelova PR, Barcaru A, Horvatovich P, Abramov AY, et al. Lipid peroxidation is involved in calcium dependent upregulation of mitochondrial metabolism in skeletal muscle. Biochim Biophys Acta Gen Subj 1864;2020(3):129487.
[85] Calbet JAL, Martin-Rodriguez S, Martin-Rincon M, Morales-Alamo D. An integrative approach to the regulation of mitochondrial respiration during exercise: focus on high-intensity exercise. Redox Biol 2020;35:101478.

[86] Dollerup OL, Chubanava S, Agerholm M, Sondergard SD, Altintas A, Moller AB, et al. Nicotinamide riboside does not alter mitochondrial respiration, content or morphology in skeletal muscle from obese and insulin-resistant men. J Physiol 2020;598(4):731–54.

[87] Robin JD, Jacome Burbano MS, Peng H, Croce O, Thomas JL, Laberthonniere C, et al. Mitochondrial function in skeletal myofibers is controlled by a TRF2-SIRT3 axis over lifetime. Aging Cell 2020;19(3):e13097.

[88] Canugovi C, Stevenson MD, Vendrov AE, Hayami T, Robidoux J, Xiao H, et al. Increased mitochondrial NADPH oxidase 4 (NOX4) expression in aging is a causative factor in aortic stiffening. Redox Biol 2019;26:101288.

[89] Ungvari Z, Labinskyy N, Gupte S, Chander PN, Edwards JG, Csiszar A. Dysregulation of mitochondrial biogenesis in vascular endothelial and smooth muscle cells of aged rats. Am J Physiol Heart Circ Physiol 2008;294(5):H2121–8.

[90] Huang DD, Fan SD, Chen XY, Yan XL, Zhang XZ, Ma BW, et al. Nrf2 deficiency exacerbates frailty and sarcopenia by impairing skeletal muscle mitochondrial biogenesis and dynamics in an age-dependent manner. Exp Gerontol 2019;119:61–73.

[91] Potes Y, Perez-Martinez Z, Bermejo-Millo JC, Rubio-Gonzalez A, Fernandez-Fernandez M, Bermudez M, et al. Overweight in the elderly induces a switch in energy metabolism that undermines muscle integrity. Aging Dis 2019;10(2):217–30.

[92] Taylor RW, Turnbull DM. Mitochondrial DNA mutations in human disease. Nat Rev Genet 2005;6(5):389–402.

[93] Hood DA. Invited review: contractile activity-induced mitochondrial biogenesis in skeletal muscle. J Appl Physiol (1985) 2001;90(3):1137–57.

[94] Wallace DC. A mitochondrial paradigm for degenerative diseases and ageing. Novartis Found Symp 2001;235:247–63 [discussion 63–6].

[95] Freyssenet D, Irrcher I, Connor MK, Di Carlo M, Hood DA. Calcium-regulated changes in mitochondrial phenotype in skeletal muscle cells. Am J Physiol Cell Physiol 2004;286(5):C1053–61.

[96] Xu Y, Shen J, Ran Z. Emerging views of mitophagy in immunity and autoimmune diseases. Autophagy 2020;16(1):3–17.

[97] Picca A, Guerra F, Calvani R, Bucci C, Lo Monaco MR, Bentivoglio AR, et al. Mitochondrial dysfunction and aging: insights from the analysis of extracellular vesicles. Int J Mol Sci 2019;20(4).

[98] Martensson CU, Priesnitz C, Song J, Ellenrieder L, Doan KN, Boos F, et al. Mitochondrial protein translocation-associated degradation. Nature 2019;569(7758):679–83.

[99] Hathaway QA, Roth SM, Pinti MV, Sprando DC, Kunovac A, Durr AJ, et al. Machine-learning to stratify diabetic patients using novel cardiac biomarkers and integrative genomics. Cardiovasc Diabetol 2019;18(1):78.

[100] Geng J, Wei M, Yuan X, Liu Z, Wang X, Zhang D, et al. TIGAR regulates mitochondrial functions through SIRT1-PGC1alpha pathway and translocation of TIGAR into mitochondria in skeletal muscle. FASEB J 2019;33(5):6082–98.

[101] Goody MF, Henry CA. A need for NAD+ in muscle development, homeostasis, and aging. Skelet Muscle 2018;8(1):9.

[102] Miller BF, Robinson MM, Bruss MD, Hellerstein M, Hamilton KL. A comprehensive assessment of mitochondrial protein synthesis and cellular proliferation with age and caloric restriction. Aging Cell 2012;11(1):150–61.

[103] Distefano G, Standley RA, Dube JJ, Carnero EA, Ritov VB, Stefanovic-Racic M, et al. Chronological age does not influence ex-vivo mitochondrial respiration and quality control in skeletal muscle. J Gerontol A Biol Sci Med Sci 2017;72(4):535–42.

[104] Picard M, Ritchie D, Wright KJ, Romestaing C, Thomas MM, Rowan SL, et al. Mitochondrial functional impairment with aging is exaggerated in isolated mitochondria compared to permeabilized myofibers. Aging Cell 2010;9(6):1032–46.

[105] Konopka AR, Laurin JL, Schoenberg HM, Reid JJ, Castor WM, Wolff CA, et al. Metformin inhibits mitochondrial adaptations to aerobic exercise training in older adults. Aging Cell 2019;18(1):e12880.

[106] Konopka AR, Castor WM, Wolff CA, Musci RV, Reid JJ, Laurin JL, et al. Skeletal muscle mitochondrial protein synthesis and respiration in response to the energetic stress of an ultra-endurance race. J Appl Physiol (1985) 2017;123(6):1516–24.

[107] Konopka AR, Suer MK, Wolff CA, Harber MP. Markers of human skeletal muscle mitochondrial biogenesis and quality control: effects of age and aerobic exercise training. J Gerontol A Biol Sci Med Sci 2014;69(4):371–8.

[108] Lanza IR, Nair KS. Mitochondrial function as a determinant of life span. Pflugers Arch 2010;459(2):277–89.

[109] Drake JC, Peelor 3rd FF, Biela LM, Watkins MK, Miller RA, Hamilton KL, et al. Assessment of mitochondrial biogenesis and mTORC1 signaling during chronic rapamycin feeding in male and female mice. J Gerontol A Biol Sci Med Sci 2013;68(12):1493–501.

[110] Monaco CMF, Bellissimo CA, Hughes MC, Ramos SV, Laham R, Perry CGR, et al. Sexual dimorphism in human skeletal muscle mitochondrial bioenergetics in response to type 1 diabetes. Am J Physiol Endocrinol Metab 2020;318(1):E44–51.

[111] Mohajeri M, Martin-Jimenez C, Barreto GE, Sahebkar A. Effects of estrogens and androgens on mitochondria under normal and pathological conditions. Prog Neurobiol 2019;176:54–72.

[112] Samouri G, Stouffs A, Essen LV, Simonet O, De Kock M, Forget P. What can we learn from sarcopenia with Curarisation in the context of Cancer surgery? A review of the literature. Curr Pharm Des 2019;25(28):3005–10.

[113] Drey M. Sarcopenia—pathophysiology and clinical relevance. Wien Med Wochenschr 2011;161(17–18):402–8.

[114] Joseph AM, Adhihetty PJ, Wawrzyniak NR, Wohlgemuth SE, Picca A, Kujoth GC, et al. Dysregulation of mitochondrial quality control processes contribute to sarcopenia in a mouse model of premature aging. PLoS One 2013;8(7):e69327.

[115] Picard M, Ritchie D, Wright KJ, Romestaing C, Thomas MM, Rowan SL, et al. Mitochondrial functional impairment with aging is exaggerated in isolated mitochondria compared to permeabilized myofibers. Aging Cell 2010;9(6):1032–46.

[116] Picard M, Ritchie D, Thomas MM, Wright KJ, Hepple RT. Alterations in intrinsic mitochondrial function with aging are fiber type-specific and do not explain differential atrophy between muscles. Aging Cell 2011;10(6):1047–55.

[117] Powers S, Ozdemir M, Hyatt H. Redox control of proteolysis during inactivity-induced skeletal muscle atrophy. Antioxid Redox Signal 2020;33(8):559–69. https://doi.org/10.1089/ars.2019.8000.

[118] Hyatt H, Deminice R, Yoshihara T, Powers SK. Mitochondrial dysfunction induces muscle atrophy during prolonged inactivity: a review of the causes and effects. Arch Biochem Biophys 2019;662:49–60.

[119] Dos Santos JM, de Oliveira DS, Moreli ML, Benite-Ribeiro SA. The role of mitochondrial DNA damage at skeletal muscle oxidative stress on the development of type 2 diabetes. Mol Cell Biochem 2018;449(1–2):251–5.

[120] Klaus S, Ost M. Mitochondrial uncoupling and longevity—a role for mitokines? Exp Gerontol 2020;130:110796.

[121] Baldelli S, Aquilano K, Ciriolo MR. PGC-1alpha buffers ROS-mediated removal of mitochondria during myogenesis. Cell Death Dis 2014;5:e1515.

[122] Brand MD. Mitochondrial generation of superoxide and hydrogen peroxide as the source of mitochondrial redox signaling. Free Radic Biol Med 2016;100:14–31.

[123] Sriram S, Subramanian S, Sathiakumar D, Venkatesh R, Salerno MS, McFarlane CD, et al. Modulation of reactive oxygen species in skeletal muscle by myostatin is mediated through NF-kappaB. Aging Cell 2011;10(6):931–48.

[124] Sriram S, Subramanian S, Juvvuna PK, Ge X, Lokireddy S, McFarlane CD, et al. Myostatin augments muscle-specific ring finger protein-1 expression through an NF-kB independent mechanism in SMAD3 null muscle. Mol Endocrinol 2014;28(3):317–30.

[125] Munro D, Banh S, Sotiri E, Tamanna N, Treberg JR. The thioredoxin and glutathione-dependent H2O2 consumption pathways in muscle mitochondria: involvement in H2O2 metabolism and consequence to H2O2 efflux assays. Free Radic Biol Med 2016;96:334–46.

[126] Sataranatarajan K, Qaisar R, Davis C, Sakellariou GK, Vasilaki A, Zhang Y, et al. Neuron specific reduction in CuZnSOD is not sufficient to initiate a full sarcopenia phenotype. Redox Biol 2015;5:140–8.

[127] Su Y, Ahn B, Macpherson PCD, Ranjit R, Claflin DR, Van Remmen H, et al. Transgenic expression of SOD1 specifically in neurons of Sod1 deficient mice prevents defects in muscle mitochondrial function and calcium handling. Free Radic Biol Med 2021;165:299–311. https://doi.org/10.1016/j.freeradbiomed.2021.01.047.

[128] Pharaoh G, Owen D, Yeganeh A, Premkumar P, Farley J, Bhaskaran S, et al. Disparate central and peripheral effects of circulating IGF-1 deficiency on tissue mitochondrial function. Mol Neurobiol 2020;57(3):1317–31.

[129] Munro D, Baldy C, Pamenter ME, Treberg JR. The exceptional longevity of the naked mole-rat may be explained by mitochondrial antioxidant defenses. Aging Cell 2019;18(3):e12916.

[130] Serino A, Salazar G. Protective role of polyphenols against vascular inflammation, aging and cardiovascular disease. Nutrients 2018;11(1).

[131] Salazar G, Huang J, Feresin RG, Zhao Y, Griendling KK. Zinc regulates Nox1 expression through a NF-kappaB and mitochondrial ROS dependent mechanism to induce senescence of vascular smooth muscle cells. Free Radic Biol Med 2017;108:225–35.

[132] Garcia-Prat L, Martinez-Vicente M, Munoz-Canoves P. Methods for mitochondria and mitophagy flux analyses in stem cells of resting and regenerating skeletal muscle. Methods Mol Biol 2016;1460:223–40.

[133] Ryan MJ, Jackson JR, Hao Y, Leonard SS, Alway SE. Inhibition of xanthine oxidase reduces oxidative stress and improves skeletal muscle function in response to electrically stimulated isometric contractions in aged mice. Free Radic Biol Med 2011;51(1):38–52.

[134] Jackson JR, Ryan MJ, Hao Y, Alway SE. Mediation of endogenous antioxidant enzymes and apoptotic signaling by resveratrol following muscle disuse in the gastrocnemius muscles of young and old rats. Am J Physiol Regul Integr Comp Physiol 2010;299(6):R1572–81.

[135] Ryan MJ, Jackson JR, Hao Y, Williamson CL, Dabkowski ER, Hollander JM, et al. Suppression of oxidative stress by resveratrol after isometric contractions in gastrocnemius muscles of aged mice. J Gerontol A Biol Sci Med Sci 2010;65(8):815–31.

[136] Nascimento CM, Ingles M, Salvador-Pascual A, Cominetti MR, Gomez-Cabrera MC, Vina J. Sarcopenia, frailty and their prevention by exercise. Free Radic Biol Med 2019;132:42–9.

[137] Coen PM, Musci RV, Hinkley JM, Miller BF. Mitochondria as a target for mitigating sarcopenia. Front Physiol 2018;9:1883.

[138] Pollock RD, O'Brien KA, Daniels LJ, Nielsen KB, Rowlerson A, Duggal NA, et al. Properties of the vastus lateralis muscle in relation to age and physiological function in master cyclists aged 55–79 years. Aging Cell 2018;17(2).

[139] Ryan MJ, Dudash HJ, Docherty M, Geronilla KB, Baker BA, Haff GG, et al. Vitamin E and C supplementation reduces oxidative stress, improves antioxidant enzymes and positive muscle work in chronically loaded muscles of aged rats. Exp Gerontol 2010;45(11):882–95.

[140] Ryan MJ, Dudash HJ, Docherty M, Geronilla KB, Baker BA, Cutlip RG, et al. Aging-dependent regulation of antioxidant enzymes and redox status in chronically loaded rat dorsiflexor muscles. J Gerontol A Biol Sci Med Sci 2008;63:1015–26.

[141] Javadov S, Jang S, Rodriguez-Reyes N, Rodriguez-Zayas AE, Soto Hernandez J, Krainz T, et al. Mitochondria-targeted antioxidant preserves contractile properties and mitochondrial function of skeletal muscle in aged rats. Oncotarget 2015;6(37):39469–81.

[142] Spendiff S, Vuda M, Gouspillou G, Aare S, Perez A, Morais JA, et al. Denervation drives mitochondrial dysfunction in skeletal muscle of octogenarians. J Physiol 2016;594(24):7361–79.

[143] Picca A, Lezza AMS, Leeuwenburgh C, Pesce V, Calvani R, Bossola M, et al. Circulating mitochondrial DNA at the crossroads of mitochondrial dysfunction and inflammation during aging and muscle wasting disorders. Rejuvenation Res 2018;21(4):350–9.

[144] Gomez-Cabrera MC, Sanchis-Gomar F, Garcia-Valles R, Pareja-Galeano H, Gambini J, Borras C, et al. Mitochondria as sources and targets of damage in cellular aging. Clin Chem Lab Med 2012;50(8):1287–95.

[145] Bua E, Johnson J, Herbst A, Delong B, McKenzie D, Salamat S, et al. Mitochondrial DNA-deletion mutations accumulate intracellularly to detrimental levels in aged human skeletal muscle fibers. Am J Hum Genet 2006;79(3):469–80.

[146] Cheema N, Herbst A, McKenzie D, Aiken JM. Apoptosis and necrosis mediate skeletal muscle fiber loss in age-induced mitochondrial enzymatic abnormalities. Aging Cell 2015;14(6):1085–93.

[147] McKenzie D, Bua E, McKiernan S, Cao Z, Aiken JM, Jonathan W. Mitochondrial DNA deletion mutations: a causal role in sarcopenia. Eur J Biochem 2002;269(8):2010–5.

[148] Pak JW, Herbst A, Bua E, Gokey N, McKenzie D, Aiken JM. Mitochondrial DNA mutations as a fundamental mechanism in physiological declines associated with aging. Aging Cell 2003;2(1):1–7.

[149] Aiken J, Bua E, Cao Z, Lopez M, Wanagat J, McKenzie D, et al. Mitochondrial DNA deletion mutations and sarcopenia. Ann N Y Acad Sci 2002;959:412–23.

[150] Herbst A, Widjaja K, Nguy B, Lushaj EB, Moore TM, Hevener AL, et al. Digital PCR quantitation of muscle mitochondrial DNA: age, fiber type, and mutation-induced changes. J Gerontol A Biol Sci Med Sci 2017;72(10):1327–33.

[151] Aiken J, Roudier E, Ciccone J, Drouin G, Stromberg A, Vojnovic J, et al. Phosphorylation of murine double minute-2 on Ser166 is downstream of VEGF-A in exercised skeletal muscle and regulates primary endothelial cell migration and FoxO gene expression. FASEB J 2016;30(3):1120–34.

[152] Herbst A, Wanagat J, Cheema N, Widjaja K, McKenzie D, Aiken JM. Latent mitochondrial DNA deletion mutations drive muscle fiber loss at old age. Aging Cell 2016;15:1132–9.

[153] Woo M, Choi HI, Park SH, Ahn J, Jang YJ, Ha TY, et al. The unc-51 like autophagy activating kinase 1-autophagy related 13 complex has distinct functions in tunicamycin-treated cells. Biochem Biophys Res Commun 2020.

[154] Herrington CS, Poulsom R, Coates PJ. Recent advances in pathology: the 2019 annual review issue of the journal of pathology. J Pathol 2019;247(5):535–8.

[155] Nilsson MI, Tarnopolsky MA. Mitochondria and aging—the role of exercise as a countermeasure. Biology (Basel) 2019;8(2).

[156] Son JM, Lee C. Mitochondria: multifaceted regulators of aging. BMB Rep 2019;52(1):13–23.

[157] Kokubun T, Saitoh SI, Miura S, Ishida T, Takeishi Y. Telomerase plays a pivotal role in collateral growth under ischemia by suppressing age-induced oxidative stress, expression of p53, and pro-apoptotic proteins. Int Heart J 2019;60(3):736–45.

[158] Jacinto TA, Meireles GS, Dias AT, Aires R, Porto ML, Gava AL, et al. Increased ROS production and DNA damage in monocytes are biomarkers of aging and atherosclerosis. Biol Res 2018;51(1):33.

[159] Martin LJ, Wong M. Enforced DNA repair enzymes rescue neurons from apoptosis induced by target deprivation and axotomy in mouse models of neurodegeneration. Mech Ageing Dev 2017;161:149–62.

[160] Mercer JR, Cheng KK, Figg N, Gorenne I, Mahmoudi M, Griffin J, et al. DNA damage links mitochondrial dysfunction to atherosclerosis and the metabolic syndrome. Circ Res 2010;107(8):1021–31.

[161] Rygiel KA, Picard M, Turnbull DM. The ageing neuromuscular system and sarcopenia: a mitochondrial perspective. J Physiol 2016;594(16):4499–512.

[162] Wanagat J, Cao Z, Pathare P, Aiken JM. Mitochondrial DNA deletion mutations colocalize with segmental electron transport system abnormalities, muscle fiber atrophy, fiber splitting, and oxidative damage in sarcopenia. FASEB J 2001;15(2):322–32.

[163] Wanagat J, Ahmadieh N, Bielas JH, Ericson NG, Van Remmen H. Skeletal muscle mitochondrial DNA deletions are not increased in CuZn-superoxide dismutase deficient mice. Exp Gerontol 2015;61:15–9.

[164] Hiona A, Sanz A, Kujoth GC, Pamplona R, Seo AY, Hofer T, et al. Mitochondrial DNA mutations induce mitochondrial dysfunction, apoptosis and sarcopenia in skeletal muscle of mitochondrial DNA mutator mice. PLoS One 2010;5(7):e11468.

[165] Hiona A, Leeuwenburgh C. The role of mitochondrial DNA mutations in aging and sarcopenia: implications for the mitochondrial vicious cycle theory of aging. Exp Gerontol 2008;43(1):24–33.

[166] Cheema N, Herbst A, McKenzie D, Aiken JM. Apoptosis and necrosis mediate skeletal muscle fiber loss in age-induced mitochondrial enzymatic abnormalities. Aging Cell 2015;14(6):1085–93.

[167] McKiernan SH, Colman RJ, Aiken E, Evans TD, Beasley TM, Aiken JM, et al. Cellular adaptation contributes to calorie restriction-induced preservation of skeletal muscle in aged rhesus monkeys. Exp Gerontol 2012;47(3):229–36.

[168] McKiernan SH, Colman R, Lopez M, Beasley TM, Weindruch R, Aiken JM. Longitudinal analysis of early stage sarcopenia in aging rhesus monkeys. Exp Gerontol 2009;44(3):170–6.

[169] Stoll EA, Karapavlovic N, Rosa H, Woodmass M, Rygiel K, White K, et al. Naked mole-rats maintain healthy skeletal muscle and complex IV mitochondrial enzyme function into old age. Aging (Albany NY) 2016;8(12):3468–85.

[170] Vincent AE, Rosa HS, Alston CL, Grady JP, Rygiel KA, Rocha MC, et al. Dysferlin mutations and mitochondrial dysfunction. Neuromuscul Disord 2016;26(11):782–8.

[171] Vincent AE, Grady JP, Rocha MC, Alston CL, Rygiel KA, Barresi R, et al. Mitochondrial dysfunction in myofibrillar myopathy. Neuromuscul Disord 2016;26(10):691–701.

[172] Reeve A, Meagher M, Lax N, Simcox E, Hepplewhite P, Jaros E, et al. The impact of pathogenic mitochondrial DNA mutations on substantia nigra neurons. J Neurosci 2013;33(26):10790–801.

[173] Reeve AK, Park TK, Jaros E, Campbell GR, Lax NZ, Hepplewhite PD, et al. Relationship between mitochondria and alpha-synuclein: a study of single substantia nigra neurons. Arch Neurol 2012;69(3):385–93.

[174] Cenini G, Lloret A, Cascella R. Oxidative stress in neurodegenerative diseases: from a mitochondrial point of view. Oxid Med Cell Longev 2019;2019:2105607.

[175] Chen FZ, Zhao Y, Chen HZ. MicroRNA-98 reduces amyloid beta-protein production and improves oxidative stress and mitochondrial dysfunction through the notch signaling pathway via HEY2 in Alzheimer's disease mice. Int J Mol Med 2019;43(1):91–102.

[176] Chabi B, Ljubicic V, Menzies KJ, Huang JH, Saleem A, Hood DA. Mitochondrial function and apoptotic susceptibility in aging skeletal muscle. Aging Cell 2008;7(1):2–12.

[177] Adhihetty PJ, Ljubicic V, Menzies KJ, Hood DA. Differential susceptibility of subsarcolemmal and intermyofibrillar mitochondria to apoptotic stimuli. Am J Physiol Cell Physiol 2005;289(4):C994–C1001.

[178] Primeau AJ, Adhihetty PJ, Hood DA. Apoptosis in heart and skeletal muscle. Can J Appl Physiol 2002;27(4):349–95.

[179] Crescenzo R, Bianco F, Mazzoli A, Giacco A, Liverini G, Iossa S. Skeletal muscle mitochondrial energetic efficiency and aging. Int J Mol Sci 2015;16(5):10674–85.

[180] Crescenzo R, Bianco F, Coppola P, Mazzoli A, Liverini G, Iossa S. Subsarcolemmal and intermyofibrillar mitochondrial responses to short-term high-fat feeding in rat skeletal muscle. Nutrition 2014;30(1):75–81.

[181] Leduc-Gaudet JP, Picard M, St-Jean Pelletier F, Sgarioto N, Auger MJ, Vallee J, et al. Mitochondrial morphology is altered in atrophied skeletal muscle of aged mice. Oncotarget 2015;6(20):17923–37.

[182] Vincent AE, White K, Davey T, Philips J, Ogden RT, Lawless C, et al. Quantitative 3D mapping of the human skeletal muscle mitochondrial network. Cell Rep 2019;26(4):996–1009.e4.

[183] Gouspillou G, Godin R, Piquereau J, Picard M, Mofarrahi M, Mathew J, et al. Protective role of Parkin in skeletal muscle contractile and mitochondrial function. J Physiol 2018;596(13):2565–79.

[184] Morrow RM, Picard M, Derbeneva O, Leipzig J, McManus MJ, Gouspillou G, et al. Mitochondrial energy deficiency leads to hyperproliferation of skeletal muscle mitochondria and enhanced insulin sensitivity. Proc Natl Acad Sci USA 2017;114(10):2705–10.

[185] Rygiel KA, Picard M, Turnbull DM. The ageing neuromuscular system and sarcopenia: a mitochondrial perspective. J Physiol 2016;594(16):4499–512.

[186] Picard M, Shirihai OS, Gentil BJ, Burelle Y. Mitochondrial morphology transitions and functions: implications for retrograde signaling? Am J Physiol Regul Integr Comp Physiol 2013;304(6):R393–406.

[187] Jian B, Yang S, Chen D, Zou L, Chatham JC, Chaudry I, et al. Aging influences cardiac mitochondrial gene expression and cardiovascular function following hemorrhage injury. Mol Med 2011;17(5–6):542–9.

[188] Chen B, Zhong Y, Peng W, Sun Y, Kong WJ. Age-related changes in the central auditory system: comparison of D-galactose-induced aging rats and naturally aging rats. Brain Res 2010;1344:43–53.

[189] Chen H, Vermulst M, Wang YE, Chomyn A, Prolla TA, McCaffery JM, et al. Mitochondrial fusion is required for mtDNA stability in skeletal muscle and tolerance of mtDNA mutations. Cell 2010;141(2):280–9.

[190] Zhuo Y, Li SH, Chen MS, Wu J, Kinkaid HY, Fazel S, et al. Aging impairs the angiogenic response to ischemic injury and the activity of implanted cells: combined consequences for cell therapy in older recipients. J Thorac Cardiovasc Surg 2010;139(5):1286–94. 94 e1–2.

[191] Wu JJ, Quijano C, Chen E, Liu H, Cao L, Fergusson MM, et al. Mitochondrial dysfunction and oxidative stress mediate the physiological impairment induced by the disruption of autophagy. Aging (Albany NY) 2009;1(4):425–37.

[192] Ibebunjo C, Chick JM, Kendall T, Eash JK, Li C, Zhang Y, et al. Genomic and proteomic profiling reveals reduced mitochondrial function and disruption of the neuromuscular junction driving rat sarcopenia. Mol Cell Biol 2013;33(2):194–212.

[193] Arribat Y, Broskey NT, Greggio C, Boutant M, Conde Alonso S, Kulkarni SS, et al. Distinct patterns of skeletal muscle mitochondria fusion, fission and mitophagy upon duration of exercise training. Acta Physiol (Oxf) 2019;225(2):e13179.

[194] Iqbal S, Hood DA. The role of mitochondrial fusion and fission in skeletal muscle function and dysfunction. Front Biosci (Landmark Ed) 2015;20:157–72.

[195] Iqbal S, Hood DA. Cytoskeletal regulation of mitochondrial movements in myoblasts. Cytoskeleton (Hoboken) 2014;71(10):564–72.

[196] Faitg J, Leduc-Gaudet JP, Reynaud O, Ferland G, Gaudreau P, Gouspillou G. Effects of aging and caloric restriction on fiber type composition, mitochondrial morphology and dynamics in rat oxidative and glycolytic muscles. Front Physiol 2019;10:420.

[197] Joseph AM, Joanisse DR, Baillot RG, Hood DA. Mitochondrial dysregulation in the pathogenesis of diabetes: potential for mitochondrial biogenesis-mediated interventions. Exp Diabetes Res 2012;2012:642038.

[198] Iqbal S, Ostojic O, Singh K, Joseph AM, Hood DA. Expression of mitochondrial fission and fusion regulatory proteins in skeletal muscle during chronic use and disuse. Muscle Nerve 2013;48(6):963–70.

[199] Oliveira JRS, Mohamed JS, Myers MJ, Brooks MJ, Alway SE. Effects of hindlimb suspension and reloading on gastrocnemius and soleus muscle mass and function in geriatric mice. Exp Gerontol 2019;115:19–31.

[200] Haramizu S, Asano S, Butler DC, Stanton DA, Hajira A, Mohamed JS, et al. Dietary resveratrol confers apoptotic resistance to oxidative stress in myoblasts. J Nutr Biochem 2017;50:103–15.

[201] Alway SE, Bennett BT, Wilson JC, Sperringer J, Mohamed JS, Edens NK, et al. Green tea extract attenuates muscle loss and improves muscle function during disuse, but fails to improve muscle recovery following unloading in aged rats. J Appl Physiol (1985) 2015;118(3):319–30.

[202] Alway SE, Bennett BT, Wilson JC, Edens NK, Pereira SL. Epigallocatechin-3-gallate improves plantaris muscle recovery after disuse in aged rats. Exp Gerontol 2014;50:82–94.

[203] Sebastian D, Sorianello E, Segales J, Irazoki A, Ruiz-Bonilla V, Sala D, et al. Mfn2 deficiency links age-related sarcopenia and impaired autophagy to activation of an adaptive mitophagy pathway. EMBO J 2016;35(15):1677–93.

[204] Bori Z, Zhao Z, Koltai E, Fatouros IG, Jamurtas AZ, Douroudos II, et al. The effects of aging, physical training, and a single bout of exercise on mitochondrial protein expression in human skeletal muscle. Exp Gerontol 2012;47(6):417–24.

[205] Koltai E, Bori Z, Osvath P, Ihasz F, Peter S, Toth G, et al. Master athletes have higher miR-7, SIRT3 and SOD2 expression in skeletal muscle than age-matched sedentary controls. Redox Biol 2018;19:46–51.

[206] Billingsley KJ, Barbosa IA, Bandres-Ciga S, Quinn JP, Bubb VJ, Deshpande C, et al. Mitochondria function associated genes contribute to Parkinson's disease risk and later age at onset. NPJ Parkinsons Dis 2019;5:8.

[207] Shao Q, Yang M, Liang C, Ma L, Zhang W, Jiang Z, et al. C9orf72 and smcr8 mutant mice reveal MTORC1 activation due to impaired lysosomal degradation and exocytosis. Autophagy 2019;1–16.

[208] Jiang Z, Wang W, Perry G, Zhu X, Wang X. Mitochondrial dynamic abnormalities in amyotrophic lateral sclerosis. Transl Neurodegener 2015;4:14.

[209] Qi Z, Huang Z, Xie F, Chen L. Dynamin-related protein 1: a critical protein in the pathogenesis of neural system dysfunctions and neurodegenerative diseases. J Cell Physiol 2019;234(7):10032–46.

[210] Zhou J, Li A, Li X, Yi J. Dysregulated mitochondrial Ca(2+) and ROS signaling in skeletal muscle of ALS mouse model. Arch Biochem Biophys 2019;663:249–58.

[211] Xu Z, Jung C, Higgins C, Levine J, Kong J. Mitochondrial degeneration in amyotrophic lateral sclerosis. J Bioenerg Biomembr 2004;36(4):395–9.
[212] Wang W, Zhang F, Li L, Tang F, Siedlak SL, Fujioka H, et al. MFN2 couples glutamate excitotoxicity and mitochondrial dysfunction in motor neurons. J Biol Chem 2015;290(1):168–82.
[213] Abrigo J, Simon F, Cabrera D, Vilos C, Cabello-Verrugio C. Mitochondrial dysfunction in skeletal muscle pathologies. Curr Protein Pept Sci 2019;20(6):536–46.
[214] Agnihotri A, Aruoma OI. Alzheimer's disease and Parkinson's disease: a nutritional toxicology perspective of the impact of oxidative stress, mitochondrial dysfunction, nutrigenomics and environmental chemicals. J Am Coll Nutr 2020;39(1):16–27.
[215] Kestenbaum B, Gamboa J, Liu S, Ali AS, Shankland E, Jue T, et al. Impaired skeletal muscle mitochondrial bioenergetics and physical performance in chronic kidney disease. JCI Insight 2020;5(5).
[216] Safdar A, Khrapko K, Flynn JM, Saleem A, De Lisio M, Johnston AP, et al. Exercise-induced mitochondrial p53 repairs mtDNA mutations in mutator mice. Skelet Muscle 2016;6:7.
[217] Lee S, Kim M, Lim W, Kim T, Kang C. Strenuous exercise induces mitochondrial damage in skeletal muscle of old mice. Biochem Biophys Res Commun 2015;461(2):354–60.
[218] Rygiel KA, Picard M, Turnbull DM. The ageing neuromuscular system and sarcopenia—a mitochondrial perspective. J Physiol 2016;594(16):4499–512.
[219] Aiken J, Bua E, Cao Z, Lopez M, Wanagat J, McKenzie D, et al. Mitochondrial DNA deletion mutations and sarcopenia. Ann NY Acad Sci 2002;959:412–23.
[220] McKenzie D, Bua E, McKiernan S, Cao Z, Aiken JM. Mitochondrial DNA deletion mutations: a causal role in sarcopenia. Eur J Biochem 2002;269(8):2010–5.
[221] Wallace DC, Fan W. The pathophysiology of mitochondrial disease as modeled in the mouse. Genes Dev 2009;23(15):1714–36.
[222] Herbst A, Pak JW, McKenzie D, Bua E, Bassiouni M, Aiken JM. Accumulation of mitochondrial DNA deletion mutations in aged muscle fibers: evidence for a causal role in muscle fiber loss. J Gerontol A Biol Sci Med Sci 2007;62(3):235–45.
[223] Marzetti E, Calvani R, Cesari M, Buford TW, Lorenzi M, Behnke BJ, et al. Mitochondrial dysfunction and sarcopenia of aging: from signaling pathways to clinical trials. Int J Biochem Cell Biol 2013;45(10):2288–301.
[224] Yuzefovych LV, LeDoux SP, Wilson GL, Rachek LI. Mitochondrial DNA damage via augmented oxidative stress regulates endoplasmic reticulum stress and autophagy: crosstalk, links and signaling. PLoS One 2013;8(12):e83349.
[225] Wang PW, Lin TK, Weng SW, Liou CW. Mitochondrial DNA variants in the pathogenesis of type 2 diabetes—relevance of asian population studies. Rev Diabet Stud 2009;6(4):237–46.
[226] Trifunovic A, Larsson NG. Mitochondrial dysfunction as a cause of ageing. J Intern Med 2008;263(2):167–78.
[227] Meissner C. Mutations of mitochondrial DNA—cause or consequence of the ageing process? Z Gerontol Geriatr 2007;40(5):325–33.
[228] Sinha KM, Tseng C, Guo P, Lu A, Pan H, Gao X, et al. Hypoxia-inducible factor 1alpha (HIF-1alpha) is a major determinant in the enhanced function of muscle-derived progenitors from MRL/MpJ mice. FASEB J 2019;33(7):8321–34.
[229] McKiernan SH, Colman RJ, Lopez M, Beasley TM, Aiken JM, Anderson RM, et al. Caloric restriction delays aging-induced cellular phenotypes in rhesus monkey skeletal muscle. Exp Gerontol 2011;46(1):23–9.
[230] Bua E, McKiernan SH, Aiken JM. Calorie restriction limits the generation but not the progression of mitochondrial abnormalities in aging skeletal muscle. FASEB J 2004;18(3):582–4.
[231] Liu HW, Chang YC, Chan YC, Hu SH, Liu MY, Chang SJ. Dysregulations of mitochondrial quality control and autophagic flux at an early age lead to progression of sarcopenia in SAMP8 mice. Biogerontology 2020;21(3):367–80.
[232] Seo DY, Lee SR, Kim N, Ko KS, Rhee BD, Han J. Age-related changes in skeletal muscle mitochondria: the role of exercise. Integr Med Res 2016;5(3):182–6.
[233] Del Campo A. Mitophagy as a new therapeutic target for sarcopenia. Acta Physiol (Oxf) 2019;225(2):e13219.
[234] Broskey NT, Greggio C, Boss A, Boutant M, Dwyer A, Schlueter L, et al. Skeletal muscle mitochondria in the elderly: effects of physical fitness and exercise training. J Clin Endocrinol Metab 2014;99(5):1852–61.

[235] Powers SK, Wiggs MP, Duarte JA, Zergeroglu AM, Demirel HA. Mitochondrial signaling contributes to disuse muscle atrophy. Am J Physiol Endocrinol Metab 2012;303(1):E31–9.
[236] Peterson CM, Johannsen DL, Ravussin E. Skeletal muscle mitochondria and aging: a review. J Aging Res 2012;2012:194821.
[237] Pietrangelo L, Michelucci A, Ambrogini P, Sartini S, Guarnier FA, Fusella A, et al. Muscle activity prevents the uncoupling of mitochondria from Ca(2+) release units induced by ageing and disuse. Arch Biochem Biophys 2019;663:22–33.
[238] Zampieri S, Mammucari C, Romanello V, Barberi L, Pietrangelo L, Fusella A, et al. Physical exercise in aging human skeletal muscle increases mitochondrial calcium uniporter expression levels and affects mitochondria dynamics. Physiol Rep 2016;4(24).
[239] Alway SE, Sale DG, MacDougall JD. Twitch contractile adaptations are not dependent on the intensity of isometric exercise in the human triceps surae. Eur J Appl Physiol 1990;60(5):346–52.
[240] Alway SE, MacDougall JD, Sale DG. Contractile adaptations in the human triceps surae after isometric exercise. J Appl Physiol (1985) 1989;66(6):2725–32.
[241] Roux E, Marhl M. Role of sarcoplasmic reticulum and mitochondria in Ca2+ removal in airway myocytes. Biophys J 2004;86(4):2583–95.
[242] Umanskaya A, Santulli G, Xie W, Andersson DC, Reiken SR, Marks AR. Genetically enhancing mitochondrial antioxidant activity improves muscle function in aging. Proc Natl Acad Sci USA 2014;111(42):15250–5.
[243] Andersson DC, Betzenhauser MJ, Reiken S, Meli AC, Umanskaya A, Xie W, et al. Ryanodine receptor oxidation causes intracellular calcium leak and muscle weakness in aging. Cell Metab 2011;14(2):196–207.
[244] Wescott AP, Kao JPY, Lederer WJ, Boyman L. Voltage-energized calcium-sensitive ATP production by mitochondria. Nat Metab 2019;1(10):975–84.
[245] Mammucari C, Rizzuto R. Signaling pathways in mitochondrial dysfunction and aging. Mech Ageing Dev 2010;131(7–8):536–43.
[246] Mammucari C, Raffaello A, Vecellio Reane D, Gherardi G, De Mario A, Rizzuto R. Mitochondrial calcium uptake in organ physiology: from molecular mechanism to animal models. Pflugers Arch 2018;470(8):1165–79.
[247] Raffaello A, Mammucari C, Gherardi G, Rizzuto R. Calcium at the center of cell signaling: interplay between endoplasmic reticulum, mitochondria, and lysosomes. Trends Biochem Sci 2016;41(12):1035–49.
[248] Rizzuto R, Marchi S, Bonora M, Aguiari P, Bononi A, De Stefani D, et al. Ca(2+) transfer from the ER to mitochondria: when, how and why. Biochim Biophys Acta 2009;1787(11):1342–51.
[249] Rizzuto R, De Stefani D, Raffaello A, Mammucari C. Mitochondria as sensors and regulators of calcium signalling. Nat Rev Mol Cell Biol 2012;13(9):566–78.
[250] Georgiadou E, Haythorne E, Dickerson MT, Lopez-Noriega L, Pullen TJ, da Silva Xavier G, et al. The pore-forming subunit MCU of the mitochondrial Ca(2+) uniporter is required for normal glucose-stimulated insulin secretion in vitro and in vivo in mice. Diabetologia 2020;63(7):1368–81. https://doi.org/10.1007/s00125-020-05148-x.
[251] Doghman-Bouguerra M, Granatiero V, Sbiera S, Sbiera I, Lacas-Gervais S, Brau F, et al. FATE1 antagonizes calcium- and drug-induced apoptosis by uncoupling ER and mitochondria. EMBO Rep 2016;17(9):1264–80.
[252] Granatiero V, Giorgio V, Cali T, Patron M, Brini M, Bernardi P, et al. Reduced mitochondrial Ca(2+) transients stimulate autophagy in human fibroblasts carrying the 13514A>G mutation of the ND5 subunit of NADH dehydrogenase. Cell Death Differ 2016;23(2):231–41.
[253] Granatiero V, De Stefani D, Rizzuto R. Mitochondrial calcium handling in physiology and disease. Adv Exp Med Biol 2017;982:25–47.
[254] Granatiero V, Pacifici M, Raffaello A, De Stefani D, Rizzuto R. Overexpression of mitochondrial calcium uniporter causes neuronal death. Oxid Med Cell Longev 2019;2019:1681254.
[255] Penna E, Espino J, De Stefani D, Rizzuto R. The MCU complex in cell death. Cell Calcium 2018;69:73–80.
[256] Mijares M, Allen PD, Lopez JR. Senescence is associated with elevated intracellular resting [Ca(2+)] in mice skeletal muscle fibers. An in vivo study. Front Physiol 2021;11:601189. https://doi.org/10.3389/fphys.2020.601189. 601189.

[257] Watanabe D, Hatakeyama K, Ikegami R, Eshima H, Yagishita K, Poole DC, et al. Sex differences in mitochondrial Ca(2+) handling in mouse fast-twitch skeletal muscle in vivo. J Appl Physiol (1985) 2020;128(2):241–51.
[258] Mammucari C, Patron M, Granatiero V, Rizzuto R. Molecules and roles of mitochondrial calcium signaling. Biofactors 2011;37(3):219–27.
[259] Mammucari C, Gherardi G, Zamparo I, Raffaello A, Boncompagni S, Chemello F, et al. The mitochondrial calcium uniporter controls skeletal muscle trophism in vivo. Cell Rep 2015;10(8):1269–79.
[260] Kwong JQ, Huo J, Bround MJ, Boyer JG, Schwanekamp JA, Ghazal N, et al. The mitochondrial calcium uniporter underlies metabolic fuel preference in skeletal muscle. JCI Insight 2018;3(22), e121689.
[261] Protasi F. Mitochondria association to calcium release units is controlled by age and muscle activity. Eur J Transl Myol 2015;25(4):257–62.
[262] Nichols CE, Shepherd DL, Knuckles TL, Thapa D, Stricker JC, Stapleton PA, et al. Cardiac and mitochondrial dysfunction following acute pulmonary exposure to mountaintop removal mining particulate matter. Am J Physiol Heart Circ Physiol 2015;309(12):H2017–30.
[263] Alway SE, Myers MJ, Mohamed JS. Regulation of satellite cell function in sarcopenia. Front Aging Neurosci 2014;6:246.
[264] Alway SE, Pereira SL, Edens NK, Hao Y, Bennett BT. B-Hydroxy-B-methylbutyrate (HMB) enhances the proliferation of satellite cells in fast muscles of aged rats during recovery from disuse atrophy. Exp Gerontol 2013;48(9):973–84.
[265] Wang Y, Hao Y, Alway SE. Suppression of GSK-3beta activation by M-cadherin protects myoblasts against mitochondria-associated apoptosis during myogenic differentiation. J Cell Sci 2011;124(Pt 22):3835–47.
[266] Yoo SZ, No MH, Heo JW, Park DH, Kang JH, Kim SH, et al. Role of exercise in age-related sarcopenia. J Exerc Rehabil 2018;14(4):551–8.
[267] Ji LL, Kang C. Role of PGC-1alpha in sarcopenia: etiology and potential intervention—a mini-review. Gerontology 2015;61(2):139–48.
[268] Alway SE, Myers MJ, Mohamed JS. Regulation of satellite cell function in sarcopenia. Front Aging Neurosci 2014;6(9):1–15.
[269] Gouspillou G, Sgarioto N, Kapchinsky S, Purves-Smith F, Norris B, Pion CH, et al. Increased sensitivity to mitochondrial permeability transition and myonuclear translocation of endonuclease G in atrophied muscle of physically active older humans. FASEB J 2014;28(4):1621–33.
[270] Marzetti E, Calvani R, Bernabei R, Leeuwenburgh C. Apoptosis in skeletal myocytes: a potential target for interventions against sarcopenia and physical frailty—a mini-review. Gerontology 2012;58(2):99–106.
[271] Gomez-Cabrera MC, Sanchis-Gomar F, Garcia-Valles R, Pareja-Galeano H, Gambini J, Borras C, et al. Mitochondria as sources and targets of damage in cellular aging. Clin Chem Lab Med 2012;50(8):1287–95.
[272] Marzetti E, Hwang JC, Lees HA, Wohlgemuth SE, Dupont-Versteegden EE, Carter CS, et al. Mitochondrial death effectors: relevance to sarcopenia and disuse muscle atrophy. Biochim Biophys Acta 2010;1800(3):235–44.
[273] Degens H. The role of systemic inflammation in age-related muscle weakness and wasting. Scand J Med Sci Sports 2010;20(1):28–38.
[274] Hiona A, Sanz A, Kujoth GC, Pamplona R, Seo AY, Hofer T, et al. Mitochondrial DNA mutations induce mitochondrial dysfunction, apoptosis and sarcopenia in skeletal muscle of mitochondrial DNA mutator mice. PLoS One 2010;5(7):e11468.
[275] Marzetti E, Lees HA, Wohlgemuth SE, Leeuwenburgh C. Sarcopenia of aging: underlying cellular mechanisms and protection by calorie restriction. Biofactors 2009;35(1):28–35.
[276] Siu PM, Alway SE. Response and adaptation of skeletal muscle to denervation stress: the role of apoptosis in muscle loss. Front Biosci (Landmark Ed) 2009;14:432–52.
[277] Triolo M, Hood DA. Mitochondrial breakdown in skeletal muscle and the emerging role of the lysosomes. Arch Biochem Biophys 2019;661:66–73.
[278] Kim Y, Triolo M, Erlich AT, Hood DA. Regulation of autophagic and mitophagic flux during chronic contractile activity-induced muscle adaptations. Pflugers Arch 2019;471(3):431–40.

[279] Parousis A, Carter HN, Tran C, Erlich AT, Mesbah Moosavi ZS, Pauly M, et al. Contractile activity attenuates autophagy suppression and reverses mitochondrial defects in skeletal muscle cells. Autophagy 2018;14(11):1886–97.

[280] Vainshtein A, Hood DA. The regulation of autophagy during exercise in skeletal muscle. J Appl Physiol (1985) 2016;120(6):664–73.

[281] Hood DA, Tryon LD, Vainshtein A, Memme J, Chen C, Pauly M, et al. Exercise and the regulation of mitochondrial turnover. Prog Mol Biol Transl Sci 2015;135:99–127.

[282] Tryon LD, Vainshtein A, Memme JM, Crilly MJ, Hood DA. Recent advances in mitochondrial turnover during chronic muscle disuse. Integr Med Res 2014;3(4):161–71.

[283] Hood DA, Iqbal S. Muscle mitochondrial ultrastructure: new insights into morphological divergences. J Appl Physiol (1985) 2013;114(2):159–60.

[284] O'Leary MF, Vainshtein A, Iqbal S, Ostojic O, Hood DA. Adaptive plasticity of autophagic proteins to denervation in aging skeletal muscle. Am J Physiol Cell Physiol 2013;304(5):C422–30.

[285] Hood DA, Tryon LD, Vainshtein A, Memme J, Chen C, Pauly M, et al. Exercise and the regulation of mitochondrial turnover. Prog Mol Biol Transl Sci 2015;135:99–127.

[286] Carter HN, Chen CC, Hood DA. Mitochondria, muscle health, and exercise with advancing age. Physiology (Bethesda) 2015;30(3):208–23.

[287] Saleem A, Adhihetty PJ, Hood DA. Role of p53 in mitochondrial biogenesis and apoptosis in skeletal muscle. Physiol Genomics 2009;37(1):58–66.

[288] Saleem A, Hood DA. Acute exercise induces tumour suppressor protein p53 translocation to the mitochondria and promotes a p53-Tfam-mitochondrial DNA complex in skeletal muscle. J Physiol 2013;591(14):3625–36.

[289] Saleem A, Carter HN, Hood DA. p53 is necessary for the adaptive changes in cellular milieu subsequent to an acute bout of endurance exercise. Am J Physiol Cell Physiol 2014;306(3):C241–9.

[290] Carnio S, Serena E, Rossi CA, De Coppi P, Elvassore N, Vitiello L. Three-dimensional porous scaffold allows long-term wild-type cell delivery in dystrophic muscle. J Tissue Eng Regen Med 2011;5(1):1–10.

[291] Carnio S, LoVerso F, Baraibar MA, Longa E, Khan MM, Maffei M, et al. Autophagy impairment in muscle induces neuromuscular junction degeneration and precocious aging. Cell Rep 2014;8(5):1509–21.

[292] O'Leary MF, Hood DA. Effect of prior chronic contractile activity on mitochondrial function and apoptotic protein expression in denervated muscle. J Appl Physiol (1985) 2008;105(1):114–20.

[293] O'Leary MF, Hood DA. Denervation-induced oxidative stress and autophagy signaling in muscle. Autophagy 2009;5(2):230–1.

[294] Adhihetty PJ, O'Leary MF, Chabi B, Wicks KL, Hood DA. Effect of denervation on mitochondrially mediated apoptosis in skeletal muscle. J Appl Physiol 2007;102(3):1143–51.

[295] Iqbal S, Ostojic O, Singh K, Joseph AM, Hood DA. Expression of mitochondrial fission and fusion regulatory proteins in skeletal muscle during chronic use and disuse. Muscle Nerve 2013;48(6):963–70.

[296] Hao Y, Jackson JR, Wang Y, Edens N, Pereira SL, Alway SE. B-Hydroxy-B-methylbutyrate reduces myonuclear apoptosis during recovery from hind limb suspension-induced muscle fiber atrophy in aged rats. Am J Physiol Regul Integr Comp Physiol 2011;301(3):R701–15.

[297] Biala AK, Dhingra R, Kirshenbaum LA. Mitochondrial dynamics: orchestrating the journey to advanced age. J Mol Cell Cardiol 2015;83:37–43.

[298] Alway SE, Bennett BT, Wilson JC, Sperringer J, Mohamed JS, Edens NK, et al. Green tea extract attenuates muscle loss and improves muscle function during disuse, but fails to improve muscle recovery following unloading in aged rats. J Appl Physiol (1985) 2015;118(3):319–30.

[299] Bennett BT, Mohamed JS, Alway SE. Effects of resveratrol on the recovery of muscle mass following disuse in the plantaris muscle of aged rats. PLoS One 2013;8(12):e83518.

[300] Krajnak K, Waugh S, Miller R, Baker B, Geronilla K, Alway SE, et al. Proapoptotic factor Bax is increased in satellite cells in the tibialis anterior muscles of old rats. Muscle Nerve 2006;34(6):720–30.

[301] Pistilli EE, Siu PM, Alway SE. Molecular regulation of apoptosis in fast plantaris muscles of aged rats. J Gerontol A Biol Sci Med Sci 2006;61(3):245–55.

[302] Dirks-Naylor AJ, Lennon-Edwards S. Cellular and molecular mechanisms of apoptosis in age-related muscle atrophy. Curr Aging Sci 2011;4(3):269–78.
[303] Dirks Naylor AJ, Leeuwenburgh C. Sarcopenia: the role of apoptosis and modulation by caloric restriction. Exerc Sport Sci Rev 2008;36(1):19–24.
[304] Dirks AJ, Hofer T, Marzetti E, Pahor M, Leeuwenburgh C. Mitochondrial DNA mutations, energy metabolism and apoptosis in aging muscle. Ageing Res Rev 2006;5(2):179–95.
[305] Dirks A, Leeuwenburgh C. Apoptosis in skeletal muscle with aging. Am J Physiol Regul Integr Comp Physiol 2002;282(2):R519–27.
[306] Marzetti E, Leeuwenburgh C. Skeletal muscle apoptosis, sarcopenia and frailty at old age. Exp Gerontol 2006;41(12):1234–8.
[307] Marzetti E, Wohlgemuth SE, Lees HA, Chung HY, Giovannini S, Leeuwenburgh C. Age-related activation of mitochondrial caspase-independent apoptotic signaling in rat gastrocnemius muscle. Mech Ageing Dev 2008;129(9):542–9.
[308] Marzetti E, Lawler JM, Hiona A, Manini T, Seo AY, Leeuwenburgh C. Modulation of age-induced apoptotic signaling and cellular remodeling by exercise and calorie restriction in skeletal muscle. Free Radic Biol Med 2008;44(2):160–8.
[309] Pistilli EE, Jackson JR, Alway SE. Death receptor-associated pro-apoptotic signaling in aged skeletal muscle. Apoptosis 2006;11(12):2115–26.
[310] Alway SE, Degens H, Krishnamurthy G, Chaudhrai A. Denervation stimulates apoptosis but not Id2 expression in hindlimb muscles of aged rats. J Gerontol A Biol Sci Med Sci 2003;58(8):687–97.
[311] Jejurikar SS, Marcelo CL, Kuzon Jr WM. Skeletal muscle denervation increases satellite cell susceptibility to apoptosis. Plast Reconstr Surg 2002;110(1):160–8.
[312] Jin H, Wu Z, Tian T, Gu Y. Apoptosis in atrophic skeletal muscle induced by brachial plexus injury in rats. J Trauma 2001;50(1):31–5.
[313] Siu PM, Alway SE. Mitochondria-associated apoptotic signalling in denervated rat skeletal muscle. J Physiol 2005;565(Pt 1):309–23.
[314] Siu PM, Alway SE. Deficiency of the Bax gene attenuates denervation-induced apoptosis. Apoptosis 2006;11(6):967–81.
[315] Caiozzo VJ, Wu YZ, Baker MJ, Crumley R. Effects of denervation on cell cycle control in laryngeal muscle. Arch Otolaryngol Head Neck Surg 2004;130(9):1056–68.
[316] Jejurikar SS, Kuzon Jr WM. Satellite cell depletion in degenerative skeletal muscle. Apoptosis 2003;8(6):573–8.
[317] O'Leary MF, Vainshtein A, Carter HN, Zhang Y, Hood DA. Denervation-induced mitochondrial dysfunction and autophagy in skeletal muscle of apoptosis-deficient animals. Am J Physiol Cell Physiol 2012;303(4):C447–54.
[318] Jang JH, Surh YJ. Protective effects of resveratrol on hydrogen peroxide-induced apoptosis in rat pheochromocytoma (PC12) cells. Mutat Res 2001;496(1–2):181–90.
[319] Jang YC, Lustgarten MS, Liu Y, Muller FL, Bhattacharya A, Liang H, et al. Increased superoxide in vivo accelerates age-associated muscle atrophy through mitochondrial dysfunction and neuromuscular junction degeneration. FASEB J 2010;24(5):1376–90.
[320] Jang YC, Van Remmen H. Age-associated alterations of the neuromuscular junction. Exp Gerontol 2011;46(2–3):193–8.
[321] Fulle S, Sancilio S, Mancinelli R, Gatta V, Di Pietro R. Dual role of the caspase enzymes in satellite cells from aged and young subjects. Cell Death Dis 2013;4:e955.
[322] Marzetti E, Lees HA, Manini TM, Buford TW, Aranda Jr JM, Calvani R, et al. Skeletal muscle apoptotic signaling predicts thigh muscle volume and gait speed in community-dwelling older persons: an exploratory study. PLoS One 2012;7(2):e32829.
[323] Alway SE, Siu PM. Nuclear apoptosis contributes to sarcopenia. Exerc Sport Sci Rev 2008;36(2):51–7.
[324] Siu PM, Pistilli EE, Alway SE. Age-dependent increase in oxidative stress in gastrocnemius muscle with unloading. J Appl Physiol (1985) 2008;105(6):1695–705.

[325] Rajabian N, Asmani M, Shahini A, Vydiam K, Choudhury D, Nguyen T, et al. Bioengineered skeletal muscle as a model of muscle aging and regeneration. Tissue Eng Part A 2021;27(1–2):74–86. https://doi.org/10.1089/ten.TEA.2020.0005.

[326] Chang YC, Chen YT, Liu HW, Chan YC, Liu MY, Hu SH, et al. Oligonol alleviates sarcopenia by regulation of signaling pathways involved in protein turnover and mitochondrial quality. Mol Nutr Food Res 2019;63(10):e1801102.

[327] Cruz-Jentoft AJ. Beta-hydroxy-beta-methyl butyrate (HMB): from experimental data to clinical evidence in sarcopenia. Curr Protein Pept Sci 2018;19(7):668–72.

[328] Dalle S, Rossmeislova L, Koppo K. The role of inflammation in age-related sarcopenia. Front Physiol 2017;8:1045.

[329] Brioche T, Lemoine-Morel S. Oxidative stress, sarcopenia, antioxidant strategies and exercise: molecular aspects. Curr Pharm Des 2016;22(18):2664–78.

[330] Ji LL, Kang C. Role of PGC-1alpha in sarcopenia: etiology and potential intervention—a mini-review. Gerontology 2015;61(2):139–48.

[331] Joseph AM, Malamo AG, Silvestre J, Wawrzyniak N, Carey-Love S, Nguyen LM, et al. Short-term caloric restriction, resveratrol, or combined treatment regimens initiated in late-life alter mitochondrial protein expression profiles in a fiber-type specific manner in aged animals. Exp Gerontol 2013;48(9):858–68.

[332] Wohlgemuth SE, Lees HA, Marzetti E, Manini TM, Aranda JM, Daniels MJ, et al. An exploratory analysis of the effects of a weight loss plus exercise program on cellular quality control mechanisms in older overweight women. Rejuvenation Res 2011;14(3):315–24.

[333] Aagaard P, Suetta C, Caserotti P, Magnusson SP, Kjaer M. Role of the nervous system in sarcopenia and muscle atrophy with aging: strength training as a countermeasure. Scand J Med Sci Sports 2010;20(1):49–64.

[334] Kovacheva EL, Hikim AP, Shen R, Sinha I, Sinha-Hikim I. Testosterone supplementation reverses sarcopenia in aging through regulation of myostatin, c-Jun NH2-terminal kinase, notch, and Akt signaling pathways. Endocrinology 2010;151(2):628–38.

[335] Meng SJ, Yu LJ. Oxidative stress, molecular inflammation and sarcopenia. Int J Mol Sci 2010;11(4):1509–26.

[336] Ogata T, Machida S, Oishi Y, Higuchi M, Muraoka I. Differential cell death regulation between adult-unloaded and aged rat soleus muscle. Mech Ageing Dev 2009;130(5):328–36.

[337] Hood DA. Mechanisms of exercise-induced mitochondrial biogenesis in skeletal muscle. Appl Physiol Nutr Metab 2009;34(3):465–72.

[338] Kujoth GC, Hiona A, Pugh TD, Someya S, Panzer K, Wohlgemuth SE, et al. Mitochondrial DNA mutations, oxidative stress, and apoptosis in mammalian aging. Science 2005;309(5733):481–4.

[339] Leeuwenburgh C. Role of apoptosis in sarcopenia. J Gerontol A Biol Sci Med Sci 2003;58(11):999–1001.

[340] Leeuwenburgh C, Gurley CM, Strotman BA, Dupont-Versteegden EE. Age-related differences in apoptosis with disuse atrophy in soleus muscle. Am J Physiol Regul Integr Comp Physiol 2005;288(5):R1288–96.

[341] Gouspillou G, Hepple RT. Editorial: mitochondria in skeletal muscle health, aging and diseases. Front Physiol 2016;7:446.

[342] Whitman SA, Wacker MJ, Richmond SR, Godard MP. Contributions of the ubiquitin-proteasome pathway and apoptosis to human skeletal muscle wasting with age. Pflugers Arch 2005;450(6):437–46.

[343] Chabi B, Adhihetty PJ, Ljubicic V, Hood DA. How is mitochondrial biogenesis affected in mitochondrial disease? Med Sci Sports Exerc 2005;37(12):2102–10.

[344] Ziaaldini MM, Marzetti E, Picca A, Murlasits Z. Biochemical pathways of sarcopenia and their modulation by physical exercise: a narrative review. Front Med (Lausanne) 2017;4:167.

[345] Ziaaldini MM, Koltai E, Csende Z, Goto S, Boldogh I, Taylor AW, et al. Exercise training increases anabolic and attenuates catabolic and apoptotic processes in aged skeletal muscle of male rats. Exp Gerontol 2015;67:9–14.

[346] Hepple RT. Impact of aging on mitochondrial function in cardiac and skeletal muscle. Free Radic Biol Med 2016;98:177–86.

[347] Hepple RT. Mitochondrial involvement and impact in aging skeletal muscle. Front Aging Neurosci 2014;6:211.
[348] Lee JD, Fry CS, Mula J, Kirby TJ, Jackson JR, Liu F, et al. Aged muscle demonstrates fiber-type adaptations in response to mechanical overload, in the absence of myofiber hypertrophy, independent of satellite cell abundance. J Gerontol A Biol Sci Med Sci 2016;71(4):461–7.
[349] Nilwik R, Snijders T, Leenders M, Groen BB, van Kranenburg J, Verdijk LB, et al. The decline in skeletal muscle mass with aging is mainly attributed to a reduction in type II muscle fiber size. Exp Gerontol 2013;48(5):492–8.
[350] Lee DE, Bareja A, Bartlett DB, White JP. Autophagy as a therapeutic target to enhance aged muscle regeneration. Cells 2019;8(2).
[351] Snijders T, Nederveen JP, Bell KE, Lau SW, Mazara N, Kumbhare DA, et al. Prolonged exercise training improves the acute type II muscle fibre satellite cell response in healthy older men. J Physiol 2019;597(1):105–19.
[352] Deschenes MR, Sherman EG, Roby MA, Glass EK, Harris MB. Effect of resistance training on neuromuscular junctions of young and aged muscles featuring different recruitment patterns. J Neurosci Res 2015;93(3):504–13.
[353] Korhonen MT, Cristea A, Alen M, Hakkinen K, Sipila S, Mero A, et al. Aging, muscle fiber type, and contractile function in sprint-trained athletes. J Appl Physiol (1985) 2006;101(3):906–17.
[354] McPhee JS, Cameron J, Maden-Wilkinson T, Piasecki M, Yap MH, Jones DA, et al. The contributions of fiber atrophy, fiber loss, in situ specific force, and voluntary activation to weakness in sarcopenia. J Gerontol A Biol Sci Med Sci 2018;73(10):1287–94.
[355] Pansarasa O, Felzani G, Vecchiet J, Marzatico F. Antioxidant pathways in human aged skeletal muscle: relationship with the distribution of type II fibers. Exp Gerontol 2002;37(8–9):1069–75.
[356] McMillan EM, Quadrilatero J. Differential apoptosis-related protein expression, mitochondrial properties, proteolytic enzyme activity, and DNA fragmentation between skeletal muscles. Am J Physiol Regul Integr Comp Physiol 2011;300(3):R531–43.
[357] Pak JW, Aiken JM. Low levels of mtDNA deletion mutations in ETS normal fibers from aged rats. Ann N Y Acad Sci 2004;1019:289–93.
[358] Braga M, Sinha Hikim AP, Datta S, Ferrini MG, Brown D, Kovacheva EL, et al. Involvement of oxidative stress and caspase 2-mediated intrinsic pathway signaling in age-related increase in muscle cell apoptosis in mice. Apoptosis 2008;13(6):822–32.
[359] Chabi B, Adhihetty PJ, O'Leary MF, Menzies KJ, Hood DA. Relationship between Sirt1 expression and mitochondrial proteins during conditions of chronic muscle use and disuse. J Appl Physiol (1985) 2009;107(6):1730–5.
[360] McMillan EM, Quadrilatero J. Differential apoptosis-related protein expression, mitochondrial properties, proteolytic enzyme activity, and DNA fragmentation between skeletal muscles. Am J Physiol Regul Integr Comp Physiol 2011;300(3):R531–43.
[361] Carnio S, LoVerso F, Baraibar MA, Longa E, Khan MM, Maffei M, et al. Autophagy impairment in muscle induces neuromuscular junction degeneration and precocious aging. Cell Rep 2014;8(5):1509–21.
[362] Vainshtein A, Hood DA. The regulation of autophagy during exercise in skeletal muscle. J Appl Physiol (1985) 2016;120(6):664–73.
[363] Vainshtein A, Desjardins EM, Armani A, Sandri M, Hood DA. PGC-1alpha modulates denervation-induced mitophagy in skeletal muscle. Skelet Muscle 2015;5:9.
[364] Wang B, Cai Z, Tao K, Zeng W, Lu F, Yang R, et al. Essential control of mitochondrial morphology and function by chaperone-mediated autophagy through degradation of PARK7. Autophagy 2016;12(8):1215–28.
[365] Jiang X, Li L, Ying Z, Pan C, Huang S, Li L, et al. A small molecule that protects the integrity of the Electron transfer chain blocks the mitochondrial apoptotic pathway. Mol Cell 2016;63(2):229–39.
[366] Luo S, Rubinsztein DC. BCL2L11/BIM: a novel molecular link between autophagy and apoptosis. Autophagy 2013;9(1):104–5.

[367] Luo L, Lu AM, Wang Y, Hong A, Chen Y, Hu J, et al. Chronic resistance training activates autophagy and reduces apoptosis of muscle cells by modulating IGF-1 and its receptors, Akt/mTOR and Akt/FOXO3a signaling in aged rats. Exp Gerontol 2013;48(4):427–36.

[368] Luo G, Yi J, Ma C, Xiao Y, Yi F, Yu T, et al. Defective mitochondrial dynamics is an early event in skeletal muscle of an amyotrophic lateral sclerosis mouse model. PLoS One 2013;8(12):e82112.

[369] Wang X, Zhang Q, Bao R, Zhang N, Wang Y, Polo-Parada L, et al. Deletion of Nampt in projection neurons of adult mice leads to motor dysfunction, neurodegeneration, and death. Cell Rep 2017;20(9):2184–200.

[370] Wen D, Cui C, Duan W, Wang W, Wang Y, Liu Y, et al. The role of insulin-like growth factor 1 in ALS cell and mouse models: a mitochondrial protector. Brain Res Bull 2019;144:1–13.

[371] Rygiel KA, Grady JP, Turnbull DM. Respiratory chain deficiency in aged spinal motor neurons. Neurobiol Aging 2014;35(10):2230–8.

[372] Santoro B, Bigini P, Levandis G, Nobile V, Biggiogera M, Botti F, et al. Evidence for chronic mitochondrial impairment in the cervical spinal cord of a murine model of motor neuron disease. Neurobiol Dis 2004;17(2):349–57.

[373] Yeo D, Kang C, Gomez-Cabrera MC, Vina J, Ji LL. Data on in vivo PGC-1alpha overexpression model via local transfection in aged mouse muscle. Data Brief 2019;22:199–203.

[374] Arany Z, Lebrasseur N, Morris C, Smith E, Yang W, Ma Y, et al. The transcriptional coactivator PGC-1beta drives the formation of oxidative type IIX fibers in skeletal muscle. Cell Metab 2007;5(1):35–46.

[375] Calvo JA, Daniels TG, Wang X, Paul A, Lin J, Spiegelman BM, et al. Muscle-specific expression of PPARgamma coactivator-1alpha improves exercise performance and increases peak oxygen uptake. J Appl Physiol (1985) 2008;104(5):1304–12.

[376] Liu JF, Chang WY, Chan KH, Tsai WY, Lin CL, Hsu MC. Blood lipid peroxides and muscle damage increased following intensive resistance training of female weightlifters. Ann N Y Acad Sci 2005;1042:255–61.

[377] Kang C, Goodman CA, Hornberger TA, Ji LL. PGC-1alpha overexpression by in vivo transfection attenuates mitochondrial deterioration of skeletal muscle caused by immobilization. FASEB J 2015;29(10):4092–106.

[378] Kang C, Lim W. Data on mitochondrial function in skeletal muscle of old mice in response to different exercise intensity. Data Brief 2016;7:1519–23.

[379] Brault JJ, Jespersen JG, Goldberg AL. Peroxisome proliferator-activated receptor gamma coactivator 1alpha or 1beta overexpression inhibits muscle protein degradation, induction of ubiquitin ligases, and disuse atrophy. J Biol Chem 2010;285(25):19460–71.

[380] Sandri M, Lin J, Handschin C, Yang W, Arany ZP, Lecker SH, et al. PGC-1alpha protects skeletal muscle from atrophy by suppressing FoxO3 action and atrophy-specific gene transcription. Proc Natl Acad Sci USA 2006;103(44):16260–5.

[381] Lu JJ, Wang Q, Xie LH, Zhang Q, Sun SH. Tumor necrosis factor-like weak inducer of apoptosis regulates quadriceps muscle atrophy and fiber-type alteration in a rat model of chronic obstructive pulmonary disease. Tob Induc Dis 2017;15:43.

[382] Hindi SM, Mishra V, Bhatnagar S, Tajrishi MM, Ogura Y, Yan Z, et al. Regulatory circuitry of TWEAK-Fn14 system and PGC-1alpha in skeletal muscle atrophy program. FASEB J 2014;28(3):1398–411.

[383] Leick L, Lyngby SS, Wojtaszewski JF, Pilegaard H. PGC-1alpha is required for training-induced prevention of age-associated decline in mitochondrial enzymes in mouse skeletal muscle. Exp Gerontol 2010;45(5):336–42.

[384] Adhihetty PJ, Uguccioni G, Leick L, Hidalgo J, Pilegaard H, Hood DA. The role of PGC-1alpha on mitochondrial function and apoptotic susceptibility in muscle. Am J Physiol Cell Physiol 2009;297(1):C217–25.

[385] Leick L, Wojtaszewski JF, Johansen ST, Kiilerich K, Comes G, Hellsten Y, et al. PGC-1alpha is not mandatory for exercise- and training-induced adaptive gene responses in mouse skeletal muscle. Am J Physiol Endocrinol Metab 2008;294(2):E463–74.

[386] Wenz T. Mitochondria and PGC-1alpha in aging and age-associated diseases. J Aging Res 2011;2011:810619.
[387] Wenz T, Rossi SG, Rotundo RL, Spiegelman BM, Moraes CT. Increased muscle PGC-1alpha expression protects from sarcopenia and metabolic disease during aging. Proc Natl Acad Sci USA 2009;106(48):20405–10.
[388] Formosa LE, Hofer A, Tischner C, Wenz T, Ryan MT. Translation and assembly of radiolabeled mitochondrial DNA-encoded protein subunits from cultured cells and isolated mitochondria. Methods Mol Biol 2016;1351:115–29.
[389] Ascenzi F, Barberi L, Dobrowolny G, Villa Nova Bacurau A, Nicoletti C, Rizzuto E, et al. Effects of IGF-1 isoforms on muscle growth and sarcopenia. Aging Cell 2019;18(3):e12954.
[390] Arnold AS, Gill J, Christe M, Ruiz R, McGuirk S, St-Pierre J, et al. Morphological and functional remodelling of the neuromuscular junction by skeletal muscle PGC-1alpha. Nat Commun 2014;5:3569.
[391] Garcia S, Nissanka N, Mareco EA, Rossi S, Peralta S, Diaz F, et al. Overexpression of PGC-1alpha in aging muscle enhances a subset of young-like molecular patterns. Aging Cell 2018;17(2).
[392] Mills R, Taylor-Weiner H, Correia JC, Agudelo LZ, Allodi I, Kolonelou C, et al. Neurturin is a PGC-1alpha1-controlled myokine that promotes motor neuron recruitment and neuromuscular junction formation. Mol Metab 2018;7:12–22.
[393] Islam MT. Oxidative stress and mitochondrial dysfunction-linked neurodegenerative disorders. Neurol Res 2017;39(1):73–82.
[394] Da CS, Parone PA, Lopes VS, Lillo C, McAlonis-Downes M, Lee SK, et al. Elevated PGC-1alpha activity sustains mitochondrial biogenesis and muscle function without extending survival in a mouse model of inherited ALS. Cell Metab 2012;15(5):778–86.
[395] Zhao W, Varghese M, Yemul S, Pan Y, Cheng A, Marano P, et al. Peroxisome proliferator activator receptor gamma coactivator-1alpha (PGC-1alpha) improves motor performance and survival in a mouse model of amyotrophic lateral sclerosis. Mol Neurodegener 2011;6(1):51.
[396] de Castro GS, Simoes E, Lima J, Ortiz-Silva M, Festuccia WT, Tokeshi F, et al. Human cachexia induces changes in mitochondria, autophagy and apoptosis in the skeletal muscle. Cancers (Basel) 2019;11(9).
[397] Penna F, Ballaro R, Martinez-Cristobal P, Sala D, Sebastian D, Busquets S, et al. Autophagy exacerbates muscle wasting in cancer cachexia and impairs mitochondrial function. J Mol Biol 2019;431(15):2674–86. https://doi.org/10.1016/j.jmb.2019.05.032.
[398] Hirano K, Fujimaki M, Sasazawa Y, Yamaguchi A, Ishikawa KI, Miyamoto K, et al. Neuroprotective effects of memantine via enhancement of autophagy. Biochem Biophys Res Commun 2019;518(1):161–70.
[399] Pryde KR, Smith HL, Chau KY, Schapira AH. PINK1 disables the anti-fission machinery to segregate damaged mitochondria for mitophagy. J Cell Biol 2016;213(2):163–71.
[400] Wang W, Esbensen Y, Kunke D, Suganthan R, Rachek L, Bjoras M, et al. Mitochondrial DNA damage level determines neural stem cell differentiation fate. J Neurosci 2011;31(26):9746–51.
[401] Yoshii SR, Mizushima N. Autophagy machinery in the context of mammalian mitophagy. Biochim Biophys Acta 2015;1853(10 Pt B):2797–801.
[402] Yoshii SR, Kishi C, Ishihara N, Mizushima N. Parkin mediates proteasome-dependent protein degradation and rupture of the outer mitochondrial membrane. J Biol Chem 2011;286(22):19630–40.
[403] Yeo D, Kang C, Gomez-Cabrera MC, Vina J, Ji LL. Intensified mitophagy in skeletal muscle with aging is downregulated by PGC-1alpha overexpression in vivo. Free Radic Biol Med 2019;130:361–8.
[404] Yan J, Feng Z, Liu J, Shen W, Wang Y, Wertz K, et al. Enhanced autophagy plays a cardinal role in mitochondrial dysfunction in type 2 diabetic Goto-Kakizaki (GK) rats: ameliorating effects of (−)-epigallocatechin-3-gallate. J Nutr Biochem 2012;23(7):716–24.
[405] Wang K, Klionsky DJ. Mitochondria removal by autophagy. Autophagy 2011;7(3):297–300.
[406] Fallaize D, Chin LS, Li L. Differential submitochondrial localization of PINK1 as a molecular switch for mediating distinct mitochondrial signaling pathways. Cell Signal 2015;27(12):2543–54.
[407] Eid N, Ito Y, Horibe A, Otsuki Y. Ethanol-induced mitophagy in liver is associated with activation of the PINK1-Parkin pathway triggered by oxidative DNA damage. Histol Histopathol 2016;11747.

[408] Berezhnov AV, Soutar MP, Fedotova EI, Frolova MS, Plun-Favreau H, Zinchenko VP, et al. Intracellular pH modulates autophagy and mitophagy. J Biol Chem 2016;291(16):8701–8.
[409] McArthur K, Whitehead LW, Heddleston JM, Li L, Padman BS, Oorschot V, et al. BAK/BAX macropores facilitate mitochondrial herniation and mtDNA efflux during apoptosis. Science 2018;359(6378).
[410] Lazarou M, Sliter DA, Kane LA, Sarraf SA, Wang C, Burman JL, et al. The ubiquitin kinase PINK1 recruits autophagy receptors to induce mitophagy. Nature 2015;524(7565):309–14.
[411] Kane LA, Lazarou M, Fogel AI, Li Y, Yamano K, Sarraf SA, et al. PINK1 phosphorylates ubiquitin to activate Parkin E3 ubiquitin ligase activity. J Cell Biol 2014;205(2):143–53.
[412] Heo K, Lim SM, Nahm M, Kim YE, Oh KW, Park HT, et al. A de novo RAPGEF2 variant identified in a sporadic amyotrophic lateral sclerosis patient impairs microtubule stability and axonal mitochondria distribution. Exp Neurobiol 2018;27(6):550–63.
[413] Vial G, Coudy-Gandilhon C, Pinel A, Wauquier F, Chevenet C, Bechet D, et al. Lipid accumulation and mitochondrial abnormalities are associated with fiber atrophy in the skeletal muscle of rats with collagen-induced arthritis. Biochim Biophys Acta Mol Cell Biol Lipids 1865;2020(2):158574.
[414] Favaro G, Romanello V, Varanita T, Andrea Desbats M, Morbidoni V, Tezze C, et al. DRP1-mediated mitochondrial shape controls calcium homeostasis and muscle mass. Nat Commun 2019;10(1):2576.
[415] Ju JS, Jeon SI, Park JY, Lee JY, Lee SC, Cho KJ, et al. Autophagy plays a role in skeletal muscle mitochondrial biogenesis in an endurance exercise-trained condition. J Physiol Sci 2016;66(5):417–30.
[416] O'Leary MF, Vainshtein A, Iqbal S, Ostojic O, Hood DA. Adaptive plasticity of autophagic proteins to denervation in aging skeletal muscle. Am J Physiol Cell Physiol 2013;304(5):C422–30.
[417] O'Leary MF, Vainshtein A, Carter HN, Zhang Y, Hood DA. Denervation-induced mitochondrial dysfunction and autophagy in skeletal muscle of apoptosis-deficient animals. Am J Physiol Cell Physiol 2012;303(4):C447–54.
[418] Chen CCW, Erlich AT, Crilly MJ, Hood DA. Parkin is required for exercise-induced mitophagy in muscle: impact of aging. Am J Physiol Endocrinol Metab 2018;315(3):E404–15.
[419] Garcia-Prat L, Martinez-Vicente M, Perdiguero E, Ortet L, Rodriguez-Ubreva J, Rebollo E, et al. Autophagy maintains stemness by preventing senescence. Nature 2016;529(7584):37–42.
[420] Garcia-Prat L, Munoz-Canoves P, Martinez-Vicente M. Dysfunctional autophagy is a driver of muscle stem cell functional decline with aging. Autophagy 2016;12(3):612–3.
[421] Herst PM, Rowe MR, Carson GM, Berridge MV. Functional mitochondria in health and disease. Front Endocrinol (Lausanne) 2017;8:296.
[422] Mercken EM, Capri M, Carboneau BA, Conte M, Heidler J, Santoro A, et al. Conserved and species-specific molecular denominators in mammalian skeletal muscle aging. NPJ Aging Mech Dis 2017;3:8.
[423] Tohma H, Hepworth AR, Shavlakadze T, Grounds MD, Arthur PG. Quantification of ceroid and lipofuscin in skeletal muscle. J Histochem Cytochem 2011;59(8):769–79.
[424] Prajapati P, Dalwadi P, Gohel D, Singh K, Sripada L, Bhatelia K, et al. Enforced lysosomal biogenesis rescues erythromycin- and clindamycin-induced mitochondria-mediated cell death in human cells. Mol Cell Biochem 2019;481(1–2):23–36. https://doi.org/10.1007/s11010-019-03585-w.
[425] Schaaf GJ, Canibano-Fraile R, van Gestel TJM, van der Ploeg AT, Pijnappel W. Restoring the regenerative balance in neuromuscular disorders: satellite cell activation as therapeutic target in Pompe disease. Ann Transl Med 2019;7(13):280.
[426] Jannig PR, Moreira JB, Bechara LR, Bozi LH, Bacurau AV, Monteiro AW, et al. Autophagy signaling in skeletal muscle of infarcted rats. PLoS One 2014;9(1):e85820.
[427] Terman A, Kurz T, Navratil M, Arriaga EA, Brunk UT. Mitochondrial turnover and aging of long-lived postmitotic cells: the mitochondrial-lysosomal axis theory of aging. Antioxid Redox Signal 2010;12(4):503–35.
[428] Navratil M, Terman A, Arriaga EA. Giant mitochondria do not fuse and exchange their contents with normal mitochondria. Exp Cell Res 2008;314(1):164–72.
[429] Sarparanta J, Garcia-Macia M, Singh R. Autophagy and mitochondria in obesity and type 2 diabetes. Curr Diabetes Rev 2017;13(4):352–69.

[430] Chen Y, Dorn GW. PINK1-phosphorylated mitofusin 2 is a Parkin receptor for culling damaged mitochondria. Science 2013;340(6131):471–5.

[431] Sebastian S, Sreenivas P, Sambasivan R, Cheedipudi S, Kandalla P, Pavlath GK, et al. MLL5, a trithorax homolog, indirectly regulates H3K4 methylation, represses cyclin A2 expression, and promotes myogenic differentiation. Proc Natl Acad Sci USA 2009;106(12):4719–24.

[432] Sebastian D, Palacin M, Zorzano A. Mitochondrial dynamics: coupling mitochondrial fitness with healthy aging. Trends Mol Med 2017;23(3):201–15.

[433] He L, Zhou Q, Huang Z, Xu J, Zhou H, Lv D, et al. PINK1/Parkin-mediated mitophagy promotes apelin-13-induced vascular smooth muscle cell proliferation by AMPKalpha and exacerbates atherosclerotic lesions. J Cell Physiol 2019;234(6):8668–82.

[434] Cilenti L, Ambivero CT, Ward N, Alnemri ES, Germain D, Zervos AS. Inactivation of Omi/HtrA2 protease leads to the deregulation of mitochondrial Mulan E3 ubiquitin ligase and increased mitophagy. Biochim Biophys Acta 2014;1843(7):1295–307.

[435] Fornai F, Longone P, Ferrucci M, Lenzi P, Isidoro C, Ruggieri S, et al. Autophagy and amyotrophic lateral sclerosis: the multiple roles of lithium. Autophagy 2008;4(4):527–30.

[436] Natale LC, Rodrigues MC, Alania Y, MDS C, Vilela HS, Vieira DN, et al. Development of calcium phosphate/ethylene glycol dimethacrylate particles for dental applications. J Biomed Mater Res B Appl Biomater 2019;107(3):708–15. https://doi.org/10.1002/jbm.b.34164.

[437] Natale G, Lenzi P, Lazzeri G, Falleni A, Biagioni F, Ryskalin L, et al. Compartment-dependent mitochondrial alterations in experimental ALS, the effects of mitophagy and mitochondriogenesis. Front Cell Neurosci 2015;9:434.

[438] Fedorowicz MA, de Vries-Schneider RL, Rub C, Becker D, Huang Y, Zhou C, et al. Cytosolic cleaved PINK1 represses Parkin translocation to mitochondria and mitophagy. EMBO Rep 2014;15(1):86–93.

[439] Luo C, Li Y, Wang H, Feng Z, Li Y, Long J, et al. Mitochondrial accumulation under oxidative stress is due to defects in autophagy. J Cell Biochem 2013;114(1):212–9.

[440] Vainshtein A, Tryon LD, Pauly M, Hood DA. Role of PGC-1alpha during acute exercise-induced autophagy and mitophagy in skeletal muscle. Am J Physiol Cell Physiol 2015;308(9):C710–9.

[441] Aguilar-Agon KW, Capel AJ, Martin NRW, Player DJ, Lewis MP. Mechanical loading stimulates hypertrophy in tissue-engineered skeletal muscle: molecular and phenotypic responses. J Cell Physiol 2019;234(12):23547–58.

[442] Joseph GA, Wang SX, Jacobs CE, Zhou W, Kimble GC, Tse HW, et al. Partial inhibition of mTORC1 in aged rats counteracts the decline in muscle mass and reverses molecular signaling associated with sarcopenia. Mol Cell Biol 2019;39(19).

[443] Tan KT, Ang STJ, Tsai SY. Sarcopenia: tilting the balance of protein homeostasis. Proteomics 2020;20(5–6):e1800411. https://doi.org/10.1002/pmic.201800411.

[444] Tang H, Inoki K, Lee M, Wright E, Khuong A, Khuong A, et al. mTORC1 promotes denervation-induced muscle atrophy through a mechanism involving the activation of FoxO and E3 ubiquitin ligases. Sci Signal 2014;7(314):ra18.

[445] Castets P, Rion N, Theodore M, Falcetta D, Lin S, Reischl M, et al. mTORC1 and PKB/Akt control the muscle response to denervation by regulating autophagy and HDAC4. Nat Commun 2019;10(1):3187.

[446] Castets P, Lin S, Rion N, Di Fulvio S, Romanino K, Guridi M, et al. Sustained activation of mTORC1 in skeletal muscle inhibits constitutive and starvation-induced autophagy and causes a severe, late-onset myopathy. Cell Metab 2013;17(5):731–44.

[447] Castets P, Ruegg MA. MTORC1 determines autophagy through ULK1 regulation in skeletal muscle. Autophagy 2013;9(9):1435–7.

[448] Koga A, Notohara M, Hirai H. Evolution of subterminal satellite (StSat) repeats in hominids. Genetica 2011;139(2):167–75.

[449] Fernando R, Drescher C, Nowotny K, Grune T, Castro JP. Impaired proteostasis during skeletal muscle aging. Free Radic Biol Med 2019;132:58–66.

[450] Matteucci A, Patron M, Vecellio Reane D, Gastaldello S, Amoroso S, Rizzuto R, et al. Parkin-dependent regulation of the MCU complex component MICU1. Sci Rep 2018;8(1):14199.

[451] Rivera-Reyes A, Ye S, Marino GE, Egolf S, Ciotti GE, Chor S, et al. YAP1 enhances NF-kappaB-dependent and independent effects on clock-mediated unfolded protein responses and autophagy in sarcoma. Cell Death Dis 2018;9(11):1108.

[452] Al-Khalili L, de Castro BT, Ostling J, Massart J, Cuesta PG, Osler ME, et al. Proteasome inhibition in skeletal muscle cells unmasks metabolic derangements in type 2 diabetes. Am J Physiol Cell Physiol 2014;307(9):C774–87.

[453] Hwee DT, Baehr LM, Philp A, Baar K, Bodine SC. Maintenance of muscle mass and load-induced growth in Muscle RING Finger 1 null mice with age. Aging Cell 2014;13(1):92–101.

[454] Assereto S, Piccirillo R, Baratto S, Scudieri P, Fiorillo C, Massacesi M, et al. The ubiquitin ligase tripartite-motif-protein 32 is induced in Duchenne muscular dystrophy. Lab Invest 2016;96(8):862–71.

[455] Gomes AV, Waddell DS, Siu R, Stein M, Dewey S, Furlow JD, et al. Upregulation of proteasome activity in muscle RING finger 1-null mice following denervation. FASEB J 2012;26(7):2986–99.

[456] Kapadia MR, Eng JW, Jiang Q, Stoyanovsky DA, Kibbe MR. Nitric oxide regulates the 26S proteasome in vascular smooth muscle cells. Nitric Oxide 2009;20(4):279–88.

[457] Gardrat F, Montel V, Raymond J, Azanza JL. Degradation of an ubiquitin-conjugated protein is associated with myoblast differentiation in primary cell culture. Biochem Mol Biol Int 1999;47(3):387–96.

[458] Newman DJ, Schultz KU, Rochlis JL. Closed-loop, estimator-based model of human posture following reduced gravity exposure. J Guid Control Dynam 1996;19(5):1102–8.

[459] Newman AB, Lee JS, Visser M, Goodpaster BH, Kritchevsky SB, Tylavsky FA, et al. Weight change and the conservation of lean mass in old age: the health, aging and body composition study. Am J Clin Nutr 2005;82(4):872–8. quiz 915–6.

[460] Bodine-Fowler S. Skeletal muscle regeneration after injury: an overview. J Voice 1994;8(1):53–62.

[461] Cong J, Zhang L, Li J, Wang S, Gao F, Zhou G. Effects of dietary supplementation with carnosine on growth performance, meat quality, antioxidant capacity and muscle fiber characteristics in broiler chickens. J Sci Food Agric 2017;97(11):3733–41.

[462] Lagirand-Cantaloube J, Cornille K, Csibi A, Batonnet-Pichon S, Leibovitch MP, Leibovitch SA. Inhibition of atrogin-1/MAFbx mediated MyoD proteolysis prevents skeletal muscle atrophy in vivo. PLoS One 2009;4(3):e4973.

[463] Zhao K, Liang G, Sun X, Guan le L. Comparative miRNAome analysis revealed different miRNA expression profiles in bovine sera and exosomes. BMC Genomics 2016;17(1):630.

[464] Cai D, Lee KK, Li M, Tang MK, Chan KM. Ubiquitin expression is up-regulated in human and rat skeletal muscles during aging. Arch Biochem Biophys 2004;425(1):42–50.

[465] Abu-Baker A, Laganiere J, Gaudet R, Rochefort D, Brais B, Neri C, et al. Lithium chloride attenuates cell death in oculopharyngeal muscular dystrophy by perturbing Wnt/beta-catenin pathway. Cell Death Dis 2013;4:e821.

[466] Henderson DM, Nicholls R. Balance and strength—estimating the maximum prey-lifting potential of the large predatory dinosaur Carcharodontosaurus saharicus. Anat Rec (Hoboken) 2015;298(8):1367–75.

[467] Altun M, Besche HC, Overkleeft HS, Piccirillo R, Edelmann MJ, Kessler BM, et al. Muscle wasting in aged, sarcopenic rats is associated with enhanced activity of the ubiquitin proteasome pathway. J Biol Chem 2010;285(51):39597–608.

[468] Loubiere C, Clavel S, Gilleron J, Harisseh R, Fauconnier J, Ben-Sahra I, et al. The energy disruptor metformin targets mitochondrial integrity via modification of calcium flux in cancer cells. Sci Rep 2017;7(1):5040.

[469] Edstrom E, Altun M, Bergman E, Johnson H, Kullberg S, Ramirez-Leon V, et al. Factors contributing to neuromuscular impairment and sarcopenia during aging. Physiol Behav 2007;92(1–2):129–35.

[470] Edstrom E, Altun M, Hagglund M, Ulfhake B. Atrogin-1/MAFbx and MuRF1 are downregulated in aging-related loss of skeletal muscle. J Gerontol A Biol Sci Med Sci 2006;61(7):663–74.

[471] Jong CJ, Ito T, Schaffer SW. The ubiquitin-proteasome system and autophagy are defective in the taurine-deficient heart. Amino Acids 2015;47(12):2609–22.

[472] Sulkshane P, Duek I, Ram J, Thakur A, Reis N, Ziv T, et al. Inhibition of proteasome reveals basal mitochondrial ubiquitination. J Proteomics 2020;229:103949. https://doi.org/10.1016/j.jprot.2020.103949.103949.

[473] Wu H, Dridi S, Ferrando A, Wolfe R, Kim II Y, Baum J. Net protein balance correlates with expression of autophagy, mitochondrial biogenesis, and fat metabolism-related genes in skeletal muscle from older adults. Physiol Rep 2020;8:e147575. https://doi.org/10.14814/phy2.14575. e147575.
[474] Ferrington DA, Husom AD, Thompson LV. Altered proteasome structure, function, and oxidation in aged muscle. FASEB J 2005;19(6):644–6.
[475] Husom AD, Peters EA, Kolling EA, Fugere NA, Thompson LV, Ferrington DA. Altered proteasome function and subunit composition in aged muscle. Arch Biochem Biophys 2004;421(1):67–76.
[476] Strucksberg KH, Tangavelou K, Schroder R, Clemen CS. Proteasomal activity in skeletal muscle: a matter of assay design, muscle type, and age. Anal Biochem 2010;399(2):225–9.
[477] Hepple RT. Sarcopenia—a critical perspective. Sci Aging Knowledge Environ 2003;2003(46):pe31.
[478] Rom O, Reznick AZ. The role of E3 ubiquitin-ligases MuRF-1 and MAFbx in loss of skeletal muscle mass. Free Radic Biol Med 2016;98:218–30. https://doi.org/10.1016/j.freeradbiomed.2015.12.031 [Epub ahead of print].
[479] Castets P, Ruegg MA. MTORC1 determines autophagy through ULK1 regulation in skeletal muscle. Autophagy 2013;9(9):1435–7.
[480] Koga H, Kaushik S, Cuervo AM. Protein homeostasis and aging: the importance of exquisite quality control. Ageing Res Rev 2011;10(2):205–15.
[481] Riederer BM, Leuba G, Vernay A, Riederer IM. The role of the ubiquitin proteasome system in Alzheimer's disease. Exp Biol Med (Maywood) 2011;236(3):268–76.
[482] Riederer BM, Leuba G, Elhajj Z. Oxidation and ubiquitination in neurodegeneration. Exp Biol Med (Maywood) 2013;238(5):519–24.
[483] Riederer P, Berg D, Casadei N, Cheng F, Classen J, Dresel C, et al. alpha-Synuclein in Parkinson's disease: causal or bystander? J Neural Transm (Vienna) 2019;126(7):815–40.
[484] Shamoto-Nagai M, Maruyama W, Akao Y, Osawa T, Tribl F, Gerlach M, et al. Neuromelanin inhibits enzymatic activity of 26S proteasome in human dopaminergic SH-SY5Y cells. J Neural Transm (Vienna) 2004;111(10−11):1253–65.
[485] Larabee CM, Georgescu C, Wren JD, Plafker SM. Expression profiling of the ubiquitin conjugating enzyme UbcM2 in murine brain reveals modest age-dependent decreases in specific neurons. BMC Neurosci 2015;16:76.
[486] Liu W, Duan X, Fang X, Shang W, Tong C. Mitochondrial protein import regulates cytosolic protein homeostasis and neuronal integrity. Autophagy 2018;14(8):1293–309.
[487] Jung S, Chung Y, Oh YJ. Breaking down autophagy and the ubiquitin proteasome system. Parkinsonism Relat Disord 2018;46(Suppl 1):S97–S100.
[488] Tanaka K, Matsuda N. Proteostasis and neurodegeneration: the roles of proteasomal degradation and autophagy. Biochim Biophys Acta 2014;1843(1):197–204.
[489] Papa L, Rockwell P. Persistent mitochondrial dysfunction and oxidative stress hinder neuronal cell recovery from reversible proteasome inhibition. Apoptosis 2008;13(4):588–99.
[490] Hohn A, Konig J, Grune T. Protein oxidation in aging and the removal of oxidized proteins. J Proteomics 2013;92:132–59.
[491] Bobkova NV, Evgen'ev M, Garbuz DG, Kulikov AM, Morozov A, Samokhin A, et al. Exogenous Hsp70 delays senescence and improves cognitive function in aging mice. Proc Natl Acad Sci USA 2015;112(52):16006–11.
[492] Chen PC, Qin LN, Li XM, Walters BJ, Wilson JA, Mei L, et al. The proteasome-associated deubiquitinating enzyme Usp14 is essential for the maintenance of synaptic ubiquitin levels and the development of neuromuscular junctions. J Neurosci 2009;29(35):10909–19.
[493] Hohn A, Tramutola A, Cascella R. Proteostasis failure in neurodegenerative diseases: focus on oxidative stress. Oxid Med Cell Longev 2020;2020:5497046.
[494] Cattaud V, Bezzina C, Rey CC, Lejards C, Dahan L, Verret L. Early disruption of parvalbumin expression and perineuronal nets in the hippocampus of the Tg2576 mouse model of Alzheimer's disease can be rescued by enriched environment. Neurobiol Aging 2018;72:147–58.
[495] Opoku-Nsiah KA, Gestwicki JE. Aim for the core: suitability of the ubiquitin-independent 20S proteasome as a drug target in neurodegeneration. Transl Res 2018;198:48–57.

[496] Colell A, Ricci JE, Tait S, Milasta S, Maurer U, Bouchier-Hayes L, et al. GAPDH and autophagy preserve survival after apoptotic cytochrome c release in the absence of caspase activation. Cell 2007;129(5):983–97.
[497] Liu H, He Z, Germic N, Ademi H, Frangez Z, Felser A, et al. ATG12 deficiency leads to tumor cell oncosis owing to diminished mitochondrial biogenesis and reduced cellular bioenergetics. Cell Death Differ 2019.
[498] Rubinstein AD, Eisenstein M, Ber Y, Bialik S, Kimchi A. The autophagy protein Atg12 associates with antiapoptotic Bcl-2 family members to promote mitochondrial apoptosis. Mol Cell 2011;44(5):698–709.
[499] Haller M, Hock AK, Giampazolias E, Oberst A, Green DR, Debnath J, et al. Ubiquitination and proteasomal degradation of ATG12 regulates its proapoptotic activity. Autophagy 2014;10(12):2269–78.
[500] Nichenko AS, Southern WM, Tehrani KF, Qualls AE, Flemington AB, Mercer GH, et al. Mitochondrial-specific autophagy linked to mitochondrial dysfunction following traumatic freeze injury in mice. Am J Physiol Cell Physiol 2020;318(2):C242–52.
[501] Nichenko AS, Southern WM, Atuan M, Luan J, Peissig KB, Foltz SJ, et al. Mitochondrial maintenance via autophagy contributes to functional skeletal muscle regeneration and remodeling. Am J Physiol Cell Physiol 2016;311(2):C190–200.
[502] Watson EL, Baker LA, Wilkinson TJ, Gould DW, Graham-Brown MPM, Major RW, et al. Reductions in skeletal muscle mitochondrial mass are not restored following exercise training in patients with chronic kidney disease. FASEB J 2020;34(1):1755–67.
[503] Kasai S, Shimizu S, Tatara Y, Mimura J, Itoh K. Regulation of Nrf2 by mitochondrial reactive oxygen species in physiology and pathology. Biomolecules 2020;10(2).
[504] Ahn B, Pharaoh G, Premkumar P, Huseman K, Ranjit R, Kinter M, et al. Nrf2 deficiency exacerbates age-related contractile dysfunction and loss of skeletal muscle mass. Redox Biol 2018;17:47–58.
[505] Moussa CE, Fu Q, Kumar P, Shtifman A, Lopez JR, Allen PD, et al. Transgenic expression of beta-APP in fast-twitch skeletal muscle leads to calcium dyshomeostasis and IBM-like pathology. FASEB J 2006;20(12):2165–7.
[506] Hoffmann-Conaway S, Brockmann MM, Schneider K, Annamneedi A, Rahman KA, Bruns C, et al. Parkin contributes to synaptic vesicle autophagy in bassoon-deficient mice. Elife 2020;9.
[507] Ham SJ, Lee D, Yoo H, Jun K, Shin H, Chung J. Decision between mitophagy and apoptosis by Parkin via VDAC1 ubiquitination. Proc Natl Acad Sci USA 2020;117(8):4281–91.
[508] Safiulina D, Kuum M, Choubey V, Gogichaishvili N, Liiv J, Hickey MA, et al. Miro proteins prime mitochondria for Parkin translocation and mitophagy. EMBO J 2019;38(2).
[509] Reddy PH, Oliver DM. Amyloid beta and phosphorylated tau-induced defective autophagy and mitophagy in Alzheimer's disease. Cells 2019;8(5).
[510] Cornelissen T, Vilain S, Vints K, Gounko N, Verstreken P, Vandenberghe W. Deficiency of parkin and PINK1 impairs age-dependent mitophagy in Drosophila. Elife 2018;7.
[511] Kaarniranta K, Uusitalo H, Blasiak J, Felszeghy S, Kannan R, Kauppinen A, et al. Mechanisms of mitochondrial dysfunction and their impact on age-related macular degeneration. Prog Retin Eye Res 2020;79:100858.
[512] Jannuzzi AT, Arslan S, Yilmaz AM, Sari G, Beklen H, Mendez L, et al. Higher proteotoxic stress rather than mitochondrial damage is involved in higher neurotoxicity of bortezomib compared to carfilzomib. Redox Biol 2020;32:101502.
[513] Romanello V, Scalabrin M, Albiero M, Blaauw B, Scorrano L, Sandri M. Inhibition of the fission machinery mitigates OPA1 impairment in adult skeletal muscles. Cells 2019;8(6):597.
[514] Ruas JL, White JP, Rao RR, Kleiner S, Brannan KT, Harrison BC, et al. A PGC-1alpha isoform induced by resistance training regulates skeletal muscle hypertrophy. Cell 2012;151(6):1319–31.
[515] Martinez-Redondo V, Jannig PR, Correia JC, Ferreira DM, Cervenka I, Lindvall JM, et al. Peroxisome proliferator-activated receptor gamma coactivator-1 alpha isoforms selectively regulate multiple splicing events on target genes. J Biol Chem 2016;291(29):15169–84.
[516] Brault JJ, Jespersen JG, Goldberg AL. Peroxisome proliferator-activated receptor gamma coactivator 1alpha or 1beta overexpression inhibits muscle protein degradation, induction of ubiquitin ligases, and disuse atrophy. J Biol Chem 2010;285(25):19460–71.
[517] Rodriguez-Nuevo A, Diaz-Ramos A, Noguera E, Diaz-Saez F, Duran X, Munoz JP, et al. Mitochondrial DNA and TLR9 drive muscle inflammation upon Opa1 deficiency. EMBO J 2018;37(10).

[518] Molero J, Moize V, Flores L, De Hollanda A, Jimenez A, Vidal J. The impact of age on the prevalence of Sarcopenic obesity in bariatric surgery candidates. Obes Surg 2020;30(6):2158–64.

[519] Chan W, Chin SH, Whittaker AC, Jones D, Kaur O, Bosch JA, et al. The associations of muscle strength, muscle mass, and adiposity with clinical outcomes and quality of life in prevalent kidney transplant recipients. J Ren Nutr 2019;29(6):536–47.

[520] Rasaei N, Kashavarz SA, Yekaninejad MS, Mirzaei K. The association between sarcopenic obesity (SO) and major dietary patterns in overweight and obese adult women. Diabetes Metab Syndr 2019;13(4):2519–24.

[521] Batsis JA, Gilbert-Diamond D, McClure AC, Weintraub A, Sette D, Mecchella JN, et al. Prevalence of sarcopenia obesity in patients treated at a rural, multidisciplinary weight and wellness center. Clin Med Insights Arthritis Musculoskelet Disord 2019;12. 1179544119862288.

[522] Gutierrez-Casado E, Khraiwesh H, Lopez-Dominguez JA, Montero-Guisado J, Lopez-Lluch G, Navas P, et al. The impact of aging, calorie restriction and dietary fat on autophagy markers and mitochondrial ultrastructure and dynamics in mouse skeletal muscle. J Gerontol A Biol Sci Med Sci 2019;74(6):760–9.

[523] Boengler K, Kosiol M, Mayr M, Schulz R, Rohrbach S. Mitochondria and ageing: role in heart, skeletal muscle and adipose tissue. J Cachexia Sarcopenia Muscle 2017;8(3):349–69.

[524] Fan J, Kou X, Jia S, Yang X, Yang Y, Chen N. Autophagy as a potential target for sarcopenia. J Cell Physiol 2016;231(7):1450–9.

[525] Rhoads TW, Clark JP, Gustafson GE, Miller KN, Conklin MW, DeMuth TM, et al. Molecular and functional networks linked to sarcopenia prevention by caloric restriction in rhesus monkeys. Cell Syst 2020;10(2). 156–68.e5.

[526] Lu J, McKinsey TA, Zhang CL, Olson EN. Regulation of skeletal myogenesis by association of the MEF2 transcription factor with class II histone deacetylases. Mol Cell 2000;6(2):233–44.

[527] Tang H, Goldman D. Activity-dependent gene regulation in skeletal muscle is mediated by a histone deacetylase (HDAC)-Dach2-myogenin signal transduction cascade. Proc Natl Acad Sci USA 2006;103(45):16977–82.

[528] Walsh ME, Bhattacharya A, Sataranatarajan K, Qaisar R, Sloane L, Rahman MM, et al. The histone deacetylase inhibitor butyrate improves metabolism and reduces muscle atrophy during aging. Aging Cell 2015;14(6):957–70.

[529] Selman C, Gredilla R, Phaneuf S, Kendaiah S, Barja G, Leeuwenburgh C. Short-term caloric restriction and regulatory proteins of apoptosis in heart, skeletal muscle and kidney of Fischer 344 rats. Biogerontology 2003;4(3):141–7.

[530] White JP, Billin AN, Campbell ME, Russell AJ, Huffman KM, Kraus WE. The AMPK/p27(Kip1) axis regulates autophagy/apoptosis decisions in aged skeletal muscle stem cells. Stem Cell Reports 2018;11(2):425–39.

[531] Anton SD, Hida A, Mankowski R, Layne A, Solberg LM, Mainous AG, et al. Nutrition and exercise in sarcopenia. Curr Protein Pept Sci 2018;19(7):649–67.

[532] Sakuma K, Yamaguchi A. Molecular mechanisms in aging and current strategies to counteract sarcopenia. Curr Aging Sci 2010;3(2):90–101.

[533] Ramirez-Velez R, Perez-Sousa MA, Garcia-Hermoso A, Zambom-Ferraresi F, Martinez-Velilla N, Saez de Asteasu ML, et al. Relative handgrip strength diminishes the negative effects of excess adiposity on dependence in older adults: a moderation analysis. J Clin Med 2020;(4):9.

[534] Hepple RT, Qin M, Nakamoto H, Goto S. Caloric restriction optimizes the proteasome pathway with aging in rat plantaris muscle: implications for sarcopenia. Am J Physiol Regul Integr Comp Physiol 2008;295(4):R1231–7.

[535] Baker DJ, Betik AC, Krause DJ, Hepple RT. No decline in skeletal muscle oxidative capacity with aging in long-term calorically restricted rats: effects are independent of mitochondrial DNA integrity. J Gerontol A Biol Sci Med Sci 2006;61(7):675–84.

[536] Lopez-Dominguez JA, Khraiwesh H, Gonzalez-Reyes JA, Lopez-Lluch G, Navas P, Ramsey JJ, et al. Dietary fat modifies mitochondrial and plasma membrane apoptotic signaling in skeletal muscle of calorie-restricted mice. Age (Dordr) 2013;35(6):2027–44.

[537] Pattanakuhar S, Sutham W, Sripetchwandee J, Minta W, Mantor D, Palee S, et al. Combined exercise and calorie restriction therapies restore contractile and mitochondrial functions in skeletal muscle of obese-insulin resistant rats. Nutrition 2019;62:74–84.

[538] Limanjaya A, Song KM, Choi MJ, Ghatak K, Minh NN, Kang DH, et al. Calorie restriction reverses age-related alteration of cavernous neurovascular structure in the rat. Andrology 2017;5(5):1023–31.

[539] Hord JM, Botchlett R, Lawler JM. Age-related alterations in the sarcolemmal environment are attenuated by lifelong caloric restriction and voluntary exercise. Exp Gerontol 2016;83:148–57.

[540] Dutta D, Xu J, Dirain ML, Leeuwenburgh C. Calorie restriction combined with resveratrol induces autophagy and protects 26-month-old rat hearts from doxorubicin-induced toxicity. Free Radic Biol Med 2014;74:252–62.

[541] Alugoju P, Swamy K, Periyasamy L. Effect of short-term quercetin, caloric restriction and combined treatment on age-related oxidative stress markers in the rat cerebral cortex. CNS Neurol Disord Drug Targets 2018;17(2):119–31.

[542] Chen Y, Hagopian K, Bibus D, Villalba JM, Lopez-Lluch G, Navas P, et al. The influence of dietary lipid composition on skeletal muscle mitochondria from mice following eight months of calorie restriction. Physiol Res 2014;63(1):57–71.

[543] Rohrbach S, Aslam M, Niemann B, Schulz R. Impact of caloric restriction on myocardial ischaemia/reperfusion injury and new therapeutic options to mimic its effects. Br J Pharmacol 2014;171(12):2964–92.

[544] Gouspillou G, Hepple RT. Facts and controversies in our understanding of how caloric restriction impacts the mitochondrion. Exp Gerontol 2013;48(10):1075–84.

[545] Bevilacqua L, Ramsey JJ, Hagopian K, Weindruch R, Harper ME. Long-term caloric restriction increases UCP3 content but decreases proton leak and reactive oxygen species production in rat skeletal muscle mitochondria. Am J Physiol Endocrinol Metab 2005;289(3):E429–38.

[546] Sohal RS, Forster MJ. Caloric restriction and the aging process: a critique. Free Radic Biol Med 2014;73:366–82.

[547] Sohal RS. Role of oxidative stress and protein oxidation in the aging process. Free Radic Biol Med 2002;33(1):37–44.

[548] Hepple RT. Why eating less keeps mitochondria working in aged skeletal muscle. Exerc Sport Sci Rev 2009;37(1):23–8.

[549] Barbat-Artigas S, Garnier S, Joffroy S, Riesco E, Sanguignol F, Vellas B, et al. Caloric restriction and aerobic exercise in sarcopenic and non-sarcopenic obese women: an observational and retrospective study. J Cachexia Sarcopenia Muscle 2016;7(3):284–9.

[550] Kim JH, Lee Y, Kwak HB, Lawler JM. Lifelong wheel running exercise and mild caloric restriction attenuate nuclear EndoG in the aging plantaris muscle. Exp Gerontol 2015;69:122–8.

[551] Yang L, Licastro D, Cava E, Veronese N, Spelta F, Rizza W, et al. Long-term calorie restriction enhances cellular quality-control processes in human skeletal muscle. Cell Rep 2016;14(3):422–8.

[552] Kim JH, Kwak HB, Leeuwenburgh C, Lawler JM. Lifelong exercise and mild (8%) caloric restriction attenuate age-induced alterations in plantaris muscle morphology, oxidative stress and IGF-1 in the Fischer-344 rat. Exp Gerontol 2008;43(4):317–29.

[553] Civitarese AE, Carling S, Heilbronn LK, Hulver MH, Ukropcova B, Deutsch WA, et al. Calorie restriction increases muscle mitochondrial biogenesis in healthy humans. PLoS Med 2007;4(3):e76.

[554] Chen CN, Liao YH, Tsai SC, Thompson LV. Age-dependent effects of caloric restriction on mTOR and ubiquitin-proteasome pathways in skeletal muscles. GeroScience 2019;41(6):871–80.

[555] Chen K, Kobayashi S, Xu X, Viollet B, Liang Q. AMP activated protein kinase is indispensable for myocardial adaptation to caloric restriction in mice. PLoS One 2013;8(3):e59682.

[556] Joseph AM, Malamo AG, Silvestre J, Wawrzyniak N, Carey-Love S, Nguyen LM, et al. Short-term caloric restriction, resveratrol, or combined treatment regimens initiated in late-life alter mitochondrial protein expression profiles in a fiber-type specific manner in aged animals. Exp Gerontol 2013;48(9):858–68.

[557] Kume S, Uzu T, Kashiwagi A, Koya D. SIRT1, a calorie restriction mimetic, in a new therapeutic approach for type 2 diabetes mellitus and diabetic vascular complications. Endocr Metab Immune Disord Drug Targets 2010;10(1):16–24.

[558] Wohlgemuth SE, Seo AY, Marzetti E, Lees HA, Leeuwenburgh C. Skeletal muscle autophagy and apoptosis during aging: effects of calorie restriction and life-long exercise. Exp Gerontol 2010;45(2):138–48.

[559] Marzetti E, Carter CS, Wohlgemuth SE, Lees HA, Giovannini S, Anderson B, et al. Changes in IL-15 expression and death-receptor apoptotic signaling in rat gastrocnemius muscle with aging and life-long calorie restriction. Mech Ageing Dev 2009;130(4):272–80.

[560] Villalba JM, Lopez-Dominguez JA, Chen Y, Khraiwesh H, Gonzalez-Reyes JA, Del Rio LF, et al. The influence of dietary fat source on liver and skeletal muscle mitochondrial modifications and lifespan changes in calorie-restricted mice. Biogerontology 2015;16(5):655–70.

[561] Pae M, Meydani SN, Wu D. The role of nutrition in enhancing immunity in aging. Aging Dis 2012;3(1):91–129.

[562] Faulks SC, Turner N, Else PL, Hulbert AJ. Calorie restriction in mice: effects on body composition, daily activity, metabolic rate, mitochondrial reactive oxygen species production, and membrane fatty acid composition. J Gerontol A Biol Sci Med Sci 2006;61(8):781–94.

[563] Rodriguez-Bies E, Tung BT, Navas P, Lopez-Lluch G. Resveratrol primes the effects of physical activity in old mice. Br J Nutr 2016;116(6):979–88.

[564] Patel BP, Safdar A, Raha S, Tarnopolsky MA, Hamadeh MJ. Caloric restriction shortens lifespan through an increase in lipid peroxidation, inflammation and apoptosis in the G93A mouse, an animal model of ALS. PLoS One 2010;5(2):e9386.

[565] Keipert S, Ost M, Chadt A, Voigt A, Ayala V, Portero-Otin M, et al. Skeletal muscle uncoupling-induced longevity in mice is linked to increased substrate metabolism and induction of the endogenous antioxidant defense system. Am J Physiol Endocrinol Metab 2013;304(5):E495–506.

[566] Pamplona R, Naudi A, Gavin R, Pastrana MA, Sajnani G, Ilieva EV, et al. Increased oxidation, glycoxidation, and lipoxidation of brain proteins in prion disease. Free Radic Biol Med 2008;45(8):1159–66.

[567] Civitarese AE, Carling S, Heilbronn LK, Hulver MH, Ukropcova B, Deutsch WA, et al. Calorie restriction increases muscle mitochondrial biogenesis in healthy humans. PLoS Med 2007;4(3):e76.

[568] Myers MJ, Shepherd DL, Durr AJ, Stanton DS, Mohamed JS, Hollander JM, et al. The role of SIRT1 in skeletal muscle function and repair of older mice. J Cachexia Sarcopenia Muscle 2019;10(4):929–49.

[569] Zhang Q, Zheng J, Qiu J, Wu X, Xu Y, Shen W, et al. ALDH2 restores exhaustive exercise-induced mitochondrial dysfunction in skeletal muscle. Biochem Biophys Res Commun 2017;485(4):753–60.

[570] Zheng Q, Zhao K, Han X, Huff AF, Cui Q, Babcock SA, et al. Inhibition of AMPK accentuates prolonged caloric restriction-induced change in cardiac contractile function through disruption of compensatory autophagy. Biochim Biophys Acta 2015;1852(2):332–42.

[571] Amigo I, Menezes-Filho SL, Luevano-Martinez LA, Chausse B, Kowaltowski AJ. Caloric restriction increases brain mitochondrial calcium retention capacity and protects against excitotoxicity. Aging Cell 2017;16(1):73–81.

[572] Fang H, Chen M, Ding Y, Shang W, Xu J, Zhang X, et al. Imaging superoxide flash and metabolism-coupled mitochondrial permeability transition in living animals. Cell Res 2011;21(9):1295–304.

[573] Dutta D, Xu J, Dirain ML, Leeuwenburgh C. Calorie restriction combined with resveratrol induces autophagy and protects 26-month-old rat hearts from doxorubicin-induced toxicity. Free Radic Biol Med 2014;74:252–62.

[574] Calvani R, Joseph AM, Adhihetty PJ, Miccheli A, Bossola M, Leeuwenburgh C, et al. Mitochondrial pathways in sarcopenia of aging and disuse muscle atrophy. Biol Chem 2013;394(3):393–414.

[575] Seo AY, Joseph AM, Dutta D, Hwang JC, Aris JP, Leeuwenburgh C. New insights into the role of mitochondria in aging: mitochondrial dynamics and more. J Cell Sci 2010;123(Pt 15):2533–42.

[576] Buford TW, Anton SD, Judge AR, Marzetti E, Wohlgemuth SE, Carter CS, et al. Models of accelerated sarcopenia: critical pieces for solving the puzzle of age-related muscle atrophy. Ageing Res Rev 2010;9(4):369–83.

[577] Marzetti E, Privitera G, Simili V, Wohlgemuth SE, Aulisa L, Pahor M, et al. Multiple pathways to the same end: mechanisms of myonuclear apoptosis in sarcopenia of aging. ScientificWorldJournal 2010;10:340–9.

[578] Oost LJ, Kustermann M, Armani A, Blaauw B, Romanello V. Fibroblast growth factor 21 controls mitophagy and muscle mass. J Cachexia Sarcopenia Muscle 2019;10(3):630–42.

[579] Karim MR, Fisher CR, Kapphahn RJ, Polanco JR, Ferrington DA. Investigating AKT activation and autophagy in immunoproteasome-deficient retinal cells. PLoS One 2020;15(4):e0231212.

CHAPTER 2

The role of the neuromuscular junction in sarcopenia

Michael R. Deschenes, Jeongeun Oh, and Hannah Tufts
Department of Health Sciences, College of William & Mary, Williamsburg, VA, United States

Abstract
The neuromuscular junction (NMJ) is the synapse joining the motor neuron with the myofiber(s) that are innervated by an excitatory neuron, enabling the proper function of the neuromuscular system. Since sarcopenia is currently defined mainly by age-related declines in muscle function, rather than mass, the importance of understanding age-related degeneration of the NMJ has grown in importance. Morphological and physiological disruptions of the NMJ significantly contribute to, and are at the core of, age-related decrements in muscle strength and power, and thus, the larger phenomenon of sarcopenia. Opposing explanations of "dying forward" and "dying back" have been proposed to explain the beginning and progression of sarcopenia. Likely, both play roles, but in distinct components of the neuromuscular system. Here, we examine the effects of age-related deterioration of the NMJ on muscle function, and thus sarcopenia, an increasingly common malady that imposes severe health and financial burdens on societies throughout the world.

Keywords: Synapse, Acetylcholine, Endplate, Nerve terminal, Apoptosis

Introduction

Sarcopenia is an age-related affliction characterized by loss of skeletal muscle mass that was first described by Dr. I.H. Rosenberg in 1989 at a conference on the epidemiology of aging [1], who later published his description in detail in 1997 [2]. The term sarcopenia is derived from the Greek words "sarx" for flesh, and "penia" for loss, and until recently, the condition of sarcopenia was defined as a loss of skeletal muscle leaving the individual at least two standard deviations below the average muscle mass observed in young adults. Recently, however, the presence of sarcopenia has been assessed by age-related loss of skeletal muscle function, and in particular, muscle strength [3]. The main reason for changing the principal criterion for the determination of sarcopenia from the loss of muscle mass to the decline in muscle strength is that strength decrements are more closely related to the health concerns associated with sarcopenia, e.g., osteoporosis, heart disease, diabetes, stroke, accidental falls, and even mortality, than the loss of muscle mass [4–6]. Because of these widespread comorbidities, the estimated health care costs associated with sarcopenia are more than $10 billion each year [4]. This staggering burden can be at least partly explained by the prevalence of sarcopenia in the United States where it affects roughly 45% of the country's aged (≥ 65 years) population [4]. Sarcopenia is a progressive condition beginning from the age of 40 years with people losing ~ 1.5% of muscle mass annually so that, by the age of 70 years, up to 30% of the total muscle mass has been lost, with an even greater decline of muscle strength, i.e., 40% [7]. Because of the many negative health consequences associated with sarcopenia, the European Working Group on Sarcopenia in Older People recently upgraded the severity of its outcomes and has labeled sarcopenia a muscle disease, as opposed to a condition as it had previously been categorized [3]. Thus, age-related loss of muscle mass, and particularly strength, is now viewed as a disease and one that is different from, yet in many ways overlapping with, the more broadly based syndrome of frailty, which, unlike sarcopenia, also encompasses social dimensions such as loneliness and socioeconomic support [8, 9].

For some time now, the NMJ's role in generating optimal muscular force has been known [10, 11]. However, if using the strict, technical definition of strength as being the maximal amount of force exerted in a single attempt, the NMJ is not as critical as is the capacity to optimally recruit motor units, particularly large, high threshold ones. Instead, evidence reveals that proper function of the NMJ is essential to maintaining muscle force overtime, or a sequence of maximal efforts, rather than during a single effort in a rested state. For example, in a well-rested muscle, neural (indirect) stimulation of muscle results in the production of almost all of the force that is generated when directly stimulating the muscle by way of its sarcolemma. However, following a series of maximal contractile events, the same muscle produces a significantly smaller fraction of that which occurs at the onset of the train of contractions, indicating greater blockage of the neural signal at the NMJ (see Fig. 1).

It has been determined that such neuromuscular blockage is more pronounced in aged muscles and that this age-related discrepancy can be located in one of four potential sites [12]: (1) at axonal branch points of presynaptic nerve terminals, (2) at presynaptic vesicular release sites of nerve terminal endings, (3) disruption of optimal apposition orientation between presynaptic ACh release sites and postsynaptic binding sites, and (4) desensitization of postsynaptic ACh receptors.

Although historically the initial examination into the causes and consequences of sarcopenia focused on disturbances in muscle tissue, it is now recognized that the age-related loss of muscle function can also be ascribed to neurological factors [13–16]. In particular, these alterations are most easily viewed as maladaptations of the neuromuscular junction (NMJ), which is the vital synapse connecting motor neurons with the skeletal myofibers which they innervate [15, 17, 18]. Perhaps, the recent attention to the critical role that the NMJ plays in the onset of sarcopenia is best captured by a landmark review on the subject titled "The neuromuscular junction: aging at the crossroad between nerves and muscle" by Gonzalez-Freire et al. appearing in 2014 in the journal *Frontiers in Aging Neuroscience* [19]. More recently, it

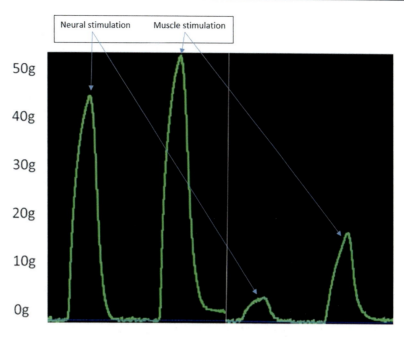

Fig. 1

Recording of ex vivo muscle stimulation technique showing the difference between muscle force produced by indirect (neural) stimulation and direct (muscle) stimulation at the start *(left panel)* and end *(right panel)* of 5 min of stimulation. The difference is considered neuromuscular transmission failure at the NMJ. Note that the difference increases over the 5-min train of stimuli.

has been reported that alterations at the NMJ serve as the most useful biomarker for the onset and progression of sarcopenia [20]. On investigating the etiology and effects of sarcopenia, the focus has changed from issues solely within the skeletal muscle system to disruptions within the more comprehensive and integrated neuromuscular system. In this chapter, the role of the NMJ in both developing and combatting sarcopenia will be addressed.

Age-related structural adaptations of the NMJ

In brief, the structural features of the NMJ include the presynaptic nerve terminals of the motor neuron and the postsynaptic endplate (features of the NMJ are shown in Fig. 2). The function of the nerve terminals is to deliver excitatory electrical impulses from the motor neuron emanating from the central nervous system (CNS) and traveling down the axon to the myofibers [21]. After leaving the spinal cord, these axons become components of the peripheral nervous system (PNS). As the axons arrive at the myofibers, they branch out to form several nerve terminal endings while losing their myelin sheath. The termination of myelin coverings is important so that calcium channels can be expressed in the membranes of

62   Chapter 2

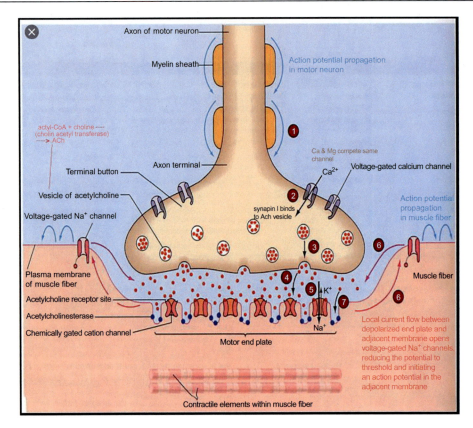

Fig. 2
Illustration of the pre- and postsynaptic features of a young, healthy NMJ, and events occurring during neuromuscular transmission. *Reproduced with permission from McGraw-Hill Higher Education.*

the nerve terminal endings. Upon the arrival of the action potential at the nerve terminal, these voltage-gated calcium channels open permitting a rapid influx of calcium into the cytoplasm of the nerve terminal triggering the release of vesicles containing the neurotransmitter acetylcholine (ACh) from their "docked" positions at the "active zones" of the terminals. Thus, untethered, ACh-containing vesicles can then dispense their contents into the synaptic cleft separating terminals from postsynaptic myofibers via exocytosis. It is important to note that several terminal branches originate from a single motor axon, thus amplifying the excitatory potential of that axon.

Typically, the vesicles participating in the release of ACh into the synaptic cleft come from the "readily releasable" pool of presynaptic vesicles, which represents only a small fraction (< 10%) of the total number of vesicles residing at the nerve terminal ending [22, 23]. During periods of high use, however, a larger reserve pool of vesicles can also participate in neurotransmitter release into the synapse [23, 24]. Once released into the synapse, ACh can only passively diffuse across that gap and bind to postsynaptic ACh receptors expressed on the postsynaptic endplate, which is a specialized segment of the postsynaptic myofiber's sarcolemma. Since this binding is governed solely by the elements of probability, it is no surprise that these binding sites are lined up in direct "apposition," or across from, presynaptic transmitter release sites. It is a measure of the importance of this coupling of the location of presynaptic release sites with postsynaptic binding sites (receptors) that this colocalization is sustained even though the overall structure of the NMJ might be altered as a result of changes in neuromuscular activity or even the long-term process of aging [25, 26].

The endplate occurs in the middle third of the length of the myofiber and is slightly elevated relative to the rest of the sarcolemma's surface [27]. Within this swollen endplate are deeply etched grooves; at the crest of these grooves reside ACh receptors, which feature sodium/potassium channels. The ionic channels that are embedded as constituents of the ACh receptors are ligand-gated, rather than voltage, channels allowing cations to enter the myofiber, causing a brief depolarization of the membrane referred to as the "endplate potential" (EPP). This EPP then diffuses into the depths of the grooves, or "junctional folds," arriving at voltage-gated sodium channels. Research has shown that, with aging, these junctional folds are shallower and that there are ACh receptors located not just at the crests of the folds but also in extra-synaptic locations, resulting in problems with optimal excitation (see Fig. 3).

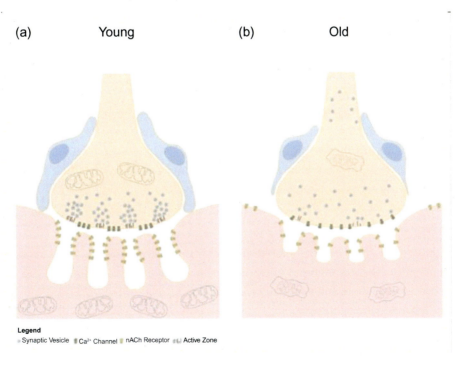

Fig. 3
Illustration of age-related signs of damage at the NMJ. Note the shallow postsynaptic gutters, the greater dispersion of postsynaptic receptors, and damaged mitochondria. The terminal Schwann cells around the terminals can also be seen. *From Taetzsch T, Valdez G. NMJ maintenance and repair in aging. Curr Opin Physiol 2018;4:57–64.*

However, in young, healthy NMJs, the local depolarization caused by the arriving EPP is typically of sufficient intensity—in fact, having a "safety factor" of three- to fivefold—to open those voltage-gated sodium channels beyond the endplate region, allowing a sharp influx of sodium resulting in an action potential. This electrical impulse then traverses the entirety of the myofiber's sarcolemma and ultimately causes a single contractile event to occur, which is termed a muscle "twitch." In effect, a single action potential stimulates a single muscle twitch. The process of postsynaptic excitation is almost immediately terminated by the chemical breakdown of ACh bound to the receptor by the enzyme acetylcholinesterase. In short, the postsynaptic component of the NMJ is responsible for the excitation-contraction event that lies at the core of the neuromuscular system; however, it is triggered by actions occurring at the nerve terminal ending.

For decades, it has been known that throughout the lifespan, the pre- and postsynaptic components of the NMJ undergo a continual, but subtle degree of plasticity, or structural remodeling [28–30]. Microscopic analysis has revealed that presynaptic nerve terminal branches exhibit a gradual, ongoing process of retraction from their postsynaptic target sites, reprobing, and establishing a new area of synaptic contact with the endplate without altering its overall shape and dimensions. This natural, relentless exercise of retraction and probing noted among presynaptic nerve terminal endings is matched by postsynaptic ACh receptor reconfiguration, first by deterioration and then by the expression of new binding sites within the existing endplate to enable proper synaptic function. Indeed, it has been demonstrated that this nuanced structural remodeling of the NMJ has little effect on its synaptic performance [31].

The reorganization of the coupling of pre- and postsynaptic sites points to the importance of soluble factors in maintaining NMJ function and how aging can alter the secretion of those molecules. As but one example, our laboratory has confirmed that aged NMJs express more of the potent synaptogenic agent neural cell adhesion molecule (NCAM) than young adult synapses, signifying a greater degree of NMJ plasticity among aged muscles [32, 33]. Similarly, aging is linked to a decline in IGF-1 levels; such a change has been found to contribute to NMJ degeneration [19, 34].

Even though this minor degree of synaptic plasticity is evident throughout life, it becomes greater in magnitude and more rapid in its manifestation later in life, particularly as the senescent, or aged, stage of life is entered [35, 36]. With advanced aging and greater NMJ remodeling, maintenance of proper pre- to postsynaptic coupling becomes more of a challenge, and the endplate becomes more fragmented (see Fig. 4). To that point, in aged muscle, it is not uncommon to detect nerve terminal branches leading to postsynaptic regions that are bereft of ACh receptors or clusters of receptors that appear to have been abandoned by presynaptic nerve terminal branches [35, 37]. In addition, these newly abandoned ACh receptors show alterations of the subunit composition whereby the Epsilon subunit, which is

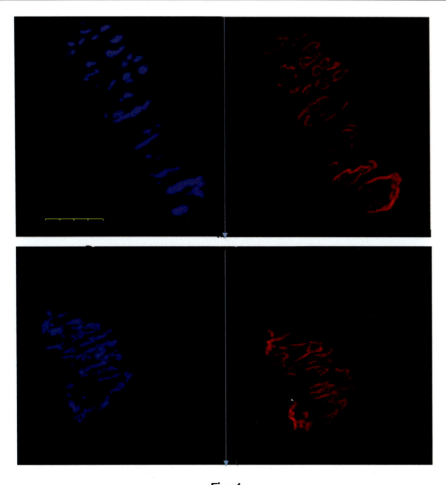

Fig. 4
Micrograph of immunofluorescent staining of aged *(top panels)* and young *(bottom panels)* NMJs. Presynaptic ACh vesicles are stained *blue*, and postsynaptic ACh receptors are stained *red*. Note the greater dispersion of vesicles and receptors in the aged NMJ. Scale bar = 20 μm.

normally expressed before the innervation of the myofiber and adult formation of the NMJ, begins to once again be expressed providing proof of local denervation [38, 39]. Functionally, this natural event in the development of the NMJ is important as the step of replacing the ACh receptor's fetal gamma subunit with the mature epsilon subunit has a direct impact on muscle function. Indeed, a muscle's capacity to maximally generate muscle force occurs only after the subunit replacement process has been completed among all NMJs of the muscle [40]. It is likely then that sarcopenic declines in muscle strength are at least partly accounted for by increased gamma subunit expression at the expense of epsilon subunit expression at the ACh receptor [39].

In more closely examining the effects of aging on presynaptic components of the NMJ, it has been revealed that nerve terminal branching patterns adapt such that aged NMJs have a greater total length of nerve terminal branching, which is due mainly to a larger number of branches, but at times also to the extended length of existing branches [31, 41]. Recall that neurotransmitter-containing vesicles reside in those nerve terminal endings and that it appears that the density of vesicles supported per unit length of the branch is constant, meaning that if branch length increases, so does the number of presynaptic vesicles [26]. Moreover, aging has been associated with a smaller number of vesicles per NMJ, eliciting a more scattered dispersion of these vesicles, which, in turn, mirrors the greater complexity of branching found among aged NMJs [42]. Additionally, the total area accounted for by vesicle expression is expanded in aged compared to young adult NMJs [43, 44], and the length of the perimeter that all vesicles may be encircled within is greater in aged NMJs. Yet, when quantifying the number of vesicles per given length of terminal branching, aging shows no effect [45]. This suggests that the relative, if not the absolute capacity of branches to support vesicles is resistant to the effects of aging. At the same time, there is evidence that aging elicits a decrease in the number of active zones of terminal endings where vesicles are docked awaiting release [46].

In accounting for postsynaptic morphological remodeling with aging, it appears that the total number of ACh receptors per endplate is reduced and that there is a more dispersed distribution of them [14, 39]. Again, this leads to a greater area of the endplate region, but with a reduced density of receptor expression per given postsynaptic area [33, 47]. As with presynaptic nerve terminals, aging is associated with a decrease in mitochondrial content, with a greater degree of mitochondrial damage, at subsarcolemmal areas of the postsynaptic endplate region [48–50]. All told, morphological adaptations of the aged NMJ reveal an overall state of instability, thus creating an environment for further NMJ degeneration. Such reconfiguration eventually results in denervation of myofibers, which ultimately causes atrophy or even death if those myofibers are not reinnervated by another motor axon in close proximity [42, 51]. Morphological adaptations of the NMJ to aging are presented in Table 1.

Age-related functional adaptations of the NMJ

A fundamental biological tenet is that form and function are inexorably and tightly interwoven. This premise applies to age-related adaptations of the NMJ, although a recent investigation of the diaphragm suggested that structural changes may be unaccompanied by alterations in NMJ function [52]. In general, however, the current knowledge base points to a robust relationship between form and function within the neuromuscular system, as indicated by a recent review of the literature [53]. For example, recall that it was previously mentioned that one of the morphological adaptations to aging expressed presynaptically was an increase in total nerve terminal branching length and number. In turn, this was

Table 1: Age-related anatomical adaptations of the neuromuscular junction.

Presynaptic
• Increased complexity of nerve terminal branching • Increased number of nerve terminal branches • Increased total length of nerve terminal branching • Increased area occupied by ACh vesicles • Increased circumference surrounding vesicles • Increased dispersion of vesicles • Decreased total number of vesicles • Decreased mitochondrial content
Postsynaptic
• Increased number of abandoned synaptic gutters • Decreased depth of synaptic grooves • Decreased number of ACh receptors • Increased number of extrasynaptic receptors • Increased dispersion of receptors • Increased circumference surrounding vesicles • Decreased colocalization of ACh vesicles and receptors • Decreased concentration of acetylcholinesterase • Increased expression of N-CAM • Decreased mitochondrial content • Decreased expression of terminal Schwann cells

accompanied by a more dispersed and smaller number of ACh-containing vesicles resulting in more release sites with the amplified distance separating them [37, 42, 45]. In accord with this, electrophysiological and functional procedures have established that, upon stimulation, the initial quantal content, or amount of neurotransmitter released, is embellished in aged NMJs compared to young adult ones [31, 41, 54]. However, upon continual stimulation, there is a more severe drop-off in the amplitude of the postsynaptic endplate potential in those same aged NMJs [31, 54]. This is likely attributed not only to the smaller density of ACh vesicles observed among aged synapses, but also an age-related slowing of the rate of presynaptic vesicular recycling [55]. This impaired rate of vesicular turnover might well be related to diminished ATP production by mitochondria located in presynaptic nerve terminal endings, which commonly exhibit signs of damage [17, 56]. Similarly, with prolonged electrical stimulation of motor neurons, there is a greater incidence of "drop outs" where the arriving action potential is of insufficient strength to open voltage-gated calcium channels embedded in nerve terminal membranes and thus trigger the untethering of vesicles from their docked positions at active zones [57, 58]. To that point, it is known that the relationship between nerve terminal calcium channels and docked vesicles affects the rate and amount of ACh released upon the arrival of an electrical impulse at the nerve terminal end. Preliminary evidence, however, suggests that at least in moderately aged systems, i.e., roughly the equivalent of 70-year-old human beings, the relationship between the ionic channels and the active zones docking vesicles is unaffected by the impact of age [59], although the nanostructure of the active zone itself may be slightly altered with aging [46].

Another factor that may play a role in age-related differences in NMJ function is the slowed axonal transport rate noted among aged motor neurons [18, 39]. This results in diminished delivery of the proteins, e.g., enzymes, channels, to terminal endings that are required for effective neuromuscular transmission.

Electrophysiological procedures have also been used to demonstrate that aging increases the frequency of mini-endplate potentials (MEPP) or the spontaneous release of the contents of a single presynaptic vesicle from its docked site into the synaptic cleft. When this occurs, it causes a small postsynaptic depolarization, suggesting less tightly controlled synaptic function [60, 61]. Similar procedures have provided evidence that at least under rested conditions, individual vesicles from aged NMJs contain larger amounts of neurotransmitter, i.e., quantal size, than younger synapses [31, 54, 62]. It is quite possible, though, that the impaired rate of vesicular recycling noted in aged nerve terminal endings also includes incomplete filling of newly formed vesicles with Ach, resulting in a lower amplitude of endplate potentials among aged muscles during a train of stimulus events.

Recall that acetylcholinesterase (AChE) is the enzyme located postsynaptically near binding sites for the neurotransmitter ACh. This enzyme's function is not only to destroy transmitter bound at the receptor but also to remove its destroyed remnants from the synaptic cleft, thus providing clear binding sites for newly released neurotransmitters [27]. Aging has been found to result in decrements in AChE at postsynaptic sites, resulting in less efficient neurotransmission [27].

While discussing neurotransmission across the NMJ, it is important to note that evidence suggests that what is rate-limiting to synaptic function during continuous stimulation is not the maximal rate of vesicular recycling, i.e., retaking vesicular membrane from terminal membrane release sites, repackaging with ACh, and inserting into docked positions, but the ability to provide vacant release sites at nerve terminal endings [63]. Yet, aging may also have deleterious effects on this process, thus hindering prolonged neurotransmission at the NMJ.

Using the method of ex vivo muscle stimulation, a recent report indicates that aging influences the rate of recovery of neuromuscular transmission and force production following a 5-min train of stimuli [64]. Accordingly, it appears that aging not only has unfavorable consequences on neurotransmission across the NMJ but also on the rate and efficacy of recovery following cessation of its activity. A summary of the functional alterations of the NMJ associated with aging is displayed in Table 2.

Table 2: Age-related functional adaptations of the neuromuscular junction.

Presynaptic
• Increased quantal content (amount of ACh released per stimulus) • Increased MEPP amplitude • Increased quantal size (amount of ACh per vesicle) • Increased calcium influx upon stimulation • Decreased rate of calcium clearance following stimulation • Increased incidence of neuromuscular transmission failure • Greater susceptibility to partial denervation (less ACh release upon stimulation)
Postsynaptic
• Increased endplate potential amplitude • Decreased safety factor of endplate potential, especially during the train of stimuli • Increases synaptic depression during the train of stimuli • Increased number of "drop-outs" during the train of stimuli • Decreased neuromuscular transmission efficiency • Increased latency between stimulus and muscle twitch

Preventing and managing the effects of aging on the NMJ

To date, very few effective interventions have been identified to defend against the onset and progressive deterioration of NMJ function and structure that has been attributed to age. This is true despite the fact that the scientific community has gained substantial insight concerning the physiological mechanisms involved in aging-induced neuromuscular dysfunction. Indeed, current knowledge suggests that only dietary restriction and habitual physical exercise may be capable of slowing the onset of age-related alterations in the function and structure of the NMJ. In short, according to the current database, only behavioral modification has been shown to provide antiaging effects to the NMJ. For example, adult mice allowed to age naturally demonstrate an increase in the incidence of nerve terminal sprouting, denervation of myofibers, and fragmentation of postsynaptic motor endplates. However, when aging mice are placed on a diet restricting daily caloric intake by 40%, the incidence and magnitude of those markers of denervation and aging are significantly reduced, albeit still being significantly greater than in young adult mice [37]. More recently, it was reported that consumption of an agent that mimics the effects of caloric restriction—resveratrol—also effectively offsets signs of aging on NMJ structure [65]. It is important to note, however, that caloric restriction is known to slow the detrimental effects of aging in many physiological variables, including myofiber morphology [66–68], indicating that the beneficial effect of reduced caloric intake on the degenerative effects of aging is not necessarily specific to myoneural synapses. Another concern regarding the utilization of dietary measures to control the aging of the NMJ is the feasibility of asking men and women to voluntarily reduce their caloric intake to what is almost half of normal and maintaining such self-discipline in the long-term. More encouraging, however, is evidence that when combined with exercise training, daily caloric decreases of only 8% showed positive consequences to muscle morphology; unfortunately, NMJs were not examined in that study [69].

Similar to restricted caloric intake, habitual physical activity, or exercise, also bestows antiaging benefits on many of the body's physiological systems [68, 70]. This includes the neuromuscular system, acting to preserve skeletal muscle mass and function [71] and also mitigating age-related deterioration of the NMJ [72, 73]. Physiologically, exercise among aged animals has been found to attenuate, sometimes even fully alleviate, age-related increases in MEPP frequency and amplitude as assessed with electrophysiology, returning those values to what was recorded in young, untrained neuromuscular systems. Equivalent results were noted in recordings of quantal content during neuronal firing and membrane resistance to electrical current [54].

As another example of the linkage between form and function within the body, exercise among aged animals also was found to significantly mitigate, but not completely offset, age-related morphological remodeling of the NMJ. More specifically, age-related increases in presynaptic nerve terminal branch number, length, and complexity, and even sprouting were significantly less in aged, trained muscles, than in aged, untrained muscles while still being greater than in young controls [54, 74]. Postsynaptically, exercise in aged animals resulted in diminished evidence of the denervation observed in aged controls such as endplate fragmentation, increased perimeter length surrounding endplates, and total area occupied by ACh receptors, i.e., endplate regions [59, 75]. Thus, exercise among the aged can mitigate the deleterious consequences of senescence on NMJ structure and function, as well as promote overall health benefits, even being viewed by some as a form of medicine [76, 77].

Role of NMJ in sarcopenia

Because of the heavy financial and health burdens of sarcopenia, factors causing the disease have been a subject of intense investigation for the last 20–25 years. Despite this, the precise mechanisms involved in its onset and progression have yet to be clearly and fully elucidated. Perhaps, this is why that to date no pharmacological agent(s) has been developed that can effectively prevent the onset of sarcopenia or effectively recover from it. It has been revealed that in human beings as well as rodents, sarcopenia shows its most pronounced effects, both in terms of strength and muscle mass, in muscles of the lower body [78, 79]. At first glance, this may seem counterintuitive as the legs in human beings are activated to a greater extent than the upper body, and exercise has been shown to be effective in staving off the loss of muscle mass [37, 54, 59].

The reason for this discrepancy between the incidence of sarcopenia between upper and lower body musculature may be explained by a recent report confirming that it is the muscles whose motor neurons emanate from the brain stem and cervical regions of the CNS that display the most resistance to the negative effects of sarcopenia [80]. Research has also showed us that there are two distinct phases apparent when examining the progression of sarcopenia. The first stage typically begins at about 40 years of age in human beings and is characterized by slow and moderate declines in muscle mass and strength [7, 81]. This can generally be ascribed to the atrophy of skeletal muscles and their constituent myofibers. Yet, at approximately 60 years old, there ensues the second stage of sarcopenia during which we see a more rapid decline in muscle mass and strength. In a landmark investigation by Lexell and colleagues [82], examining human cadavers, it was ascertained that this more rapid progression of the disease was due to a loss of motor neurons detected during examination of spinal cord tissue. Aged spinal cords were found to have up to 50% fewer motor neurons than young adult ones [82–84].

In brief, the slower rate of muscle and strength loss occurring with sarcopenia between the ages of 40 and 60 is mainly a result of the atrophy of myofibers. In contrast, the more rapid losses occurring beyond the age of 60 are principally a result of the death, or apoptosis, of motor neurons, even while the process of myofiber and whole muscle atrophy continues. Indeed, a recent investigation determined that sarcopenic-induced whole muscle loss was, in roughly equal proportion, explained by myofiber atrophy and loss, i.e., death, of myofibers [85].

The processes of myofiber atrophy and death are linked together mechanistically. That is, it has been known for some time—as mentioned earlier—that throughout life there is an ongoing and subtle process of denervation and reinnervation occurring with myofibers [28, 29]. This process is gradual and hardly detectable; yet, pioneering work by Robbins and his coworkers established that presynaptic nerve terminals are consistently reconfiguring and probing within the overall postsynaptic endplate domains of the myofibers they innervate [41]. Normally, this process begins with individual nerve terminal branches—constituents of the larger nerve terminal arborization—retreating from specific sections of the endplate and reaching out to nearby regions of that same endplate. This is presented by some nerve terminal branches that are found to be unaccompanied by endplate receptors. Conversely, the same NMJ may display clusters of ACh receptors that are bereft of accompanying nerve terminal innervation points. Because this modest plasticity occurs only at small sections of the NMJ, the synapse functions adequately, and this ongoing process of probing and retracting is considered a very natural, healthful phenomenon ensuring the fidelity of the nerve to muscle communicative system. However, as the neuromuscular system ages, this denervation-reinnervation process becomes both more prevalent throughout the NMJ and occurs at a faster rate until a threshold is reached where the rate of denervation exceeds the ability of the nerve terminal branches to reinnervate leading to an overall state of denervation of the myofiber [86, 87]. Consequently, the myofiber eventually receives such a sparse amount of nerve terminal excitation that it becomes functionally denervated. This is evident in the dispersion or fragmentation observed among the clusters of ACh receptors expressed at the endplate.

At that point, the newly abandoned myofiber may be reinnervated by a nearby motor neuron by its sprouting of a new nerve terminal branch point allowing the myofiber to survive, albeit of a smaller size, i.e., atrophied. This reinnervation process usually also leads to an increase in type I or slow-twitch muscle fibers in the affected muscle. Often, these newly innervated myofibers can be identified by the expression of embryonic and/or neonatal myosin heavy chain, and also at the NMJ as it reverts, at least temporarily, to expressing the gamma, or immature, ACh receptor subunit rather than the adult epsilon subunit [38]. This whole process then increases the size—number of myofibers—of that motor unit and increases metabolic demands placed upon the innervating motor neuron [51, 88]. It has been postulated that this increased metabolic demand that is coupled with the expanded size of the motor unit can exceed the capacity of the motor neuron to meet its energy requirements, thus exhausting the motor neuron leading to its death [7, 89, 90]. Of course, these outcomes would then contribute to sarcopenia. This phenomenon would explain both the atrophy and loss of motor neurons, which result in sarcopenia.

While the failure of the natural denervation/reinnervation cycling process does play a role in sarcopenia, other factors are also at play. In trying to determine the etiology of sarcopenia and the NMJ's role in that process, there has been an ongoing debate as to whether this is a "die forward" or "die backward" occurrence [14, 91, 92]. In the former, sarcopenia has its beginning in the spinal cord and is carried out by programmed cell death—apoptosis—which first destroys the soma, or cell body, of aging motor neurons. This degeneration then continues down the axon in an anterograde fashion—indeed, there is evidence of damaged myelination in aged motor neurons—where it would then destabilize the nerve terminals, before resulting in fragmentation of the postsynaptic endplate. The cessation of receiving electrical impulses ultimately leads to deterioration, including atrophy, and death of the myofibers innervated by the nonfunctional motor neuron. This may, in part, be accounted for by data showing that aging is accompanied by impaired cholesterol production. This limited cholesterol synthesis obstructs motor neuron function related to decreased myelination of the neuron's axon. This disruption provokes disturbed neuromuscular function, including problems at the NMJ [83].

On the other side of the debate, the "die back" supporters point to the many similarities between sarcopenia and other degenerative neurological diseases such as amyotrophic lateral sclerosis (ALS), Parkinson's disease, and Huntington's disease [93, 94]. In each of these maladies, there appears to be evidence of damage at the NMJ before there are indications of similar disruption and functional impairment at the cell body of the motor neuron. More specifically, it appears that the NMJ first suffers damage, which then continues up the axon in a retrograde fashion, ultimately resulting in damage to the neuron's controlling soma within the CNS. Etiological causes of such a "die back" progression of sarcopenia remain to be fully elucidated, but a primary candidate is impaired mitophagy or the natural process of removal and cleaning-up of mitochondrial waste products, resulting in the accumulation of DNA and protein damaging reactive oxygen species (ROS). The areas beneath both the surface of the postsynaptic endplate and the presynaptic nerve terminal endings of the NMJ display richly embellished mitochondrial content making them targets for ROS production, and thus damage to both protein and DNA. Indeed, due to the increasing fragility of mitochondrial membranes, which is detected in aging cells [95], ROS particles are found leaked into the cytoplasm of nerve terminals and endplate regions of myofibers where they accumulate and cause damage. This damage then progresses both up the axon in a retrograde fashion, as well as down and throughout the myofiber causing first muscle and neuronal damage, and then eventually death. In a recent encouraging study, however, it was discovered that in aged rodents, caloric restriction offset both age-related increases in ROS production and physical disruption of the NMJ [37]. This suggests that such ROS-related damage to aged muscle and nervous tissue is not necessarily inevitable.

Similar to how aging weakens the outer membranes of mitochondria, so does it compromise the nuclear envelope of the nuclei located in the endplate region of the postsynaptic myofiber, which has been specialized to transcribe proteins of the NMJ [96]. This weakening of the nuclear envelope allows the release of acidic enzymes, i.e., calpains, from the nuclei into the cytoplasm of the myofiber where they have destructive effects on the metabolic enzymes and contractile proteins that are essential to the myofiber's function, and as such, resulting in sarcopenia [96, 97]. In addition to those destructive effects, aged NMJs are known to have less genetic transcriptional activity of not only nuclear DNA but also mitochondrial DNA culminating in impaired oxidative energy synthesis [14, 98].

Another potential mediator of sarcopenia is the constant state of low-grade inflammation, termed "inflammaging," that is observed among the aged [99–101]. This inflammatory state is characterized by an enhanced production and release of cytokines, including TNF-α, and interleukins such as IL-6 and IL-1, which have harmful interactions with the metabolic and contractile machinery that is essential to the function of the neuromuscular system [102, 103]. Adding support to the "die back" argument for the onset of sarcopenia are recent reports asserting that damage to the NMJ itself precedes any disruptions to the motor neurons' cell bodies within the spinal cord [104]. Moreover, it has been reported that the NMJ exhibits signs of age-related decay before any evidence of sarcopenia can be detected in the myofibers on which those synapses reside [104, 105]. These data indicate that the NMJ may be uniquely susceptible to the deleterious consequences of aging and the onset of sarcopenia. After instability to the NMJ is manifested, the age-related disturbance appears to spread in both retrograde and anterograde directions to affect both motor neurons and myofibers, respectively.

In shedding more light on the relationship between the NMJ and sarcopenia, it has been demonstrated that many of the molecules playing a role in the initial postnatal assembly of the NMJ are also necessary to maintain the health of adult myoneural synapses. More specifically, aging is associated with disturbances in the expression of these molecules, which, in turn, have been linked to age-related fragmentation of NMJs. Experimentation has shown, however, that restoring these synaptogenic factors can alleviate age-related disruptions in NMJ function and structure. For example, Agrin is a factor released by presynaptic nerve terminal endings onto postsynaptic endplate regions during the initial natural assembly of NMJs causing concentrations of receptors to be aligned across from the presynaptic terminal endings [106, 107]. Yet with aging, fragments of Agrin resulting from natural proteolytic activity can be found near the NMJ. It is interesting to note that this proteolysis of Agrin at young adult NMJs results in what has been referred to as "precocious sarcopenia" [108]. Equally informative of the potency of Agrin is evidence that if it is supplied to those affected muscles, the destabilization of the NMJ is mitigated, as is the decrement in muscle function [108, 109]. These findings present an intriguing line of future research for countering or even preventing the onset of sarcopenia.

Insulin-like growth factor-1 (IGF-1) mainly functions as an anabolic hormone being produced principally by the liver but also to a lesser extent by skeletal muscle [99, 110, 111]. Most of the research conducted on IGF-1 has investigated its anabolic and reparative effects on skeletal muscle [112, 113], but it has also been reported that IGF-1 has potent effects on the NMJ by maintaining its structural integrity, particularly in the face of aging. Indeed, Messi and Delbono [114] documented that delivering IGF-1 to aging muscle inhibits the NMJ alterations typically seen with aging and prevents the loss of muscle force production commonly found with aging [34].

Furthermore, giving credence to the view that age-related degeneration of the NMJ is coupled with and precipitated by the fragility of pre- and postsynaptic mitochondria is evidence of the efficacy of PGC1-α in neutralizing the effects of aging on the NMJ. PGC-1α is an important cofactor in the transcriptional activities of mitochondria helping maintain the normal, healthy function of mitochondria, i.e., ATP production and calcium buffering [115, 116]. As with most physiological variables, however, aging is coupled with altered, i.e., decreased, production of this potent regulator of ROS accumulation leading to increased free radical concentrations in aged neuromuscular systems. Given this, it has been determined that adding PGC-1α to aged muscle effectively counters NMJ instability and as a consequence re-establishes healthy and effective NMJ structure and function [116, 117], even offsetting sarcopenia [118, 119]. This also represents a significant and meaningful potential for future research into developing interventions that might act robustly in combatting sarcopenia.

To conclude, sarcopenia presents a very real health threat to the growing aged fraction of our society. Much has been learned about the negative consequences of this progressive disease since it was first defined in the late 20th century. However, the causes and the physiological mechanisms accounting for the onset and progression of sarcopenia are only now beginning to be revealed. To date, there has been little success in treating it pharmacologically, while behavior modification, i.e., controlled caloric intake and exercise, has been shown to successfully ameliorate its pathological symptomology. Importantly, there has been, and remains, an ongoing dispute as to whether sarcopenia is a retrograde or anterograde phenomenon. Increasingly, the retrograde or "dying back" concept suggests that degeneration of the NMJ is observed first, and only subsequently is damage seen at the motor neurons and then followed by damage to muscle tissue is becoming more convincing. That said, it could be reasonably argued that sarcopenia features both "dying forward" or anterograde and "dying backward" or retrograde characteristics, leading to myofiber and neuronal death, respectively. Regardless of the merit of the anterograde vs. the retrograde debate, a growing body of evidence suggests that not only is the NMJ a critical player in the onset and progression of sarcopenia, but that it is an early and formative element in the costly outcomes of that disease.

References

[1] Rosenberg IH. Summary contents. Am J Nutr 1989;50:1231–3.
[2] Rosenberg IH. Sarcopenia: origins and clinical relevance. J Nutr 1997;127(5 Suppl):990S–1S.
[3] Cruz-Jentoft AJ, Bahat G, Bauer J, Boirie Y, Bruyere O, Cederholm T, et al. Sarcopenia: revised European consensus on definition and diagnosis. Age Ageing 2019;48(1):16–31.
[4] Janssen I, Shepard DS, Katzmarzyk PT, Roubenoff R. The healthcare costs of sarcopenia in the United States. J Am Geriatr Soc 2004;52(1):80–5.
[5] Beaudart C, Zaaria M, Pasleau F, Reginster JY, Bruyere O. Health outcomes of sarcopenia: a systematic review and meta-analysis. PLoS One 2017;12(1), e0169548.
[6] Lindle RS, Metter EJ, Lynch NA, Fleg JL, Fozard JL, Tobin J, et al. Age and gender comparisons of muscle strength in 654 women and men aged 20-93 yr. J Appl Physiol (1985) 1997;83(5):1581–7.
[7] Vandervoort AA. Aging of the human neuromuscular system. Muscle Nerve 2002;25(1):17–25.
[8] Langlois F, Vu TT, Kergoat MJ, Chasse K, Dupuis G, Bherer L. The multiple dimensions of frailty: physical capacity, cognition, and quality of life. Int Psychogeriatr 2012;24(9):1429–36.
[9] Sieber CC. Frailty—from concept to clinical practice. Exp Gerontol 2017;87(Pt B):160–7.
[10] Hennig R, Lomo T. Firing patterns of motor units in normal rats. Nature 1985;314(6007):164–6.
[11] Pagala MK, Namba T, Grob D. Failure of neuromuscular transmission and contractility during muscle fatigue. Muscle Nerve 1984;7(6):454–64.
[12] Fogarty MJ, Gonzalez Porras MA, Mantilla CB, Sieck GC. Diaphragm neuromuscular transmission failure in aged rats. J Neurophysiol 2019;122(1):93–104.
[13] Kwan P. Sarcopenia, a neurogenic syndrome? J Aging Res 2013;2013:791679.
[14] Anagnostou ME, Hepple RT. Mitochondrial mechanisms of neuromuscular junction degeneration with aging. Cell 2020;9(1). https://doi.org/10.3390/cells9010197.
[15] Manini TM, Hong SL, Clark BC. Aging and muscle: a neuron's perspective. Curr Opin Clin Nutr Metab Care 2013;16(1):21–6.
[16] Ham DJ, Ruegg MA. Causes and consequences of age-related changes at the neuromusscualr junction. Curr Opin Physio 2018;4:32–9.
[17] Jang YC, Lustgarten MS, Liu Y, Muller FL, Bhattacharya A, Liang H, et al. Increased superoxide in vivo accelerates age-associated muscle atrophy through mitochondrial dysfunction and neuromuscular junction degeneration. FASEB J 2010;24(5):1376–90.
[18] Deschenes MR. Motor unit and neuromuscular junction remodeling with aging. Curr Aging Sci 2011;4(3):209–20.
[19] Gonzalez-Freire M, de Cabo R, Studenski SA, Ferrucci L. The neuromuscular junction: aging at the crossroad between nerves and muscle. Front Aging Neurosci 2014;6:208.

[20] Casati M, Costa AS, Capitanio D, Ponzoni L, Ferri E, Agostini S, et al. The biological foundations of sarcopenia: established and promising markers. Front Med (Lausanne) 2019;6:184.
[21] Slater CR. The functional organization of motor nerve terminals. Prog Neurobiol 2015;134:55–103.
[22] Denker A, Bethani I, Krohnert K, Korber C, Horstmann H, Wilhelm BG, et al. A small pool of vesicles maintains synaptic activity in vivo. Proc Natl Acad Sci U S A 2011;108(41):17177–82.
[23] Rizzoli SO, Betz WJ. Synaptic vesicle pools. Nat Rev Neurosci 2005;6(1):57–69.
[24] Kaeser PS, Regehr WG. The readily releasable pool of synaptic vesicles. Curr Opin Neurobiol 2017;43:63–70.
[25] Deschenes MR, Hurst TE, Ramser AE, Sherman EG. Presynaptic to postsynaptic relationships of the neuromuscular junction are held constant across age and muscle fiber type. Dev Neurobiol 2013;73(10):744–53.
[26] Deschenes MR, Kressin KA, Garratt RN, Leathrum CM, Shaffrey EC. Effects of exercise training on neuromuscular junction morphology and pre- to post-synaptic coupling in young and aged rats. Neuroscience 2016;316:167–77.
[27] Boaro SN, Soares JC, Konig Jr B. Comparative structural analysis of neuromuscular junctions in mice at different ages. Ann Anat 1998;180(2):173–9.
[28] Cardasis CA, Padykula HA. Ultrastructural evidence indicating reorganization at the neuromuscular junction in the normal rat soleus muscle. Anat Rec 1981;200(1):41–59.
[29] Wigston DJ. Repeated in vivo visualization of neuromuscular junctions in adult mouse lateral gastrocnemius. J Neurosci 1990;10(6):1753–61.
[30] Balice-Gordon RJ, Lichtman JW. In vivo visualization of the growth of pre- and postsynaptic elements of neuromuscular junctions in the mouse. J Neurosci 1990;10(3):894–908.
[31] Banker BQ, Kelly SS, Robbins N. Neuromuscular transmission and correlative morphology in young and old mice. J Physiol 1983;339:355–77.
[32] Rosenheimer JL, Smith DO. Age-related increase in soluble and cell surface-associated neurite-outgrowth factors from rat muscle. Brain Res 1990;509(2):309–20.
[33] Deschenes MR, Wilson MH. Age-related differences in synaptic plasticity following muscle unloading. J Neurobiol 2003;57(3):246–56.
[34] Gonzalez E, Messi ML, Zheng Z, Delbono O. Insulin-like growth factor-1 prevents age-related decrease in specific force and intracellular Ca^{2+} in single intact muscle fibres from transgenic mice. J Physiol 2003;552(Pt 3):833–44.
[35] Robbins N. Compensatory plasticity of aging at the neuromuscular junction. Exp Gerontol 1992;27(1):75–81.
[36] Chugh D, Iyer CC, Wang X, Bobbili P, Rich MM, Arnold WD. Neuromuscular junction transmission failure is a late phenotype in aging mice. Neurobiol Aging 2020;86:182–90.
[37] Valdez G, Tapia JC, Kang H, Clemenson Jr GD, Gage FH, Lichtman JW, et al. Attenuation of age-related changes in mouse neuromuscular synapses by caloric restriction and exercise. Proc Natl Acad Sci U S A 2010;107(33):14863–8.
[38] Witzemann V, Brenner HR, Sakmann B. Neural factors regulate AChR subunit mRNAs at rat neuromuscular synapses. J Cell Biol 1991;114(1):125–41.
[39] Soendenbroe C, Heisterberg MF, Schjerling P, Karlsen A, Kjaer M, Andersen JL, et al. Molecular indicators of denervation in aging human skeletal muscle. Muscle Nerve 2019;60(4):453–63.
[40] Missias AC, Mudd J, Cunningham JM, Steinbach JH, Merlie JP, Sanes JR. Deficient development and maintenance of postsynaptic specializations in mutant mice lacking an 'adult' acetylcholine receptor subunit. Development 1997;124(24):5075–86.
[41] Robbins N, Fahim MA. Progression of age changes in mature mouse motor nerve terminals and its relation to locomotor activity. J Neurocytol 1985;14(6):1019–36.
[42] Andonian MH, Fahim MA. Nerve terminal morphology in C57BL/6NNia mice at different ages. J Gerontol 1989;44(2):B43–51.
[43] Prakash YS, Sieck GC. Age-related remodeling of neuromuscular junctions on type-identified diaphragm fibers. Muscle Nerve 1998;21(7):887–95.

[44] Deschenes MR, Sherman EG, Roby MA, Glass EK, Harris MB. Effect of resistance training on neuromuscular junctions of young and aged muscles featuring different recruitment patterns. J Neurosci Res 2015;93(3):504–13.

[45] Deschenes MR, Adan MA, Kapral MC, Kressin KA, Leathrum CM, Seo A, et al. Neuromuscular adaptability of male and female rats to muscle unloading. J Neurosci Res 2018;96(2):284–96.

[46] Badawi Y, Nishimune H. Presynaptic active zones of mammalian neuromuscular junctions: nanoarchitecture and selective impairments in aging. Neurosci Res 2018;127:78–88.

[47] Fahim MA, Robbins N. Ultrastructural studies of young and old mouse neuromuscular junctions. J Neurocytol 1982;11(4):641–56.

[48] Meier T, Wallace BG. Formation of the neuromuscular junction: molecules and mechanisms. Bioessays 1998;20(10):819–29.

[49] Rosenheimer JL. Ultraterminal sprouting in innervated and partially denervated adult and aged rat muscle. Neuroscience 1990;38(3):763–70.

[50] Cheng A, Morsch M, Murata Y, Ghazanfari N, Reddel SW, Phillips WD. Sequence of age-associated changes to the mouse neuromuscular junction and the protective effects of voluntary exercise. PLoS One 2013;8(7), e67970.

[51] Piasecki M, Ireland A, Piasecki J, Stashuk DW, Swiecicka A, Rutter MK, et al. Failure to expand the motor unit size to compensate for declining motor unit numbers distinguishes sarcopenic from non-sarcopenic older men. J Physiol 2018;596(9):1627–37.

[52] Willadt S, Nash M, Slater CR. Age-related fragmentation of the motor endplate is not associated with impaired neuromuscular transmission in the mouse diaphragm. Sci Rep 2016;6:24849.

[53] Jones RA, Reich CD, Dissanayake KN, Kristmundsdottir F, Findlater GS, Ribchester RR, et al. NMJ-morph reveals principal components of synaptic morphology influencing structure-function relationships at the neuromuscular junction. Open Biol 2016;6(12). https://doi.org/10.1098/rsob.160240.

[54] Fahim MA. Endurance exercise modulates neuromuscular junction of C57BL/6NNia aging mice. J Appl Physiol (1985) 1997;83(1):59–66.

[55] VanGuilder HD, Yan H, Farley JA, Sonntag WE, Freeman WM. Aging alters the expression of neurotransmission-regulating proteins in the hippocampal synaptoproteome. J Neurochem 2010;113(6):1577–88.

[56] Dupuis L, Gonzalez de Aguilar JL, Echaniz-Laguna A, Eschbach J, Rene F, Oudart H, et al. Muscle mitochondrial uncoupling dismantles neuromuscular junction and triggers distal degeneration of motor neurons. PLoS One 2009;4(4):e5390.

[57] Dittrich M, Homan AE, Meriney SD. Presynaptic mechanisms controlling calcium-triggered transmitter release at the neuromuscular junction. Curr Opin Physio 2018;4:15–24.

[58] Homan AE, Laghaei R, Dittrich M, Meriney SD. Impact of spatiotemporal calcium dynamics within presynaptic active zones on synaptic delay at the frog neuromuscular junction. J Neurophysiol 2018;119:688–99.

[59] Deschenes MR, Tufts HL, Oh J, Li S, Noronha A, Adan MA. Effects of exercise training on neuromuscular junctions and their active zones in young and aged muscles. Neurobiol Aging 2020;95:1–8.

[60] Smith DO. Acetylcholine storage, release and leakage at the neuromuscular junction of mature adult and aged rats. J Physiol 1984;347:161–76.

[61] Smith DO, Weiler MH. Acetylcholine metabolism and choline availability at the neuromuscular junction of mature adult and aged rats. J Physiol 1987;383:693–709.

[62] Kelly SS, Robbins N. Progression of age changes in synaptic transmission at mouse neuromuscular junctions. J Physiol 1983;343:375–83.

[63] Neher E. What is rate-limiting during sustained synaptic activity: vesicle supply or the availability of release sites. Front Synaptic Neurosci 2010;2:144.

[64] Deschenes MR, Tufts HL, Noronha AL, Li S. Both aging and exercise training alter the rate of recovery of neuromuscular performance of male soleus muscles. Biogerontology 2019;20(2):213–23.

[65] Stockinger J, Maxwell N, Shapiro D, de Cabo R, Valdez G. Caloric restriction mimetics slow aging of neuromuscular synapses and muscle fibers. J Gerontol A Biol Sci Med Sci 2017;73(1):21–8.

[66] Hepple RT, Baker DJ, Kaczor JJ, Krause DJ. Long-term caloric restriction abrogates the age-related decline in skeletal muscle aerobic function. FASEB J 2005;19(10):1320–2.
[67] McKiernan SH, Bua E, McGorray J, Aiken J. Early-onset calorie restriction conserves fiber number in aging rat skeletal muscle. FASEB J 2004;18(3):580–1.
[68] Stekovic S, Hofer SJ, Tripolt N, Aon MA, Royer P, Pein L, et al. Alternate day fasting improves physiological and molecular markers of aging in healthy, non-obese humans. Cell Metab 2019;30(3):462–76. e6.
[69] Kim JH, Kwak HB, Leeuwenburgh C, Lawler JM. Lifelong exercise and mild (8%) caloric restriction attenuate age-induced alterations in plantaris muscle morphology, oxidative stress and IGF-1 in the Fischer-344 rat. Exp Gerontol 2008;43(4):317–29.
[70] Shetty AK, Kodali M, Upadhya R, Madhu LN. Emerging anti-aging strategies—scientific basis and efficacy. Aging Dis 2018;9(6):1165–84.
[71] Miyazaki R, Takeshima T, Kotani K. Exercise intervention for anti-sarcopenia in community-dwelling older people. J Clin Med Res 2016;8(12):848–53.
[72] Krause Neto W, Ciena AP, Anaruma CA, de Souza RR, Gama EF. Effects of exercise on neuromuscular junction components across age: systematic review of animal experimental studies. BMC Res Notes 2015;8:713. https://doi.org/10.1186/s13104-015-1644-4.
[73] Taetzsch T, Valdez G. NMJ maintenance and repair in aging. Curr Opin Physiol 2018;4:57–64.
[74] Andonian MH, Fahim MA. Effects of endurance exercise on the morphology of mouse neuromuscular junctions during ageing. J Neurocytol 1987;16(5):589–99.
[75] Nishimune H, Stanford JA, Mori Y. Role of exercise in maintaining the integrity of the neuromuscular junction. Muscle Nerve 2014;49(3):315–24.
[76] Sallis R. Exercise is medicine: a call to action for physicians to assess and prescribe exercise. Phys Sportsmed 2015;43(1):22–6.
[77] Swisher AK. Yes, "Exercise is Medicine"…but It Is So Much More! Cardiopulm Phys Ther J 2010;21(4):4.
[78] Abe T, Loenneke JP, Thiebaud RS, Fukunaga T. Age-related site-specific muscle wasting of upper and lower extremities and trunk in Japanese men and women. Age (Dordr) 2014;36(2):813–21.
[79] Thiebaud RS, Loenneke JP, Abe T, Fahs CA, Rossow LM, Kim D, et al. Appendicular lean mass and site-specific muscle loss in the extremities correlate with dynamic strength. Clin Physiol Funct Imaging 2017;37(3):328–31.
[80] Valdez G, Tapia JC, Lichtman JW, Fox MA, Sanes JR. Shared resistance to aging and ALS in neuromuscular junctions of specific muscles. PLoS One 2012;7(4), e34640.
[81] Hakkinen K, Pastinen UM, Karsikas R, Linnamo V. Neuromuscular performance in voluntary bilateral and unilateral contraction and during electrical stimulation in men at different ages. Eur J Appl Physiol Occup Physiol 1995;70(6):518–27.
[82] Lexell J. Human aging, muscle mass, and fiber type composition. J Gerontol A Biol Sci Med Sci 1995;50 Spec No:11–6.
[83] Pannerec A, Springer M, Migliavacca E, Ireland A, Piasecki M, Karaz S, et al. A robust neuromuscular system protects rat and human skeletal muscle from sarcopenia. Aging (Albany NY) 2016;8(4):712–29.
[84] Tomlinson BE, Irving D. The numbers of limb motor neurons in the human lumbosacral cord throughout life. J Neurol Sci 1977;34(2):213–9.
[85] McPhee JS, Cameron J, Maden-Wilkinson T, Piasecki M, Yap MH, Jones DA, et al. The contributions of fiber atrophy, fiber loss, in situ specific force, and voluntary activation to weakness in sarcopenia. J Gerontol A Biol Sci Med Sci 2018;73(10):1287–94.
[86] Cardasis CA. Ultrastructural evidence of continued reorganization at the aging (11-26 months) rat soleus neuromuscular junction. Anat Rec 1983;207(3):399–415.
[87] Courtney J, Steinbach JH. Age changes in neuromuscular junction morphology and acetylcholine receptor distribution on rat skeletal muscle fibres. J Physiol 1981;320:435–47.
[88] Porter MM, Vandervoort AA, Lexell J. Aging of human muscle: structure, function and adaptability. Scand J Med Sci Sports 1995;5(3):129–42.
[89] Agre JC, Rodriquez AA, Tafel JA. Late effects of polio: critical review of the literature on neuromuscular function. Arch Phys Med Rehabil 1991;72(11):923–31.

[90] Agre JC, Rodriquez AA. Neuromuscular function in polio survivors. Orthopedics 1991;14(12):1343–7.
[91] Chung T, Park JS, Kim S, Montes N, Walston J, Hoke A. Evidence for dying-back axonal degeneration in age-associated skeletal muscle decline. Muscle Nerve 2017;55(6):894–901.
[92] van den Bos MAJ, Geevasinga N, Higashihara M, Menon P, Vucic S. Pathophysiology and diagnosis of ALS: insights from advances in neurophysiological techniques. Int J Mol Sci 2019;20(11). https://doi.org/10.3390/ijms20112818.
[93] Drey M, Hasmann SE, Krenovsky JP, Hobert MA, Straub S, Elshehabi M, et al. Associations between early markers of Parkinson's disease and sarcopenia. Front Aging Neurosci 2017;9:53.
[94] Vetrano DL, Pisciotta MS, Laudisio A, Lo Monaco MR, Onder G, Brandi V, et al. Sarcopenia in parkinson disease: comparison of different criteria and association with disease severity. J Am Med Dir Assoc 2018;19(6):523–7.
[95] Lemeshko VV, Shekh VE. Hypotonic fragility of outer membrane and activation of external pathway of NADH oxidation in rat liver mitochondria are increased with age. Mech Ageing Dev 1993;68(1–3):221–33.
[96] Gillon A, Nielsen K, Steel C, Cornwall J, Sheard P. Exercise attenuates age-associated changes in motoneuron number, nucleocytoplasmic transport proteins and neuromuscular health. Geroscience 2018;40(2):177–92.
[97] Alway SE, Siu PM. Nuclear apoptosis contributes to sarcopenia. Exerc Sport Sci Rev 2008;36(2):51–7.
[98] Rygiel KA, Picard M, Turnbull DM. The ageing neuromuscular system and sarcopenia: a mitochondrial perspective. J Physiol 2016;594(16):4499–512.
[99] Mankhong S, Kim S, Moon S, Kwak HB, Park DH, Kang JH. Experimental models of sarcopenia: bridging molecular mechanism and therapeutic strategy. Cell 2020;9(6). https://doi.org/10.3390/cells9061385.
[100] Livshits G, Kalinkovich A. Inflammaging as a common ground for the development and maintenance of sarcopenia, obesity, cardiomyopathy and dysbiosis. Ageing Res Rev 2019;56:100980.
[101] Fougere B, Boulanger E, Nourhashemi F, Guyonnet S, Cesari M. Chronic inflammation: accelerator of biological aging. J Gerontol A Biol Sci Med Sci 2017;72(9):1218–25.
[102] Vatic M, von Haehling S, Ebner N. Inflammatory biomarkers of frailty. Exp Gerontol 2020;133:110858.
[103] Marzetti E, Picca A, Marini F, Biancolillo A, Coelho-Junior HJ, Gervasoni J, et al. Inflammatory signatures in older persons with physical frailty and sarcopenia: the frailty "cytokinome" at its core. Exp Gerontol 2019;122:129–38.
[104] Maxwell N, Castro RW, Sutherland NM, Vaughan KL, Szarowicz MD, de Cabo R, et al. alpha-Motor neurons are spared from aging while their synaptic inputs degenerate in monkeys and mice. Aging Cell 2018;17(2). https://doi.org/10.1111/acel.12726 [Epub 2018 Feb 4].
[105] Tamaki T, Hirata M, Uchiyama Y. Qualitative alteration of peripheral motor system begins prior to appearance of typical sarcopenia syndrome in middle-aged rats. Front Aging Neurosci 2014;6:296.
[106] Barik A, Zhang B, Sohal GS, Xiong WC, Mei L. Crosstalk between Agrin and Wnt signaling pathways in development of vertebrate neuromuscular junction. Dev Neurobiol 2014;74(8):828–38.
[107] Belotti E, Schaeffer L. Regulation of gene expression at the neuromuscular junction. Neurosci Lett 2020;735:135163.
[108] Butikofer L, Zurlinden A, Bolliger MF, Kunz B, Sonderegger P. Destabilization of the neuromuscular junction by proteolytic cleavage of agrin results in precocious sarcopenia. FASEB J 2011;25(12):4378–93.
[109] Hettwer S, Lin S, Kucsera S, Haubitz M, Oliveri F, Fariello RG, et al. Injection of a soluble fragment of neural agrin (NT-1654) considerably improves the muscle pathology caused by the disassembly of the neuromuscular junction. PLoS One 2014;9(2), e88739.
[110] Herbst R. MuSk function during health and disease. Neurosci Lett 2020;716:134676.
[111] Swenarchuk LE. Nerve, muscle, and synaptogenesis. Cell 2019;8(11). https://doi.org/10.3390/cells8111448.
[112] Hamarneh SR, Murphy CA, Shih CW, Frontera W, Torriani M, Irazoqui JE, et al. Relationship between serum IGF-1 and skeletal muscle IGF-1 mRNA expression to phosphocreatine recovery after exercise in obese men with reduced GH. J Clin Endocrinol Metab 2015;100(2):617–25.
[113] Barclay RD, Burd NA, Tyler C, Tillin NA, Mackenzie RW. The role of the IGF-1 signaling cascade in muscle protein synthesis and anabolic resistance in aging skeletal muscle. Front Nutr 2019;6:146.

[114] Messi ML, Delbono O. Target-derived trophic effect on skeletal muscle innervation in senescent mice. J Neurosci 2003;23(4):1351–9.

[115] Austin S, St-Pierre J. PGC1alpha and mitochondrial metabolism—emerging concepts and relevance in ageing and neurodegenerative disorders. J Cell Sci 2012;125(Pt 21):4963–71.

[116] St-Pierre J, Drori S, Uldry M, Silvaggi JM, Rhee J, Jager S, et al. Suppression of reactive oxygen species and neurodegeneration by the PGC-1 transcriptional coactivators. Cell 2006;127(2):397–408.

[117] Wareski P, Vaarmann A, Choubey V, Safiulina D, Liiv J, Kuum M, et al. PGC-1{alpha} and PGC-1{beta} regulate mitochondrial density in neurons. J Biol Chem 2009;284(32):21379–85.

[118] Handschin C, Kobayashi YM, Chin S, Seale P, Campbell KP, Spiegelman BM. PGC-1alpha regulates the neuromuscular junction program and ameliorates Duchenne muscular dystrophy. Genes Dev 2007;21(7):770–83.

[119] Da Cruz S, Parone PA, Lopes VS, Lillo C, McAlonis-Downes M, Lee SK, et al. Elevated PGC-1alpha activity sustains mitochondrial biogenesis and muscle function without extending survival in a mouse model of inherited ALS. Cell Metab 2012;15(5):778–86.

CHAPTER 3

Dietary approaches to maintaining muscle mass

Rafael A. Alamilla[a], Kevin J.M. Paulussen[a], Andrew T. Askow[a], and Nicholas A. Burd[a,b]

[a]Department of Kinesiology and Community Health, University of Illinois at Urbana-Champaign, Urbana, IL, United States, [b]Division of Nutritional Sciences, University of Illinois at Urbana-Champaign, Urbana, IL, United States

Abstract
Skeletal muscle is a vital tissue for the maintenance of physical independence and quality of life across the lifespan. Skeletal muscle mass is regulated by net protein balance—the difference between muscle protein synthesis and muscle protein breakdown rates—and can be maximized by resistance exercise and consuming adequate amounts of high-quality dietary protein at strategic times across the day. The age-related decline in skeletal muscle mass has been coined sarcopenia. The preservation of skeletal muscle becomes vital as we age, as the loss of skeletal muscle mass can contribute to impairments in functional capacity and an increased risk of chronic metabolic diseases. In turn, individuals with anabolic resistance, such as those with sarcopenia, should attempt to preserve lean mass by consuming dietary protein intakes above the recommended dietary allowance and couple these feeding strategies with a resistance training program that caters to their physical limitations.

Keywords: Aging, Anabolic resistance, Dietary protein, Amino acids, Leucine, Sarcopenia, Older adults

Introduction

The aging process is associated with a progressive decline of muscular function and skeletal muscle mass. Characteristic of muscle mass and strength decrements with aging is a reduction in the ability to conduct activities of daily living and ultimately be active in family and community life. From this standpoint, it is clear that attenuating the age-related loss of muscle mass is important. However, it is also relevant to protect against losses of muscle mass to ensure optimal metabolic health. For example, skeletal muscle mass is an important determinate of postprandial glucose disposal, fat oxidation, and is the primary contributor to basal metabolic rate and, as such, total daily energy expenditure. As such, identifying strategies to preserve and maintain skeletal muscle quantity and quality (the ability to produce force relative to its protein mass) throughout the lifespan is of vital importance to maximize both longevity and quality of life.

Modifiable lifestyle factors such as regular exercise and healthy eating patterns are often implicated as a means to promote skeletal muscle maintenance or deposition. When considering a healthy diet from a muscle-centric perspective, it is clear that protein has a central role. This is because dietary amino acids serve as both anabolic signals and substrate for the stimulation of skeletal muscle protein turnover. Fundamentally, skeletal muscle protein content is subject to regulation by two distinct processes—muscle protein synthesis (MPS) and muscle protein breakdown (MPB). The difference between MPS and MPB is referred to as net protein balance (i.e., MPS-MPB). A net positive balance results in skeletal muscle accretion; a net negative balance results in skeletal muscle degradation [1, 2]. While both MPS and MPB are responsive to stimuli, the magnitude of change in MPS has been generally shown to be more responsive to elevations in dietary amino acid availability when compared to changes in MPB. Hence, it is common for a scientist to probe MPS in response to various nutritional manipulations to understand changes in 24 h net protein balance with youth and old age. Interestingly, studies that have compared changes in MPS after eating protein or exercise have generally shown aging muscles to be less responsive when compared to their youthful counterparts. This age-related anabolic resistance of MPS to these main anabolic stimuli (dietary protein and exercise) to human skeletal muscle is believed to be the primary mechanism underpinning muscle mass and strength loss. Therefore, identifying strategies that maximize MPS in older adults could aid in the prevention and treatment of sarcopenia and its deleterious effects [3].

The purpose of this chapter is to discuss dietary strategies that may be most effective at offsetting risk factors that contribute to sarcopenia (i.e., the progressive loss of muscle mass and strength with advancing age). Dietary protein is central to our discussion given its potency toward stimulating MPS, and the amount of protein in the diet is associated with overall muscle mass with aging. When considering dietary protein and aging, protein quality, amount, and distribution are likely important factors in the development of optimal feeding strategies for older people. These topics will also be the highlight within this chapter.

Dietary protein quality

The quality of a dietary protein source is dependent on its constituent amino acids, and several scoring systems have been developed to determine food protein quality.

Defining high-quality protein sources

Between 1989 and 2011, the Food and Agricultural Organization (FAO) of the United Nations recommended the use of the Protein Digestibility Corrected Amino Acid Score (PDCAAS) as the "gold standard" method of measuring protein quality. PDCAAS determines protein quality in terms of the potential capacity of the food protein to provide the appropriate pattern of dietary EAAs [4]. However, the calculation of PDCAAS has several shortcomings that limit its ability to effectively differentiate between high(er) quality proteins [4, 5]. Specifically, PDCAAS uses fecal protein digestibility to calculate the absorption rates of amino acids, which can falsely increase values of true protein digestibility and thus falsely enhance values of true protein digestibility [6]. Additionally, PDCAAS uses a truncated scoring system whereby PDCAAS values are cut off at 1.0, which fails to distinguish high-quality proteins from one another [5, 6]. Finally, PDCAAS derives fecal protein digestibility values from rodent models with different amino acid requirements for growth and repair compared to human beings [6].

To address the shortcoming of PDCAAS and distinguish the rates of digestibility among high-quality proteins, the FAO promotes the Digestible Indispensable Amino Acid Score (DIAAS). The DIAAS method requires the absolute protein content and levels of EAAs for a given food to be calculated (Table 1). Once this is determined, the DIAAS uses the ileal digestibility coefficients of each amino acid to calculate the true ileal digestibility of the EAAs present within a protein or food mixture [4]. Finally, the proportion of each digestible

Table 1: Digestible indispensable amino acid score (DIAAS) and protein digestibility-corrected amino acid score (PDCAAS) for selected isolated and whole-food animal and plant protein sources.

Food Item	DIAAS score	PDCAAS score
Animal-based proteins		
Whey protein isolate	1.00	0.99
Skimmed milk protein	1.05	1.00
Whole milk powder	1.16	1.00
Cow milk	1.16	–
Whole egg, boiled	1.13	1.00
Beef	1.12	1.00
Pork	1.14	1.00
Chicken breast	1.08	1.00
Plant-based proteins		
Soy protein isolate	0.84	0.93
Cooked peas	0.58	0.60
Raw almonds	0.40	0.39
Tofu	0.52	0.56
Cooked rice[a]	0.60	0.62
Cooked kidney beans[a]	0.59	0.65
Roasted peanuts[a]	0.43	0.51

Unless indicated, all values were measured in growing pigs.
[a] Value obtained in growing rats.
Values obtained from the following sources: Huang S, Wang LM, Sivendiran T, Bohrer BM. Review: amino acid concentration of high protein food products and an overview of the current methods used to determine protein quality. Crit Rev Food Sci Nutr 2018;58(15):2673-2678. https://doi.org/10.1080/10408398.2017.1396202, Wolfe RR, Rutherfurd S.M., Kim I.Y., Moughan P.J. Protein quality as determined by the Digestible Indispensable Amino Acid Score: evaluation of factors underlying the calculation. Nutr Rev 2016;74(9):584-599. https://doi.org/10.1093/nutrit/nuw022., and Burd NA, McKenna CF, Salvador AF, Paulussen KJM, Moore DR. Dietary protein quantity, quality, and exercise are key to healthy living: a muscle-centric perspective across the lifespan. Front Nutr 2019;6:83. https://doi.org/10.3389/fnut.2019.00083; Burd NA, Beals JW, Martinez IG, Salvador AF, Skinner SK. Food-first approach to enhance the regulation of post-exercise skeletal muscle protein synthesis and remodeling. Sport Med 2019;49:59-68. https://doi.org/10.1007/s40279-018-1009-y.

amino acid is calculated relative to a reference amino acid pattern. The DIAAS score for a protein or food mixture is based on the lowest value across the amino acid profile of the tested protein expressed as a percentage [4, 7, 8]. On top of the methodological advantages of this calculation, the DIAAS calculation is useful for investigators because the scoring system does not have a cut-off point, allowing for comparison between high-protein food items. Moreover, the DIAAS scoring method accounts for the amount of protein provided per a specific amount of food [7, 9]. Although concerns have been raised about the methodology of the DIAAS scoring system [10], it is a considerable step forward for the determination of the digestibility of dietary protein sources.

Despite this, the invasive nature of DIAAS assessment makes this measurement challenging to apply in human research. Moreover, while the digestibility of a dietary protein source is an important index of its ability to support protein turnover, DIAAS scoring does not describe any downstream processes related to the target tissues. As such, stable isotope amino acid tracers in metabolic research have been widely incorporated to estimate the degree and rate at which dietary protein-derived amino acids are released into circulation and the rate of their subsequent incorporation into skeletal muscle tissue (i.e., MPS). Stable isotope tracers have proven to be a versatile tool for researchers aiming to assess both protein quality and relevant physiological correlates such as protein metabolism in vivo in human beings. In the subsequent sections, we will discuss protein quality in the context of plant vs. animal protein sources and their ability to deliver target amounts of essential amino acids into circulation for the stimulation of MPS.

Plant-based protein sources

The source of our dietary protein intake has been of increasing interest. While the merit of claims from both animal- and plant-based dieters are outside of the scope of this chapter, the popularity of plant-based meat alternatives has increased against the backdrop of a push to reduce our reliance on animal-based protein foods. While some countries have reduced their consumption of meat products [11], most of the developed world continues to increase its reliance on animal-based protein sources [12, 13]. National Data from the National Health and Nutrition Examination Survey demonstrated that total protein intake derived from animal protein was 46% and was primarily consumed via chicken, red meat (beef and cold cuts), and egg. Protein intake from dairy and plant protein sources represented 16% and 30%, respectively, of daily protein intake. Primary sources of dairy included cheese, reduced-fat milk, and ice cream/dairy desserts, while primary sources of plant protein included yeast breads, rolls/buns, and nuts/seeds [14]. Studies in the French [15] and Belgian [16] populations have reported similar trends in animal and plant protein intakes, alluding to a reliance on animal protein in the western world.

Previous reports have reported that primarily plant-based diets (e.g., lacto-ovo-vegetarian, vegan) were able to meet intake recommendations for dietary protein and other key nutrients

[17, 18]. Several large-scale investigations have demonstrated the benefit of consuming nuts as part of a balanced diet. Data from 24,385 participants demonstrated that individuals who consume nuts regularly had greater coingestion of key micronutrients as well as lower intakes of carbohydrates, cholesterol, and sodium than those who did not consume nuts regularly [19]. Additionally, diet quality was higher in regular nut consumers and was accompanied by a more favorable metabolic panel (e.g., greater high-density lipoprotein cholesterol, lower plasma insulin, and C-reactive protein levels). Regular nut consumers also had a lower prevalence of two risk factors for metabolic syndrome (hypertension and dyslipidemia) [19]. Other investigations have also reported similar benefits of regular nut or bean consumption on micronutrient intake and overall diet quality [20–22]—further supporting the incorporation of nuts into a healthy eating pattern to maximize diet quality.

Soy protein may have the greatest potential as a substitute for animal-based protein sources because (1) it contains a similar EAA profile to high-quality animal protein sources, and (2) soy protein maintains high PDCAAS and DIAAS scores [5, 23]. The ability of soy protein to support dietary protein needs has been demonstrated as early as the 1980s when investigators conducted several studies to determine the nutritional value of soy protein when compared to milk and beef protein. Results demonstrated that soy was capable of sustaining nitrogen balance across a 10-day experimental period to the same degree as milk and beef protein [24–26]. More recent investigations have focused specifically on the capacity of soy protein to increase rates of MPS and promote a positive net protein balance. Consumption of 18 g of soy protein after resistance exercise significantly increased FSR and total plasma amino acid concentrations [27]. Further, supplementation of soy protein has proven effective in supporting resistance training-induced gains in muscle fiber cross-sectional area, skeletal muscle mass, muscular strength, and postprandial plasma amino acid concentrations [28–30].

While high-quality nonanimal-derived proteins in the diet are potentially sufficient to support hypertrophic protein remodeling, it is important to note that plant-based protein foods yield lower DIAAS scores when compared to animal-based proteins. For example, no nonanimal-derived protein foods score yields a DIAAS score greater than 100 while a variety of animal-based protein foods (e.g., cow milk, beef, pork, chicken breast, and tilapia) score 100 or greater [31, 32]. Thus, it is clear that many plant-based protein sources lack the EAA content present in animal-based sources and should be considered when constructing a dietary plan.

Considering the suboptimal quantity of EAA in plant-based proteins, consuming larger quantities of these sources is a potential way of consuming enough protein to sustain muscle mass maintenance [33]. However, achieving sufficient protein intake while relying primarily on plant-based foods will come at the expense of higher energy intakes. In turn, individuals consuming lower caloric intakes—such as individuals undergoing weight loss, and older adults—should take this into consideration when selecting plant-based protein sources [34]. This drawback could be addressed by fortifying food sources with EAAs (specifically lysine, methionine, and leucine) to achieve optimal intakes while also keeping caloric intake down [33]. Moreover, many plant-based protein sources do not have complete EAA profiles to maximize a positive net protein balance. However, multiple plant-based food items can achieve a complete EAA profile when consumed together (e.g., pinto beans and rice) [9].

Animal-based protein sources

An emphasis on red meat, poultry, and fish consumption across various cultures is not completely unwarranted, as animal-based protein sources have a higher protein density as plant-based sources [14]. Importantly, animal and fish protein sources contain all nine EAAs, making them a high-quality source of protein [4] High-quality animal-derived protein sources often contribute substantially to the daily intake of a number of other nutrients such as calcium, vitamin D, potassium, iron, and folate [34], several of which are often lacking in the diets of older persons [35]. Indeed, consumption of animal protein sources is an effective means for stimulating rates of MPS in acute studies and promoting deposition of lean body mass in longitudinal human interventions. In an acute, randomized crossover trial, 12 participants consumed 30 g of either beef or milk protein following a bout of lower body exercise. Both conditions increased amino acid availability across a 5-h postprandial period. Interestingly, milk produced a twofold increase in FSR over the first 2 h of recovery when compared to beef, but had a similar FSR between the 2–5 h recovery period [36]. In a similarly designed investigation (randomized crossover design, acute lower-body resistance exercise), skim milk was demonstrated to significantly increase plasma amino acid concentrations and FSR while also producing a greater positive net protein balance compared to soy protein [27].

Additionally, multiple investigations providing animal-based protein over extended periods have proven effective in improving body composition and increasing muscular strength. After completing a 12-week progressive resistance exercise program, young women consuming fat-free milk immediately after exercise had significant increases in lean mass and muscular strength and decreases in fat mass when compared to a carbohydrate control [37]. Consuming fat-free milk (17.5 g protein) immediately after and 1 h after resistance exercise across a 12-week training study produced increases in type I and II muscle fibers, but failed to increase muscular strength [28]. Moreover, ingesting whey protein at a dose of $1.2\,g\,kg^{-1}\,day^{-1}$ before exercise, after exercise, and before sleep for 6 weeks increased lean mass and muscular strength. However, these results did not differ from participants consuming an isonitrogenous and calorically matched dose of soy protein [38].

From these data, it is evident that animal-based protein is capable of supporting increases in skeletal muscle mass and strength among healthy adults. Although concerns have been raised about the impact of long-term animal protein intake on systemic inflammation and development of metabolic disease, the current body of evidence is inconclusive and sometimes contradictory.

It must be noted that the impact of whole food sources on skeletal muscle remodeling in vivo in human beings has been understudied. Recent evidence suggests that a whole food source may be superior to an isolated protein source. Ten young men completed a crossover study where they consumed either whole eggs (18 g protein, 17 g fat) or egg whites (18 g protein, 0 g fat) immediately after exercise. While both conditions produced similar degrees of protein signaling expression, the whole egg condition produced a higher MPS rate [39]. These findings suggest that a food's matrix (i.e., the food structure and nutrient-nutrient interaction) may play a role in the stimulation of muscle protein remodeling. Ultimately, both the protein quality and density of a food item is an important factor to consider when constructing an individual's diet.

Leucine as a determinant of protein quality

Of the nine EAAs, leucine has been demonstrated to be of particular importance in human metabolism due to its ability to stimulate endogenous insulin release, inhibit MPB, and directly stimulate MPS by acting as an anabolic signaling molecule in both healthy and diseased populations [40]. As such, leucine is often considered a marker of protein quality whereby food proteins with higher leucine by total amino acid content are considered to be more anabolic for MPS. Studies describing the effects of leucine on the mechanisms underpinning muscle protein turnover were first conducted as far back as the 1970s when researchers isolated rat hemidiaphragm with leucine and demonstrated that leucine stimulated the incorporation of amino acids into muscle protein [41]. When compared to a mixture of branched-chain amino acids (BCAA), leucine promoted greater incorporation of amino acids. Other early works demonstrated that isolation of food-deprived rat leg muscle supplemented with leucine increased protein synthesis rates compared to controls [42].

These early papers [41, 43] were some of the first investigations to suggest that leucine has an impact on the initiation phase of protein translation. Over time, multiple investigations would highlight leucine's impact on specific downstream proteins in the protein synthetic machinery. Specifically, leucine ingestion increases phosphorylation of ribosomal protein S6 kinase (p70S6K), a downstream target of mammalian target of rapamycin complex 1 (mTORC1) [44]. Leucine has also been demonstrated to have a direct impact on other proteins in the mTOR signaling pathway, such as the 4E-BP1-eIF4E complex (Fig. 1). Here, mTORC1 phosphorylates 4E-BP1, reducing the affinity of 4E-BP1 for initiation factor 4E (eIF4E) leading to the formation of an active eIF4F, which subsequently allows for translation initiation [45]. Further leucine ingestion can increase phosphorylation of 4E-BP1 and p70S6K phosphorylation, resulting in elevated rates of protein synthesis [46].

Later investigations would demonstrate that leucine can stimulate MPS in an mTOR-independent manner by increasing eIF4G phosphorylation, leading to increased formation of the eIF4E-eIF4G complex [47]. Similarly, rats supplemented with leucine had increased eIF4G phosphorylation and increased MPS rates [48]. Finally, Atherton et al. [49]

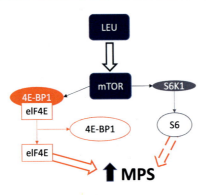

Fig. 1
Leucine's impact on the mTOR signaling pathway has been well investigated and established. Leucine has been shown to directly activate mTOR, in turn increasing the phosphorylation of ribosomal protein S6 kinase 1 (S6K1) and the eukaryotic initiation factor 4E-binding protein (4E-BP1). Phosphorylation of 4E-BP1 prevents binding with eIF4E, thereby enhancing the assembly of the eIF4F complex. Both these processes result in the stimulation of muscle protein synthesis.

investigated the anabolic signaling activity induced by amino acids in cell-cultured Murine C2C12 myocytes. Investigators determined that leucine stimulated a threefold increase in the phosphorylation of p70S6K1 and RPS6. Moreover, they also demonstrated that leucine is unique in its capacity to stimulate mTORC1 and 4E-BP1 phosphorylation, suggesting that leucine is the most potent stimulator of anabolic signaling in skeletal muscle cells. Collectively, these studies suggest that leucine is a potent anabolic stimulator of the mTOR signaling pathway and its downstream targets.

In addition to stimulation of anabolic signaling and muscle protein synthesis, cell and animal models suggest that leucine may exert control over protein breakdown as well, further increasing its effect on net protein balance [50]. In one such study, mouse C2C12 myotubes were starved of either leucine or all amino acids for up to 21 h [51]. Leucine starvation accounted for 30%–40% of L-[35^S]Met release—a proxy measure of total protein breakdown. Moreover, leucine concentrations below the average physiological plasma concentrations had an impact on MPB in a dose-dependent manner—a lower leucine concentration resulted in higher rates of protein breakdown. A separate investigation reported that skeletal muscle protein degradation—measured via NT-methyl histidine release—was suppressed in rats who were fed isolated leucine. After an 18-h starvation period, rats refed with a leucine-enriched diet had similar reductions in protein degradation when compared to rats fed either a 20% casein diet, an amino acid mixture, and an EAA diet.

Similar findings demonstrating proteolysis inhibition were obtained when studying chick skeletal muscle. Researchers incubated chick myotubes with leucine at different doses (0.2, 0.4, or 1 mM) for 2 or 6 h and measured the concentration of NT-methyl histidine in the incubation medium. In addition, a second experiment was conducted in which chicks were starved for 24 h and then fed 225 mg/100 g of leucine. Leucine suppressed myofibrillar proteolysis both in chick myotubes (in a dose-dependent manner) and in live chicks. Leucine was also reported to inhibit the PI3K and PKC pathways—both of which are responsible for preventing ubiquitin and proteasome C2 subunit mRNA expression and hence decrease protein degradation [52].

The potency of leucine to stimulate rates of MPS in vivo in human beings has been demonstrated across a broad range of populations. One group [53] reported that 1.8 g of leucine—a dose typically found in high-quality protein sources—was sufficient to stimulate MPS when part of an EAA mixture when compared to a high leucine dose of 3.5 g. A separate investigation providing 3.4 g of leucine reported a 110% increase in MPS rates over a 2.5-h postprandial period [54]. Similarly, another group [55] reported that an EAA mixture containing ~ 2.8 g of leucine was able to stimulate increases in mixed MPS rates in both young and elderly adults—suggesting that leucine, when combined with the other EAAs, can similarly stimulate an anabolic response in both younger and older adults.

Despite the promising literature suggesting that leucine is the primary amino acid responsible for stimulating MPS, other studies have shown that leucine is unable to significantly increase MPS rates in aging populations [56–58]. However, this may partially be attributed to the investigators providing an insufficient dose to stimulate a robust MPS response, as highlighted by the leucine threshold hypothesis. Investigators have determined that there is not an absolute blood leucine concentration that serves as an "on switch" for the MPS response. Rather, increasing blood leucine concentrations results in a step-wise increase in MPS rates and ultimately results in an eventual plateau in MPS rates when high leucine-containing proteins are consumed [59, 60].

Dietary protein quantity

Current protein recommendations are defined by the Recommended Dietary Allowance (RDA) in the United States, and the Population Reference Intake (PRI) in Europe. These recommendations were originally established using nitrogen balance methodologies and were thereafter adopted by their respective governments to reduce disease risk/malnourishment in nearly all individuals [61]. Current protein intake recommendations for the RDA and PRI are set at 0.80 and 0.83 g kg^{-1} day^{-1}, respectively. While the role of these recommendations in preventing deficiencies is clear, their adequacy in support of an active lifestyle or maintenance of muscle mass with age is the subject of debate. Increasing evidence suggests that a variety of populations (e.g., active individuals and older adults) might require higher protein intakes. As such, individual characteristics and lifestyle habits need to be considered when assessing protein intake. Regular exercise has been shown to directly affect nutrient utilization and dietary protein requirements when compared to the sedentary state [62, 63]. Furthermore, different forms of exercise (e.g., resistance training and endurance training) have different effects on protein metabolism [64, 65], further complicating the identification of an "optimal" protein recommendation to maintain skeletal muscle mass.

Resistance exercise has been shown to enhance the dietary amino acid sensitivity of MPS such that lower protein amounts are needed to elicit a robust anabolic stimulus compared to the sedentary state [9]. In addition, skeletal muscle tissue is more responsive to and can absorb more dietary amino acids after a resistance exercise bout [66], resulting in increased whole-body nitrogen retention [67]. Overall, these exercise-mediated anabolic effects can subsist for up to 2 days [64]. This is evidenced by investigations demonstrating an improved net muscle protein balance (e.g., shift to a net positive protein balance) in the immediate postprandial period (0–5h) [68] and prolonged recovery period (1–2 days) [69]. As an example, in the sedentary state, about 25 g of high-quality protein is required to maximize net muscle protein balance. However, only about 20 g of high-quality protein is required to maximize net muscle protein balance in the postresistance exercise state [70]. These findings suggest that regular strength training leads to the optimization of dietary protein utilization and directly alters dietary protein requirements.

When considering the other side of the exercise spectrum, endurance exercise seems to have inherently different effects on muscle protein metabolism when compared to strength training. Nonendurance trained individuals have endogenous protein oxidation rates that represent only a fraction of the body's required energy production (~ 2%–10%). Interestingly, seminal work performed in the 1970s found that performing endurance exercise increases amino acid utilization, as apparent by their appearance in blood circulation with increasing exercise intensity [71]. Separate work building on this topic demonstrated that performing endurance exercise results in increased breakdown of amino acids, and this occurs to a higher extent with increased exercise duration [72]. That said, protein oxidation, and more specifically leucine oxidation, becomes blunted as an individual becomes familiarized with endurance exercise [73]. As a result of the increased oxidation rate associated with endurance exercise, the protein intake recommendations aimed toward those performing resistance exercise fail to meet those for endurance training individuals [9]. Moreover, postprandial net protein balance after endurance exercise seems to be dependent on the duration and intensity of the exercise performed. Consequently, the available data suggest that dietary protein requirements are higher in individuals who regularly partake in endurance exercise when compared to resistance exercise [74]. More importantly, health professionals should consider the type, frequency, duration, and intensity of activity performed when determining optimal protein intakes.

Protein intake above the RDA

Increasing dietary protein intake above the RDA/PRI is an effective strategy for combatting diminished muscle protein synthetic responses present in various populations. Of note, higher protein intakes have been demonstrated to promote a positive protein balance in older adults, a population shown to have anabolic resistance [75]. Moreover, a protein intake higher than the RDA or PRI protein intake can increase muscle mass retention during weight loss [76]. During a caloric deficit, we not only lose body fat but also skeletal muscle mass, which is important for maintaining functional capacity and metabolic health. Increasing protein intake above the RDA may be beneficial for decreasing the loss of skeletal muscle during weight loss. Protein intakes up to $2.4\,g\,kg^{-1}\,day^{-1}$ have been shown beneficial when compared to lower intakes [77]. Metaanalyses on the topic show that high protein diets ranging from ~ 1.2 to $1.6\,g\,kg^{-1}\,day^{-1}$ are more effective in inducing weight loss, fat mass loss, and retention of skeletal muscle mass when compared to normal protein diets [62]. However, it may take an anabolic (resistance training) or catabolic (energy restriction) stressor for the benefits of protein intakes above the RDA to manifest—as protein intake greater than the RDA appears to have no benefit on lean mass in studies without a resistance training or energy restriction component [78].

The importance of protein distribution across the day

The suggestion to distribute protein intake equally at each meal to favor protein anabolism stems from two main concepts [79]. First, because EAAs (leucine, in particular) themselves stimulate muscle protein synthesis [80], a threshold of high-quality protein intake must be reached at each meal. Second, excess dietary amino acids (i.e., beyond the capacity to maximally stimulate protein synthesis) are oxidized at an increasingly higher rate [62]. With this information as a foundation, it can be speculated that a skewed protein distribution (i.e., eating a low-protein meal at breakfast and a high-protein meal at dinnertime) could result in a suboptimal net protein balance. In turn, it has been proposed that the anabolic response to protein intake would be improved if skewed feeding patterns (e.g., American diet) were adjusted to distribute protein intake more evenly across daily meals. This idea gains support from findings that suggest that a high-quality protein dose of 25–30 g is sufficient to maximally stimulate MPS [79]. Research in healthy young men revealed that ingesting intact protein above 20 g fails to further stimulate MPS [70]. Interestingly, 40 g did not result in greater MPS rates while also resulting in higher rates of irreversible protein oxidation. Regarding an even protein distribution, one investigation found that providing ~ 30 g of protein evenly distributed across the day resulted in higher rates of 24-h MPS compared to a skewed feeding pattern [81]. This difference in MPS rate was maintained both at the beginning and the end of the 7-day period, suggesting that habituation to an even distribution does not attenuate the observed differential effect.

Work counter to the idea of an even protein distribution has been primarily conducted in the older adult population. One such study reported no significant differences in whole-body protein synthesis and breakdown when distributing dietary protein equally over three meals as compared to a skewed intake. The lack of impact of protein distribution of dietary protein was evident at relative dietary protein intakes of 0.8 and 1.5 g kg^{-1} day^{-1} [82]. A separate investigation came to a similar conclusion after feeding 1.1 g kg^{-1} day^{-1} of dietary protein as either a part of a skewed or balanced distribution. Evenly distributed protein intake did not result in significant differences in lean body mass, muscle strength, and other functional outcomes when compared to a skewed distribution [83]. It is evident from the conflicting literature on protein distribution that further work is needed to gain a better understanding of the limits of anabolic potential across the lifespan. We can, however, conclude that there is a practical limit of protein to stimulate MPS on a meal-to-meal basis.

Dietary considerations for older adults

Aging is associated with an inevitable loss of skeletal muscle mass. This marked decrease in skeletal muscle with aging has been a key point of concern for investigators and clinicians, as loss of skeletal muscle can ultimately lead to decreased physical activity, metabolic disease, loss of independence, and an increased risk for mortality. However, the etiology of this age-related muscle mass is complex and can result from a variety of issues, including modified dietary habits via loss of appetite, gastrointestinal issues, reduced energy need, and/or changes in food preference [84]. More alarmingly, aging is also associated with a blunted response to well-establish proanabolic stimuli. This blunted response is generally defined as a reduced stimulation of muscle protein synthesis in response to the provision of dietary protein/amino acids when compared to younger adults and contributes to a decline in skeletal muscle mass [85].

The underlying mechanism for anabolic resistance in older adults is currently not fully understood. Researchers have suggested that anabolic resistance can be attributed to several factors such as systemic age-related inflammation or prolonged skeletal muscle disuse stemming from reductions in physical activity [2, 85, 86]. Studies elucidating the impact of inflammation on MPS suggest that systemic low-grade inflammation blunts the phosphorylation of anabolic signaling targets within the mTOR signaling cascade and, thus, reduces the protein synthetic response. Moreover, a proinflammatory environment may also induce a higher rate of muscle protein breakdown, resulting in a net negative protein balance [2]. However, data from in vivo human studies are currently lacking and require further investigation before a causal relationship between systemic inflammation and blunted MPS can be established in human beings.

Other investigators have suggested that the main cause of anabolic resistance in older adults is a lack of physical activity. This can prove to be problematic, as chronic physical inactivity has been shown to lead to the development of obesity and type-2 diabetes—which can promote insulin resistance and further potentiate anabolic resistance [85]. Numerous studies have demonstrated the anabolic potency of exercise in the older adult population. Human trials have shown that older adults were able to increase rates of MPS by simply walking on a treadmill. Additionally, habitual exercise has been shown to augment the MPS response when combined with a bolus of protein, implying that older adults need to partake in habitual exercise if they are to offset the anabolic resistance [75]. With this in mind, several studies have demonstrated that older adults fail to respond to higher load resistance exercise in the same way that younger adults do. However, resistance training strategies that include low-load, high volume training, and blood flow restriction training have been proven effective at stimulating MPS in older adults [2] and may be a safer alternative for long-term adherence to resistance exercise.

Anabolic resistance can be attributed to either blunted basal MPS, blunted postprandial MPS, or a combination of the two. One such study, a secondary analysis of 215 young and older adults, demonstrated that basal MPS rates did not differ between young and older adults [87]. Interestingly, the authors also reported higher mechanistic signaling within the mTOR signaling pathway in older adults. Collectively, these data suggest that anabolic resistance is not attributable to impaired basal MPS rates, but rather to the way that older adults handle dietary amino acids in the postprandial state.

One of the key studies in support of the idea that older adults are anabolically resistant to dietary protein was conducted by Cuthbertson et al. [88]. Investigators sought to assess the differential anabolic signaling and MPS response of young and old adults to incremental doses of EAAs (0, 2.5, 5, 10, and 20 with an additional dose of 40 g for older adults). Investigators reported that 10 g of EAAs was sufficient to maximally stimulate myofibrillar and sarcoplasmic FSR in both young and old adults with no further increases observed with larger doses. However, the degree of stimulation above basal rates was blunted in older adults. A reduction in the phosphorylation of the mTOR signaling proteins p70S6K, 4E-BP1, and eIF2B were also reported in older adults, leading this team of investigators to suggest that these decrements in the mTOR-mediated signaling may contribute to anabolic resistance [88]. Later, a retrospective analysis compiling in vivo postabsorptive and postprandial mixed muscle MPS rates from young and old adult males determined that (1) young and old adults did not differ in postabsorptive MPS rates, (2) postprandial MPS rates were 16% lower in old adults when compared with the young adults, and (3) young adults had a threefold higher responsiveness dietary protein ingestion in the young, further supporting the theory of anabolic resistance [89].

Dietary protein intake consideration for older adults

There is a considerable degree of evidence to suggest that the RDA for protein is insufficient to support skeletal muscle mass in older adults. Some of the first data to support this idea came from a study of 54–78-year-old men and women who consumed diets that provided the RDA for protein and either remained sedentary or performed lower-body or whole-body resistance exercise 3 days per week for 12 weeks. At the end of the 12-week intervention, midthigh muscle mass was maintained in the resistance training group and decreased (− 2%) in the sedentary group [90, 91]. This idea is further supported by the findings of a review conducted by Campbell that analyzed the finding of nutritional intervention studies targeting older adults from 1998 to 2007. From this review, the author concluded that older adults require daily protein ingestion above the RDA to maintain muscle mass [92].

Considerable data in favor of dietary protein intake above the RDA have also been reported by the investigators leading the Health, Aging, and Body Composition study [93]. Dietary protein intake was assessed by using an interviewer-administered 108-item food-frequency questionnaire in men and women aged 70–79 years. Participants in the highest quintile of protein intake ($1.2\,g\,kg^{-1}\,day^{-1}$) lost 40% less lean mass and appendicular lean mass than those in the lowest quintile of protein intake ($0.8\,g\,kg^{-1}\,day^{-1}$) across a 3-year span. Interestingly, despite consuming less protein than those in the highest quintile, those consuming more than $0.8\,g\,kg^{-1}\,day^{-1}$ still preserved more skeletal muscle mass than those in the lowest quintile [93]. Protein intake at twice the RDA ($1.6\,g\,kg^{-1}\,day^{-1}$) for 10 weeks has been demonstrated to increase LBM and isokinetic knee strength in older males [94]. Additionally, providing an EAA-enriched diet is effective to support increases in basal MPS rates [95] and LBM in older women [95, 96]. Together, these data suggest that dietary protein intake, especially across a multiyear span, may be a modifiable factor for the preservation of skeletal muscle mass.

The quantity of protein consumed per meal, as well as the frequency of high-quantity protein consumption across a day, is correlated with the preservation of lean mass and strength. Twenty-four-hour dietary recall and isokinetic dynamometry data compiled from 1081 middle-aged and older adults from 1998 to 2002 determined that consuming two or more meals containing 30–45 g of protein was associated with higher lean mass and strength. A single 30–45 g bolus of protein proved to be beneficial for the preservation of lean mass across all sampled participants [97]. In addition to consuming a higher quantity of protein per meal, older adults should strive to maintain an even protein distribution across the day. In a longitudinal cohort investigation of free-living older adults, all participants lost lean body mass across the 2-year follow-up period. However, those who distributed their protein intake evenly across meals maintained more total and appendicular lean mass across the 2-year follow-up period. This remained true after adjusting for study confounders (e.g., BMI, age, and physical activity) [98]. A second investigation from this group also demonstrated that even mealtime distribution was associated with the preservation of muscular strength across a 3-year follow-up period in both men and women [99]. More recent work has also supported the association between protein distribution and preservation of LBM and physical functioning, reporting that a distributed protein intake resulted in higher gait speed compared to a skewed protein intake. Despite these promising findings, these investigations have reported that an even mealtime distribution of protein was unable to ameliorate losses in muscle mass.

The digestibility, amino acid profile, and leucine content of high-quality protein sources may be particularly important in older when compared to younger adults for stimulating MPS. In a randomized, counterbalanced single-trial investigation, older men were assigned to consume 0, 20, or 40 g of whey or soy protein isolate after a bout of lower-body unilateral resistance exercise. Interestingly, 20 g soy protein was insufficient to stimulate MPS above basal rates despite having similar total amino acid concentrations as 20 g of whey protein (which was able to stimulate MPS above basal rates) [100]. As mentioned previously, plant-based protein sources contain lower quantities of EAA compared to animal-based sources (in this case, the 20 and 40 g doses of soy protein have considerably less total EAA than whey), which partially explain the discrepancy in MPS stimulation. Moreover, elevations in blood leucine concentrations following both doses of soy protein were significantly less than the respective doses of whey protein. This data allude to the importance of protein digestibility and leucine/EAA content of consumed dietary proteins for older adults.

To date, there is minimal data regarding effective strategies to preserve muscle mass in the very old (those aged > 85 years). Franzke et al. [101] conducted a literature review on this and tentatively suggested that much older adults do not have significantly different MPS rates from older adults (those aged 55–85 years). Of note, these authors stress the interaction between a higher protein intake and regular physical activity for the preservation of physical function in this age group [101].

Impact of leucine on muscle mass maintenance in older adults

In conjunction with the increased protein requirements, older adults require a greater amount of leucine to stimulate MPS. One group reported that while 6.7 g EAAs with 1.7 g leucine did not result in significant stimulation of MPS above basal rates, the same total EAA dose with a higher proportion of leucine (2.7 g) resulted in elevations in MPS rates and muscle protein balance similar to those achieved by younger adults [102]. Moreover, a similar dose of 20 g protein bolus enriched with 2.5 g leucine further stimulated rates of MPS above that observed without the leucine enrichment older adults [103]. These findings are further supported by Koopman et al. [58], who reported similar high-dose leucine ingestion among younger and older adults.

While acute coingestion of leucine has been demonstrated to support increases in MPS, chronic ingestion does not appear to support longitudinal increases in muscle mass and strength. For example, a 24-week intervention providing $7.5\,g\,day^{-1}$ (2.5 g provided at each meal) of leucine was unable to augment muscle mass or strength in older adults with type-2 diabetes [104]. Other investigations lasting between 3 and 6 months among healthy and diseased older populations have also reported no increases in LBM after chronic leucine supplementation at doses ranging from 2.3 to $16.1\,g\,day^{-1}$ [105]. These longitudinal data allude to the idea that EAA supplementation—while the key to supporting LBM—is limited in its capacity to support lean mass changes in free-living older adults, particularly when a healthy eating pattern with adequate quantities of high-quality protein is consumed. Comprehensive approaches that include regular physical activity and minimizing sedentary behavior should be considered in conjunction with higher protein intake to supporting muscle mass maintenance.

Dietary approaches to preserving and gaining muscle mass in those with sarcopenia

Having addressed the primary dietary variables that influence muscle protein turnover and how this is altered in older adults, it is important to understand strategies implemented for preservation in people with sarcopenia. Depending on the definition and screening criteria used, the prevalence of sarcopenia in older adults between 65 and 70 years can range from 5% to 13% and increases considerably to 11%–50% in those ≥ 80 years of age [3, 106]. To date, several definitions for sarcopenia have been proposed and used by investigators and clinicians. Consensus papers from the European Working Group on Sarcopenia in Older People (EWGSOP) [107], the European Society for Clinical Nutrition and Metabolism Special Interest Groups (ESPEN-SIG) [108], and the International Working Group on Sarcopenia (IWGS) [109] have all published a definition of sarcopenia and testing methods for screening for the onset of sarcopenia. More recently, the EWGSOP has published a revised definition of sarcopenia with associated resources to assess and diagnose sarcopenia [110]. Generally speaking, sarcopenia is a syndrome characterized by the progressive and generalized loss of skeletal muscle mass and strength with a risk of adverse outcomes, such as the increased chance of falls, physical disability, and loss of autonomy [3]. Interest groups have demonstrated that sarcopenia is preceded by low levels of measures of muscle strength (i.e., low handgrip, muscle quantity/quality, and slow gait speed) [110, 111]. Furthermore, sarcopenia can lead to the development of, or be exacerbated by, other comorbidities such as obesity, osteoporosis, type-2 diabetes, and insulin resistance.

Strategies to treat and prevent sarcopenia can depend on how the individual developed sarcopenia. To assist clinicians in distinguishing the different variations of sarcopenia, EWGSOP has developed definitions of primary and secondary classifications of sarcopenia. Primary sarcopenia is present when the syndrome is developed solely due to the result of aging, while secondary sarcopenia is the result of other comorbidities not associated with aging (e.g., obesity and osteoporosis) [107]. Moreover, the EWGSOP has published conceptual staging criteria for investigators and clinicians to assess the progression of sarcopenia in a patient. The first stage, presarcopenia, is characterized by low muscle mass without the impact on muscle strength or physical performance. The second and third stages are characterized by low muscle mass and either low muscle strength or low physical performance (sarcopenia) or both (severe sarcopenia) [107]. Ultimately, these stages and categorizations of the sarcopenia spectrum may help clinicians and investigators select treatments and set appropriate and achievable recovery goals [3].

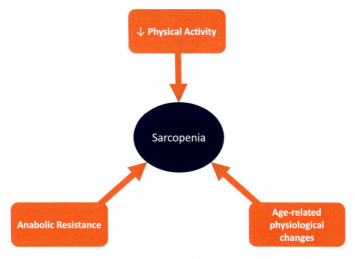

Fig. 2
The development of sarcopenia is multifactorial and can develop from numerous lifestyle changes. Older adults have been shown to reduce their habitual exercise regimens and consume a lower quantity of protein, further exacerbating anabolic resistance. Sarcopenia can also result from inflammatory disease, disuse, or endocrine disorders. These conditions may further accelerate the onset of age-related sarcopenia.

The etiology of sarcopenia is not currently well understood, but can be attributed to numerous changes in skeletal muscle physiology that include (1) a reduction in muscle fiber count, (2) a loss of type-II (fast-twitch) muscle fibers, (3) a decline in satellite cell quality and function, (4) an increase in skeletal muscle protein breakdown rate, and (5) a decrease in the production of anabolic hormones [30]. Sarcopenia is also believed to be accelerated by the decline of physical activity and changes in lifestyle that negatively impact mass maintenance (Fig. 2) [3, 106]. Indeed, a review conducted by Janssen [106] determined that the association between sarcopenia and the decline in physical function is moderate to strong. Moreover, older adults have been shown to consume inadequate amounts of dietary protein to sustain and preserve skeletal muscle mass [112]. In turn, investigators have dedicated efforts to using dietary approaches to offset the loss of skeletal muscle mass and preserve physical functioning.

Dietary protein and amino acid interventions in older adults with sarcopenia

Dietary approaches to offset skeletal muscle mass losses from sarcopenia have primarily focused on implementing short- and long-term interventions that primarily provide protein and EAA mixtures. In a double-blind, randomized control trial, adults aged above 65 years consumed either a placebo drink (no protein, 7.1 g lactose, 0.4 g calcium) or a protein supplement (15 g protein, 7.1 g lactose, 0.4 g calcium) twice per day for 24 weeks and completed resistance exercise twice per week. Protein supplementation did not increase skeletal muscle mass or change skeletal muscle fiber type composition. However, investigators did observe an improvement in muscular strength and physical performance [113]. A separate study supplementing a habitual diet with 210 g day^{-1} of ricotta cheese (17.8 g protein, 18.4 g fat, 10.4 g carbohydrates) for 3 months was successful at increasing lean body mass, muscle strength, and insulin sensitivity in sarcopenic older adults aged > 60 years [114]. Similar results in muscular strength and body composition were also achieved in sarcopenic Malaysian older adults consuming a soy protein-enriched diet (20 g for women, 40 g for men) for 12 weeks [115].

In another study, participants were randomized to four groups: (1) amino acid supplementation only, (2) exercise training only, (3) supplementation plus exercise, or (4) health education (once per month, three times total). Results from this investigation found that participants in the exercise/EAA group increased skeletal muscle mass, muscular strength, and walking speed, while EAA supplementation alone failed to yield any benefit [116]. A leucine- and vitamin D-enriched whey protein supplement has also been shown to be effective at promoting lean body mass [117].

In addition to the supplementing with leucine, investigators have attempted to elicit favorable lean mass changes with the leucine metabolite β-hydroxy-β-methyl butyrate (HMB). Healthy older men and women < 70 years old in a double-blind, randomized trial were assigned to consume either HMB or a placebo supplement containing rice flour for 8 weeks. Supplement capsules were consumed three times per day, resulting in an intake of 3 g day^{-1} of either HMB or placebo. All participants completed a multicomponent exercise intervention consisting of walking, stretching, and strength training. Results in this investigation suggest that HMB is capable of producing favorable changes in body composition, as participants increased skeletal muscle mass and reduced body fat percentage [118].

Despite the promising findings of these investigations, the current body of literature is not in consensus about the impact of protein/EAA on skeletal muscle mass preservation and improvement. A metaanalysis of studies using dietary and exercise interventions together found that studies using dietary protein interventions are inconsistent in their methods, dietary interventions, and intervention durations [119]. Indeed, the interventions included in this metaanalysis used protein supplement intakes of varying doses and EAA compositions. Additionally, there is no standardized intake protocol among these studies—some studies provided the supplement immediately after exercise, while others provide the supplements at breakfast and lunch. Moreover, the majority of these investigations did not make an effort to standardize the nutritional intake of participants (i.e., participants were allowed to consume their habitual intake).

Despite these discrepancies in the literature, it is abundantly clear that dietary protein intake is a key factor in the maintenance of skeletal muscle mass for individuals with sarcopenia. To this end, special interest groups have synthesized these findings and produced nutritional and exercise interventions for patients with sarcopenia. The Society of Sarcopenia, Cachexia, and Wasting disorders recommend protein intakes of 1.0–1.5 g kg^{-1} day^{-1} [120].

Conclusions and future work

The evidence presented in this chapter has highlighted the complexities and variables involved with maintaining skeletal muscle mass at all stages of life, but particularly those in the later stages of life and those with sarcopenia. Investigators and clinicians must overcome the metabolic limitations faced by older adults, which included systemic low-grade inflammation, impaired anabolic signaling, and increased rates of MPB. Work conducted by various research teams has clarified the role that dietary protein digestibility, leucine/EAA content, protein quantity, and the role of protein distribution on net protein balance and muscle mass preservation. When implemented individually, each feeding variable has produced positive results in both younger and older adults. That said, certain feeding variables play a more significant role in the older adult population. It is clear that the RDA is not optimal to support muscle mass in all older adults. It is also clear that the digestibility of the protein, quality of protein consumed (e.g., greater leucine and EAA content), and maintaining an even protein distribution across the day play a significant role in preserving skeletal muscle mass and quality of life in this population. Many investigations have demonstrated limited gains in muscle mass, muscular strength, and functional capacity when intervening with diet alone.

Dietary habits are only part of the equation. Investigations implementing exercise interventions in addition to the dietary interventions promoted greater stimulation of MPS and contributed more substantial long-term gains in LBM and functional capacity. As such, it is imperative that investigators and healthcare professionals promote the adoption of regular, structured exercise (e.g., resistance exercise) to maintain and preserve skeletal muscle in older adults and those with sarcopenia. Doing so would preserve functional capacity and independence in the later stages of life. More importantly, the data presented in this chapter allude to the importance of building and maintaining as much LBM as possible in the early stages of life. Those with poor dietary protein intake and low physical activity levels during the first portion of life are more likely to experience greater muscle mass losses into advanced age, placing them at greater risk for chronic disease and loss of functional capacity.

Despite the considerable knowledgebase obtained on the topic of skeletal muscle mass preservation over the last few decades, there are still gaps in our understanding that require further investigation. First, our current understanding of dietary protein quality is largely founded on isolated protein sources (e.g., whey and casein). Future work should explore the impact of whole-food protein sources on rates of muscle protein synthesis and breakdown in young and older adults. Doing so would provide more translatable dietary recommendations. Our current understanding of the muscle protein synthetic and breakdown response at rest and after an anabolic trigger is limited in those with sarcopenia. If the current methods used to directly measure MPS and MPB can be safely implemented in this special population, future studies should directly measure MPS/MPB, as well as muscle fiber composition, in those with sarcopenia. A considerable limitation to the current body of literature is the various feeding and exercise methodologies used. In turn, the lack of standardization can complicate the dissemination and implementation of these findings into the clinical and general populations. Researchers should consider standardizing the experimental methods used for feed protein/EAA and assess protein quality. Finally, future work should aim to clarify the underlying causes of anabolic resistance in older adults.

These data presented have encouraging implications for future strategies aimed at enhancing skeletal muscle mass and quality across general and clinical populations. Particularly, dietary protein quantity and quality is an easily modifiable variable that can be adapted to anabolically resistant populations and patients who suffer from muscle wasting. That said, maintaining sound nutritional and exercise habits is a key factor for the preservation of skeletal muscle mass across the lifespan. Both have the potential to improve the quality of life and general well-being.

References

[1] Kim IY, Suh SH, Lee IK, Wolfe RR. Applications of stable, nonradioactive isotope tracers in in vivo human metabolic research. Exp Mol Med 2016;48. https://doi.org/10.1038/emm.2015.97, e203.

[2] Breen L, Phillips SM. Skeletal muscle protein metabolism in the elderly: interventions to counteract the "anabolic resistance" of ageing. Nutr Metab (Lond) 2011;8:68. https://doi.org/10.1186/1743-7075-8-68.

[3] Santilli V, Bernetti A, Mangone M, Paoloni M. Clinical definition of sarcopenia. Clin Cases Miner Bone Metab 2014;11:177–80. https://doi.org/10.11138/ccmbm/2014.11.3.177.

[4] Anon. Dietary protein quality evaluation in human nutrition. Report of an FAQ Expert Consultation. FAO Food Nutr Pap 2013;92:1–66.

[5] Huang S, Wang LM, Sivendiran T, Bohrer BM. Review: amino acid concentration of high protein food products and an overview of the current methods used to determine protein quality. Crit Rev Food Sci Nutr 2018;58:2673–8. https://doi.org/10.1080/10408398.2017.1396202.

[6] Phillips SM. Current concepts and unresolved questions in dietary protein requirements and supplements in adults. Front Nutr 2017;4:13. https://doi.org/10.3389/fnut.2017.00013.

[7] Hodgkinson SM, Montoya CA, Scholten PT, Rutherfurd SM, Moughan PJ. Cooking conditions affect the true ileal digestible amino acid content and digestible indispensable amino acid score (DIAAS) of bovine meat as determined in pigs. J Nutr 2018;148:1564–9. https://doi.org/10.1093/jn/nxy153.

[8] Marinangeli CPF, House JD. Potential impact of the digestible indispensable amino acid score as a measure of protein quality on dietary regulations and health. Nutr Rev 2017;75:658–67. https://doi.org/10.1093/nutrit/nux025.

[9] Burd NA, McKenna CF, Salvador AF, Paulussen KJM, Moore DR. Dietary protein quantity, quality, and exercise are key to healthy living: a muscle-centric perspective across the lifespan. Front Nutr 2019;6:83. https://doi.org/10.3389/fnut.2019.00083.

[10] Wolfe RR, Rutherfurd SM, Kim IY, Moughan PJ. Protein quality as determined by the digestible indispensable amino acid score: evaluation of factors underlying the calculation. Nutr Rev 2016;74:584–99. https://doi.org/10.1093/nutrit/nuw022.

[11] Leitzmann C. Vegetarian nutrition: past, present, future. Am J Clin Nutr 2014;100:496S–502S. https://doi.org/10.3945/ajcn.113.071365.

[12] Daniel CR, Cross AJ, Koebnick C, Sinha R. Trends in meat consumption in the USA. Public Health Nutr 2011;14:575–83. https://doi.org/10.1017/S1368980010002077.

[13] Delgado CL. Rising consumption of meat and milk in developing countries has created a new food revolution. J Nutr 2003;133:3907S–10S. https://doi.org/10.1093/jn/133.11.3907S.

[14] Pasiakos SM, Agarwal S, Lieberman HR, Fulgoni VL. Sources and amounts of animal, dairy, and plant protein intake of US adults in 2007–2010. Nutrients 2015;7:7058–69. https://doi.org/10.3390/nu7085322.

[15] Camilleri GM, Verger EO, Huneau JF, Carpentier F, Dubuisson C, Mariotti F. Plant and animal protein intakes are differently associated with nutrient adequacy of the diet of French adults. J Nutr 2013;143:1466–73. https://doi.org/10.3945/jn.113.177113.

[16] Lin Y, Bolca S, Vandevijvere S, De Vriese S, Mouratidou T, De Neve M, et al. Plant and animal protein intake and its association with overweight and obesity among the Belgian population. Br J Nutr 2011;105:1106–16. https://doi.org/10.1017/S0007114510004642.

[17] U.S. Department of Health and Human Services and U.S. Department of Agriculture. Dietary guidelines for Americans. 8th ed. U.S. Government Printing Office; 2015.

[18] U.S. Department of Health and Human Services and U.S. Department of Agriculture. Dietary guidelines for Americans. 7th ed. Washington, DC: U.S. Government Printing Office; 2010.

[19] O'Neil CE, Keast DR, Nicklas TA, Fulgoni VL. Out-of-hand nut consumption is associated with improved nutrient intake and health risk markers in US children and adults: National Health and Nutrition Examination Survey 1999-2004. Nutr Res 2012;32:185–94. https://doi.org/10.1016/j.nutres.2012.01.005.

[20] O'Neil CE, Nicklas TA, Fulgoni VL. Tree nut consumption is associated with better nutrient adequacy and diet quality in adults: National Health and Nutrition Examination Survey 2005–2010. Nutrients 2015;7:595–607. https://doi.org/10.3390/nu7010595.

[21] Bibiloni MDM, Julibert A, Bouzas C, Martínez-González MA, Corella D, Salas-Salvadó J, et al. Nut consumptions as a marker of higher diet quality in a mediterranean population at high cardiovascular risk. Nutrients 2019;11:754. https://doi.org/10.3390/nu11040754.

[22] Papanikolaou Y, Fulgoni VL. Bean consumption is associated with greater nutrient intake, reduced systolic blood pressure, lower body weight, and a smaller waist circumference in adults: results from the National Health and Nutrition Examination Survey 1999-2002. J Am Coll Nutr 2008;27:569–76. https://doi.org/10.1080/07315724.2008.10719740.

[23] Wolfe RR, Baum JI, Starck C, Moughan PJ. Factors contributing to the selection of dietary protein food sources. Clin Nutr 2018;37:130–8. https://doi.org/10.1016/j.clnu.2017.11.017.

[24] Istfan N, Murray E, Janghorbani M, Young VR. An evaluation of the nutritional value of a soy protein concentrate in young adult men using the short-term N-balance method. J Nutr 1983;113:2516–23. https://doi.org/10.1093/jn/113.12.2516.

[25] Wayler A, Queiroz E, Scrimshaw NS, Steinke FH, Rand WM, Young VR. Nitrogen balance studies in young men to assess the protein quality of an isolated soy protein in relation to meat proteins. J Nutr 1983;113:2485–91. https://doi.org/10.1093/jn/113.12.2485.

[26] Scrimshaw NS, Wayler A, Murray E, Steinke FH, Rand WM, Young VR. Nitrogen balance response in young men given one of two isolated soy proteins or milk proteins. J Nutr 1983;113:2492–7. https://doi.org/10.1093/jn/113.12.2492.

[27] Wilkinson SB, Tarnopolsky MA, MacDonald MJ, MacDonald JR, Armstrong D, Phillips SM. Consumption of fluid skim milk promotes greater muscle protein accretion after resistance exercise than does consumption of an isonitrogenous and isoenergetic soy-protein beverage. Am J Clin Nutr 2007;85:1031–40. https://doi.org/10.1093/ajcn/85.4.1031.

[28] Hartman JW, Tang JE, Wilkinson SB, Tarnopolsky MA, Lawrence RL, Fullerton AV, et al. Consumption of fat-free fluid milk after resistance exercise promotes greater lean mass accretion than does consumption of soy or carbohydrate in young, novice, male weightlifters. Am J Clin Nutr 2007;86:373–81. https://doi.org/10.1093/ajcn/86.2.373.

[29] Volek JS, Volk BM, Gómez AL, Kunces LJ, Kupchak BR, Freidenreich DJ, et al. Whey protein supplementation during resistance training augments lean body mass. J Am Coll Nutr 2013;32:122–35. https://doi.org/10.1080/07315724.2013.793580.

[30] Candow DG. Sarcopenia: current theories and the potential beneficial effect of creatine application strategies. Biogerontology 2011;12:273–81. https://doi.org/10.1007/s10522-011-9327-6.

[31] Mathai JK, Liu Y, Stein HH. Values for digestible indispensable amino acid scores (DIAAS) for some dairy and plant proteins may better describe protein quality than values calculated using the concept for protein digestibility-corrected amino acid scores (PDCAAS). Br J Nutr 2017;117:490–9. https://doi.org/10.1017/S0007114517000125.

[32] Ertl P, Steinwidder A, Schönauer M, Krimberger K, Knaus W, Zollitsch W. Net food production of different livestock: a national analysis for Austria including relative occupation of different land categories/Netto-Lebensmittelproduktion der Nutztierhaltung: Eine nationale Analyse für Österreich inklusive relativer Flächenbea. Die Bodenkultur J L Manage Food Environ 2016;67:91–103. https://doi.org/10.1515/boku-2016-0009.

[33] van Vliet S, Burd NA, van Loon LJC. The skeletal muscle anabolic response to plant- versus animal-based protein consumption. J Nutr 2015;145:1981–91. https://doi.org/10.3945/jn.114.204305.

[34] Phillips SM, Fulgoni VL, Heaney RP, Nicklas TA, Slavin JL, Weaver CM. Commonly consumed protein foods contribute to nutrient intake, diet quality, and nutrient adequacy. Am J Clin Nutr 2015;101:1346S–52S. https://doi.org/10.3945/ajcn.114.084079.

[35] ter Borg S, Verlaan S, Hemsworth J, Mijnarends DM, Schols JMGA, Luiking YC, et al. Micronutrient intakes and potential inadequacies of community-dwelling older adults: a systematic review. Br J Nutr 2015;113:1195–206. https://doi.org/10.1017/S0007114515000203.

[36] Burd NA, Gorissen SH, Van Vliet S, Snijders T, Van Loon LJC. Differences in postprandial protein handling after beef compared with milk ingestion during postexercise recovery: a randomized controlled trial. Am J Clin Nutr 2015;102:828–36. https://doi.org/10.3945/ajcn.114.103184.

[37] Josse AR, Tang JE, Tarnopolsky MA, Phillips SM. Body composition and strength changes in women with milk and resistance exercise. Med Sci Sports Exerc 2010;42:1122–30. https://doi.org/10.1249/MSS.0b013e3181c854f6.

[38] Candow DG, Burke NC, Smith-Palmer T, Burke DG. Effect of whey and soy protein supplementation combined with resistance training in young adults. Int J Sport Nutr Exerc Metab 2006;16:233–44. https://doi.org/10.1123/ijsnem.16.3.233.

[39] Van Vliet S, Shy EL, Sawan SA, Beals JW, West DWD, Skinner SK, et al. Consumption of whole eggs promotes greater stimulation of postexercise muscle protein synthesis than consumption of isonitrogenous amounts of egg whites in young men. Am J Clin Nutr 2017;106:1401–12. https://doi.org/10.3945/ajcn.117.159855.

[40] Leenders M, van Loon LJ. Leucine as a pharmaconutrient to prevent and treat sarcopenia and type 2 diabetes. Nutr Rev 2011;69:675–89. https://doi.org/10.1111/j.1753-4887.2011.00443.x.

[41] Buse MG, Reid SS. Leucine. A possible regulator of protein turnover in muscle. J Clin Invest 1975;56:1250–61. https://doi.org/10.1172/JCI108201.

[42] Chang Hong S-O, Layman DK. Effects of leucine on in vitro protein synthesis and degradation in rat skeletal muscles. J Nutr 1984;114:1204–12. https://doi.org/10.1093/jn/114.7.1204.

[43] Li JB, Jefferson LS. Influence of amino acid availability on protein turnover in perfused skeletal muscle. BBA-Gen Subjects 1978;544:351–9. https://doi.org/10.1016/0304-4165(78)90103-4.

[44] Burnett PE, Barrow RK, Cohen NA, Snyder SH, Sabatini DM. RAFT1 phosphorylation of the translational regulators p70 S6 kinase and 4E-BP1. Proc Natl Acad Sci U S A 1998;95:1432–7. https://doi.org/10.1073/pnas.95.4.1432.

[45] Anthony JC, Anthony TG, Kimball SR, Vary TC, Jefferson LS. Orally administered leucine stimulates protein synthesis in skeletal muscle of postabsorptive rats in association with increased eIF4F formation. J Nutr 2000;130:139–45. https://doi.org/10.1093/jn/130.2.139.

[46] Anthony JC, Yoshizawa F, Anthony TG, Vary TC, Jefferson LS, Kimball SR. Leucine stimulates translation initiation skeletal muscle of postabsorptive rats via a rapamycin-sensitive pathway. J Nutr 2000;130:2413–9. https://doi.org/10.1093/jn/130.10.2413.

[47] Bolster DR, Vary TC, Kimball SR, Jefferson LS. Leucine regulates translation initiation in rat skeletal muscle via enhanced eIF4G phosphorylation. J Nutr 2004;134:1704–10. https://doi.org/10.1093/jn/134.7.1704.

[48] Crozier SJ, Kimball SR, Emmert SW, Anthony JC, Jefferson LS. Oral leucine administration stimulates protein synthesis in rat skeletal muscle. J Nutr 2005;135:376–82. https://doi.org/10.1093/jn/135.3.376.

[49] Atherton PJ, Smith K, Etheridge T, Rankin D, Rennie MJ. Distinct anabolic signalling responses to amino acids in C2C12 skeletal muscle cells. Amino Acids 2010;38:1533–9. https://doi.org/10.1007/s00726-009-0377-x.

[50] Garlick PJ. The role of leucine in the regulation of protein metabolism. J Nutr 2005;135:1553S–6S. https://doi.org/10.1093/jn/135.6.1553s.

[51] Mordier S, Deval C, Béchet D, Tassa A, Ferrara M. Leucine limitation induces autophagy and activation of lysosome-dependent proteolysis in C2C12 myotubes through a mammalian target of rapamycin-independent signaling pathway. J Biol Chem 2000;275:29900–6. https://doi.org/10.1074/jbc.M003633200.

[52] Nakashima K, Ishida A, Yamazaki M, Abe H. Leucine suppresses myofibrillar proteolysis by down-regulating ubiquitin-proteasome pathway in chick skeletal muscles. Biochem Biophys Res Commun 2005;336:660–6. https://doi.org/10.1016/j.bbrc.2005.08.138.

[53] Glynn EL, Fry CS, Drummond MJ, Timmerman KL, Dhanani S, Volpi E, et al. Excess leucine intake enhances muscle anabolic signaling but not net protein anabolism in young men and women. J Nutr 2010;140:1970–6. https://doi.org/10.3945/jn.110.127647.

[54] Wilkinson DJ, Hossain T, Hill DS, Phillips BE, Crossland H, Williams J, et al. Effects of leucine and its metabolite β-hydroxy-β-methylbutyrate on human skeletal muscle protein metabolism. J Physiol 2013;591:2911–23. https://doi.org/10.1113/jphysiol.2013.253203.

[55] Paddon-Jones D, Sheffield-Moore M, Zhang XJ, Volpi E, Wolf SE, Aarsland A, et al. Amino acid ingestion improves muscle protein synthesis in the young and elderly. Am J Physiol Endocrinol Metab 2004;286:E321–8. https://doi.org/10.1152/ajpendo.00368.2003.

[56] Katsanos CS, Kobayashi H, Sheffield-Moore M, Aarsland A, Wolfe RR. Aging is associated with diminished accretion of muscle proteins after the ingestion of a small bolus of essential amino acids. Am J Clin Nutr 2005;82:1065–73. https://doi.org/10.1093/ajcn/82.5.1065.

[57] van Vliet S, Smith GI, Porter L, Ramaswamy R, Reeds DN, Okunade AL, et al. The muscle anabolic effect of protein ingestion during a hyperinsulinaemic euglycaemic clamp in middle-aged women is not caused by leucine alone. J Physiol 2018;596:4681–92. https://doi.org/10.1113/JP276504.

[58] Koopman R, Verdijk L, Manders RJF, Gijsen AP, Gorselink M, Pijpers E, et al. Co-ingestion of protein and leucine stimulates muscle protein synthesis rates to the same extent in young and elderly lean men. Am J Clin Nutr 2006;84:623–32. https://doi.org/10.1093/ajcn/84.3.623.

[59] Burd NA, Phillips SM. Fast whey protein and the leucine trigger. Nutrafoods 2010;9:7–11. https://doi.org/10.1007/bf03223343.

[60] Burd NA, Beals JW, Martinez IG, Salvador AF, Skinner SK. Food-first approach to enhance the regulation of post-exercise skeletal muscle protein synthesis and remodeling. Sports Med 2019;49:59–68. https://doi.org/10.1007/s40279-018-1009-y.

[61] WHO. Protein and amino acid requirements in human nutrition [Report of a Joint WHO/FAO/UNU Expert Consultation]. Geneva: WHO; 2007.

[62] Phillips SM, Chevalier S, Leidy HJ. Protein "requirements" beyond the RDA: implications for optimizing health. Appl Physiol Nutr Metab 2016;41:565–72. https://doi.org/10.1139/apnm-2015-0550.

[63] Phillips SM, van Loon LJC. Dietary protein for athletes: from requirements to optimum adaptation. J Sports Sci 2011;29:S29–38. https://doi.org/10.1080/02640414.2011.619204.

[64] Phillips SM, Tipton KD, Aarsland A, Wolf SE, Wolfe RR. Mixed muscle protein synthesis and breakdown after resistance exercise in humans. Am J Physiol Endocrinol Metab 1997;273. https://doi.org/10.1152/ajpendo.1997.273.1.e99.

[65] Moore DR, Camera DM, Areta JL, Hawley JA. Beyond muscle hypertrophy: why dietary protein is important for endurance athletes. Appl Physiol Nutr Metab 2014;39:987–97. https://doi.org/10.1139/apnm-2013-0591.

[66] Pennings B, Koopman R, Beelen M, Senden JMG, Saris WHM, Van Loon LJC. Exercising before protein intake allows for greater use of dietary protein-derived amino acids for de novo muscle protein synthesis in both young and elderly men. Am J Clin Nutr 2011;93:322–31. https://doi.org/10.3945/ajcn.2010.29649.

[67] Moore DR, Del Bel NC, Nizi KI, Hartman JW, Tang JE, Armstrong D, et al. Resistance training reduces fasted- and fed-state leucine turnover and increases dietary nitrogen retention in previously untrained young men. J Nutr 2007;137:985–91. https://doi.org/10.1093/jn/137.4.985.

[68] Biolo G, Tipton KD, Klein S, Wolfe RR. An abundant supply of amino acids enhances the metabolic effect of exercise on muscle protein. Am J Physiol Endocrinol Metab 1997;273. https://doi.org/10.1152/ajpendo.1997.273.1.e122.

[69] Wall BT, Burd NA, Franssen R, Gorissen SHM, Snijders T, Senden JM, et al. Presleep protein ingestion does not compromise the muscle protein synthetic response to protein ingested the following morning. Am J Physiol Endocrinol Metab 2016;311:E964–73. https://doi.org/10.1152/ajpendo.00325.2016.

[70] Moore DR, Robinson MJ, Fry JL, Tang JE, Glover EI, Wilkinson SB, et al. Ingested protein dose response of muscle and albumin protein synthesis after resistance exercise in young men. Am J Clin Nutr 2009;89:161–8. https://doi.org/10.3945/ajcn.2008.26401.

[71] Felig P, Wahren J. Amino acid metabolism in exercising man. J Clin Invest 1971;50:2703–14. https://doi.org/10.1172/JCI106771.

[72] Haralambie G, Berg A. Serum urea and amino nitrogen changes with exercise duration. Eur J Appl Physiol Occup Physiol 1976;36:39–48. https://doi.org/10.1007/BF00421632.

[73] McKenzie S, Phillips SM, Carter SL, Lowther S, Gibala MJ, Tarnopolsky MA. Endurance exercise training attenuates leucine oxidation and BCOAD activation during exercise in humans. Am J Physiol Endocrinol Metab 2000;278:E580–7. https://doi.org/10.1152/ajpendo.2000.278.4.e580.

[74] American College of Sports Medicine, American Dietetics Association, Dietitians of Canada. Nutrition and athletic performance. Med Sci Sports Exerc 2009;41:709–31. https://doi.org/10.1249/MSS.0b013e31890eb86.

[75] Burd NA, Gorissen SH, Van Loon LJC. Anabolic resistance of muscle protein synthesis with aging. Exerc Sport Sci Rev 2013;41:169–73. https://doi.org/10.1097/JES.0b013e318292f3d5.

[76] Jäger R, Kerksick CM, Campbell BI, Cribb PJ, Wells SD, Skwiat TM, et al. International society of sports nutrition position stand: protein and exercise. J Int Soc Sports Nutr 2017;14:20. https://doi.org/10.1186/s12970-017-0177-8.

[77] Helms ER, Zinn C, Rowlands DS, Brown SR. A systematic review of dietary protein during caloric restriction in resistance trained lean athletes: a case for higher intakes. Int J Sport Nutr Exerc Metab 2014;24:127–38. https://doi.org/10.1123/ijsnem.2013-0054.

[78] Hudson JL, Wang Y, Bergia III RE, Campbell WW. Protein intake greater than the RDA differentially influences whole-body lean mass responses to purposeful catabolic and anabolic stressors: a systematic review and meta-analysis. Adv Nutr 2020;11:548–58. https://doi.org/10.1093/advances/nmz106.

[79] Paddon-Jones D, Rasmussen BB. Dietary protein recommendations and the prevention of sarcopenia. Curr Opin Clin Nutr Metab Care 2009;12:86–90. https://doi.org/10.1097/MCO.0b013e32831cef8b.

[80] Volpi E, Kobayashi H, Sheffield-Moore M, Mittendorfer B, Wolfe RR. Essential amino acids are primarily responsible for the amino acid stimulation of muscle protein anabolism in healthy elderly adults. Am J Clin Nutr 2003;78:250–8. https://doi.org/10.1093/ajcn/78.2.250.

[81] Mamerow MM, Mettler JA, English KL, Casperson SL, Arentson-Lantz E, Sheffield-Moore M, et al. Dietary protein distribution positively influences 24-h muscle protein synthesis in healthy adults. J Nutr 2014;144:876–80. https://doi.org/10.3945/jn.113.185280.

[82] Kim IY, Schutzler S, Schrader A, Spencer H, Kortebein P, Deutz NEP, et al. Quantity of dietary protein intake, but not pattern of intake, affects net protein balance primarily through differences in protein synthesis in older adults. Am J Physiol Endocrinol Metab 2015;308:E21–8. https://doi.org/10.1152/ajpendo.00382.2014.

[83] Kim IY, Schutzler S, Schrader AM, Spencer HJ, Azhar G, Wolfe RR, et al. Protein intake distribution pattern does not affect anabolic response, lean body mass, muscle strength or function over 8 weeks in older adults: a randomized-controlled trial. Clin Nutr 2018;37:488–93. https://doi.org/10.1016/j.clnu.2017.02.020.

[84] Deer RR, Volpi E. Protein intake and muscle function in older adults. Curr Opin Clin Nutr Metab Care 2015;18:248–53. https://doi.org/10.1097/MCO.0000000000000162.

[85] Morton RW, Traylor DA, Weijs PJM, Phillips SM. Defining anabolic resistance: implications for delivery of clinical care nutrition. Curr Opin Crit Care 2018;24:124–30. https://doi.org/10.1097/MCC.0000000000000488.

[86] Haran PH, Rivas DA, Fielding RA. Role and potential mechanisms of anabolic resistance in sarcopenia. J Cachexia Sarcopenia Muscle 2012;3:157–62. https://doi.org/10.1007/s13539-012-0068-4.

[87] Markofski MM, Dickinson JM, Drummond MJ, Fry CS, Fujita S, Gundermann DM, et al. Effect of age on basal muscle protein synthesis and mTORC1 signaling in a large cohort of young and older men and women. Exp Gerontol 2015;65:1–7. https://doi.org/10.1016/j.exger.2015.02.015.

[88] Cuthbertson D, Smith K, Babraj J, Leese G, Waddell T, Atherton P, et al. Anabolic signaling deficits underlie amino acid resistance of wasting, aging muscle. FASEB J 2005;19:1–22. https://doi.org/10.1096/fj.04-2640fje.

[89] Wall BT, Gorissen SH, Pennings B, Koopman R, Groen BBL, Verdijk LB, et al. Aging is accompanied by a blunted muscle protein synthetic response to protein ingestion. PLoS One 2015;10. https://doi.org/10.1371/journal.pone.0140903, e0140903.

[90] Campbell WW, Trappe TA, Jozsi AC, Kruskall LJ, Wolfe RR, Evans WJ. Dietary protein adequacy and lower body versus whole body resistive training in older humans. J Physiol 2002;542:631–42. https://doi.org/10.1113/jphysiol.2002.020685.

[91] Campbell WW, Trappe TA, Wolfe RR, Evans WJ. The recommended dietary allowance for protein may not be adequate for older people to maintain skeletal muscle. J Gerontol A: Biol Sci Med Sci 2001;56:M373–80. https://doi.org/10.1093/gerona/56.6.M373.

[92] Campbell WW. Synergistic use of higher-protein diets or nutritional supplements with resistance training to counter sarcopenia. Nutr Rev 2008;65:416–22. https://doi.org/10.1111/j.1753-4887.2007.tb00320.x.

[93] Houston DK, Nicklas BJ, Ding J, Harris TB, Tylavsky FA, Newman AB, et al. Dietary protein intake is associated with lean mass change in older, community-dwelling adults: the Health, Aging, and Body Composition (Health ABC) study. Am J Clin Nutr 2008;87:150–5. https://doi.org/10.1093/ajcn/87.1.150.

[94] Mitchell CJ, Milan AM, Mitchell SM, Zeng N, Ramzan F, Sharma P, et al. The effects of dietary protein intake on appendicular lean mass and muscle function in elderly men: a 10-wk randomized controlled trial. Am J Clin Nutr 2017;106:1375–83. https://doi.org/10.3945/ajcn.117.160325.

[95] Dillon EL, Sheffield-Moore M, Paddon-Jones D, Gilkison C, Sanford AP, Casperson SL, et al. Amino acid supplementation increases lean body mass, basal muscle protein synthesis, and insulin-like growth factor-I expression in older women. J Clin Endocrinol Metab 2009;94:1630–7. https://doi.org/10.1210/jc.2008-1564.

[96] Børsheim E, Bui QUT, Tissier S, Kobayashi H, Ferrando AA, Wolfe RR. Effect of amino acid supplementation on muscle mass, strength and physical function in elderly. Clin Nutr 2008;27:189–95. https://doi.org/10.1016/j.clnu.2008.01.001.

[97] Loenneke JP, Loprinzi PD, Murphy CH, Phillips SM. Per meal dose and frequency of protein consumption is associated with lean mass and muscle performance. Clin Nutr 2016;35:1506–11. https://doi.org/10.1016/j.clnu.2016.04.002.

[98] Farsijani S, Morais JA, Payette H, Gaudreau P, Shatenstein B, Gray-Donald K, et al. Relation between mealtime distribution of protein intake and lean mass loss in free-living older adults of the NuAge study. Am J Clin Nutr 2016;104:694–703. https://doi.org/10.3945/ajcn.116.130716.

[99] Farsijani S, Payette H, Morais JA, Shatenstein B, Gaudreau P, Chevalier S. Even mealtime distribution of protein intake is associated with greater muscle strength, but not with 3-y physical function decline, in free-living older adults: the Quebec longitudinal study on Nutrition as a Determinant of Successful Aging (NuAge study). Am J Clin Nutr 2017;106:113–24. https://doi.org/10.3945/ajcn.116.146555.

[100] Yang Y, Churchward-Venne TA, Burd NA, Breen L, Tarnopolsky MA, Phillips SM. Myofibrillar protein synthesis following ingestion of soy protein isolate at rest and after resistance exercise in elderly men. Nutr Metab 2012;9:57. https://doi.org/10.1186/1743-7075-9-57.

[101] Franzke B, Neubauer O, Cameron-Smith D, Wagner KH. Dietary protein, muscle and physical function in the very old. Nutrients 2018;10:935. https://doi.org/10.3390/nu10070935.

[102] Katsanos CS, Kobayashi H, Sheffield-Moore M, Aarsland A, Wolfe RR. A high proportion of leucine is required for optimal stimulation of the rate of muscle protein synthesis by essential amino acids in the elderly. Am J Physiol Endocrinol Metab 2006;291:E381–7. https://doi.org/10.1152/ajpendo.00488.2005.

[103] Wall BT, Hamer HM, de Lange A, Kiskini A, Groen BBL, Senden JMG, et al. Leucine co-ingestion improves post-prandial muscle protein accretion in elderly men. Clin Nutr 2013;32:412–9. https://doi.org/10.1016/j.clnu.2012.09.002.

[104] Leenders M, Verdijk LB, van der Hoeven L, van Kranenburg J, Hartgens F, Wodzig WKWH, et al. Prolonged leucine supplementation does not augment muscle mass or affect glycemic control in elderly type 2 diabetic men. J Nutr 2011;141:1070–6. https://doi.org/10.3945/jn.111.138495.

[105] Xu ZR, Tan ZJ, Zhang Q, Gui QF, Yang YM. The effectiveness of leucine on muscle protein synthesis, lean body mass and leg lean mass accretion in older people: a systematic review and meta-analysis. Br J Nutr 2015;113:25–34. https://doi.org/10.1017/S0007114514002475.

[106] Janssen I. The epidemiology of sarcopenia. Clin Geriatr Med 2011;27:355–63. https://doi.org/10.1016/j.cger.2011.03.004.

[107] Cruz-Jentoft AJ, Baeyens JP, Bauer JM, Boirie Y, Cederholm T, Landi F, et al. Sarcopenia: European consensus on definition and diagnosis. Age Ageing 2010;39:412–23. https://doi.org/10.1093/ageing/afq034.

[108] Muscaritoli M, Anker SD, Argilés J, Aversa Z, Bauer JM, Biolo G, et al. Consensus definition of sarcopenia, cachexia and pre-cachexia: joint document elaborated by Special Interest Groups (SIG) "cachexia-anorexia in chronic wasting diseases" and " nutrition in geriatrics". Clin Nutr 2010;29:154–9. https://doi.org/10.1016/j.clnu.2009.12.004.

[109] Fielding RA, Vellas B, Evans WJ, Bhasin S, Morley JE, Newman AB, et al. Sarcopenia: an undiagnosed condition in older adults. Current consensus definition: prevalence, etiology, and consequences. International working group on sarcopenia. J Am Med Dir Assoc 2011;12:249–56. https://doi.org/10.1016/j.jamda.2011.01.003.

[110] Cruz-Jentoft AJ, Bahat G, Bauer J, Boirie Y, Bruyère O, Cederholm T, et al. Sarcopenia: revised European consensus on definition and diagnosis. Age Ageing 2019;48:16–31. https://doi.org/10.1093/ageing/afy169.

[111] Bhasin S, Travison TG, Manini TM, Patel S, Pencina KM, Fielding RA, et al. Sarcopenia definition: the position statements of the sarcopenia definition and outcomes consortium. J Am Geriatr Soc 2020;68:1410–8. https://doi.org/10.1111/jgs.16372.

[112] Yanai H. Nutrition for sarcopenia. J Clin Med Res 2015;7:926–31. https://doi.org/10.14740/jocmr2361w.

[113] Tieland M, van de Rest O, Dirks ML, van der Zwaluw N, Mensink M, van Loon LJC, et al. Protein supplementation improves physical performance in frail elderly people: a randomized, double-blind, placebo-controlled trial. J Am Med Dir Assoc 2012;13:720–6. https://doi.org/10.1016/j.jamda.2012.07.005.

[114] Alemán-Mateo H, Macías L, Esparza-Romero J, Astiazaran-García H, Blancas AL. Physiological effects beyond the significant gain in muscle mass in sarcopenic elderly men: evidence from a randomized clinical trial using a protein-rich food. Clin Interv Aging 2012;7:225–34. https://doi.org/10.2147/CIA.S32356.

[115] Shahar S, Kamaruddin NS, Badrasawi M, Mohamed Sakian NI, Manaf ZA, Yassin Z, et al. Effectiveness of exercise and protein supplementation intervention on body composition, functional fitness, and oxidative stress among elderly Malays with sarcopenia. Clin Interv Aging 2013;8:1365–75. https://doi.org/10.2147/CIA.S46826.

[116] Kim HK, Suzuki T, Saito K, Yoshida H, Kobayashi H, Kato H, et al. Effects of exercise and amino acid supplementation on body composition and physical function in community-dwelling elderly Japanese sarcopenic women: a randomized controlled trial. J Am Geriatr Soc 2012;60:16–23. https://doi.org/10.1111/j.1532-5415.2011.03776.x.

[117] Bauer JM, Verlaan S, Bautmans I, Brandt K, Donini LM, Maggio M, et al. Effects of a vitamin D and leucine-enriched whey protein nutritional supplement on measures of sarcopenia in older adults, the PROVIDE study: a randomized, double-blind, placebo-controlled trial. J Am Med Dir Assoc 2015;16:740–7. https://doi.org/10.1016/j.jamda.2015.05.021.

[118] Vukovich MD, Stubbs NB, Bohlken RM. Body composition in 70-year-old adults responds to dietary β-hydroxy-β-methylbutyrate similarly to that of young adults. J Nutr 2001;131:2049–52. https://doi.org/10.1093/jn/131.7.2049.

[119] Denison HJ, Cooper C, Sayer AA, Robinson SM. Prevention and optimal management of sarcopenia: a review of combined exercise and nutrition interventions to improve muscle outcomes in older people. Clin Interv Aging 2015;10:859–69. https://doi.org/10.2147/CIA.S55842.

[120] Bauer J, Morley JE, Schols AMWJ, Ferrucci L, Cruz-Jentoft AJ, Dent E, et al. Sarcopenia: a time for action. An SCWD position paper. J Cachexia Sarcopenia Muscle 2019;10:956–61. https://doi.org/10.1002/jcsm.12483.

CHAPTER 4

Role of muscle stem cells in sarcopenia

Ryo Fujita
Division of Regenerative Medicine, Transborder Medical Research Center, University of Tsukuba, Tsukuba City, Ibaraki, Japan

Abstract
Sarcopenia, the progressive loss of skeletal muscle strength and mass with age, has a detrimental effect on the quality of life, including impaired mobility, increased risk of metabolic diseases, and even death. Although skeletal muscle fibers are postmitotic, skeletal muscle has a remarkable potential to regenerate after injury, which is mainly achieved by the resident muscle stem cells, called satellite cells. Although satellite cells are required for adult muscle regeneration and postnatal muscle growth, whether they are indispensable during skeletal muscle homeostasis and adaptations, including hypertrophy, atrophy and age-related sarcopenia, remains unclear. To fully understand the impact of satellite cells on sarcopenia, it is essential to understand their potential role in muscle fiber regeneration, homeostatic hypertrophy, and atrophy. In this chapter, we will provide an update on recent advances in research on the role of satellite cells during skeletal muscle adaptations and the development of age-related sarcopenia.

Keywords: Muscle stem cell, Satellite cell, Sarcopenia, Hypertrophy, Atrophy, Muscle regeneration

Introduction

Skeletal muscle is the most abundant tissue in the body, with remarkable diversity and plasticity, and is responsible for locomotion, energy storage, and metabolism. In recent decades, muscular dystrophies have been intensively studied and characterized with the aim of developing new therapies. Among these, Duchenne muscular dystrophy (DMD), a severe type of muscular dystrophy, is characterized by progressive muscle degeneration and muscle weakness due to the mutation of a protein called dystrophin, which stabilizes the plasma membrane of skeletal muscle fibers [1–3]. Skeletal muscle dysfunction is also associated with several multifactorial conditions, including cancer, arthritis, heart failure, diabetes mellitus, and aging [4, 5]. Skeletal muscle wasting is a significant factor in the loss of independence, eventually leading to the hospitalization of affected individuals, and is associated with an elevation of morbidity and mortality. According to the World Health Organization (WHO), the number of people aged 65 years and older will be around 1.5 billion by the year 2050, making disorders associated with muscle wasting an economic and societal burden across the world.

Sarcopenia is an age-related muscle disease associated with the loss of both skeletal muscle mass and muscle strength, compromising the well-being and life span of affected individuals [6]. During sarcopenia, muscle mass is lost due to both a loss of myofibers and a decrease in myofiber mass, with type II (fast-twitch) myofibers being particularly vulnerable [6, 7]. These changes are linked to alterations in mitochondrial energy metabolism and function, with the potential to affect the whole body metabolism, associated with type II diabetes [8–10]. Sarcopenic muscles also exhibit an accumulation of intramuscular connective tissues and excessive fat deposition with increased inflammation. The mechanisms responsible for the onset and development of sarcopenia are highly complex, and many factors are involved in this process. Therefore, understanding the biological mechanisms of sarcopenia and muscle homeostasis is crucial. In particular, stem cells that are capable of maintaining tissue integrity, regeneration, and development are an area of notable interest.

Skeletal muscle has a population of stem cells called satellite cells [11] that are essential for muscle regeneration. Satellite cells are located between the sarcolemma and the basal lamina of mature multinucleated myofibers (Fig. 1A and B). Although satellite cells are generally found in a quiescent state, they can become activated in response to injury to amplify a population of myogenic progenitors that then either differentiate into new myofibers or undergo self-renewal to restore their stem cell pool for the next round of injury. Although the central role of muscle stem cells in skeletal muscle regeneration and development is evident

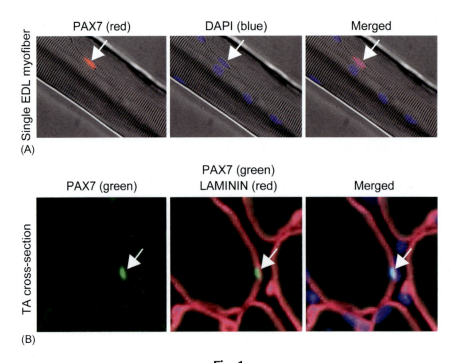

Fig. 1
Morphological and anatomical characteristics of satellite cells. (A) Quiescent satellite cell expressing Pax7 *(green)* on a myofiber. (B) Quiescent satellite cell on a transverse cross-section of tibialis anterior (TA) muscle. Satellite cells expressing Pax7 *(green)* are closely associated with myofibers, located within the basal lamina *(red)*. Nuclei are stained by DAPI *(blue)*.

and well established in the literature, particularly in studies using genetically modified mouse models, their role in skeletal muscle homeostasis, including the development of sarcopenia, is unclear. To fully understand the role of muscle stem cells on muscle homeostasis and age-related sarcopenia, it is essential to consider their potential role in different experimental models, including hypertrophy, atrophy, growth (prenatal vs postnatal), regeneration, and muscular dystrophies.

Although the mechanisms responsible for sarcopenia are not yet well established, there are many factors, including motor neurons, hormones, immune systems, nutrition, and muscle activity, that directly or indirectly contribute to muscle failure with aging [12–16]. These conditions include a decline in muscle stem function. In this review, we present the most recent findings in muscle stem cell biology for the different types of muscle adaptive conditions and discuss the potential impact of muscle stem cells on the maintenance of skeletal muscle mass and regenerative capacity with aging. Furthermore, their potential protective action against declines in skeletal muscle function with age is also discussed.

Muscle stem cells

Despite the fact that adult muscle fibers are terminally differentiated, adult muscles retain their ability to regenerate after severe injury. This extraordinary ability of skeletal muscles is generally associated with the presence of muscle stem cells, also known as satellite cells. They were first identified in 1961 as a unique population of cells found between the sarcolemma and the basement membrane of myofibers [11, 17]. Satellite cells are derived from somites expressing the paired homeobox transcriptional factor, Pax7/Pax3, and were first detected in skeletal muscles underneath a basal lamina between E16.5 and E18.5 in mice [18]. Since cells with a similar anatomical location are absent from cardiac muscle, a muscle that does not have the ability to regenerate, Mauro [11] speculated that these cells are always prepared to reenact the development of skeletal muscle after myofiber damage in adult organisms (Fig. 2A). In addition to their peculiar anatomical location, satellite cells contain very little activated mitochondria, cytoplasm, and a high content of dense heterochromatin within the nucleus. These features reflect the subsequent observation that satellite cells, similar to other adult stem cells, are mitotically quiescent, in addition to being transcriptionally and translationally less active [13, 19–22].

Since Mauro's description of satellite cells [11], more details regarding the molecular mechanisms responsible for regulating the activity of satellite cells are coming to light. It is believed that the quiescent state is maintained to preserve key functional features in tissue-specific stem cells [19, 23]. Several studies have recently identified the intrinsic and extrinsic regulatory mechanisms that govern satellite cell quiescence [20, 22, 24–33]. Brack and colleagues made an important finding when they found that the FGF2/Sprouty-1 axis is required to return to and maintain quiescence in satellite cells [25, 34]. Similarly,

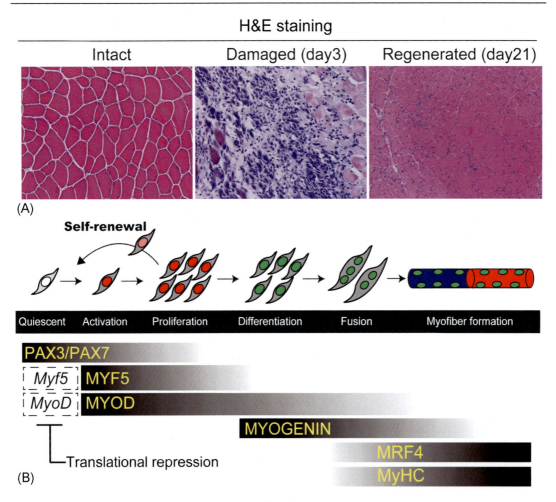

Fig. 2

Satellite cell in muscle regeneration. (A) Hematoxylin and eosin (H&E)-stained cross-section of postinjured TA muscles exhibits the ability of the skeletal muscle to undergo regeneration. (B) Schematic illustration of gene expression of satellite cells during myogenesis. Satellite cells are quiescent under normal physiological conditions and can be activated by muscle injury. Activated satellite cells enter a phase of proliferation required to expand myogenic progenitors capable of myogenic differentiation and fusion needed for new muscle formation. A small population of activated satellite cells undergo asymmetric cell divisions to generate myogenic progenitors for maintaining the satellite cell pool. The tightly controlled transcription and translation of transcription factors are necessary for successful muscle regeneration.

Yamaguchi et al. demonstrated that the impairment of the quiescent state by the loss of calcitonin receptor, highly expressed in quiescent satellite cells, was attributed to a reduction of the satellite cell pool [32]. Subsequently, Baghdadi et al. found that collagen V (COV), a possible ligand of calcitonin receptor, is produced by quiescent satellite cells themselves to create their stem cell niche [24]. Moreover, the deletion of COLV in satellite cells results in the spontaneous activation and differentiation of satellite cells, leading to the exhaustion of the stem cell pool over time. These data indicate that the quiescent state in satellite cells is actively regulated by signals from the stem cell niche.

In addition to connections in their niche, satellite cells exert cell-autonomous mechanisms to maintain their quiescence. For example, satellite cell quiescence is also maintained by microRNAs (miRNAs). Cell proliferation and growth require a substantial amount of protein synthesis, which in turn requires a lot of molecular material and energy. Therefore, posttranscriptional gene regulatory mechanisms, including miRNA, are relevant to quiescent satellite cells and have been previously shown by several research groups [20–22, 26, 28, 33, 35]. MiR-489 is highly expressed in quiescent satellite cells and represses the translation of Dek, a cell cycle promoter, to reinforce satellite cell quiescence [26]. Sato et al. previously found that miR197/497 promotes cell cycle arrest, inducing quiescence in satellite cells by targeting cell cycle genes, namely, Cdc25 and Ccnd [36]. Another interesting mechanism of miRNA-mediated satellite cell quiescence was elucidated by Crist et al. [20]. Myf5 is a critical factor for muscle cell determination during development [37]. In adult quiescent satellite cells, paradoxically, the Myf5 transcript is enriched; however, MYF5 protein is maintained at low levels, in part, due to miR-31, which targets the 3′UTR of Myf5 and prevents its translation [20].

Upon injury, satellite cells exit quiescence, enter the cell cycle, and rapidly proliferate their progenitors, which are capable of engaging the myogenic program to generate new myofibers and replace damaged muscles [13], wherein a small subpopulation of satellite cells returns to quiescence to being so-called self-renewal by asymmetric divisions [38–41], yielding uncommitted stem cells to repopulate the stem cell pool for the next round of external insults (Fig. 2B). The progression of satellite cells from quiescence to myogenic differentiation is tightly regulated by extrinsic factors from the muscle stem cell niche as well as intrinsic transcriptional factors, such as Pax7 [42] and Pax3 [18, 43], and myogenic regulatory factors (MRFs). The MRFs include myogenic differentiation 1 protein (MyoD), myogenic factor 5 (Myf5), myogenin, and muscle-specific regulatory factor 4 (Mrf4) (Fig. 2B). Quiescent satellite cells express Pax7 [42, 44], while a small subset of satellite cells express Pax3 [43, 45, 46], a paralog of Pax7. A previous study found that Pax7 mutant mice exhibited a complete loss of the muscle stem cell population, markedly decreased muscle mass, and a reduced fiber area, although the organization of the muscle fibers overall was not severely affected [42]. This suggests that Pax7 is necessary for the myogenic specification of muscle stem cells during development and the postnatal growth of skeletal muscle. During development, most satellite cells activate MRFs. However, these factors are not accumulated at the protein level in adult quiescent satellite cells. The MYOD and MYF5 protein levels increase quickly upon satellite cell activation, in part, via posttranscriptional mechanisms [20, 47]. The subsequent upregulation of myogenin is required for further differentiation, which is necessary for the formation of new myofibers and tissue regeneration. In contrast, a subfraction of satellite cells repopulates the stem cell pool by maintaining a high level of Pax7 [48, 49]. It is worth noting that the balance between the differentiation and maintenance of a satellite cell pool during regeneration is a causal factor determining successful regeneration and the life-long capacity of muscle regeneration. Therefore, the balance between quiescence and proliferation/differentiation in stem cells must be regulated carefully, since the deregulation or imbalance of quiescence and proliferation can lead to impaired tissue regeneration and the exhaustion of the stem cell population.

Satellite cells are functionally and molecularly highly heterogeneous [40, 43, 45, 46, 50, 51]. Based on label dilution assays, only a subset of satellite cells is capable of self-renewal, an important property of stem cells, with the rest committing to proliferation and differentiation. Recently, two studies [45, 46] from different research groups demonstrated that a minor subset of adult Pax7$^+$ satellite cells expressing Pax3 exhibited marked stress resistance against environmental pollutant stress or radiation stress, possessing high levels of stem cell activity and being capable of clonal expansion, which may be essential for muscle homeostasis throughout the lifecycle. However, the proportion of change in the cell populations of different conditions, such as muscle diseases and aging, is unknown and will need further investigation. Recently, Barruet et al. demonstrated functional heterogeneity in human satellite cells using single RNA sequencing [52]. In contrast to the observation in mice, human Pax7$^+$ satellite cells expressing Pax3 did not show a unique cluster of gene expression by single-cell RNA sequencing analysis. This is likely to be explained by the fact that the "stem cell" gene expression pattern appears under high-stress conditions. However, in terms of tissue homeostasis, it is still unclear why satellite cells should be heterogeneous in the tissues. Understanding the more precise role in heterogeneity in satellite cells will provide valuable insights into the etiology of sarcopenia and the development of cell-based therapies of muscular dystrophies.

Support cells that influence the satellite cell activity during regeneration

Muscle injuries can result from intense exercise, insults, disease, toxins, and ischemia. The conditional knockout of Pax7 in mice was helpful to demonstrate the role of satellite cells in adult muscle regeneration. The conditional depletion of Pax7 in adult mice severely impaired the regenerative capability of skeletal muscle, indicating that Pax7 is an essential factor for the normal function of satellite cells in adults [53]. Moreover, the conditional depletion of satellite cells using diphtheria toxin A gene under the control of Pax7 expression in mice showed a strong reduction of myofiber size and numbers accompanied by massive fibrosis and fat deposition in the intercellular region after injury [54–56]. These results established the concept that Pax7 expression and satellite cells are indispensable for adult muscle regeneration.

Muscle regeneration is largely dependent on satellite cell activity. However, it is complex and requires the properly coordinated activity of multiple cell types, such as inflammatory cells, mesenchymal fibroadipogenic progenitors, and endothelial cells, to ensure the complete restoration of muscle tissues, including nerves and vasculatures [57, 58].

At the early stage of muscle regeneration, injured muscles undergo necrosis in response to damage. The rupture of myofiber membranes results in the release of the cell contents and chemotactic factors that will be recognized by resident leukocytes. Mast cells and neutrophils are the first cell type to be activated and release cytokines, such as IL-6 and TNF-α, as well as attracting circulating inflammatory cells, such as granulocytes and monocyte/macrophages. These cytokines in the inflammatory environment are known to activate satellite cell proliferation directly. During the inflammation process, macrophage accumulation is comprised initially of proinflammatory M1 macrophages, followed by antiinflammatory M2 macrophages. M1 macrophages promote myoblast proliferation and suppress early differentiation [59, 60]. On the contrary, M2 macrophages are crucial for resolving inflammation by releasing antiinflammatory cytokines and growth factors, such as IL-4, IL-10, and IL-13, to facilitate muscle regeneration [59–62]. After a sufficient proliferation of myoblasts, myoblasts (myocytes) fuse to form immature myotubes or fuse to existing damaged fibers. During the stage of myogenesis, IL-4 has been shown to directly promote myotube formation and growth [62]. Although the source of insulin-like growth factor (IGF-1) has not yet been elucidated, IGF-1 is also able to stimulate myoblast proliferation and hypertrophic growth in myotubes via the AKt-1/mTOR pathway [57, 63, 64].

Another cell type that contributes to muscle regeneration is fibroadipogenic progenitors (FAPs). FAPs are bipotent mesenchymal cells characterized by platelet-derived growth factor receptor alpha (PDGFRα) in skeletal muscle, but which are developmentally distinct myogenic progenitors [65, 66]. Upon injury, FAPs proliferate and promote myogenic differentiation rather than proliferation [65]. Recently, the FAP-derived factor WNT1 Inducible Signaling Pathway Protein 1 (WISP1) was found to be required for efficient muscle regeneration and regulates the asymmetric division of satellite cells [67]. Other immune cells that potentially regulate muscle regeneration have also received attention, namely, eosinophils, since eosinophils secrete IL-4/IL-13 at an early phase of muscle regeneration to facilitate the proliferation of FAP [68]. In this paper, the authors demonstrated that FAPs are required for the removal of necrotic debris. Therefore, the tightly regulated function of FAPs may support the regenerative response of satellite cells. Efficient muscle regeneration is also associated with the rate of angiogenesis, since endothelial cells secrete mitogens, namely, angiopoietin-1, IGF-1, hepatocyte growth factor (HGF), and vascular endothelial growth factor (VEGF), to regulate satellite cell expansion and self-renewal [58, 69, 70]. In addition to these cells, the remodeling of the extracellular matrix (ECM) critically influences the regeneration of muscles, as well as the self-renewal and quiescence of satellite cells. The components of the ECM are produced by a variety of cells, including fibroblasts and satellite cells, during regeneration and in homeostatic condition [24, 29, 71–73].

Collectively, muscle regeneration is achieved by the interplay between satellite cells and multiple cell types and factors, including the ECM, in stem cell niches that participate in the orchestration of regeneration. Alterations of the intrinsic mechanisms of satellite cells or the extrinsic signals within the stem cell niche (myofibers, immune cells, FAPs, endothelial cells, and ECM) account a decline in muscle regenerative capacity with age. In the following section, we provide a review of how muscle stem cell aging and the aging of the stem cell niche affects muscle regeneration, muscle adaptations, and muscle homeostasis.

Satellite cell function in aging

During aging, there is a striking decline in regenerative capacity. The loss of the regenerative capacity of muscle in aged muscle has led to the hypothesis that the activity and number of satellite cells is reduced over time. The reduction of the satellite cell pool and their properties with aging are due to cell-autonomous alterations and changes in the components of the stem cell niche, including systemic proteins and localized structural and soluble factors that affect quiescence, proliferation, and differentiation. In this section, we review how muscle stem cells and their niches are altered with aging.

Intrinsic changes in muscle stem cells with aging

In mice, the nuclei of satellite cells comprise ~ 5% of the skeletal muscle nuclei in adult muscles, decreasing to 2% in older muscle, at least in some muscles [13, 74, 75]. This decline in the satellite cell pool is more evident in female mice than in male mice and may be attenuated by exercise [76]. A series of previous experiments using primary and serial transplantation models have shown that satellite cells from aged muscles accumulate intrinsic alterations that lead to reduced abilities for self-renewal, expansion, and myofiber formation. Satellite cells isolated from aged (18–26 months) and geriatric (26–32 months) mice injected into young muscles exhibited severe deficits both in self-renewal, expansion, and myogenic differentiation [77–80]. These results imply that cell-autonomous changes occur in aged satellite cells, which pose difficulties to their rejuvenation by exposure to a young milieu.

The alteration of the multiple signal transduction cascades in aged satellite cells, which converge on a set of cell cycle kinase and myogenic differentiation factors, has been previously reported. These changes include the aberrant and spontaneous activation of the FGFR-Sprouty1, the Jak-Stat3, $p16^{Ink4a}$, and the stress-associated p38a/b mitogen-activated protein kinase (MAPK) pathways [25, 77, 79–81]. The increased expression of FGF2 in aged myofibers under homeostatic conditions resulted in the downregulation of Sprouty1, which is required for the return of cells to quiescence and self-renewal [25]. Thus, the aberrant activation of FGF-Sprouty1 forces satellite cells out of quiescence and leads to the loss of their self-renewal capacity, resulting in the depletion of the satellite cell pool. Furthermore, aberrant p38a/b activity and Jak-Stat3 negatively regulate the self-renewal of satellite cells by promoting myogenic differentiation via the activation of myogenin [78] and the suppression of Pax7 [82].

Notably, the pharmacological inhibition of p38 [77, 78] and Jak-Stat3 [79] was found to result in the successful rejuvenation of aged satellite cells for their regeneration capacity and serial transplantation, as well as for the strengthening of damaged muscle in aged mice. Senescence-associated markers, such as p16^{Ink4a}, a cyclin-dependent kinase (CDK) inhibitor, were also upregulated in satellite cells isolated from geriatric mice [80]. Indeed, silencing p16^{Ink4a} was sufficient to restore the self-renewal capacity, resulting in the reconstitution of the satellite cell compartment after muscle injury. Intriguingly, considering that the pharmacological inhibition of p38 dramatically reduces the population of p16^{Ink4a}-expressing satellite cells, future studies should aim to elucidate the molecular relationships between p38 MAPK pathway and p16^{Ink4a} in satellite cells during aging.

In addition to the loss of stem cell function with aging, the loss of satellite cell content in aged muscles can also be explained by increased apoptosis signals associated with an increased production of reactive oxygen species (ROS), the accumulation of oxidative damage, the impairment of genome stability, the reduction in mitochondrial biogenesis and oxidative phosphorylation, and the failure of protein turnover (proteostasis), associated with reduced levels of autophagy activity [75, 83–85], a process of self-degradation of cellular components [86]. The impairment of autophagy results in the accumulation of damaged mitochondria, which induces ROS and DNA damage as a result, and ultimately senescence and apoptosis in satellite cells [83]. Consistent with this, mice subjected to caloric restriction showed increased mitochondrial basal oxygen consumption and mitochondria content, leading to enhanced satellite cell functionality and regenerative capacity [87]. These findings indicate that the regulation of proteostasis through autophagy plays a role in preserving the integrity of stemness and prevents the accumulation of damaged proteins in quiescent satellite cells throughout their lifecycle.

Other studies have showed that telomere shortening due to multiple rounds of cell division may contribute to the reduced proliferative potential of aged satellite cells [88–90]. However, skeletal muscle and satellite cells have a low turnover in the absence of damage. As such, the contribution of telomere shortening to satellite cell aging may occur with aging accompanied by genetic muscle diseases, such as DMD, rather than with homeostatic aging. In addition, aged satellite cells show dysregulation of gene expression associated with muscle regeneration. Moreover, a decrease in delta 1 expression was found in human muscle biopsies from elderly men compared with younger men [91]. Cumulatively, these cell-autonomous changes may restrict the self-renewal/expansion and formation of mature myofibers, the two hallmarks of stem cell function.

Extrinsic changes in muscle stem cells with aging

While intrinsic changes in satellite cells have been observed in aging, multiple studies have also indicated that impaired stem cell activities could be related to the deterioration of the tissue microenvironment and systemic mediators. Satellite cells are inseparable from their niche since the definition of satellite cell is a mononucleated cell that resides adjacent to the muscle fiber membrane and under the basal lamina [11]. In addition to muscle fibers and extracellular components as satellite cell niche components, there are other types of niches, including interstitial cells, endothelial cells, and inflammatory cells, which regulate the functions of satellite cells under both physiological and pathological conditions. In this context, understanding how age-related changes in the niches influence the function of satellite cells, ultimately resulting in reduced muscle regeneration activity in aged muscles, is crucial.

The idea that extrinsic factors from the niches influence the functionality of satellite cells has been clearly demonstrated by the heterochronic parabiosis model, in which old and young mice are surgically pared to share their blood circulation [92, 93]. The muscle regenerative capacity of aged mice sharing their blood with younger mice exhibited a robust regenerative response to injury than aged mice of isochronic pairs, in which mice were exposed to the blood of other aged mice. Conversely, the satellite cells of young mice paired with old mice showed a decline in their regenerative capacity. These studies raise the following question: What are critical contributors in aged and young cellular environments that mediate the functions of satellite cells? The heterochronic parabiosis experiments identified some systemic factors as key regulators for muscle stem cell function associated with aging. These include Wnt3A [92], complement C1q [94], and oxytocin, a hormone known for its role in lactation [95]. Increased Wnt signaling driven by the complement C1q could induce the undesirable fibrogenic conversion of satellite cells [92, 94]. On the contrary, a reduction in the levels of oxytocin in plasma with age and the systemic administration of oxytocin was found to improve satellite cell activity in aged mice [95]. Recently, both Collins et al. [96] and ourselves [97] demonstrated that the female sex hormone estrogen may be a systemic hormonal regulator of satellite cell activities under both physiological and pathological conditions. Furthermore, another circulatory factor recently identified as affecting satellite cell function and the life span of aged mice is apelin, an exercise-induced myokine [98, 99]. The synthesis of apelin in muscles was found to be reduced in an age-dependent manner in both humans and mice. It has been successfully demonstrated that the genetic inactivation of apelin or its receptor accelerated the senescence program in skeletal muscle and other tissues. Interestingly, satellite cells are targeted by apelin supplementation, enhancing satellite cell proliferation and differentiation, which is normally reduced in aged mice.

In addition to systemic factors, age-related alterations in localized factors have also emerged as significant contributors in the regulation of satellite cell homeostasis and satellite cell activity during regeneration, including the FGF2-FGFR1 [25] and Delta1-Notch pathways [100]. As discussed in the previous section, aged muscle fibers in mice aberrantly express FGF2. This subsequently activates FGFR1 in satellite cells, which in turn induces downregulation of Sprouty1 in satellite cells, resulting in anomalous satellite cell activation under physiological conditions [25]. Notch signaling is required for satellite cell self-renewal, proliferation, and differentiation [101, 102]. However, aged muscles fail to upregulate Delta 1, one of the Notch ligands, which results in the insufficient activation of Notch signaling in satellite cells after injury, reducing proliferation and impairing muscle regeneration [100].

The basal lamina is a highly complex and integrated structure composed of collagen, laminin, fibronectin, perlecan, and several proteoglycans and glycoproteins. Recently, several studies have demonstrated that the interaction of satellite cells with ECM proteins is essential for regulating their quiescence, proliferation, differentiation, and self-renewal. Bentzinger et al. found that fibronectin stimulates the symmetric expansion of satellite stem cells through Syndecan-4 and Frizzled-7 to maintain the satellite cell pool [71]. Recently, Baghdadi et al. demonstrated that the Notch-mediated expression of COLV in satellite cells results in the formation of their niche to maintain their quiescent state via the calcitonin receptor [24], which is highly expressed in quiescent satellite cells [32]. However, it remains unclear whether these ECM proteins, essential for homeostasis in satellite cells, are compromised with aging. The accumulation of by-products derived from the ECM proteins, such as elastin and cleaved fibronectin, may induce a necrotic reaction [103]. In 2010, Gilbert et al. engineered a culture model to mimic the adult skeletal muscle elasticity and found that satellite cells seeded on soft matrix maintained their stemness properties, as evidenced by increased Pax7 expression and a better extent and rate of engraftment [104]. Conversely, satellite cells seeded on ECM derived from aged muscles have been found to display decreased myogenic activity and increased levels of fibrogenic marker expression [105]. Furthermore, the authors also demonstrated that, as muscles age, the collagen fibrils become tauter and increasingly deformed, resulting in stiffer muscles. As a result, the increased nuclear translocation of YAP/TAZ in fibroblast triggers the expression of fibrogenic genes, which are unfavorable to satellite cell behavior [105].

There has been an interest in the interaction of fibroadipogenic progenitors (FAPs) with satellite cells [65–67, 106]. Under physiological conditions, FAPs remain quiescent, but proliferate rapidly in response to stimuli, mediating muscle regeneration [65, 67, 68, 106]. More directly, the genetic ablation of fibroblasts in muscle using Tcf4$^{\text{CreERT2}}$-mediated diphtheria toxic expression system was found to results in premature satellite cell differentiation [55], suggesting the interaction between fibroblasts, including FAPs, and satellite cells via a direct or an indirect mechanism. A recent report by Lukjanenko et al. found that FAPs secrete WNT1 Inducible Signaling Pathway Protein 1 (WISP1) in young muscles; however, this is lost during aging [67]. WISP1 regulates the asymmetric division of satellite cells for efficient muscle regeneration, and the administration of WISP1 restores the myogenic capacity of satellite cells in aged mice. FAPs are also known as a source of IGF-1 and IL-33, a critical anabolic mediator and a T-reg mediator, respectively [68, 107]. FAPs are beneficial for muscle homeostatic maintenance under both physiological and pathological conditions when they are finely regulated. During aging, the dysregulation of type 2 innate immune response, accompanied by the overproduction of TGF-β1, may promote their differentiation into adipocytes or fibroblasts, which likely inhibits muscle regeneration [12]. These results suggest that multiple extrinsic factors and pathways are deregulated in both local and systemic levels in aged mice. These findings indicate that targeting the dysregulated pathways in aged mice could be used to develop strategies to rejuvenate the regenerative capacity of satellite cells in sarcopenic muscles.

Satellite cells and muscle adaptation

To fully understand the impact of satellite cells on the onset and development of age-related sarcopenia, it is also essential to review their potential role in muscle adaptation without severe injury. Satellite cells are indispensable for skeletal muscle regeneration after severe injuries, such as in the cardiotoxin-injury model. However, their involvement in regulating muscle adaptation under physiological conditions, including hypertrophy and atrophy without massive injury, is complex. Recently, several papers have tried to show whether satellite cells are indispensable or not for muscle hypertrophy. However, the results remain a topic of debate. In this section, we review these conflicting findings and highlight the differences between these studies and their results.

Satellite cell in muscle hypertrophy

The satellite cell population represents a large proportion of muscle nuclei, up to 30% in rodent neonates. During the first week after birth, a substantial proportion of satellite cells proliferates and is incorporated into myofibers [108]. It is thought that myonuclear accretion by satellite cells is required for myofiber hypertrophy in postnatal muscle growth [42, 109]. In addition to the postnatal period, Bachman et al. recently clearly demonstrated the need for satellite cell-dependent myonuclei accretion during myofiber hypertrophy in the prepubertal period, using a Pax7^{CreERT2}-diphtheria toxin A (Pax7-DTA) mouse model that allows for the conditional deletion of Pax7$^+$ satellite cells [110]. Pax7$^+$ satellite cell depletion during the prepubertal period exhibited a significant reduction of myofiber hypertrophic growth, as evidenced by a reduced muscle cross-sectional area (CSA), which is associated with a loss of myonuclei. Taken together, these data suggest that satellite cell-dependent myonuclear accretion is vital for postnatal and prepubertal hypertrophic muscle growth.

However, muscle growth is not restricted to the early stage of life. The size of myofibers can be enhanced by hypertrophic stimuli, such as resistance training in adults. However, the mechanisms of increased myofiber size in adults may be different from those in the postnatal and prepubertal periods. White et al. identified two stages in postnatal muscle growth. In the first stage (up to 3 weeks after birth), the number of myonuclei is correlated with an increased volume of the cytoplasm [109]. In a later stage (after P21), the size of the myofibers continues to increase without the addition of new myonuclei. This study raises two important potential mechanisms of muscle fiber hypertrophy, namely, that myofiber hypertrophy is mediated via either a myonuclear accretion-dependent mechanism or a myonuclear accretion-independent mechanism.

According to the "myonuclear domain hypothesis," to maintain the ratio of cytoplasm to the nucleus, the addition of new nuclei into growing myofibers is necessary to maintain a constant myonuclear domain ratio. Although previous studies have shown evidence of activation, the proliferation of satellite cells, as well as an increased number of myonuclei after a synergistic ablation (SA) (compensatory overload model) [111, 112], it has been shown that the size of myofibers could increase without satellite cell contribution after SA in the Pax7-DTA mouse model [113]. It has also been demonstrated that the number of myonuclei after 2 weeks of SA did not increase in satellite cell-depleted matured mice (16 weeks old), while the size of muscle fibers increased [113]. These data suggest that muscle fiber hypertrophy in matured mice does not require the addition of new nuclei and that adult muscle fiber is capable of increasing the cytoplasmic volume without the contribution of satellite cells. This is also supported by other studies using an atrophy-regrowth model [114].

In contrast, two recent independent studies support the "myonuclear domain hypothesis." Egner et al. [111] essentially repeated the experiments conducted by McCarthy et al. [113], showing that myofiber hypertrophy was not induced in satellite cell-depleted matured mice, which is in contrast to their findings. In agreement with Egner et al. [111], Goh et al. reported that the genetic deletion of myomaker, a muscle-specific membrane protein essential for cell fusion, in satellite cells resulted in the absence of myofiber hypertrophy after SA, supporting the hypothesis that myonuclear accretion by satellite cells is necessary for adult myofiber hypertrophy [115]. Although the discrepancies between these results are not yet apparent, these could be explained by the different strategies used to evaluate the CSA. Namely, McCarthy et al. excluded myofibers with central nuclei (sign of damage) [113], while Egner et al. included these fibers in their analysis [111]. However, in a follow-up study by the Peterson group, muscle fiber hypertrophy was found to be slightly compromised concomitantly with excessive ECM accumulation in skeletal muscles after 8 weeks of SA, suggesting that satellite cells may inhibit the accumulation of ECM and regulate a microenvironment favorable for muscle growth in a long-term hypertrophic model of adult mice [116]. These results suggest that satellite cells are required for long-term muscle hypertrophic adaptation. In a subsequent study, Fry et al. demonstrated a more precise mechanism of ECM deposition in skeletal muscles when satellite cells are depleted. They demonstrated that satellite cell-derived exosomes containing miR-206 could inhibit fibrogenic gene expression, providing protection from ECM accumulation and indicating a new role for satellite cells in skeletal muscle hypertrophy [117]. Taken together, whether the introduction of satellite cell-derived new myonuclei to excising myofibers is necessary for adult myofiber hypertrophy remains controversial. However, it is highly likely that satellite cells positively regulate the hypertrophic responses in adults. In a physiological context, satellite cells do proliferate or fuse to existing myofibers after overload or exercise. As such, satellite cells may contribute to functional hypertrophy. Nevertheless, further experiments investigating whether satellite cells are functionally necessary for the myofiber hypertrophy in aged mice are required to show the beneficial impact of satellite cell-targeted therapies on age-related sarcopenia (Fig. 3A).

Satellite cells in muscle atrophy

The mechanisms of muscle atrophy associated with disuse muscle atrophy and sarcopenia are complex and involve the regulation of protein synthesis/degradation and the integrity of neuromuscular junction (NMJ), as well as the levels of hormones, nutrition, and physical activity [6]. Frequently used atrophy models in rodents include hindlimb suspension, immobilization, denervation, cancer-cachexia, and aging. Several studies have reported that atrophic models induce a reduction in the number of satellite cells via apoptosis and precocious activation/differentiation [96, 118]. Moreover, Kadi et al. reported that individuals aged 70–83 years exhibited a significant reduction in the population of satellite cells compared with younger, active individuals aged 20–32 years [119]. Satellite cells are essential for skeletal muscle formation/regeneration. However, whether satellite cells directly influence the onset and progression of sarcopenia is still under debate, and multiple studies have shown that satellite cells may or may not contribute to developing muscle atrophy in different mouse models [120–124].

Numerous studies have suggested that muscle atrophy is accompanied by the loss of myonuclei through apoptosis [125]. Thus, an increase in the size of myonuclear domains could trigger cytoplasmic atrophy in muscle fibers. Therefore, the prevention of satellite cells or the replenishment of new nuclei from satellite cells represents a potential therapeutic intervention for muscle atrophy, including sarcopenia. However, whether myonuclei loss occurs in an atrophic setting in rodents also remains controversial [6]. For example, Bruusgaard et al. developed in vivo time-lapse imaging system of myonuclei on a single myofiber, which showed no loss of myonuclei and no sign of apoptosis during disuse atrophy, despite more than 50% reduction of muscle CSA in mice [126]. In line with these results, it has also been reported that the number of myonuclei is not reduced in elderly individuals [119].

In 2015, Fry et al. challenged whether satellite cells contribute to sarcopenia. In their study, the authors demonstrated that the reduction of satellite cells during natural aging (up to 24 months)

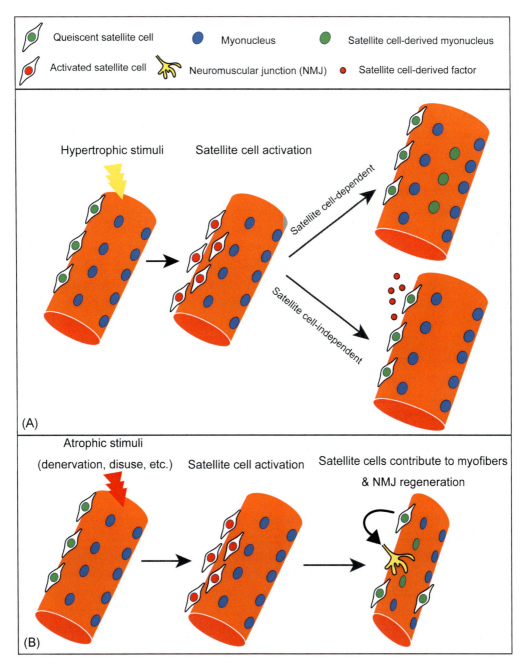

Fig. 3
Summary of the role of satellite cells in muscle hypertrophy and atrophy. (A) Satellite cells contribute to hypertrophy through both direct (fusion to the myofibers) and indirect (secrete some factors inhibiting ECM deposition in a long-term adaptation) mechanisms. (B) Satellite cells are also important for myofiber atrophy, especially when associated with NMJ degeneration. Additional studies will be needed to elucidate the mechanism by which satellite cells ameliorate muscle atrophy and NMJ regeneration. Furthermore, it is currently unclear whether satellite cells are crucial for the onset and development of sarcopenia.

neither accelerated the onset of sarcopenia nor exacerbated the progression of sarcopenia via the genetic ablation of satellite cells in mice [120]. Thus, they concluded that satellite cells are dispensable for sarcopenia. In the same year, Keefe et al. used a similar experimental model to ask two questions: whether satellite cells contribute to muscle homeostasis in sedentary adult mice, and whether a decline of satellite cell-mediated replenishment of myonuclei affects sarcopenia [121]. They first examined the contributions of satellite cells to different adult muscles, including the hind limbs, diaphragm, and extraocular (EOM) muscles. Although the rate of satellite cell contribution varies between muscles, satellite cells seem to contribute to the muscle fibers of all adult muscles (12 and 20 months), even under sedentary conditions, as evidenced by the genetic labeling of satellite cells and their lineage. The authors then investigated whether a decline in the satellite cell-mediated contribution to myofibers contributed to muscle atrophy. Although satellite cells are not globally required to maintain myofiber size in sedentary mice, the extensor digitorum longus (EDL), which is enriched in myosin heavy chain (MHC) type IIb myofibers, showed a decreased myofiber size at 20 months when the satellite cells were ablated. Type IIb myofibers are more susceptible to myonuclear apoptosis and muscle atrophy than type I fibers with aging [6]. However, according to these findings, the presence of satellite cells does not rescue the reduction of myonuclei in EDL muscles of 20-month-old mice. Recently, an interesting paper was published by Murach et al. demonstrating that satellite cells communicate with adjacent myofibers using an extracellular vesicle (EV), which contains miRNA and even cytoplasmic-localized fluorescent reporter (TdTomato) driven by Pax7^{CreERT2}, suggesting a fusion independent mechanism of satellite cell for maintaining the size of myofiber [127]. However, the role satellite cells play in maintaining muscle mass during atrophy has yet to be fully elucidated. Thus, further studies are needed to obtain conclusive results on their role in the homeostasis of muscle with aging.

Although the study by Keefe et al. is limited to 12- and 20-month-old mice, understanding the discrepancy between Fry et al. [120] and Keefe et al. [121] would be beneficial for developing a more appropriate focus on sarcopenia. Keefe et al. argued against the low frequency of satellite cell ablation performed by Fry et al. Therefore, it is possible that a small subpopulation escapes genetic deletion and prevents the development of sarcopenia. In contrast to Fry et al., Keefe et al. only examined the role of satellite cells in 20-month-old mice, but not in 24-month-old mice. In the future, it could be interesting to investigate whether the high satellite cell depletion efficiency model by Keefe et al. either accelerates or exacerbates sarcopenia. These two papers [120, 121] provide critical insights into the role of satellite cells during muscle atrophy and sarcopenia with aging. However, a caveat of these experiments is that the mice were caged without a running wheel. In this context, an additional study using lineage tracing and ablation of satellite cells, with interventions of exercise or high-fat diet, will also be necessary to translate the results to human beings.

Satellite cells are unevenly distributed along the length of myofibers, with more satellite cells found around the motor endplate [128]. The NMJ initiates the action potential required for the excitation-contraction coupling to generate force for the movement of the muscles and to maintain the homeostasis of muscles. An increased NMJ degeneration is observed in sarcopenic muscles, and the integrity of NMJ is frequently associated with muscle function [123, 129, 130]. It has been previously demonstrated that, in a sciatic nerve transection (SNT) model, where the lower limbs of NMJs are disrupted, the activation of satellite cells is induced [124, 131], suggesting that the alteration of myofiber- and motor neuron-derived trophic factors may influence the fate of satellite cells. Meanwhile, whether satellite cells directly influence the regeneration of NMJs, as well as the denervation-related muscle atrophy model, is unknown. To this question, Liu et al. [124] recently showed that satellite cells are indispensable for facilitating NMJ regeneration, and thus in preventing myofiber atrophy in response to neuromuscular disruption, using the Pax7-DTA model [55]. In their paper, the authors used an SNT model to demonstrate that satellite cell depletion further exacerbated SNT-induced atrophic phenotypes, indicated by the size of myofiber CSA, a sign of fibrosis, an increase in the proportion of type IIA/IIX hybrid myofibers, and a reduction in muscle force generation. Interestingly, they also found that SNT induced the regional activation of satellite cells around NMJs. Thus, their activity may regulate NMJ regeneration by maintaining the number of postsynaptic myonuclei. Subsequently, in 2017, the research group followed up their first study in aged mice (up to 24 months) using the same satellite cell depletion and lineage tracking strategies [123]. Remarkably, they found that satellite cell depletion was sufficient to drive age-related NMJ degeneration, a reduction in the number of postsynaptic myonuclei, and myofiber atrophy, suggesting that satellite cells are critical mediators for combating sarcopenia associated with age-related NMJ degeneration. Their findings suggest that satellite cells are a source of postsynaptic myonuclei. Therefore, the optimization of the number of satellite cells and their function in aged muscles could be a viable strategy to counteract muscle atrophy in sarcopenia (Fig. 3B).

Hormones are among the systemic factors that regulate atrophic signals, including thyroid hormone, glucocorticoid, and sex hormones. Many lines of evidence have demonstrated that hormonal regulation directly or indirectly influences muscle homeostasis and strength [132–140]. Primarily, it is well known that androgens, male sex hormones, increase muscle mass and prevent muscle atrophy [132, 139]. Conversely, a decline in circulating androgen levels in hypogonadal men and prostate cancer patients undergoing androgen deprivation therapy resulted in significant muscle atrophy and reduced muscle strength [141, 142]. Although the function of androgens in skeletal muscle homeostasis has been intensively investigated, the potential impact of female sex hormones, such as estrogens, has largely been ignored, especially in skeletal muscles. Estrogen deprivation occurs for a variety of reasons, including menopause, ovariectomy, and chemotherapy. Recent studies have clearly demonstrated that estrogens are also powerful circulating factors for the regulation of muscle mass and muscle metabolism, including the maintenance of mitochondria [133, 135, 137]. It is worth noting that female and male sex hormones have distinct functions in satellite cell activities, as shown by several studies, including our own [97, 122, 135, 143, 144]. Recently, Collins et al. [96] and ourselves [97] demonstrated that estrogen signaling via estrogen receptors (ER) regulates the proliferation and apoptosis of satellite cells, thus maintaining the muscle regenerative capacity in females. However, whether the disruption of the signal by the deletion of either ERα or ERβ in satellite cells could induce any sign of sarcopenia, including myofiber atrophy, has yet to be investigated. Many studies have independently investigated how sex hormone deprivation models, such as castration or ovariectomy, affect the muscle mass and the number and function of satellite cells, implying the importance of satellite cells in muscle atrophy. However, research focusing on the direct contribution of satellite cells to a sex hormone-deprived atrophy model is very limited. One recent report used castration and satellite cell depletion strategies to demonstrate that androgen deprivation-induced atrophy further exacerbates myofiber atrophy and functional decline in the absence of satellite cells [122]. Consistent with the role of satellite cells in contributing to the regeneration of NMJs, as shown in previous findings [123, 124], the depletion of satellite cells in young castrated mice induced the loss of NMJ-associated postsynaptic myonuclei, indicating that satellite cells can also attenuate sarcopenia in elderly men with androgen deprivation. Since this paper demonstrated a direct link between satellite cells and castration-induced atrophy in male mice using genetic tools, future studies of satellite cell functions in ovariectomy-induced atrophy in females could accelerate the development of a more precise strategy based on sex differences to prevent muscle atrophy with aging.

Satellite cells and exercise to combat sarcopenia

The use of satellite cells as a source of tissue regeneration is being actively investigated to elucidate their role in muscular dystrophies, including Duchenne muscular dystrophy. As discussed in previous sections, in addition to their primary role as stem cells for muscle regeneration following injury or degenerative conditions, satellite cells may, directly or indirectly, contribute to muscle hypertrophy and atrophy in mice models. Therefore, targeting satellite cells is a plausible strategy for combating sarcopenia and other types of muscle atrophy. In this section, we introduce a more applicable strategy, namely, exercise, for sarcopenia therapy in humans through satellite cell-mediating mechanisms.

It is widely recognized that exercise is a powerful strategy to counteract sarcopenia and other types of muscle atrophy. Several studies have found that exercise has profound effects on satellite cells, namely, by preserving their number and functions, including proliferative and differentiation, and their self-renewal capacity [145–150]. The activation of satellite cells by exercise is mediated by a number of factors, including the IGF-1, IL-6, and Wnt/β-catenin pathways [151–153]. However, whether the beneficial effect of exercise on homeostatic muscle depends on satellite cell-mediated mechanisms has not yet been fully elucidated.

Joanisse et al. found that the 8 weeks of exercise training in 22-month-old mice resulted in an increased satellite cell content without myofiber hypertrophy, compared with sedentary age-matched control mice [148]. Furthermore, the trained mice appeared to experience improved cardiotoxin-induced skeletal muscle regeneration that was comparable to that of the young sedentary mice. Sarcopenia involves the progressive loss of muscle mass without massive injury, in which the contribution of satellite cells may be limited [120, 121]. However, massive injuries, in which satellite cell activity is indispensable, happening later in life would induce secondary sarcopenia if the muscle regeneration was impaired. An important lesson provided by Joanisse et al. is that exercise can enhance the number of satellite cells and the regenerative capacity of muscle even when the training protocol is implemented at older ages [148].

Resistance-based exercise training is currently well established as an effective interventional strategy to enhance muscle mass and integrity in the elderly. Petrella et al. reported that individuals with a high satellite cell content responded well to resistance training and showed high levels of myofiber hypertrophy [154]. Even though it remains unclear whether muscle fibers experience hypertrophy to the same extent in old individuals as in younger individuals when receiving the same signals, the content of satellite cells is likely to be a crucial factor in determining the hypertrophic response in humans to exercise. Prolonged resistance training in elderly men was found to increase the satellite cell content, specifically in type II muscle fibers, following 12 and 24 weeks of training [155, 156]. This observation is particularly important for targeting satellite cell-mediated sarcopenia therapy, due to the fact that Verijk et al. found that type II-, but not type I-, associated satellite cells were significantly reduced in elderly individuals [7]. These results suggest that resistance training could target the satellite cells associated with type II muscle fibers. In addition, Fry et al. demonstrated that 12 weeks of aerobic training induced an increase in satellite cell content only in type I muscle fibers, accompanied by an increased number of myonuclei of type I fibers [147]. However, these changes were not observed in type II fibers, suggesting that the satellite cell content can be modulated by the type of exercise (resistance and endurance) in human beings. Interestingly, muscle fiber capillarization may be a causal factor regulating hypertrophic response, as well as the elevation of the satellite cell content, by exercise [155]. Since endurance training is an effective strategy for capillarization in both type I and type II muscle in humans [157], a combination of aerobic training with resistance training is likely to result in the largest benefits to both satellite cell content and muscle adaptation in elderly individuals. Taken together, these findings indicate that exercise is a potent modulator for improving muscle plasticity, in part, due to an increase in the number of satellite cells, as well as satellite cell function, in sarcopenic muscles.

Concluding remarks

Since the discovery of satellite cells by Mauro et al. over half of a century ago [11], researchers across the world have studied this unique stem cell in skeletal muscles. However, many unknowns remain regarding the properties of satellite cells. Aging is a particularly complex process associated with multiple factors, including interactions with different types of cells through systemic factors. Researchers have only just begun to start understanding the causes of aging. The past few years have seen significant progress in our understanding of satellite cell biology, thanks to advances in genetic tools, including knockout technology, the Cre/loxP system, and CRISPR-Cas9, which have enabled us to study the function of genes of the interest under temporal and tissue-specific conditions.

Many lines of evidence have clearly established that satellite cells are indispensable for muscle regeneration. In parallel, several mechanisms influencing the impaired satellite cell homeostasis and muscle regeneration associated with aging have been identified. Extrinsic factors, including systemic factors and local cytokines in stem cell niches, such as myofibers, FAP, and endothelial cells, have been found to affect the behavior of satellite cells and limit their regenerative potential. Moreover, the ECM has been found to have a significant impact on the maintenance of satellite cells during aging. Furthermore, intrinsic changes, including the accumulation of p16^{Ink4a} and the dysregulation of Sprouty-1, p38, MAPK, and Stat3, have been found to induce senescence, inhibit self-renewal, and reduce proliferation in aged satellite cells. The good news is that targeting both extrinsic and intrinsic pathways using genetic, pharmacological, or biotechnological approaches may offer opportunities to reverse aberrant phenotypes. However, future studies are needed to validate whether the extrinsic and intrinsic changes in aged satellite cells observed in mice also occur in satellite cells in human beings.

Although a number of studies have shown a significant decline in satellite cells with aging, their contribution to muscle plasticity, such as muscle hypertrophy and atrophy without massive injury, remains a topic of debate. The satellite cell depleted mouse model is currently the most promising way to prove their contribution in various experiments. However, results remain controversial, even when using similar or identical genetic tools and approaches [113, 114, 116, 120, 121]. Nevertheless, recent papers from Chakkalakal and colleagues showed the contribution of satellite cells to NMJ regeneration in SNT-induced atrophy [124], castration-induced atrophy [122], and natural aging in mice [123], opening a new avenue of therapeutic intervention through the targeting of satellite cells, especially for muscle atrophy associated with NMJ degeneration, including sarcopenia. A more comprehensive understanding of the molecular and cellular mechanisms underlying the contribution of satellite cells in various mouse models is necessary to perform more precise interventions to maximize their capacity for attenuating or reversing declines in age-related muscle plasticity, which are strongly linked to a reduced quality of life in elderly individuals.

Acknowledgment

Research conducted in our laboratory is currently supported by a MEXT Leading Initiative for Excellent Young Researchers.

References

[1] Campbell KP, Kahl SD. Association of dystrophin and an integral membrane glycoprotein. Nature 1989;338:259–62. https://doi.org/10.1038/338259a0.

[2] Hoffman EP, Brown RH, Kunkel LM. Dystrophin: the protein product of the duchenne muscular dystrophy locus. Cell 1987;51:919–28. https://doi.org/10.1016/0092-8674(87)90579-4.

[3] Yoshida M, Ozawa E. Glycoprotein complex anchoring dystrophin to sarcolemma1. J Biochem (Tokyo) 1990;108:748–52. https://doi.org/10.1093/oxfordjournals.jbchem.a123276.

[4] Cohen S, Nathan JA, Goldberg AL. Muscle wasting in disease: molecular mechanisms and promising therapies. Nat Rev Drug Discov 2015;14:58–74. https://doi.org/10.1038/nrd4467.

[5] Egerman MA, Glass DJ. Signaling pathways controlling skeletal muscle mass. Crit Rev Biochem Mol Biol 2014;49:59–68. https://doi.org/10.3109/10409238.2013.857291.

[6] Narici MV, Maffulli N. Sarcopenia: characteristics, mechanisms and functional significance. Br Med Bull 2010;95:139–59. https://doi.org/10.1093/bmb/ldq008.

[7] Verdijk LB, Koopman R, Schaart G, Meijer K, Savelberg HHCM, van Loon LJC. Satellite cell content is specifically reduced in type II skeletal muscle fibers in the elderly. Am J Physiol Endocrinol Metab 2007;292:E151–7. https://doi.org/10.1152/ajpendo.00278.2006.

[8] Fujita R, Yoshioka K, Seko D, Suematsu T, Mitsuhashi S, Senoo N, Miura S, Nishino I, Ono Y. Zmynd17 controls muscle mitochondrial quality and whole-body metabolism. FASEB J 2018;32:5012–25. https://doi.org/10.1096/fj.201701264R.

[9] Migliavacca E, Tay SKH, Patel HP, Sonntag T, Civiletto G, McFarlane C, Forrester T, Barton SJ, Leow MK, Antoun E, Charpagne A, Seng Chong Y, Descombes P, Feng L, Francis-Emmanuel P, Garratt ES, Giner MP, Green CO, Karaz S, Kothandaraman N, Marquis J, Metairon S, Moco S, Nelson G, Ngo S, Pleasants T, Raymond F, Sayer AA, Ming Sim C, Slater-Jefferies J, Syddall HE, Fang Tan P, Titcombe P, Vaz C, Westbury LD, Wong G, Yonghui W, Cooper C, Sheppard A, Godfrey KM, Lillycrop KA, Karnani N, Feige JN. Mitochondrial oxidative capacity and NAD+ biosynthesis are reduced in human sarcopenia across ethnicities. Nat Commun 2019;10:5808. https://doi.org/10.1038/s41467-019-13694-1.

[10] Yoshioka K, Fujita R, Seko D, Suematsu T, Miura S, Ono Y. Distinct roles of Zmynd17 and PGC1α in mitochondrial quality control and biogenesis in skeletal muscle. Front Cell Dev Biol 2019;7:330. https://doi.org/10.3389/fcell.2019.00330.

[11] Mauro A. Satellite cell of skeletal muscle fibers. J Biophys Biochem Cytol 1961;9:493–5. https://doi.org/10.1083/jcb.9.2.493.

[12] Blau HM, Cosgrove BD, Ho ATV. The central role of muscle stem cells in regenerative failure with aging. Nat Med 2015;21:854–62. https://doi.org/10.1038/nm.3918.

[13] Chargé SBP, Rudnicki MA. Cellular and molecular regulation of muscle regeneration. Physiol Rev 2004;84:209–38. https://doi.org/10.1152/physrev.00019.2003.

[14] Dumont NA, Wang YX, Rudnicki MA. Intrinsic and extrinsic mechanisms regulating satellite cell function. Dev Camb Engl 2015;142:1572–81. https://doi.org/10.1242/dev.114223.

[15] Shi X, Garry DJ. Muscle stem cells in development, regeneration, and disease. Genes Dev 2006;20:1692–708. https://doi.org/10.1101/gad.1419406.

[16] Sousa-Victor P, Muñoz-Cánoves P. Regenerative decline of stem cells in sarcopenia. Mol Aspects Med 2016;50:109–17. https://doi.org/10.1016/j.mam.2016.02.002.

[17] Katz B. The termination of the afferent nerve fibre in the muscle spindle of the frog. Philos Trans R Soc Lond B Biol Sci 1961;243:221–40. https://doi.org/10.1098/rstb.1961.0001.

[18] Relaix F, Rocancourt D, Mansouri A, Buckingham M. A Pax3/Pax7-dependent population of skeletal muscle progenitor cells. Nature 2005;435:948–53. https://doi.org/10.1038/nature03594.

[19] Cheung TH, Rando TA. Molecular regulation of stem cell quiescence. Nat Rev Mol Cell Biol 2013;14:329–40. https://doi.org/10.1038/nrm3591.

[20] Crist CG, Montarras D, Buckingham M. Muscle satellite cells are primed for myogenesis but maintain quiescence with sequestration of Myf5 mRNA targeted by microRNA-31 in mRNP granules. Cell Stem Cell 2012;11:118–26. https://doi.org/10.1016/j.stem.2012.03.011.

[21] Fujita R, Crist C. Translational control of the myogenic program in developing, regenerating, and diseased skeletal muscle. In: Current topics in developmental biology. Elsevier; 2018. p. 67–98. https://doi.org/10.1016/bs.ctdb.2017.08.004.

[22] Rodgers JT, King KY, Brett JO, Cromie MJ, Charville GW, Maguire KK, Brunson C, Mastey N, Liu L, Tsai C-R, Goodell MA, Rando TA. mTORC1 controls the adaptive transition of quiescent stem cells from G0 to GAlert. Nature 2014;510:393–6. https://doi.org/10.1038/nature13255.

[23] Montarras D, L'honoré A, Buckingham M. Lying low but ready for action: the quiescent muscle satellite cell. FEBS J 2013;280:4036–50. https://doi.org/10.1111/febs.12372.

[24] Baghdadi MB, Castel D, Machado L, Fukada S-I, Birk DE, Relaix F, Tajbakhsh S, Mourikis P. Reciprocal signalling by Notch-Collagen V-CALCR retains muscle stem cells in their niche. Nature 2018;557:714–8. https://doi.org/10.1038/s41586-018-0144-9.

[25] Chakkalakal JV, Jones KM, Basson MA, Brack AS. The aged niche disrupts muscle stem cell quiescence. Nature 2012;490:355–60. https://doi.org/10.1038/nature11438.

[26] Cheung TH, Quach NL, Charville GW, Liu L, Park L, Edalati A, Yoo B, Hoang P, Rando TA. Maintenance of muscle stem-cell quiescence by microRNA-489. Nature 2012;482:524–8. https://doi.org/10.1038/nature10834.

[27] Fujita R, Jamet S, Lean G, Cheng HCM, Hébert S, Kleinman CL, et al. Satellite cell expansion is mediated by P-eIF2α dependent *Tacc3* translation (preprint). Development 2021;148(2). https://doi.org/10.1242/dev.194480, dev194480.

[28] Fujita R, Zismanov V, Jacob J-M, Jamet S, Asiev K, Crist C. Fragile X mental retardation protein regulates skeletal muscle stem cell activity by regulating the stability of Myf5 mRNA. Skelet Muscle 2017;7:18. https://doi.org/10.1186/s13395-017-0136-8.

[29] Goel AJ, Rieder M-K, Arnold H-H, Radice GL, Krauss RS. Niche cadherins control the quiescence-to-activation transition in muscle stem cells. Cell Rep 2017;21:2236–50. https://doi.org/10.1016/j.celrep.2017.10.102.

[30] Machado L, Esteves de Lima J, Fabre O, Proux C, Legendre R, Szegedi A, Varet H, Ingerslev LR, Barrès R, Relaix F, Mourikis P. In situ fixation redefines quiescence and early activation of skeletal muscle stem cells. Cell Rep 2017;21:1982–93. https://doi.org/10.1016/j.celrep.2017.10.080.

[31] van Velthoven CTJ, de Morree A, Egner IM, Brett JO, Rando TA. Transcriptional profiling of quiescent muscle stem cells in vivo. Cell Rep 2017;21:1994–2004. https://doi.org/10.1016/j.celrep.2017.10.037.

[32] Yamaguchi M, Watanabe Y, Ohtani T, Uezumi A, Mikami N, Nakamura M, Sato T, Ikawa M, Hoshino M, Tsuchida K, Miyagoe-Suzuki Y, Tsujikawa K, Takeda S, Yamamoto H, Fukada S. Calcitonin receptor signaling inhibits muscle stem cells from escaping the quiescent state and the niche. Cell Rep 2015;13:302–14. https://doi.org/10.1016/j.celrep.2015.08.083.

[33] Zismanov V, Chichkov V, Colangelo V, Jamet S, Wang S, Syme A, Koromilas AE, Crist C. Phosphorylation of eIF2α is a translational control mechanism regulating muscle stem cell quiescence and self-renewal. Cell Stem Cell 2016;18:79–90. https://doi.org/10.1016/j.stem.2015.09.020.

[34] Shea KL, Xiang W, LaPorta VS, Licht JD, Keller C, Basson MA, Brack AS. Sprouty1 regulates reversible quiescence of a self-renewing adult muscle stem cell pool during regeneration. Cell Stem Cell 2010;6:117–29. https://doi.org/10.1016/j.stem.2009.12.015.

[35] Hausburg MA, Doles JD, Clement SL, Cadwallader AB, Hall MN, Blackshear PJ, Lykke-Andersen J, Olwin BB. Post-transcriptional regulation of satellite cell quiescence by TTP-mediated mRNA decay. Elife 2015;4:e03390. https://doi.org/10.7554/eLife.03390.

[36] Sato T, Yamamoto T, Sehara-Fujisawa A. miR-195/497 induce postnatal quiescence of skeletal muscle stem cells. Nat Commun 2014;5:4597. https://doi.org/10.1038/ncomms5597.

[37] Rudnicki MA, Schnegelsberg PNJ, Stead RH, Braun T, Arnold H-H, Jaenisch R. MyoD or Myf-5 is required for the formation of skeletal muscle. Cell 1993;75:1351–9. https://doi.org/10.1016/0092-8674(93)90621-V.

[38] Kuang S, Kuroda K, Le Grand F, Rudnicki MA. Asymmetric self-renewal and commitment of satellite stem cells in muscle. Cell 2007;129:999–1010. https://doi.org/10.1016/j.cell.2007.03.044.

[39] Le Grand F, Jones AE, Seale V, Scimè A, Rudnicki MA. Wnt7a activates the planar cell polarity pathway to drive the symmetric expansion of satellite stem cells. Cell Stem Cell 2009;4:535–47. https://doi.org/10.1016/j.stem.2009.03.013.

[40] Rocheteau P, Gayraud-Morel B, Siegl-Cachedenier I, Blasco MA, Tajbakhsh S. A subpopulation of adult skeletal muscle stem cells retains all template DNA strands after cell division. Cell 2012;148:112–25. https://doi.org/10.1016/j.cell.2011.11.049.

[41] Wang YX, Feige P, Brun CE, Hekmatnejad B, Dumont NA, Renaud J-M, Faulkes S, Guindon DE, Rudnicki MA. EGFR-Aurka signaling rescues polarity and regeneration defects in dystrophin-deficient muscle stem cells by increasing asymmetric divisions. Cell Stem Cell 2019;24:419–32. e6 https://doi.org/10.1016/j.stem.2019.01.002.

[42] Seale P, Sabourin LA, Girgis-Gabardo A, Mansouri A, Gruss P, Rudnicki MA. Pax7 is required for the specification of myogenic satellite cells. Cell 2000;102:777–86. https://doi.org/10.1016/S0092-8674(00)00066-0.

[43] Relaix F, Montarras D, Zaffran S, Gayraud-Morel B, Rocancourt D, Tajbakhsh S, Mansouri A, Cumano A, Buckingham M. Pax3 and Pax7 have distinct and overlapping functions in adult muscle progenitor cells. J Cell Biol 2006;172:91–102. https://doi.org/10.1083/jcb.200508044.

[44] Seale P, Ishibashi J, Scimè A, Rudnicki MA. Pax7 is necessary and sufficient for the myogenic specification of CD45+:Sca1+ stem cells from injured muscle. PLoS Biol 2004;2:e130. https://doi.org/10.1371/journal.pbio.0020130.

[45] Der Vartanian A, Quétin M, Michineau S, Auradé F, Hayashi S, Dubois C, Rocancourt D, Drayton-Libotte B, Szegedi A, Buckingham M, Conway SJ, Gervais M, Relaix F. PAX3 confers functional heterogeneity in skeletal muscle stem cell responses to environmental stress. Cell Stem Cell 2019;24:958–73. e9 https://doi.org/10.1016/j.stem.2019.03.019.

[46] Scaramozza A, Park D, Kollu S, Beerman I, Sun X, Rossi DJ, Lin CP, Scadden DT, Crist C, Brack AS. Lineage tracing reveals a subset of reserve muscle stem cells capable of clonal expansion under stress. Cell Stem Cell 2019;24:944–57. e5 https://doi.org/10.1016/j.stem.2019.03.020.

[47] de Morrée A, van Velthoven CTJ, Gan Q, Salvi JS, Klein JDD, Akimenko I, Quarta M, Biressi S, Rando TA. Staufen1 inhibits MyoD translation to actively maintain muscle stem cell quiescence. Proc Natl Acad Sci U S A 2017;114:E8996–9005. https://doi.org/10.1073/pnas.1708725114.

[48] Dick SA, Chang NC, Dumont NA, Bell RAV, Putinski C, Kawabe Y, Litchfield DW, Rudnicki MA, Megeney LA. Caspase 3 cleavage of Pax7 inhibits self-renewal of satellite cells. Proc Natl Acad Sci U S A 2015;112:E5246–52. https://doi.org/10.1073/pnas.1512869112.

[49] Olguin HC, Olwin BB. Pax-7 up-regulation inhibits myogenesis and cell cycle progression in satellite cells: a potential mechanism for self-renewal. Dev Biol 2004;275:375–88. https://doi.org/10.1016/j.ydbio.2004.08.015.

[50] Chakkalakal JV, Christensen J, Xiang W, Tierney MT, Boscolo FS, Sacco A, Brack AS. Early forming label-retaining muscle stem cells require p27kip1 for maintenance of the primitive state. Dev Camb Engl 2014;141:1649–59. https://doi.org/10.1242/dev.100842.

[51] Ono Y, Masuda S, Nam H-S, Benezra R, Miyagoe-Suzuki Y, Takeda S. Slow-dividing satellite cells retain long-term self-renewal ability in adult muscle. J Cell Sci 2012;125:1309–17. https://doi.org/10.1242/jcs.096198.

[52] Barruet E, Garcia SM, Striedinger K, Wu J, Lee S, Byrnes L, Wong A, Xuefeng S, Tamaki S, Brack AS, Pomerantz JH. Functionally heterogeneous human satellite cells identified by single cell RNA sequencing. Elife 2020;9:e51576. https://doi.org/10.7554/eLife.51576.

[53] von Maltzahn J, Jones AE, Parks RJ, Rudnicki MA. Pax7 is critical for the normal function of satellite cells in adult skeletal muscle. Proc Natl Acad Sci U S A 2013;110:16474–9. https://doi.org/10.1073/pnas.1307680110.

[54] Lepper C, Partridge TA, Fan C-M. An absolute requirement for Pax7-positive satellite cells in acute injury-induced skeletal muscle regeneration. Development 2011;138:3639–46. https://doi.org/10.1242/dev.067595.

[55] Murphy MM, Lawson JA, Mathew SJ, Hutcheson DA, Kardon G. Satellite cells, connective tissue fibroblasts and their interactions are crucial for muscle regeneration. Development 2011;138:3625–37. https://doi.org/10.1242/dev.064162.

[56] Sambasivan R, Yao R, Kissenpfennig A, Van Wittenberghe L, Paldi A, Gayraud-Morel B, Guenou H, Malissen B, Tajbakhsh S, Galy A. Pax7-expressing satellite cells are indispensable for adult skeletal muscle regeneration. Development 2011;138:3647–56. https://doi.org/10.1242/dev.067587.

[57] Forcina L, Miano C, Pelosi L, Musarò A. An overview about the biology of skeletal muscle satellite cells. Curr Genomics 2019;20:24–37. https://doi.org/10.2174/1389202920666190116094736.

[58] Wosczyna MN, Rando TA. A muscle stem cell support group: coordinated cellular responses in muscle regeneration. Dev Cell 2018;46:135–43. https://doi.org/10.1016/j.devcel.2018.06.018.

[59] Arnold L, Henry A, Poron F, Baba-Amer Y, van Rooijen N, Plonquet A, Gherardi RK, Chazaud B. Inflammatory monocytes recruited after skeletal muscle injury switch into antiinflammatory macrophages to support myogenesis. J Exp Med 2007;204:1057–69. https://doi.org/10.1084/jem.20070075.

[60] Fujita R, Kawano F, Ohira T, Nakai N, Shibaguchi T, Nishimoto N, Ohira Y. Anti-interleukin-6 receptor antibody (MR16-1) promotes muscle regeneration via modulation of gene expressions in infiltrated macrophages. Biochim Biophys Acta Gen Subj 2014;1840:3170–80. https://doi.org/10.1016/j.bbagen.2014.01.014.

[61] Deng B, Wehling-Henricks M, Villalta SA, Wang Y, Tidball JG. IL-10 triggers changes in macrophage phenotype that promote muscle growth and regeneration. J Immunol 2012;189:3669–80. https://doi.org/10.4049/jimmunol.1103180.

[62] Horsley V, Jansen KM, Mills ST, Pavlath GK. IL-4 acts as a myoblast recruitment factor during mammalian muscle growth. Cell 2003;113:483–94. https://doi.org/10.1016/S0092-8674(03)00319-2.

[63] Bodine SC, Stitt TN, Gonzalez M, Kline WO, Stover GL, Bauerlein R, Zlotchenko E, Scrimgeour A, Lawrence JC, Glass DJ, Yancopoulos GD. Akt/mTOR pathway is a crucial regulator of skeletal muscle hypertrophy and can prevent muscle atrophy in vivo. Nat Cell Biol 2001;3:1014–9. https://doi.org/10.1038/ncb1101-1014.

[64] Tonkin J, Temmerman L, Sampson RD, Gallego-Colon E, Barberi L, Bilbao D, Schneider MD, Musarò A, Rosenthal N. Monocyte/macrophage-derived IGF-1 orchestrates murine skeletal muscle regeneration and modulates autocrine polarization. Mol Ther 2015;23:1189–200. https://doi.org/10.1038/mt.2015.66.

[65] Joe AWB, Yi L, Natarajan A, Le Grand F, So L, Wang J, Rudnicki MA, Rossi FMV. Muscle injury activates resident fibro/adipogenic progenitors that facilitate myogenesis. Nat Cell Biol 2010;12:153–63. https://doi.org/10.1038/ncb2015.

[66] Uezumi A, Fukada S, Yamamoto N, Takeda S, Tsuchida K. Mesenchymal progenitors distinct from satellite cells contribute to ectopic fat cell formation in skeletal muscle. Nat Cell Biol 2010;12:143–52. https://doi.org/10.1038/ncb2014.

[67] Lukjanenko L, Karaz S, Stuelsatz P, Gurriaran-Rodriguez U, Michaud J, Dammone G, Sizzano F, Mashinchian O, Ancel S, Migliavacca E, Liot S, Jacot G, Metairon S, Raymond F, Descombes P, Palini A, Chazaud B, Rudnicki MA, Bentzinger CF, Feige JN. Aging disrupts muscle stem cell function by impairing matricellular WISP1 secretion from fibro-adipogenic progenitors. Cell Stem Cell 2019;24:433–46. e7 https://doi.org/10.1016/j.stem.2018.12.014.

[68] Heredia JE, Mukundan L, Chen FM, Mueller AA, Deo RC, Locksley RM, Rando TA, Chawla A. Type 2 innate signals stimulate fibro/adipogenic progenitors to facilitate muscle regeneration. Cell 2013;153:376–88. https://doi.org/10.1016/j.cell.2013.02.053.

[69] Christov C, Chrétien F, Abou-Khalil R, Bassez G, Vallet G, Authier F-J, Bassaglia Y, Shinin V, Tajbakhsh S, Chazaud B, Gherardi RK. Muscle satellite cells and endothelial cells: close neighbors and privileged partners. Mol Biol Cell 2007;18:1397–409. https://doi.org/10.1091/mbc.e06-08-0693.

[70] Verma M, Asakura Y, Murakonda BSR, Pengo T, Latroche C, Chazaud B, McLoon LK, Asakura A. Muscle satellite cell cross-talk with a vascular niche maintains quiescence via vegf and notch signaling. Cell Stem Cell 2018;23:530–43. e9 https://doi.org/10.1016/j.stem.2018.09.007.

[71] Bentzinger CF, Wang YX, von Maltzahn J, Soleimani VD, Yin H, Rudnicki MA. Fibronectin regulates Wnt7a signaling and satellite cell expansion. Cell Stem Cell 2013;12:75–87. https://doi.org/10.1016/j.stem.2012.09.015.

[72] Fujita R, Tamai K, Aikawa E, Nimura K, Ishino S, Kikuchi Y, Kaneda Y. Endogenous mesenchymal stromal cells in bone marrow are required to preserve muscle function in mdx mice: role of endogenous MSC population in DMD pathology. Stem Cells 2015;33:962–75. https://doi.org/10.1002/stem.1900.

[73] Urciuolo A, Quarta M, Morbidoni V, Gattazzo F, Molon S, Grumati P, Montemurro F, Tedesco FS, Blaauw B, Cossu G, Vozzi G, Rando TA, Bonaldo P. Collagen VI regulates satellite cell self-renewal and muscle regeneration. Nat Commun 2013;4:1964. https://doi.org/10.1038/ncomms2964.

[74] Alway SE, Myers MJ, Mohamed JS. Regulation of satellite cell function in sarcopenia. Front Aging Neurosci 2014;6. https://doi.org/10.3389/fnagi.2014.00246.

[75] García-Prat L, Sousa-Victor P, Muñoz-Cánoves P. Functional dysregulation of stem cells during aging: a focus on skeletal muscle stem cells. FEBS J 2013;280:4051–62. https://doi.org/10.1111/febs.12221.

[76] Day K, Shefer G, Shearer A, Yablonka-Reuveni Z. The depletion of skeletal muscle satellite cells with age is concomitant with reduced capacity of single progenitors to produce reserve progeny. Dev Biol 2010;340:330–43. https://doi.org/10.1016/j.ydbio.2010.01.006.

[77] Bernet JD, Doles JD, Hall JK, Kelly Tanaka K, Carter TA, Olwin BB. p38 MAPK signaling underlies a cell-autonomous loss of stem cell self-renewal in skeletal muscle of aged mice. Nat Med 2014;20:265–71. https://doi.org/10.1038/nm.3465.

[78] Cosgrove BD, Gilbert PM, Porpiglia E, Mourkioti F, Lee SP, Corbel SY, Llewellyn ME, Delp SL, Blau HM. Rejuvenation of the muscle stem cell population restores strength to injured aged muscles. Nat Med 2014;20:255–64. https://doi.org/10.1038/nm.3464.

[79] Price FD, von Maltzahn J, Bentzinger CF, Dumont NA, Yin H, Chang NC, Wilson DH, Frenette J, Rudnicki MA. Inhibition of JAK-STAT signaling stimulates adult satellite cell function. Nat Med 2014;20:1174–81. https://doi.org/10.1038/nm.3655.

[80] Sousa-Victor P, Gutarra S, García-Prat L, Rodriguez-Ubreva J, Ortet L, Ruiz-Bonilla V, Jardí M, Ballestar E, González S, Serrano AL, Perdiguero E, Muñoz-Cánoves P. Geriatric muscle stem cells switch reversible quiescence into senescence. Nature 2014;506:316–21. https://doi.org/10.1038/nature13013.

[81] Tierney MT, Aydogdu T, Sala D, Malecova B, Gatto S, Puri PL, Latella L, Sacco A. STAT3 signaling controls satellite cell expansion and skeletal muscle repair. Nat Med 2014;20:1182–6. https://doi.org/10.1038/nm.3656.

[82] Palacios D, Mozzetta C, Consalvi S, Caretti G, Saccone V, Proserpio V, Marquez VE, Valente S, Mai A, Forcales SV, Sartorelli V, Puri PL. TNF/p38α/polycomb signaling to Pax7 locus in satellite cells links inflammation to the epigenetic control of muscle regeneration. Cell Stem Cell 2010;7:455–69. https://doi.org/10.1016/j.stem.2010.08.013.

[83] García-Prat L, Martínez-Vicente M, Perdiguero E, Ortet L, Rodríguez-Ubreva J, Rebollo E, Ruiz-Bonilla V, Gutarra S, Ballestar E, Serrano AL, Sandri M, Muñoz-Cánoves P. Autophagy maintains stemness by preventing senescence. Nature 2016;529:37–42. https://doi.org/10.1038/nature16187.

[84] Sin J, Andres AM, Taylor DJR, Weston T, Hiraumi Y, Stotland A, Kim BJ, Huang C, Doran KS, Gottlieb RA. Mitophagy is required for mitochondrial biogenesis and myogenic differentiation of C2C12 myoblasts. Autophagy 2016;12:369–80. https://doi.org/10.1080/15548627.2015.1115172.

[85] Tang AH, Rando TA. Induction of autophagy supports the bioenergetic demands of quiescent muscle stem cell activation. EMBO J 2014;33:2782–97. https://doi.org/10.15252/embj.201488278.

[86] Takeshige K, Baba M, Tsuboi S, Noda T, Ohsumi Y. Autophagy in yeast demonstrated with proteinase-deficient mutants and conditions for its induction. J Cell Biol 1992;119:301–11. https://doi.org/10.1083/jcb.119.2.301.

[87] Cerletti M, Jang YC, Finley LWS, Haigis MC, Wagers AJ. Short-term calorie restriction enhances skeletal muscle stem cell function. Cell Stem Cell 2012;10:515–9. https://doi.org/10.1016/j.stem.2012.04.002.

[88] Sacco A, Mourkioti F, Tran R, Choi J, Llewellyn M, Kraft P, Shkreli M, Delp S, Pomerantz JH, Artandi SE, Blau HM. Short telomeres and stem cell exhaustion model duchenne muscular dystrophy in mdx/mTR mice. Cell 2010;143:1059–71. https://doi.org/10.1016/j.cell.2010.11.039.

[89] Tichy ED, Sidibe DK, Tierney MT, Stec MJ, Sharifi-Sanjani M, Hosalkar H, Mubarak S, Johnson FB, Sacco A, Mourkioti F. Single stem cell imaging and analysis reveals telomere length differences in diseased human and mouse skeletal muscles. Stem Cell Rep 2017;9:1328–41. https://doi.org/10.1016/j.stemcr.2017.08.003.

[90] Zhu C-H, Mouly V, Cooper RN, Mamchaoui K, Bigot A, Shay JW, Di Santo JP, Butler-Browne GS, Wright WE. Cellular senescence in human myoblasts is overcome by human telomerase reverse transcriptase and cyclin-dependent kinase 4: consequences in aging muscle and therapeutic strategies for muscular dystrophies. Aging Cell 2007;6:515–23. https://doi.org/10.1111/j.1474-9726.2007.00306.x.

[91] Carey KA, Farnfield MM, Tarquinio SD, Cameron-Smith D. Impaired expression of notch signaling genes in aged human skeletal muscle. J Gerontol Ser A 2007;62:9–17. https://doi.org/10.1093/gerona/62.1.9.

[92] Brack AS, Conboy MJ, Roy S, Lee M, Kuo CJ, Keller C, Rando TA. Increased Wnt signaling during aging alters muscle stem cell fate and increases fibrosis. Science 2007;317:807–10. https://doi.org/10.1126/science.1144090.

[93] Conboy IM, Conboy MJ, Wagers AJ, Girma ER, Weissman IL, Rando TA. Rejuvenation of aged progenitor cells by exposure to a young systemic environment. Nature 2005;433:760–4. https://doi.org/10.1038/nature03260.

[94] Naito AT, Sumida T, Nomura S, Liu M-L, Higo T, Nakagawa A, Okada K, Sakai T, Hashimoto A, Hara Y, Shimizu I, Zhu W, Toko H, Katada A, Akazawa H, Oka T, Lee J-K, Minamino T, Nagai T, Walsh K, Kikuchi A, Matsumoto M, Botto M, Shiojima I, Komuro I. Complement C1q activates canonical Wnt signaling and promotes aging-related phenotypes. Cell 2012;149:1298–313. https://doi.org/10.1016/j.cell.2012.03.047.

[95] Elabd C, Cousin W, Upadhyayula P, Chen RY, Chooljian MS, Li J, Kung S, Jiang KP, Conboy IM. Oxytocin is an age-specific circulating hormone that is necessary for muscle maintenance and regeneration. Nat Commun 2014;5:4082. https://doi.org/10.1038/ncomms5082.

[96] Collins BC, Arpke RW, Larson AA, Baumann CW, Xie N, Cabelka CA, Nash NL, Juppi H-K, Laakkonen EK, Sipilä S, Kovanen V, Spangenburg EE, Kyba M, Lowe DA. Estrogen regulates the satellite cell compartment in females. Cell Rep 2019;28:368–81. e6 https://doi.org/10.1016/j.celrep.2019.06.025.

[97] Seko D, Fujita R, Kitajima Y, Nakamura K, Imai Y, Ono Y. Estrogen receptor β controls muscle growth and regeneration in young female mice. Stem Cell Rep 2020. https://doi.org/10.1016/j.stemcr.2020.07.017. pii: S2213671120302940.

[98] Rai R, Ghosh AK, Eren M, Mackie AR, Levine DC, Kim S-Y, Cedernaes J, Ramirez V, Procissi D, Smith LH, Woodruff TK, Bass J, Vaughan DE. Downregulation of the apelinergic axis accelerates aging, whereas its systemic restoration improves the mammalian healthspan. Cell Rep 2017;21:1471–80. https://doi.org/10.1016/j.celrep.2017.10.057.

[99] Vinel C, Lukjanenko L, Batut A, Deleruyelle S, Pradère J-P, Le Gonidec S, Dortignac A, Geoffre N, Pereira O, Karaz S, Lee U, Camus M, Chaoui K, Mouisel E, Bigot A, Mouly V, Vigneau M, Pagano AF, Chopard A, Pillard F, Guyonnet S, Cesari M, Burlet-Schiltz O, Pahor M, Feige JN, Vellas B, Valet P, Dray C. The exerkine apelin reverses age-associated sarcopenia. Nat Med 2018;24:1360–71. https://doi.org/10.1038/s41591-018-0131-6.

[100] Conboy IM. Notch-mediated restoration of regenerative potential to aged muscle. Science 2003;302:1575–7. https://doi.org/10.1126/science.1087573.

[101] Fujimaki S, Seko D, Kitajima Y, Yoshioka K, Tsuchiya Y, Masuda S, Ono Y. Notch1 and Notch2 coordinately regulate stem cell function in the quiescent and activated states of muscle satellite cells: Notch1 and Notch2 regulate muscle stem cells. Stem Cells 2018;36:278–85. https://doi.org/10.1002/stem.2743.

[102] Mourikis P, Sambasivan R, Castel D, Rocheteau P, Bizzarro V, Tajbakhsh S. A critical requirement for notch signaling in maintenance of the quiescent skeletal muscle stem cell state. Stem Cells 2012;30:243–52. https://doi.org/10.1002/stem.775.

[103] Robert L, Labat-Robert J. Aging of connective tissues: from genetic to epigenetic mechanisms. Biogerontology 2000;1:123–31. https://doi.org/10.1023/A:1010048014925.

[104] Gilbert PM, Havenstrite KL, Magnusson KEG, Sacco A, Leonardi NA, Kraft P, Nguyen NK, Thrun S, Lutolf MP, Blau HM. Substrate elasticity regulates skeletal muscle stem cell self-renewal in culture. Science 2010;329:1078–81. https://doi.org/10.1126/science.1191035.

[105] Stearns-Reider KM, D'Amore A, Beezhold K, Rothrauff B, Cavalli L, Wagner WR, Vorp DA, Tsamis A, Shinde S, Zhang C, Barchowsky A, Rando TA, Tuan RS, Ambrosio F. Aging of the skeletal muscle extracellular matrix drives a stem cell fibrogenic conversion. Aging Cell 2017;16:518–28. https://doi.org/10.1111/acel.12578.

[106] Scott RW, Arostegui M, Schweitzer R, Rossi FMV, Underhill TM. Hic1 defines quiescent mesenchymal progenitor subpopulations with distinct functions and fates in skeletal muscle regeneration. Cell Stem Cell 2019;25:797–813. e9 https://doi.org/10.1016/j.stem.2019.11.004.

[107] Kuswanto W, Burzyn D, Panduro M, Wang KK, Jang YC, Wagers AJ, Benoist C, Mathis D. Poor repair of skeletal muscle in aging mice reflects a defect in local, interleukin-33-dependent accumulation of regulatory T cells. Immunity 2016;44:355–67. https://doi.org/10.1016/j.immuni.2016.01.009.

[108] Moss FP, Leblond CP. Satellite cells as the source of nuclei in muscles of growing rats. Anat Rec 1971;170:421–35. https://doi.org/10.1002/ar.1091700405.

[109] White RB, Biérinx A-S, Gnocchi VF, Zammit PS. Dynamics of muscle fibre growth during postnatal mouse development. BMC Dev Biol 2010;10:21. https://doi.org/10.1186/1471-213X-10-21.

[110] Bachman JF, Klose A, Liu W, Paris ND, Blanc RS, Schmalz M, Knapp E, Chakkalakal JV. Prepubertal skeletal muscle growth requires Pax7-expressing satellite cell-derived myonuclear contribution. Development 2018;145:dev167197. https://doi.org/10.1242/dev.167197.

[111] Egner IM, Bruusgaard JC, Gundersen K. Satellite cell depletion prevents fiber hypertrophy in skeletal muscle. Development 2016;143:2898–906. https://doi.org/10.1242/dev.134411.

[112] Fukuda S, Kaneshige A, Kaji T, Noguchi Y, Takemoto Y, Zhang L, Tsujikawa K, Kokubo H, Uezumi A, Maehara K, Harada A, Ohkawa Y, Fukada S. Sustained expression of HeyL is critical for the proliferation of muscle stem cells in overloaded muscle. Elife 2019;8:e48284. https://doi.org/10.7554/eLife.48284.

[113] McCarthy JJ, Mula J, Miyazaki M, Erfani R, Garrison K, Farooqui AB, Srikuea R, Lawson BA, Grimes B, Keller C, Van Zant G, Campbell KS, Esser KA, Dupont-Versteegden EE, Peterson CA. Effective fiber hypertrophy in satellite cell-depleted skeletal muscle. Development 2011;138:3657–66. https://doi.org/10.1242/dev.068858.

[114] Jackson JR, Mula J, Kirby TJ, Fry CS, Lee JD, Ubele MF, Campbell KS, McCarthy JJ, Peterson CA, Dupont-Versteegden EE. Satellite cell depletion does not inhibit adult skeletal muscle regrowth following unloading-induced atrophy. Am J Physiol Cell Physiol 2012;303:C854–61. https://doi.org/10.1152/ajpcell.00207.2012.

[115] Goh Q, Millay DP. Requirement of myomaker-mediated stem cell fusion for skeletal muscle hypertrophy. Elife 2017;6:e20007. https://doi.org/10.7554/eLife.20007.

[116] Fry CS, Lee JD, Jackson JR, Kirby TJ, Stasko SA, Liu H, Dupont-Versteegden EE, McCarthy JJ, Peterson CA. Regulation of the muscle fiber micro environment by activated satellite cells during hypertrophy. FASEB J 2014;28:1654–65. https://doi.org/10.1096/fj.13-239426.

[117] Fry CS, Kirby TJ, Kosmac K, McCarthy JJ, Peterson CA. Myogenic progenitor cells control extracellular matrix production by fibroblasts during skeletal muscle hypertrophy. Cell Stem Cell 2017;20:56–69. https://doi.org/10.1016/j.stem.2016.09.010.

[118] Brack AS. Evidence that satellite cell decrement contributes to preferential decline in nuclear number from large fibres during murine age-related muscle atrophy. J Cell Sci 2005;118:4813–21. https://doi.org/10.1242/jcs.02602.

[119] Kadi F, Charifi N, Denis C, Lexell J. Satellite cells and myonuclei in young and elderly women and men. Muscle Nerve 2004;29:120–7. https://doi.org/10.1002/mus.10510.

[120] Fry CS, Lee JD, Mula J, Kirby TJ, Jackson JR, Liu F, Yang L, Mendias CL, Dupont-Versteegden EE, McCarthy JJ, Peterson CA. Inducible depletion of satellite cells in adult, sedentary mice impairs muscle regenerative capacity without affecting sarcopenia. Nat Med 2015;21:76–80. https://doi.org/10.1038/nm.3710.

[121] Keefe AC, Lawson JA, Flygare SD, Fox ZD, Colasanto MP, Mathew SJ, Yandell M, Kardon G. Muscle stem cells contribute to myofibres in sedentary adult mice. Nat Commun 2015;6:7087. https://doi.org/10.1038/ncomms8087.

[122] Klose A, Liu W, Paris ND, Forman S, Krolewski JJ, Nastiuk KL, Chakkalakal JV. Castration induces satellite cell activation that contributes to skeletal muscle maintenance. JCSM Rapid Commun 2018;1:1–16. https://doi.org/10.1002/j.2617-1619.2018.tb00004.x.

[123] Liu W, Klose A, Forman S, Paris ND, Wei-LaPierre L, Cortés-Lopéz M, Tan A, Flaherty M, Miura P, Dirksen RT, Chakkalakal JV. Loss of adult skeletal muscle stem cells drives age-related neuromuscular junction degeneration. Elife 2017;6:e26464. https://doi.org/10.7554/eLife.26464.

[124] Liu W, Wei-LaPierre L, Klose A, Dirksen RT, Chakkalakal JV. Inducible depletion of adult skeletal muscle stem cells impairs the regeneration of neuromuscular junctions. Elife 2015;4:e09221. https://doi.org/10.7554/eLife.09221.

[125] Gundersen K, Bruusgaard JC. Nuclear domains during muscle atrophy: nuclei lost or paradigm lost?: nuclear domains during muscle atrophy. J Physiol 2008;586:2675–81. https://doi.org/10.1113/jphysiol.2008.154369.

[126] Bruusgaard JC, Gundersen K. In vivo time-lapse microscopy reveals no loss of murine myonuclei during weeks of muscle atrophy. J Clin Invest 2008;118:1450–7. https://doi.org/10.1172/JCI34022.

[127] Murach KA, Vechetti IJ, Van Pelt DW, Crow SE, Dungan CM, Figueiredo VC, Kosmac K, Fu X, Richards CI, Fry CS, McCarthy JJ, Peterson CA. Fusion-independent satellite cell communication to muscle fibers during load-induced hypertrophy. Function 2020;1:zqaa009. https://doi.org/10.1093/function/zqaa009.

[128] Zammit PS, Partridge TA, Yablonka-Reuveni Z. The skeletal muscle satellite cell: the stem cell that came in from the cold. J Histochem Cytochem 2006;54:1177–91. https://doi.org/10.1369/jhc.6R6995.2006.

[129] Chai RJ, Vukovic J, Dunlop S, Grounds MD, Shavlakadze T. Striking denervation of neuromuscular junctions without lumbar motoneuron loss in geriatric mouse muscle. PLoS One 2011;6:e28090. https://doi.org/10.1371/journal.pone.0028090.

[130] Gonzalez-Freire M, de Cabo R, Studenski SA, Ferrucci L. The neuromuscular junction: aging at the crossroad between nerves and muscle. Front Aging Neurosci 2014;6. https://doi.org/10.3389/fnagi.2014.00208.

[131] Koishi K, Zhang M, McLennan IS, Harris AJ. MyoD protein accumulates in satellite cells and is neurally regulated in regenerating myotubes and skeletal muscle fibers. Dev Dyn 1995;202:244–54. https://doi.org/10.1002/aja.1002020304.

[132] Axell A-M, MacLean HE, Plant DR, Harcourt LJ, Davis JA, Jimenez M, Handelsman DJ, Lynch GS, Zajac JD. Continuous testosterone administration prevents skeletal muscle atrophy and enhances resistance to fatigue in orchidectomized male mice. Am J Physiol Endocrinol Metab 2006;291:E506–16. https://doi.org/10.1152/ajpendo.00058.2006.

[133] Diel P. The role of the estrogen receptor in skeletal muscle mass homeostasis and regeneration. Acta Physiol 2014;212:14–6. https://doi.org/10.1111/apha.12341.

[134] Horstman AM, Dillon EL, Urban RJ, Sheffield-Moore M. The role of androgens and estrogens on healthy aging and longevity. J Gerontol A Biol Sci Med Sci 2012;67:1140–52. https://doi.org/10.1093/gerona/gls068.

[135] Kitajima Y, Ono Y. Estrogens maintain skeletal muscle and satellite cell functions. J Endocrinol 2016;229:267–75. https://doi.org/10.1530/JOE-15-0476.

[136] McClung JM, Davis JM, Wilson MA, Goldsmith EC, Carson JA. Estrogen status and skeletal muscle recovery from disuse atrophy. J Appl Physiol 2006;100:2012–23. https://doi.org/10.1152/japplphysiol.01583.2005.

[137] Ribas V, Drew BG, Zhou Z, Phun J, Kalajian NY, Soleymani T, Daraei P, Widjaja K, Wanagat J, de Aguiar Vallim TQ, Fluitt AH, Bensinger S, Le T, Radu C, Whitelegge JP, Beaven SW, Tontonoz P, Lusis AJ, Parks BW, Vergnes L, Reue K, Singh H, Bopassa JC, Toro L, Stefani E, Watt MJ, Schenk S, Akerstrom T, Kelly M, Pedersen BK, Hewitt SC, Korach KS, Hevener AL. Skeletal muscle action of estrogen receptor α is critical for the maintenance of mitochondrial function and metabolic homeostasis in females. Sci Transl Med 2016;8:334ra54. https://doi.org/10.1126/scitranslmed.aad3815.

[138] Seko D, Ogawa S, Li T, Taimura A, Ono Y. μ-Crystallin controls muscle function through thyroid hormone action. FASEB J 2016;30:1733–40. https://doi.org/10.1096/fj.15-280933.

[139] Sinha-Hikim I, Artaza J, Woodhouse L, Gonzalez-Cadavid N, Singh AB, Lee MI, Storer TW, Casaburi R, Shen R, Bhasin S. Testosterone-induced increase in muscle size in healthy young men is associated with muscle fiber hypertrophy. Am J Physiol Endocrinol Metab 2002;283:E154–64. https://doi.org/10.1152/ajpendo.00502.2001.

[140] Velders M, Schleipen B, Fritzemeier KH, Zierau O, Diel P. Selective estrogen receptor-β activation stimulates skeletal muscle growth and regeneration. FASEB J 2012;26:1909–20. https://doi.org/10.1096/fj.11-194779.

[141] Haseen F, Murray LJ, Cardwell CR, O'Sullivan JM, Cantwell MM. The effect of androgen deprivation therapy on body composition in men with prostate cancer: systematic review and meta-analysis. J Cancer Surviv 2010;4:128–39. https://doi.org/10.1007/s11764-009-0114-1.

[142] Serra C, Sandor NL, Jang H, Lee D, Toraldo G, Guarneri T, Wong S, Zhang A, Guo W, Jasuja R, Bhasin S. The effects of testosterone deprivation and supplementation on proteasomal and autophagy activity in the skeletal muscle of the male mouse: differential effects on high-androgen responder and low-androgen responder muscle groups. Endocrinology 2013;154:4594–606. https://doi.org/10.1210/en.2013-1004.

[143] Kim J-H, Han G-C, Seo J-Y, Park I, Park W, Jeong H-W, Lee SH, Bae S, Seong J, Yum M-K, Hann S-H, Kwon Y-G, Seo D, Choi MH, Kong Y-Y. Sex hormones establish a reserve pool of adult muscle stem cells. Nat Cell Biol 2016;18:930–40. https://doi.org/10.1038/ncb3401.

[144] Sinha-Hikim I, Roth SM, Lee MI, Bhasin S. Testosterone-induced muscle hypertrophy is associated with an increase in satellite cell number in healthy, young men. Am J Physiol Endocrinol Metab 2003;285:E197–205. https://doi.org/10.1152/ajpendo.00370.2002.

[145] Abreu P, Kowaltowski AJ. Satellite cell self-renewal in endurance exercise is mediated by inhibition of mitochondrial oxygen consumption. J Cachexia Sarcopenia Muscle 2020. https://doi.org/10.1002/jcsm.12601.

[146] Cisterna B, Giagnacovo M, Costanzo M, Fattoretti P, Zancanaro C, Pellicciari C, Malatesta M. Adapted physical exercise enhances activation and differentiation potential of satellite cells in the skeletal muscle of old mice. J Anat 2016;228:771–83. https://doi.org/10.1111/joa.12429.

[147] Fry CS, Noehren B, Mula J, Ubele MF, Westgate PM, Kern PA, Peterson CA. Fibre type-specific satellite cell response to aerobic training in sedentary adults: fibre type satellite cell content increases with aerobic training. J Physiol 2014;592:2625–35. https://doi.org/10.1113/jphysiol.2014.271288.

[148] Joanisse S, Nederveen JP, Baker JM, Snijders T, Iacono C, Parise G. Exercise conditioning in old mice improves skeletal muscle regeneration. FASEB J 2016;30:3256–68. https://doi.org/10.1096/fj.201600143RR.

[149] Masschelein E, D'Hulst G, Zvick J, Hinte L, Soro-Arnaiz I, Gorski T, von Meyenn F, Bar-Nur O, De Bock K. Exercise promotes satellite cell contribution to myofibers in a load-dependent manner. Skelet Muscle 2020;10:21. https://doi.org/10.1186/s13395-020-00237-2.

[150] Shefer G, Rauner G, Yablonka-Reuveni Z, Benayahu D. Reduced satellite cell numbers and myogenic capacity in aging can be alleviated by endurance exercise. PLoS One 2010;5:e13307. https://doi.org/10.1371/journal.pone.0013307.

[151] Fujimaki S, Hidaka R, Asashima M, Takemasa T, Kuwabara T. Wnt protein-mediated satellite cell conversion in adult and aged mice following voluntary wheel running. J Biol Chem 2014;289:7399–412. https://doi.org/10.1074/jbc.M113.539247.

[152] McKay BR, O'Reilly CE, Phillips SM, Tarnopolsky MA, Parise G. Co-expression of IGF-1 family members with myogenic regulatory factors following acute damaging muscle-lengthening contractions in humans: IGF-1, myogenic regulatory factors and exercise. J Physiol 2008;586:5549–60. https://doi.org/10.1113/jphysiol.2008.160176.

[153] Pedersen BK, Fischer CP. Beneficial health effects of exercise—the role of IL-6 as a myokine. Trends Pharmacol Sci 2007;28:152–6. https://doi.org/10.1016/j.tips.2007.02.002.

[154] Petrella JK, Kim J, Mayhew DL, Cross JM, Bamman MM. Potent myofiber hypertrophy during resistance training in humans is associated with satellite cell-mediated myonuclear addition: a cluster analysis. J Appl Physiol 2008;104:1736–42. https://doi.org/10.1152/japplphysiol.01215.2007.

[155] Snijders T, Nederveen JP, Joanisse S, Leenders M, Verdijk LB, van Loon LJC, Parise G. Muscle fibre capillarization is a critical factor in muscle fibre hypertrophy during resistance exercise training in older men: muscle fibre capillarization and exercise training in older men. J Cachexia Sarcopenia Muscle 2017;8:267–76. https://doi.org/10.1002/jcsm.12137.

[156] Verdijk LB, Gleeson BG, Jonkers RAM, Meijer K, Savelberg HHCM, Dendale P, van Loon LJC. Skeletal muscle hypertrophy following resistance training is accompanied by a fiber type-specific increase in satellite cell content in elderly men. J Gerontol A Biol Sci Med Sci 2009;64A:332–9. https://doi.org/10.1093/gerona/gln050.

[157] Jensen L, Bangsbo J, Hellsten Y. Effect of high intensity training on capillarization and presence of angiogenic factors in human skeletal muscle: capillarization in exercise-trained skeletal muscle. J Physiol 2004;557:571–82. https://doi.org/10.1113/jphysiol.2003.057711.

CHAPTER 5

Sarcopenia and the inflammatory cytokines

Arkadiusz Orzechowski (Bernard)
Department of Physiological Sciences, Faculty of Veterinary Medicine, Warsaw University of Life Sciences - SGGW, Warsaw, Poland

Abstract

Sarcopenia is a loss of skeletal muscle mass and strength due to a reduced number of myofibers. The atrophied muscle should not be mistaken for cachexia (muscle wasting) even though sarcopenia could accompany the latter. There are numerous causes of sarcopenia, including neuropathic (absence of nerve supply), such as loss of motor neurons (central and peripheral), and myopathic (muscle diseases). The term neuromuscular disease is addressed to disorders of both motor neurons, peripheral nerves, neuromuscular junctions, and muscle itself. Diminished input of anabolic hormones or sensitivity thereof (sex steroids, insulin), increased catabolism (glucocorticoids), and finally, the harmful effects of an imbalance between activities of anti- and proinflammatory cytokines (herewith inflammatory) contribute to sarcopenia. The clinical importance of sarcopenia in human beings becomes evident in the elderly when physical disability paralleled by greater visceral fat leads both to a higher incidence of metabolic syndrome (MS) and cardiovascular disease (CVD). The muscle–fat crosstalk points to the considerable role played by adipokines and myokines. It is clear now that some of the inflammatory cytokines stem from adipocytes and myofibers (TNF-alpha and IL-6, respectively). The consequences of sarcopenia such as physical frailty, falls, disability, abnormal deglutition together with CVD are liable for higher mortality rates. Thus, deciphering the pathogenesis of sarcopenia is of paramount significance to improve human health and wellbeing.

Keywords: Skeletal muscle, Sarcopenia, Inflammatory mediators, Adipose tissue, Inflammaging

Histology of skeletal muscle

Muscle cell (muscle fiber, myofiber) is unique (very thin and long) as its length may approach 1 m, while the diameter is on average measured in micrometers. The myofibers are postmitotic multinucleated cells with fully differentiated myonuclei (unable for mitotic division) located at the periphery of the sarcolemmal tube. Each muscle fiber is surrounded by a basal lamina and additionally protected by a membrane of connective tissue known as endomysium. Undifferentiated muscle progenitor cells (satellite cells) are found between the basal lamina and sarcolemma. These cells are responsible for the regeneration of myofibers. Generally speaking, there are three main types of muscle fibers: oxidative type I, oxidative–glycolytic type IIA, and glycolytic type IIB. Most muscles are of mixed type with a mosaic distribution of fibers (types I, IIA, and IIB).

Interestingly, solely type II fibers are subject to atrophy, which speeds up sarcopenia [1]. It points to the metabolic profile as an important determinant of skeletal muscle resistance to sarcopenia. The high antioxidative capacity of postural muscles entirely consisting of type I fibers must have some important implications for understanding why such muscles do not undergo atrophy. Overall, the oxidative balance needs special merit. The metabolic profile of myofiber(s) is controlled by the motor unit (axon of alpha motor neuron connected with myofiber(s)). The frequency of discharges sent to motor end plate(s) (neuromuscular junction) is known to affect the oxidative metabolism. The lower the frequency (5–15 Hz), the more oxidative metabolism, more mitochondria, and myoglobin. The higher the frequency (15–40 Hz for type IIA or 50–100 Hz for type IIB), the more glycolytic metabolism. The oxidative type I muscle fibers are better vascularized, resistant to fatigue, small, and slow twitching (200 ms). Low velocity of contraction results from the lower activity of step limiting enzymes (myosin ATPase, SERCA) and allows full recovery of myofibers. Of note, type I myofibers are better armed than other types (IIA, IIB) with antioxidant systems, including low molecular weight and catalytic systems [2–4]. In vitro study showed that preconditioning with low molecular weight antioxidants rescued muscle cells from experimentally induced oxidative stress [5]. Mounting evidence indicates that oxidative stress is evoked by inflammatory cytokines (TNF-α, TNF-like weak promoter of apoptosis (TWEAK)), IL-1β, interferon-γ, and IL-6 in the elderly [6–8]. The common pathway is mediated by NF-κB (nuclear factor kappa-light-chain-enhancer of activated B cells) signaling. Variety of NF-κB eukaryotic transcription factors exists [RelA (p65), RelB, c-Rel, NF-kB1 (p50), NF-kB2 (p52)], although first in line is apparently the most prominent representative of the group. As muscle wasting (cachexia) is frequently observed in chronic systemic inflammatory diseases (AIDS, CVD, COPD, cancer), it was tempting to check if NF-κB has any input to sarcopenia. A wealth of research provides compelling evidence that proinflammatory cytokines directly as well as indirectly (by repressing appetite and action of anabolic hormones) cause accelerated proteolysis, the process also linked to the generation of reactive oxygen species (ROS). The origin of elevated ROS is not clear; nevertheless, TNF-α signaling induced activity of skeletal muscle NADPH oxidase via NF-κB signaling [9]. A vicious cycle might exist between the inflammatory cytokines and NF-κB, as the latter is known to activate genes for inflammatory cytokines. Nonsteroid anti-inflammatory drugs (NSAIDs) exhibited partial inhibition of catabolic effects reported in inflammation as the increased antioxidant capacity, and lower expression of NF-κB was demonstrated upon ibuprofen administration to old rats [10]. Apparently, proinflammatory cytokine TNF-α employs myostatin (MSTN) cytokine as a decay tool because MSTN null skeletal muscles had the higher antioxidant capacity and low basal level of NF-κB [9]. The catabolic effect of TNF-α in muscle cells could be explained by activation of FOXO-dependent atrogenes [11]. Accordingly, protein catabolism overcomes protein accretion and sarcopenia might proceed [12]. Antagonism between inflammatory cytokines and anabolic hormones (i.e., insulin) targets myofibers, but at the same time, it stimulates satellite cells to proliferate and regenerate muscle fibers. The outcome is finely tuned and enables preventive measures in order to maintain muscle mass.

Composition of skeletal muscle

Fascicles of myofibers are tightened together by perimysium, while the entire muscle has a capsule known as epimysium. Epimysium does not only protect the organ, but it indirectly participates in force generation during muscle contraction (passive force). Muscle fibers are packed with myofibrils composed of actin and myosin filaments spatially organized into sarcomeres regularly attached to transverse Z bands. This regular intracellular framework of contractile apparatus is dependent on Ca^{2+} fluxes, which control the shortening of sarcomeres. Endoplasmic (also known as sarcoplasmic) reticulum sequesters Ca^{2+} in resting conditions by the action of sarco−/endoplasmic reticulum Ca^{2+}-ATPase (SERCA). When stimulated, the action potential is immediately spread through sarcolemmal invaginations known as transverse (T) tubules being in contact with terminal cisternae of adjacent sarcomeres (triad). Ca^{2+} is released, and thus, the twitch of a muscle fiber may easily proceed from the neuromuscular junction to the periphery.

Inflammatory response in skeletal muscle

Chronic low-grade inflammation has been proved to play a prominent role in the development of sarcopenia [13]. Sarcopenia is observed in many degenerative diseases, both noninfectious [chronic obstructive pulmonary disease (COPD), diabetes mellitus type 2 (DM2), congestive heart failure (CHF), chronic renal failure (CRF), rheumatoid arthritis (RA)] and infectious diseases (AIDS). Systemic surge of inflammatory cytokines (TNF-α, IL-6) and acute phase proteins [C-reactive protein (CRP), fibrinogen] causes an imbalance in muscle protein metabolism (accelerated proteolysis, a decline in protein synthesis), which results from attenuated anabolic effects (insulin, IGF-1) [14, 15].

The basic molecular mechanism of inflammation is led by an intracellular signaling platform known as inflammasome [16]. It is put together when cytosolic pattern recognition receptor, namely, nucleotide-binding oligomerization domain-like receptor (NLR) or an absent in melanoma 2 (AIM2)-like receptor, binds the adapter apoptosis-associated speck-like protein containing a C-terminal caspase recruitment domain (ASC). The assembly results in cleavage and activation of procaspase-1, which in turn triggers inflammatory cytokines into active ones [17]. Initially, inflammasome was identified in myeloid lineage cells, but nowadays, it is reported in other cell types, including myofibers [18]. The most likely type found is NOD-like receptor family pyrin domain containing 3 inflammasome (NLRP3). The principal role of intracellular NLRs is to recognize numerous different pathogen- or damage-associated molecular patterns (PAMPs or DAMPs, [19]). Once danger signals are sensed, the NLRP3 monomers oligomerize and interact with ASC to attract cysteine protease procaspase-1 via the aforementioned caspase recruitment domain (CARD). Active caspase 1 drives the processing and secretion of inflammatory cytokines IL-1β, IL-18, and IL-33 and, if overexcited, leads to programmed inflammatory cell death called pyroptosis [20]. To upregulate the expression NLPR3, which is low in number in many cell types, the first signal is induced by toll-like receptor (TLR)/nuclear factor (NF)-κB pathway (transcriptional regulation), followed by the second signal via PAMPs and DAMPs (post-translational regulation) [21]. To induce caspase-1 activation pore formation and K^+ efflux, lysosomal rupture and mitochondrial ROS generation are critical [22]. Mitochondrial damage, nuclear fragmentation, tubular aggregates formation, reduced locomotor activity, and increased frailty index are observed once NLPR3 in myofibers is stimulated [23]. This process is further exacerbated in the elderly (Fig. 1).

Myositis, the term used to describe inflammation of the skeletal muscle, is a complex process observed when this organ is subject to injury and myofibers are segmentally ruptured with the loss of integrity of plasma membrane (sarcolemma). The cytoplasm is no longer kept inside, it eventually becomes effluent [24]. At the same time, some components of the extracellular matrix enter myofibers, either [25]. Disruptions are found at the ultrastructural level as swollen and rounded necrotic fragments (segmental necrosis) of myofibers caused by increased osmotic pressure with resultant oncosis. There is a progressive loss of skeletal muscle markers located in sarcolemma (dystrophin, desmin) and structural components of sarcomeres (myosin) pointing to the extensive proteolysis [26]. In general, defects such as myofibrillar disorder and accumulation of leukocytes herald muscle damage and initiate inflammation. Some cell components present extracellularly are known as damage-associated molecular patterns (DAMPs). Leakage of proteins (creatine kinase, CK) and low-molecular-weight molecules of cellular origin (ATP and its degradation products) are appreciated chemoattractants for leukocytes. Initially (1–24 h), the muscle tissue is infiltrated with neutrophils, which is followed by proinflammatory macrophages (M1 phenotype, 24–48 h) continued with other immune-competent cells acting through toll-like receptors [27]. Finally, inflammation is resolved by M2 macrophages (anti-inflammatory), and the tissue undergoes the process of regeneration by activated satellite cells (muscle progenitor stem cells) where myofibrillar degeneration is followed by subsequent remodeling and incorporation of newly generated myoblasts, or if the damage is huge, the muscle tissue becomes fibrotic (reparation process). Satellite cell activation is stimulated by cytokines, also inflammatory series.

The overall molecular mechanisms behind the scenes of necrosis are associated with turmoil in calcium ion (Ca^{2+}) homeostasis as a rise in cytoplasmic Ca^{2+} concentration is observed in necrotic cells. The Ca^{2+} entry through the disrupted plasma membrane, which is unable to pump it out (ATP depleted cells), activates several enzymes including calpains, proteases involved in the degradation of the myofibrillar structure, and cytoskeleton [28,29]. To be recovered, myofibers need a considerable response from regenerative apparatus; otherwise, the damage is irreversible and associated with reparatory mechanisms (fibrosis).

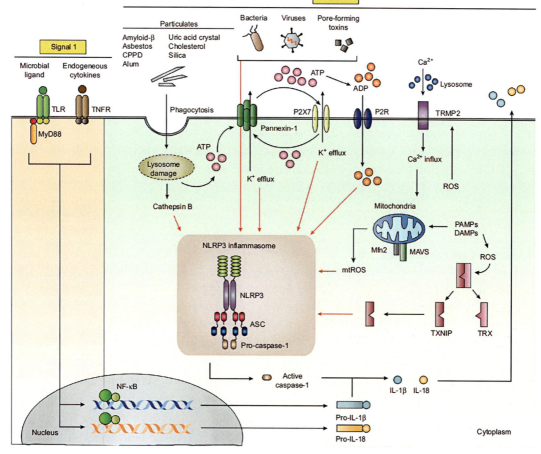

Fig. 1

Both signal 1 and signal 2 are required for NLRP3 inflammasome activation. Activation of the NLRP3 inflammasome requires at least two signals: signal 1, also known as the priming signal, is mediated by microbial ligands recognized by TLRs or cytokines such as TNF-α. Signal 1 activates the NF-κB pathway, leading to upregulation of pro-IL-1β and NLRP3 protein levels. The signal 2 is mediated by numerous PAMP or DAMP stimulation and promotes the assembly of ASC and pro-caspase-1, leading to activation of the NLRP3 inflammasome complex. Under noninfectious conditions, extracellular ATP and K$^+$ efflux leads to the activation of NLRP3 inflammasome via the P2X7 receptor and pannexin-1. Various endogenous and exogenous particulates, including MSU crystals, CPPD crystals, cholesterol crystals, amyloid β, silica crystals, asbestos, and alum, promote lysosomal damage and release cathepsin B into the cytosol, leading to the NLRP3 inflammasome activation. Particulate matters (uric acid, silica, and alum) are also able to trigger inflammasome assembly through multiple purinergic receptor signaling. Additionally, calcium influx through TRPM2 activates NLRP3 inflammasome through mitochondrial ROS. Dissociated TXNIP, which is triggered by intracellular ROS, also activates the NLRP3 inflammasome. ADP, adenosine diphosphate; ATP, adenosine triphosphate; K$^+$, potassium; ASC, the apoptosis-associated speck-like protein containing a C-terminal caspase recruitment domain; CPPD, calcium pyrophosphate dehydrate; DAMPs, damage-associated molecular patterns; NLRP3, NACHT, LRR, and PYD domains-containing protein 3; NF-κB, nuclear factor kappa-light-chain-enhancer of activated B cells; P2X7, P2X purinoceptor 7; P2R, purinergic receptor; PAMPs, pathogen-associated molecular patterns; ROS, reactive oxygen species; TLRs, toll-like receptors; TNF-α, tumor necrosis factor-α; TXNIP, thioredoxin (TRX)-interacting protein. *Adopted from Jo E-K, Kim JK, Shin D-M, Sasakawa C. Molecular mechanisms regulating NLRP3 inflammasome activation. Cell Mol Immunol 2016;13:148–59.*

Limited but various causes of skeletal muscle damage could be observed starting with the mechanical stimulus (crushing, eccentric exercise), chemical (venoms), thermal (freezing/thawing), energy deposition (electrocution), and infections (parasitic, bacterial, mycotic, viral). Eccentric exercise is the most likely cause of muscle damage as "...rapid stretching of an active muscle, beyond its optimum length, is apt to break or weaken permanently parts of contractile substance..." [30]. This could be easily achieved by downhill or downstairs running, backward cycling, and stepping or backward walking on a treadmill [31,32]. One common outcome of such damage is the so-called delayed onset muscle soreness (DOMS), which is frequently sensed if the exercise is unaccustomed and/or very vigorous [33].

Mediators of inflammation

The aforementioned damage to myofibers inevitably triggers inflammatory response both at the systemic and local level. The number of leukocytes and concentration of acute-phase proteins in peripheral blood are elevated due to the release of inflammatory cytokines, in particular, IL-1β and IL-6. Some of them are produced by immune cells, while others are secreted by injured skeletal muscle, so are called myokines or muscle-derived cytokines and chemokines [34]. Before any damage is observed in myofibers in response to exercise, these multinucleated syncytium undergoes myofibrillar disruption. Transmission electron microscopy revealed ultrastructural changes in the myofibrillar organization in the t-tubular system, sarcomeres, and sarcolemma. With more strenuous exercise or statin toxicity, myofibers could be extensively destructed, the process known as rhabdomyolysis. The latter is associated with the release of myoglobin (myoglobinuria) and CK (> 10.000 IU/L) from ruptured myofibers [35,36]. Irrespective of the severity of damage, muscle tissue is infiltrated with leukocytes. Initially, circulating leukocytes gather in the capillary vessels close to the site of injury. Next, resident and capillary monocytes/macrophages migrate to the endomysium and perimysium. Their role is to clear the cellular debris within the sarcolemmal tube confined by a basal lamina and make room for proliferating myoblasts, the progeny of satellite cells. Once the population of myoblasts is sufficient, the cells fuse to form myotubes in order to restore the integrity of injured muscle fiber. The regeneration process lasts several days and is accompanied by considerable modifications in the cytokine profile. Plasma IL-6 is elevated after exercise, and it lasts for several hours [37,38]. Next, the concentration of other cytokines is also raised [interleukin-1 receptor antagonist (IL-1ra), monocyte chemotactic protein (MCP-1), granulocyte-colony stimulating factor (G-CSF), IL-8, IL-10, IL-12, and soluble tumor necrosis factor α receptor 1 (sTNF-αR1)]. Conversely, other cytokines such as IL-1β, IL-2, IL-5, IL-13, IL-15, IL-17, TNF-α, leukemia inhibitory factor (LIF), and interferon γ are not subject to changes, even though the expression of respective genes (*IL-1β, IL-6, IL-8,*

MCP-1, TNF-α) is increased after exercise. There is scarce evidence on the role of anti-inflammatory cytokines IL-4 and IL-13 in the recovery of skeletal muscle from injury.

Myostatin

Myostatin (growth and differentiation factor 8, GDF-8) belongs to TGF-β superfamily and was initially shown to be a negative regulator of muscle growth [39]. Myostatin processing is associated with the proteolytic cleavage to form the active dimer. However, the activity of the molecule is blocked unless the dimer is released from the partner protein. Once freed, it can interact with the cognate plasma membrane activin type IIB receptor (ActRIIB), which then recruits the second receptor (coreceptor BMPR1A or ActRIB) and starts the signaling cascade through the intrinsic receptor serine–threonine kinase phosphorylation of cytosolic Smad 2/3 proteins (Fig. 2). Phosphorylated Smad2/3 binds Smad4 to form an active transcription factor, which acts on target genes [40]. The main role of myostatin was demonstrated in restraining myogenesis where it potently represses *Pax3* and *MyoD* expressions [41]. At the same time, myostatin activates *p21* in myoblasts. Altogether, myostatin inhibits the proliferation and differentiation of muscle precursor cells (myoblasts). Antagonistic interactions have been revealed between the IGF-1-Akt-mTORC1 pathway and myostatin cascade and vice versa [42,43].

Interactions between myofibers and adipocytes

Accumulation of fat (adipose tissue) is associated with accelerated loss of skeletal muscle mass and strength in the elderly. Initially described as "sarcopenic obesity" it is more suitable to use the term "obese sarcopenia" as mounting evidence points to adipocytes as a causal factor for detrimental health aftermath [45]. Functional deterioration, frailty, morbidity, and mortality rates are growing in aged obese subjects [46]. Although the molecular mechanisms are associated with increased activity of proteolytic systems such as ubiquitin–proteasome, autophagy–lysosome, and caspases, the etiology of sarcopenia is not clearly defined. Several possible inducing factors are listed: decreased anabolic stimulus (GH/IGF-I, insulin, steroid hormones), increased catabolic input (myostatin, activins, bone morphogenetic proteins), low physical activity, undernourishment, and loss of neuromuscular junctions. In aged individuals, a bulk of evidence points to immunosenescence, resulting in an altered innate and adaptive immune system [47]. The most convincing data confirm a notable rise in serum levels of inflammatory mediators, namely, C-reactive protein (CRP), IL-6, and TNF-α receptor II in the elderly [48]. Additionally, in the very old subjects (85+), the importance of inflammatory markers in frailty was confirmed as CRP, IL-6, TNF-α, and neutrophil count showed positive associations with frailty measures [49]. Besides, senior skeletal muscles expressed more innate immune receptors (MYD88, NLRX1, NAIP, TLR4, and NLR5), suggesting that myofibers are hypersensitive to signal 1 in inflammasome formation. This is indirect proof that inflammaging is driven by inflammasome and essential for secretion of inflammatory

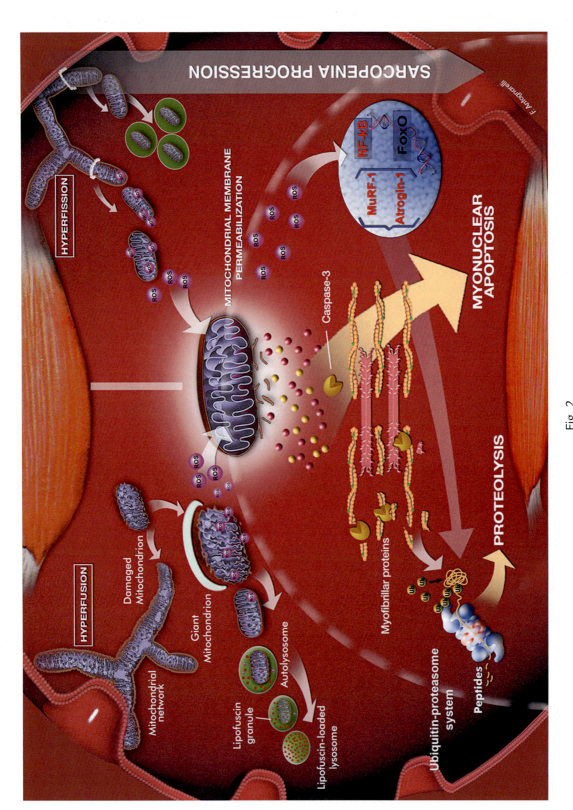

Fig. 2
see figure legend on opposite page

IL-1β. Simultaneously, an inflammasome complexed with cardiolipin and mitofusins was shown in mitochondria where ROS were extensively generated [50]. These observations clearly demonstrate the link between sarcopenia, DAMPs and PAMPs, inflammatory mediators, and aberrancy of mitochondria in old individuals [51,52]. It might be secondary to raising the number of viable senescent cells (SeCs), which are capable of secreting inflammatory cytokines and chemokines [53]. The population of SCs is metabolically active and creates a senescence-associated secretory phenotype (SASP). SeCs are the main source of TGFβ and IL-1β, which in skeletal muscle cells by autocrine/paracrine action induce cyclin-dependent kinase inhibitors p16 and p19, insulin-like growth factor binding protein 2 (IGFBP2), matrix metalloproteinase 13 (MMP13), and plasminogen activator inhibitor 1 (PAI1) [54]. Genetically engineered removal of SeCs prevented sarcopenia and restored muscle mass to nonsarcopenic level in laboratory animals [55,56] (Figs. 3 and 4).

Proresolving lipid mediators

Any injury associated with activation of phospholipase A2 (PLA2) and release of arachidonic acid from plasma membrane phospholipids start inflammatory response where lipid mediators (LM) are formed. Prostaglandins (PG) and leukotrienes (LT) recruit leukocytes to the site of damaged tissue to deactivate "intruder," clear the site of injury, adapt, and regenerate tissue. This is associated with cardinal features of inflammation: heat, redness, swelling, pain, and loss of function. Homeostasis is restored only if the inflammation is resolved; otherwise, the acute form is usually followed by chronic inflammation. For centuries, it

Fig. 2
Possible scenarios resulting from mitochondrial quality control failure during the progression of sarcopenia. An imbalance in mitochondrial dynamics toward fusion is associated with the appearance of giant mitochondria, characterized by highly interconnected networks, aberrant morphology, reduced bioenergetic efficiency, and increased ROS production. Enlarged mitochondria cannot be efficiently removed due to their larger size. The accumulation of lipofuscin within lysosomes further contributes to impairing the functionality of the autophagosomal-lysosomal axis. Oxidants generated by dysfunctional mitochondria compromise the surrounding tissue and amplify mitochondrial damage, eventually triggering apoptosis and proteolysis via ROS-mediated activation of nuclear factor κB (NF-κB) and Forkhead box O (FoxO) [44]. These transcription factors stimulate the expression of the muscle-specific ubiquitin ligases atrogin-1 and muscle-specific RING finger 1 (MuRF-1). Protein fragments derived from the action of caspase-3 on actomyosin complexes are eventually degraded by the ubiquitin–proteasome system. A shift of dynamics toward fission leads to mitochondrial network disintegration and overactivation of mitophagy. ROS generation by fragmented mitochondria is increased, which together with the upregulation of fission, stimulates muscle protein breakdown and myonuclear apoptosis through mechanisms similar to those described above. Artwork by Francesco Antognarelli. *Adopted from Marzetti E, Calvani R, Cesari M, Buford TW, Lorenzi M, Behnke BJ, Leeuwenburgh C. Mitochondrial dysfunction and sarcopenia of aging: from signaling pathways to clinical trials. J Biochem Cell Biol 2013;45:2288–301.*

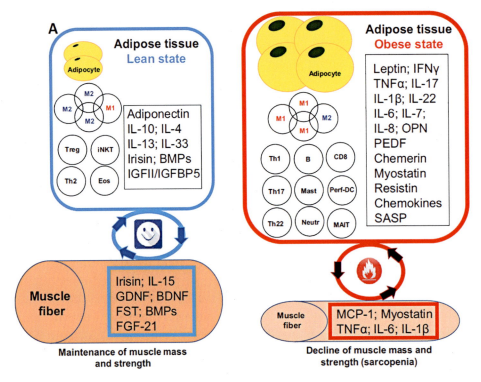

Fig. 3

Hypothesized cross-talk between adipose tissue (AT) and skeletal muscle in healthy (noninflamed) and obese (inflamed) conditions. (A) Under healthy (lean) conditions, AT is populated by macrophages in an M2-like state as well as by Th2, Tregs, iNKT, and eosinophils producing anti-inflammatory cytokines such as IL-4, IL-10, IL-13, and IL-33 [57–60]. Adipocytes secrete adipokines such as adiponectin and irisin as well as several BMPs, all capable of sustaining healthy noninflamed AT and skeletal muscle status [61–64]. Recent data suggest the ability of the AT-mediated IGFII/IGFBP5 axis to stimulate myoblast proliferation and differentiation [65]. Consequently, healthy lean skeletal muscles produce several myokines such as irisin, IL-15, FST, and FGF-21 as well as neurotrophic factors BDNF and GDNF, which collectively avert AT inflammation [66–68]. This favorable immune-metabolic pathway is capable of maintaining healthy AT and skeletal muscle status, thus preventing the development of sarcopenia. B. In an obese state, adipocytes undergo hypertrophy, hyperplasia, and activation, resulting in the accumulation of M1-skewed macrophages as well as Th1, Th17, and Th22 lymphocytes and mast cells producing proinflammatory cytokines including IFNγ, TNF-α, IL-1β, IL-6, IL-7, IL-8, IL-17, and IL-22 [60,69–71]. Other innate and adaptive immune cells, in particular, CD^{8+} T cells, B cells, perf-DCs, and MAIT cells, also play a role in obesity-induced AT inflammation [72–76]. Various chemokines, such as CCL2, CCL5, CXCL12, CXCL8, and CXCL10, which are detected in obese AT, are likely to be responsible for the recruitment of macrophages and other immune cells in obese AT [77]. Apparently, the proinflammatory milieu created (at least, partly) by these cells is the source of the senescence-associated secretory phenotype (SASP), inducing and/or exacerbating skeletal muscle mass and function decline [78]. In addition, several adipokines, such as leptin, CRP, OPN, chemerin, resistin, PEDF, and myostatin are found abundantly in obese

(Continued)

was thought that inflammation is resolved by the passive process, believed to result solely from the terminated synthesis of proinflammatory eicosanoids such as leukotrienes (LTs – LTB4) and prostaglandins (PGs – PGE2, PGD2). Recently, this view has been changed as specialized proresolving mediators (SPMs, "resolvents") have been identified (lipoxins – LX, resolvins – Rv, protectins – PD, maresins – MaR) and their respective epoxide intermediates (resolvin-, protectin-, and maresin conjugate in tissue regeneration are abbreviated as RCTR, PCTR, and MCTR, respectively) [83,84]. SPMs act through specific plasma membrane G-protein coupled receptors (GPCR) to counteract inflammatory mediators such as tumor necrosis factor-alpha (TNF-α), platelet-activating factor (PAF), PGs, LTs, chemokines, and cytokines [85,86]. These receptors could be shared by different SPMs and have variable distribution in different organs offering selective responses. Synthesis of each series of these "resolvents" (indicated by a capital letter) is dependent on access to arachidonic acid (LX) or dietary n-3 polyunsaturated fatty acid (PUFA, Rv, PD, MaR). RvE series is produced from eicosapentaenoic acid (EPA), RvD, PD, and MaR from docosahexaenoic acid (DHA). Remarkably, the foundation of some SPMs (LXA4, RvE, NPD1, RvD, MaR) is triggered by aspirin that inhibits cyclooxygenase 1/2 (COX-1/COX-2) [87–89]. Overall, the resolution process is active and initiated at the beginning of the acute inflammatory response. The timing and function played by each SPM are slightly different, and they could act sequentially and augment each other effect. SPMs attenuate the transmigration of polymorphonuclear leukocytes (PMNs) from postcapillary venules while increase phagocytosis and efferocytosis by the mononuclear leukocytes (M1 and M2). Moreover, biosynthesis of MaR and the respective epoxy intermediates occurs in macrophages, which in turn drives the conversion of M1 into M2. The latter produces even more MaR than M1. Some MaR epoxides (13S, 14S-epoxy-DHA also termed 13,14-epoxy-maresin) inhibit leukotriene hydroxylase (LTA4H)

Fig. 3—cont'd
AT in close association with AT inflammation [79-81]. Obesity is also accompanied by ectopic fat accumulation in skeletal muscle in the form of IMAT and IMCLs, which separately and/or together with muscle cells, produce myostatin, CCL2, TNF-α, IL-1β, and IL-6. All are capable of inducing IR and lipotoxicity, thus affecting, in an auto –/paracrine manner, the skeletal muscle functionality, and, in an endocrine manner, triggering and/or worsening AT inflammation [82]. This detrimental vicious circle probably maintains AT and skeletal muscle inflammation and triggers SOB development. Th, T-helper cells; Tregs, T-regulatory cells; iNKT, invariant natural killer T cells; BMPs, bone morphogenetic proteins; IGFII/IGFBP5, insulin growth factor-II (IGF-II) and its binding protein-5 (IGFBP-5); FST, follistatin; FGF-21, fibroblast growth factor-21; BDNF, brain-derived neurotrophic factor; GDNF, glial cell line-derived neurotrophic factor; perf-DCs, perforin-containing granules dendritic cells; MAIT, mucosal-associated invariant T cells; CRP, C-reactive protein; OPN, osteopontin; PEDF, pigment epithelium-derived factor; IMAT, intermuscular adipose tissue; IMCLs, intramyocellular lipids; Mast, mast cells; Eos, eosinophils; B, B-cells; Neutr, neutrophils. *Adopted from Kalinkovich A, Livshits G. Sarcopenic obesity or obese sarcopenia: a cross talk between age-associated adipose tissue and skeletal muscle inflammation as a main mechanism of the pathogenesis. Ageing Res Rev 2017;35:200–21.*

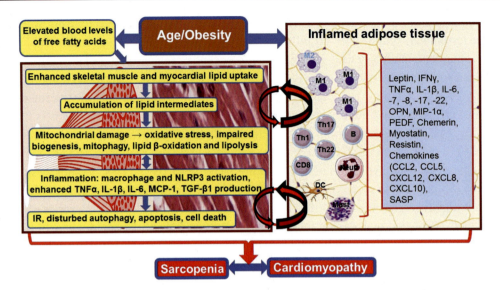

Fig. 4

Hypothesized mechanism of an age/obesity-mediated development of sarcopenia and cardiomyopathy via an inflammatory cross-talk between the skeletal muscle, myocardium, and adipose tissue (AT). Ectopically accumulated fatty acids' derivatives in the skeletal muscle and myocardium trigger a sequence of events designated on the left part of the scheme. These events mainly include mitochondrial damage, inflammation, insulin resistance (IR), and cell death via the lipotoxic effect on the skeletal muscle and myocardium. This results in reduced myocyte functionality, leading to sarcopenia and cardiomyopathy. Concomitantly, as shown on the right-hand side of the scheme, age-associated obesity is accompanied by AT inflammation, in which proinflammatory skewed M1-macrophages and other immune cells secrete a variety of proinflammatory mediators (e.g., cytokines, adipokines, chemokines, and others). In a paracrine/autocrine manner, they support ongoing AT inflammation and, in an endocrine manner, induce and support inflammation in both the skeletal muscle and myocardium. AT inflammation plays a prevailing role in this detrimental proinflammatory vicious circle, which hypothetically governs the development of sarcopenia and cardiomyopathy. Leakage of the depicted proinflammatory mediators to the circulation induces, maintains, and worsens inflammaging. Further explanations are given in the text. Th, T-helper cell; DC, dendritic cells; OPN, osteopontin; PEDF, pigment epithelium-derived factor; Mast, mast cell; Eos, eosinophils; B, B-cell; Neutr, neutrophil; MIP-1α, macrophage inflammatory protein 1 α; MCP-1, monocyte chemoattractant protein 1; NLRP3, (NLR family pyrin domain containing 3) inflammasome; SASP, senescence-associated secretory phenotype; IFNγ, interferon γ; IL, interleukin. *Adopted from Livshits G, Kalinkovich A. Inflammaging as a common ground for the development and maintenance of sarcopenia, obesity, cardiomyopathy and dysbiosis. Ageing Res. Rev. 2019;56:100980.*

and 12-lipooxygenase (12-LOX) limiting the formation of leukotrienes (LTA4, LTB4). SPMs regulate COX-2 and heme-1-oxygenase expression, counter regulate NF-κB gene targeting, and reduce inflammatory mediators (LT, PAF) but also increase anti-inflammatory IL-10 [90,91]. Regarding inflammaging, it remains to be revealed if SPMs and their synthetic analogs could be useful in combating the process. Nevertheless, muscle atrophy induced in the cell culture model of C2C12 myoblasts by lipopolysaccharide (LPS) was totally attenuated by RvE1 [92]. Inflammation and its resolving LM responses were elevated in postresistance exercise with evidence that COX1/COX2 inhibitor ibuprofen reduced both [93]. An observed decrease in blood prostanoids could be attributed to the oral dose of ibuprofen (400 mg). It would be tempting to determine if lower doses would work in favor of "resolvents" as some of their biochemical pathways are triggered by nonsteroid anti-inflammatory drugs (NSAID) (Fig. 5).

Concluding remarks

Mounting evidence indicates the general mechanism underlying the development of sarcopenia observed in the elderly. Deregulation of muscle growth, remodeling, and regeneration are possible because of repressing factors such as myostatin and increased expression of inflammatory cytokines (TNF-α, IL-1β, IL-6). These changes, found in old and very old individuals as well as laboratory animals, lead to mitochondria disruption, generation of ROS, activation of NF-κB signaling, and low-grade chronic inflammation known as "inflammaging." Long-term "inflammaging" causes muscle fiber denervation, paving the way to degeneration of myofibrils, death, and loss of type II myofibers. Not only myofibers but also adipocytes, myocardium, endothelium, and other cell types contribute to the elevated levels of inflammatory cytokines even though they may differ in the type of stimulus. For instance, mtDNA released from damaged cardiomyocytes activates inflammatory response through TLR9 and NF-κB signaling. Renin–angiotensin system activated by TNF-α and IL-1β stimulates endothelium to epithelial-mesenchymal transition (EMT), M1 macrophages resident in skeletal muscles encourage fibroblasts to differentiate into myofibroblasts, which secrete more collagen attracting more inflammatory cells (tissue infiltration). These in turn release more inflammatory mediators (vicious cycle). In obesity, adipocytes recruit M1 macrophages, lymphocytes, and mast cells, which secrete a cocktail of inflammatory cytokines, including IFNγ, TNF-α, IL-1β, IL-6, −7, −8, 17, −21, and −22. Adipocytes are also involved in "inflammaging" as they release plenty of inflammatory adipokines (osteopontin, chemerin, resistin, pigment epithelium-derived factor PEDF, CRP, leptin, and myostatin). Leptin is a potent inhibitor of myogenesis, the process directly controlling the growth of myofibers [15]. Another important issue in aging is lipotoxicity, which implicit the raise of FFA and intramuscular perilipins, lipids, and their derivatives [104,105]. The excess of FFA is deposited in tissues other than fat where this additional pool is hardly oxidized (β oxidation) and disturbs mitophagy. Fission of mitochondria, dysregulated autophagy, and

152 Chapter 5

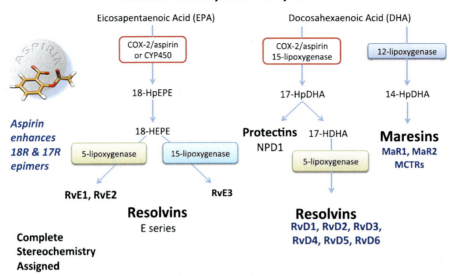

Fig. 5

Human SPM biosynthetic routes. Biosynthesis of E-series Rvs is initiated with molecular oxygen insertion at carbon-18 position of EPA, which is converted to bioactive E-series members RvE1–E3. The resolution metabolome also activates 17-lipoxygenation of DHA; 17S-HpDHA is converted to Rv-epoxide intermediates by the leukocyte 5-LOX. The intermediates are transformed to RvD1–D6, each of which carries potent actions. 17-HpDHA is also the precursor to the 16,17-epoxide-PD intermediate, which is converted to NPD1/PD1 and related PDs. MaRs are produced by macrophages via initial lipoxygenation at the carbon-14 position by lipoxygenation and insertion of molecular oxygen, producing a 13S,14S-epoxide-MaR intermediate that is enzymatically converted to the MaR family members MaR1, MaR2, and MCTRs. The stereochemistry of each bioactive SPM has been established, and SPM biosynthesis in murine exudates and human tissues is confirmed. (See refs. [94–96] for original reports, total organic synthesis, and stereochemical assignments, and the text for further details.) For complete stereochemistry of individual SPMs, see refs. [97–99]. Low dose aspirin triggers the 17R and 18R/S epimers of the Rvs [100,101] and 17R-epimer PDs [102,103]. *Adopted from Serhan CN. Treating inflammation and infection in the 21st century: new hints from decoding resolution mediators and mechanisms. FASEB J. 2017;31:1273–1288.*

ROS production all result in a higher incidence of muscle cell death by apoptosis [106]. Consequently, myofibers become resistant to insulin (IR), the primary anabolic hormone, and proteolysis takes over (disturbed proteostasis).

References

[1] Evans WJ, Campbell WW. Sarcopenia and age-related changes in body composition and functional capacity. J Nutr 1993;123:465–8.

[2] Orzechowski A, Grizard J, Jank M, Gajkowska B, Łokociejewska M, Zaron-Teperek M, Godlewski MM. Dexamethasone-mediated regulation of death and differentiation of muscle cells. Is hydrogen peroxide involved in the process? Reprod Nutr Dev 2002;42:197–216.

[3] Orzechowski A, Ostaszewski P, Brodnicka A, Wilczak J, Jank M, Bałasińska B, Grzelkowska K, Płoszaj T, Olczak J, Mrówczyńska A. Excess of glucocorticoids impairs whole body antioxidant status in young rats. Relation to the effect of dexamethasone in soleus muscle and spleen. Horm Metab Res 2000;32:174–80.

[4] Orzechowski A, Ostaszewski P, Wilczak J, Jank M, Bałasińska B, Waręski P, Fuller Jr J. Glucocorticoid-induced catabolic rats show symptoms of oxidative stress and spleen atrophy. The effect of age and recovery. J Vet Med A 2002;49:256–63.

[5] Orzechowski A, Łokociejewska M, Muras P, Hocquette, J-.F. Preconditioning with millimolar concentrations of vitamin C or N-acetylcysteine protects L6 muscle cells insulin-stimulated viability and DNA synthesis under oxidative stress. Life Sci 2002;71:1793–808.

[6] Aoi W, Sakuma K. Oxidative stress and skeletal muscle dysfunction with ageing. Curr Aging Sci 2011;4:101–9.

[7] Meng SJ, Yu LJ. Oxidative stress, molecular inflammation and sarcopenia. Int J Mol Sci 2010;11:1509–26.

[8] Thomas DR. Sarcopenia. Clin Geriatr Med 2010;26:331–46.

[9] Sriram S, Subramanian S, Sathiakumar D, Venkatesh R, Salerno MS, McFarlane CD, Kambadur R, Sharma M. Modulation of reactive oxygen species in skeletal muscle by myostatin is mediated through NF-κB. Aging Cell 2011;10:931–48.

[10] Rieu I, Magne H, Savary-Auzeloux I, Averous J, Bos C, Peyron MA, Combaret L, Dardevet D. Reduction of low grade inflammation restores blunting of postprandial muscle anabolism and limits sarcopenia in old rats. J Physiol 2009;587:5483–92.

[11] Pijet B, Pijet M, Litwiniuk A, Pajak B, Gajewska M, Orzechowski A. TNF-α and IFN-s-dependent muscle decay is linked to NF-κB and STAT-1α-stimulated *Atrogin1* and *MuRF1* genes in C2C12 myotubes. Mediat Inflamm 2013. http://www.hindawi.com/journals/mi/aip/171437.

[12] Litwiniuk A, Pijet B, Pijet-Kucicka M, Gajewska M, Pająk B, Orzechowski A. FOXO1 and GSK-3β are main targets of insulin-mediated myogenesis in C2C12 muscle cells. PLoS One 2016;11(1). https://doi.org/10.1371/journal.pone.0146726, e0146726.

[13] Berger MJ, Doherty TJ. Sarcopenia: prevalence, mechanisms, and functional consequences. Interdiscip Top Gerontol 2010;37:94–114.

[14] Degens H. The role of systemic inflammation in age-related muscle weakness and wasting. Scand J Med Sci Sports 2010;20:28–38.

[15] Pijet M, Pijet B, Litwiniuk A, Pajak B, Gajkowska B, Orzechowski A. Leptin impairs myogenesis in C2C12 cells through JAK/STAT and MEK signaling pathways. Cytokine 2013;61:445–54.

[16] Martinon F, Burns K, Tschopp J. The inflammasome: a molecular platform triggering activation of inflammatory caspases and processing of proIL-beta. Mol Cell 2002;10:417–26.

[17] Jo E-K, Kim JK, Shin D-M, Sasakawa C. Molecular mechanisms regulating NLRP3 inflammasome activation. Cell Mol Immunol 2016;13:148–59.

[18] McBride M, Foley KP, D'Souza DM, Li YE, Lau TC, Hawke TJ, Schertzer JD. The NLRP3 inflammasome contributes to sarcopenia and lower muscle glycolytic potential in old mice. Am J Physiol Endocrinol Metab 2017;313:E222–32.

[19] Mariathasan S, Weiss DS, Newton K, McBride J, O'Rourke K, Roose-Girma M, Lee WP, Weinrauch Y, Monack DM, Dixit VM. Cryopyrin activates the inflammasome in response to toxins and ATP. Nature 2006;440:228–32.

[20] Vanaja SK, Rathinam VA, Fitzgerald KA. Mechanisms of inflammasome activation: recent advances and novel insights. Trends Cell Biol 2015;25:308–15.

[21] Hornung V, Latz E. Critical functions of priming and lysosomal damage for NLRP3 activation. Eur J Immunol 2010;40:620–3. https://doi.org/10.1152/ajpendo.00060.2017.

[22] Heid ME, Keyel PA, Kamga C, Shiva S, Watkins SC, Salter RD. Mitochondrial reactive oxygen species induces NLRP3-dependent lysosomal damage and inflammasome activation. J Immunol 2013;191:5230–8.

[23] Sayed RKA, Fernández-Ortiz M, Diaz-Casado ME, Aranda-Martínez P, Fernández-Martínez J, Guerra-Librero A, Escames G, López LC, Alsaadawy RM, Acuña-Castroviejo D. Lack of NLRP3 inflammasome activation reduces age-dependent sarcopenia and mitochondrial dysfunction, favoring the prophylactic effect of melatonin. J Gerontol A Biol Sci Med Sci 2019. https://doi.org/10.1093/gerona/glz079.glz079.

[24] Sorichter S, Puschendorf B, Mair J. Skeletal muscle injury induced by eccentric muscle action: muscle proteins as markers of muscle fiber injury. Exerc Immunol Rev 1999;5:5–21.

[25] Crameri RM, Langberg H, Magnusson P, Jensen CH, Schroder HD, Olesen JL, Suetta C, Teisner B, Kjaer M. Changes in satellite cells in human skeletal muscle after a single bout of high intensity exercise. J Physiol 2004;558:333–40.
[26] Lovering RM, De Deyne PG. Contractile function, sarcolemma integrity, and the loss of dystrophin after skeletal muscle eccentric contraction-induced injury. Am J Phys Cell Phys 2004;286:C230–8.
[27] Mathes AL, Lafaytis R. Role of toll-like receptor 3 in muscle regeneration after cardiotoxin injury. Muscle Nerve 2011;43:733–40.
[28] Gissel H, Clausen T. Excitation-induced Ca2+ influx and skeletal muscle cell damage. Acta Physiol Scand 2001;171:327–34.
[29] Orzechowski A, Jank M, Gajkowska B, Sadkowski T, Godlewski MM. A novel antioxidant inhibited dexamethasone-mediated and caspase-3 independent muscle cell death. Ann N Y Acad Sci 2003;(Supplement):1–4.
[30] Katz B. The relation between force and speed in muscular contraction. J Physiol 1939;96:45–64.
[31] Friden J. Changes in human skeletal muscle induced by long-term eccentric exercise. Cell Tissue Res 1984;236:165–71.
[32] Newham DJ. The consequences of eccentric contractions and their relationship to delayed onset muscle pain. Eur J Appl Physiol Occup Physiol 1988;57:353–9.
[33] Evans WJ, Cannon JG. The metabolic effects of exercise-induced muscle damage. Exerc Sport Sci Rev 1991;19:99–125.
[34] Pedersen BK. Muscles and their myokines. J Exp Biol 2011;214:337–46.
[35] Clarkson PM, Kearns AK, Rouzier P, Rubin R, Thompson PD. Serum creatine kinase levels and renal function measures in exertional muscle damage. Med Sci Sports Exerc 2006;38:623–7.
[36] Harper CR, Jacobson TA. The broad spectrum of statin myopathy: from myalgia to rhabmomylysis. Curr Opin Lipidol 2007;18:401–8.
[37] Peake JM, Suzuki K, Hordern M, Wilson G, Nosaka K, Coombes JS. Plasma cytokine changes in relation to exercise intensity and muscle damage. Eur J Appl Physiol 2005;95:514–21.
[38] Peake JM, Suzuki K, Wilson G, Hordern M, Nosaka K, Mackinnon L, Coombes JS. Exercise-induced muscle damage, plasma cytokines, and markers of neutrophil activation. Med Sci Sports Exerc 2005;37:737–45.
[39] Lee SJ. Regulation of muscle mass by myostatin. Annu Rev Cell Dev Biol 2004;20:61–86. https://doi.org/10.1146/annurev.cellbio.20.012103.135836.
[40] Joulia-Ekaza D, Cabello G. The myostatin gene: physiology and pharmacological relevance. Curr Opin Pharmacol 2007;7:310–5.
[41] McFarlane C, Plummer E, Thomas M, Hennebry A, Ashby M, Ling N, Smith H, Sharma M, Kambadur R. Myostatin induces cachexia by activating the ubiquitin proteolytic system through an NF-κB-independent, FoxO1-dependent mechanism. J Cell Physiol 2006;209:501–14. https://doi.org/10.1002/jcp.20757.
[42] Morisette MR, Cook SA, Buranasombati C, Rosenberg MA, Rosenzweig A. Myostatin inhibits IGF-I-induced myotube hypertrophy through Akt. Am J Phys Cell Phys 2009;297:C1124–32. https://doi.org/10.1152/ajpcell.00043.2009.
[43] Trendelenburg AU, Meyer A, Rohner D, Byle J, Hatakeyama S, Glass DJ. Myostatin reduces Akt/TORC1/p70S6K signaling, inhibiting myoblasts differentiation and myotube size. Am J Phys Cell Phys 2009;296:C1258–70. https://doi.org/10.1152/ajpcell.00105.2009.
[44] Dodd SL, Gagnon BJ, Senf SM, Hain BA, Judge AR. Ros-mediated activation of NF-kappaB and Foxo during muscle disuse. Muscle Nerve 2010;41:110–3.
[45] Kalinkovich A, Livshits G. Sarcopenic obesity or obese sarcopenia: a cross talk between age-associated adipose tissue and skeletal muscle inflammation as a main mechanism of the pathogenesis. Ageing Res Rev 2017;35:200–21.
[46] Livshits G, Kalinkovich A. Inflammaging as a common ground for the development and maintenance of sarcopenia, obesity, cardiomyopathy and dysbiosis. Ageing Res Rev 2019;56:100980. https://doi.org/10.1016/j.arr.2019.100980.
[47] Pillon NJ, Krook A. Innate immune receptors in skeletal muscle metabolism. Exp Cell Res 2017;360:47–54.

[48] Marcos-Perez D, Sanchez-Flores M, Maseda A, Lorenzo-Lopez L, Millan-Calenti JC, Gostner JM, Fuchs D, Pasaro E, Laffon B, Valdiglesias V. Frailty in older adults is associated with plasma concentrations of inflammatory mediators but not with lymphocyte subpopulations. Front Immunol 2018;9:1056. https://doi.org/10.3389/fimmu.2018.01056.

[49] Collerton J, Martin-Ruiz C, Davies K, Hilkens CM, Isaacs J, Kolenda C, Parker C, Dunn M, Catt M, Jagger C, von Zglinicki T, Kirkwood TBL. Frailty and the role of inflammation, immunosenescence and cellular ageing in the very old: cross-sectional findings from the Newcastle 85+ study. Mech Ageing Dev 2012;133:456–66.

[50] Yu JW, Lee MS. Mitochondria and the NLRP3 inflammasome: physiological and pathological relevance. Arch Pharm Res 2016;39:1503–18.

[51] Huang DD, Fan SD, Chen XY, Yan XL, Zheng XZ, Ma BW, Yu DY, Xiao WY, Zhuang CL, Yu Z. Nrf2 deficiency exacerbates frailty and sarcopenia by impairing skeletal mitochondrial biogenesis and dynamics in an age-dependent manner. Exp Gerontol 2019;119:61–73.

[52] Mohan S, Gupta D. Crosstalk of toll-like receptors signaling and Nrf2 pathway for regulation of inflammation. Biomed Pharmacother 2018;108:1866–78.

[53] Sapieha P, Mallette FA. Cellular senescence in postmitotic cells: beyond growth arrest. Trends Cell Biol 2018;28:595–607.

[54] Baker D, Perez-Terzic C, Jin F, Pitel KS, Niederlander NJ, Jeganathan K, Eberhardt NL, Terzic A, van Deursen JM. Opposing roles for p16Ink4a and p19Arf in senescence and ageing caused by BubR1 insufficiency. Nat Cell Biol 2008;10:825–36.

[55] Baar MP, Perdiguero E, Monoz-Canoves P, de Keizer PL. Masculoskeletal senescence: a moving target ready to be eliminated. Curr Opin Pharmacol 2018;40:147–55.

[56] Xu M, Pirtskhalava T, Farr JN, Weigand BM, Palmer AK, Weivoda MM, Inman CL, Ogrodnik MB, Giorgadze N, LeBrasseur NK, Niederhofer LJ, Khosla S, Tchkonia T, Kirkland JL. Senolytics improve physical function and increase lifespan in old age. Nat Med 2018;24:1246–56.

[57] Brestoff JR, Artis D. Immune regulation of metabolic homeostasis in health and disease. Cell 2015;161:146–60.

[58] Han JM, Wu D, Denroche HC, Yao Y, Verchere CB, Levings MK. IL-33 reverses an obesity-induced deficit in visceral adipose tissue ST2+T regulatory cells and ameliorates adipose tissue inflammation and insulin resistance. J Immunol 2015;194:4777–83.

[59] Odegaard JI, Chawla A. Type 2 responses at the interface between immunity and fat metabolism. Curr Opin Immunol 2015;36:67–72.

[60] Wensveen FM, Valentić S, Šestan M, Turk Wensveen T, Polić B. The big bang in obese fat: events initiating obesity-induced adipose tissue inflammation. Eur J Immunol 2015;45:2446–56.

[61] Grgurevic L, Christensen GL, Schulz TJ, Vukicevic S. Bone morphogenetic proteins in inflammation: glucose homeostasis and adipose tissue energy metabolism. Cytokine Growth Factor Rev 2016;27:105–18.

[62] Sartori R, Sandri M. BMPs and the muscle-bone connection. Bone 2015;80:37–42.

[63] Schering L, Hoene M, Kanzleiter T, Jähnert M, Wimmers K, Klaus S, Eckel J, Weigert C, Schürmann A, Maak S, Jonas W, Sell H. Identification of novel putative adipomyokines by a cross-species annotation of secretomes and expression profiles. Arch Physiol Biochem 2015;121:194–205.

[64] Vaughan RA, Gannon NP, Mermier CM, Conn CA. Irisin, a unique non-inflammatory myokine in stimulating skeletal muscle metabolism. J Physiol Biochem 2015;71:679–89.

[65] Pellegrinelli V, Rouault C, Rodriguez-Cuenca S, Albert V, Edom-Vovard F, Vidal-Puig A, Clément K, Butler-Browne GS, Lacasa D. Human adipocytes induce inflammation and atrophy in muscle cells during obesity. Diabetes 2015;64:3121–34.

[66] Dong J, Dong Y, Dong Y, Chen F, Mitch WE, Zhang L. Inhibition of myostatin in mice improves insulin sensitivity via irisin-mediated cross talk between muscle and adipose tissues. Int J Obes 2016;40:434–42.

[67] Fisher FM, Maratos-Flier E. Understanding the physiology of FGF21. Annu Rev Physiol 2016;78:223–41.

[68] Mwangi SM, Nezami BG, Obukwelu B, Anitha M, Marri S, Fu P, Epperson MF, Le NA, Shanmugam M, Sitaraman SV, Tseng YH, Anania FA, Srinivasan S. Glial, cell line-derived neurotrophic factor protects against high-fat diet-induced obesity. Am J Physiol Gastrointest Liver Physiol 2014;306:G515–25.

[69] Castoldi A, Naffah de Souza C, Câmara NO, Moraes-Vieira PM. Themacrophage switch in obesity development. Front Immunol 2016;6:637.
[70] Exley MA, Hand L, O'Shea D, Lynch L. Interplay between the immune system and adipose tissue in obesity. J Endocrinol 2014;223:R41–8.
[71] Tateya S, Kim F, Tamori Y. Recent advances in obesity-induced inflammation and insulin resistance. Front Endocrinol (Lausanne) 2013;4:93.
[72] Apostolopoulos V, de Courten MP, Stojanovska L, Blatch GL, Tangalakis K, de Courten B. The complex immunological and inflammatory network of adipose tissue in obesity. Mol Nutr Food Res 2016;60:43–57.
[73] Grant RW, Dixit VD. Adipose tissue as an immunological organ. Obesity (Silver Spring) 2015;23:512–8.
[74] Magalhaes I, Kiaf B, Lehuen A. iNKT and MAIT cell alterations in diabetes. Front Immunol 2015;6:341.
[75] Magalhaes I, Pingris K, Poitou C, Bessoles S, Venteclef N, Kiaf B, Beaudoin L, Da Silva J, Allatif O, Rossjohn J, Kjer-Nielsen L, McCluskey J, Ledoux S, Genser L, Torcivia A, Soudais C, Lantz O, Boitard C, Aron-Wisnewsky J, Larger E, Clément K, Lehuen A. Mucosal-associated invariant T cell alterations in obese and type 2 diabetic patients. J Clin Invest 2015;125:1752–62.
[76] Zlotnikov-Klionsky Y, Nathansohn-Levi B, Shezen E, Rosen C, Kagan S, Bar-On L, Jung S, Shifrut E, Reich-Zeliger S, Friedman N, Aharoni R, Arnon R, Yifa O, Aronovich A, Reisner Y. Perforin-positive dendritic cells exhibit an immuno-regulatory role in metabolic syndrome and autoimmunity. Immunity 2015;43:776–87.
[77] Yao L, Herlea-Pana O, Heuser-Baker J, Chen Y, Barlic-Dicen J. Roles of the chemokine system in development of obesity, insulin resistance, and cardiovascular disease. J Immunol Res 2014;2014:181450.
[78] LeBrasseur NK, Tchkonia T, Kirkland JL. Cellular senescence and the biology of aging disease, and frailty. Nestle Nutr Inst Workshop Ser 2015;83:11–8.
[79] Gencer B, Auer R, de Rekeneire N, Butler J, Kalogeropoulos A, Bauer DC, Kritchevsky SB, Miljkovic I, Vittinghoff E, Harris T, Rodondi N. Association between resistin levels and cardiovascular disease events in older adults: the health, aging and body composition study. Atherosclerosis 2016;245:181–6.
[80] Mariani F, Roncucci L. Chemerin/chemR23 axis in inflammation onset and resolution. Inflamm Res 2015;64:85–95.
[81] Rodríguez A, Ezquerro S, Méndez-Giménez L, Becerril S, Frühbeck G. Revisiting the adipocyte: a model for integration of cytokine signaling in the regulation of energy metabolism. Am J Physiol Endocrinol Metab 2015;309:E691–714.
[82] Rivas DA, Mcdonald DJ, Rice NP, Haran PH, Dolnikowski GG, Fielding RA. Diminished anabolic signaling response to insulin induced by intramuscular lipid accumulation is associated with inflammation in aging but not obesity. Am J Phys Regul Integr Comp Phys 2016;310:R561–9.
[83] Serhan CN. Treating inflammation and infection in the 21st century: new hints from decoding resolution mediators and mechanisms. FASEB J 2017;31:1273–88.
[84] Serhan CN, Chiang N, Dalli J. The resolution code of acute inflammation: novel pro-resolving lipid mediators in resolution. Semin Immunol 2015;27:200–15.
[85] Borgeson E, McGillicuddy FC, Harford KA, Corrigan N, Higgins DF, Maderna P, Roche HM, Godson C. Lipoxin A4 attenuates adipose inflammation. FASEB J 2012;26:4287–94.
[86] Qu X, Zhang X, Xao J, Song J, Nikolic-Paterson DJ, Li J. Resolvin E1 and D1 inhibit intestinal fibrosis in the obstructed kidney via inhibition of local fibroblast proliferation. J Pathol 2012;228:506–19.
[87] Buckley CD, Gilroy DW, Serhan CN, Stockinger B, Tak PP. The resolution of inflammation. Nat Rev Immunol 2013;13:59–66.
[88] Jin S-W, Zhang L, Lian Q-Q, Liu D, Wu P, Yao S-L, Ye D-Y. Posttreatment with aspirin-triggered lipoxin A4 analog attenuates lipopolysaccharide-induced acute lung injury in mice: the role of heme oxygenase-1. Anesth Analg 2007;104:369–77.
[89] Martins V, Valenca SS, Farias-Filho FA, Molinaro R, Simoes RL, Ferreira TPT, eSilva PM, Hogaboam CM, Kunkel SL, Fierro IM, Canetti C, Benjamim CF. ATLa, an aspirin-triggered lipoxin A4 synthetic analog, prevents the inflammatory and fibrotic effects of bleomycin-induced pulmonary fibrosis. J Immunol 2009;182:5374–81.

[90] Biteman B, Hassan IR, Walker E, Leedom AJ, Dunn M, Seta F, Laniado-Schwartzman M, Gronert K. Interdependence of lipoxin A4 and heme-oxygenase in counter-regulating inflammation during corneal wound healing. FASEB J 2007;21:2257–66.

[91] Hong S, Gronert K, Devchand PR, Moussignac R-L, Serhan CN. Novel docosatrienes and 17S-resolvins generated from docosahexaenoic acid in murine brain, human blood, and glial cells. Autacoids in anti-inflammation. J Biol Chem 2003;278:1025–37.

[92] Baker DJ, Childs BG, Durik M, Wijers ME, Sieben CJ, Zhong J, et al. Resolvin E1 (Rv E1) attenuates LPS induced inflammation and subsequent atrophy in C2C12 myotubes. J Cell Biochem 2018;119:6094–103.

[93] Markworth JF, Vella LD, Lingard BS, Tull DL, Rupasinghe TW, Sinclair AJ, Maddipati KR, Cameron-Smith D. Human inflammatory and resolving lipid mediator responses to resistance exercise and ibuprofen treatment. Am J Phys Regul Integr Comp Phys 2013;305:R1281–96.

[94] Aursnes M, Tungen JE, Colas RA, Vlasakov I, Dalli J, Serhan CN, Hansen TV. Synthesis of the 16S,17Sepoxyprotectin intermediate in the biosynthesis of protectins by human macrophages. J Nat Prod 2015;78:2924–31.

[95] Serhan CN, Petasis NA. Resolvins and protectins in inflammation resolution. Chem Rev 2011;111:5922–43.

[96] Winkler JW, Orr SK, Dalli J, Cheng CY, Sanger JM, Chiang N, Petasis NA, Serhan CN. Resolvin D4 stereoassignment and its novel actions in host protection and bacterial clearance. Sci Rep 2016;6:18972.

[97] Colas RA, Shinohara M, Dalli J, Chiang N, Serhan CN. Identification and signature profiles for pro-resolving and inflammatory lipid mediators in human tissue. Am J Phys Cell Phys 2014;307:C39–54.

[98] Dalli J, Vlasakov I, Riley IR, Rodriguez AR, Spur BW, Petasis NA, Chiang N, Serhan CN. Maresin conjugates in tissue regeneration biosynthesis enzymes in human macrophages. Proc Natl Acad Sci U S A 2016;113:12232–7.

[99] Primdahl KG, Aursnes M, Walker ME, Colas RA, Serhan CN, Dalli J, Hansen TV, Vik A. Synthesis of 13(R)-hydroxy-7Z,10Z,13R,14E,16Z,19Z docosapentaenoic acid (13RHDPA) and its biosynthetic conversion to the 13-series resolvins. J Nat Prod 2016;79:2693–702.

[100] Oh SF, Pillai PS, Recchiuti A, Yang R, Serhan CN. Pro-resolving actions and stereoselective biosynthesis of 18S E-series resolvins in human leukocytes and murine inflammation. J Clin Invest 2011;121:569–81.

[101] Serhan CN, Hong S, Gronert K, Colgan SP, Devchand PR, Mirick G, Moussignac R-L. Resolvins: a family of bioactive products of omega-3 fatty acid transformation circuits initiated by aspirin treatment that counter proinflammation signals. J Exp Med 2002;196:1025–37.

[102] Bazan NG, Eady TN, Khoutorova L, Atkins KD, Hong S, Lu Y, Zhang C, Jun B, Obenaus A, Fredman G, Zhu M, Winkler JW, Petasis NA, Serhan CN, Belayev L. Novel aspirin-triggered neuroprotectin D1 attenuates cerebral ischemic injury after experimental stroke. Exp Neurol 2012;236:122–30.

[103] Serhan CN, Fredman G, Yang R, Karamnov S, Belayev LS, Bazan NG, Zhu M, Winkler JW, Petasis NA. Novel proresolving aspirin-triggered DHA pathway. Chem Biol 2011;18:976–87.

[104] Ferrara D, Montecucco F, Dallegri F, Carbone F. Impact of different ectopic fat depots on cardiovascular and metabolic diseases. J Cell Physiol 2019. https://doi.org/10.1002/jcp.28881.

[105] Shuman GI. Ectopic fat in insulin resistance, dyslipidemia, and cardiometabolic disease. N Engl J Med 2014;371:1131–41.

[106] Marzetti E, Calvani R, Cesari M, Buford TW, Lorenzi M, Behnke BJ, Leeuwenburgh C. Mitochondrial dysfunction and sarcopenia of aging: from signaling pathways to clinical trials. J Biochem Cell Biol 2013;45:2288–301.

CHAPTER 6

Molecular mechanisms of exercise providing therapeutic rationale to counter sarcopenia

Ki-Sun Kwon[a,b]

[a]Aging Research Center, Korea Research Institute of Bioscience and Biotechnology, Daejeon, Republic of Korea, [b]Aventi Inc., Daejeon, Republic of Korea

Abstract

Aging induces loss of skeletal muscle mass and function referred to as sarcopenia, which exacerbates age-related diseases. However, no medication has been FDA-approved yet. Physical exercise is the most effective strategy to improve muscle mass and strength in adults. Therefore, many studies have been focused on the molecular mechanism in exercise to develop the medication to counter sarcopenia. This chapter introduces molecular mechanisms in sarcopenia which provide therapeutic targets and suggests medication candidates such as exercise mimetics, myokines, and anabolic hormones.

Keywords: Aging, Skeletal muscle, Sarcopenia, Exercise

Introduction

Sarcopenia, the loss of skeletal muscle mass and function with age, began to be recognized as a disease with ICD-10-CM (M62.84) and has recently attracted attention as the aged population increases. Sarcopenia complicates many aging-associated diseases including cognitive disorders and metabolic diseases, lowers life quality, and increases mortality. Although there are standard diagnostic criteria of EWGSOP and AWGS [1, 2], no medications for sarcopenia have been FDA-approved yet. Myostatin/ActR2 signaling inhibitors, anabolic hormones, and natural compounds are under development. Combined nondrug therapies with exercise and nutritional supplements are needed for more effective intervention strategies against sarcopenia [3].

The etiologies of sarcopenia are not fully understood. An imbalance between muscle protein synthesis (anabolism) and degradation (catabolism) may cause the onset of sarcopenia and various mechanisms are potentially involved in the pathogenesis of sarcopenia. Both intrinsic factors within skeletal muscle (e.g., inflammation, apoptosis, autophagy, mitochondria, neuromuscular junction, and calcium metabolism) and extrinsic factors in systemic environments (e.g., endocrine, nutrition, immobility) [4–9] contribute to defective satellite cell maintenance, myogenesis, and myotube atrophy, as well as neuromuscular coordination.

Therefore, understanding the mechanisms in sarcopenia is essential to identify a variety of molecular targets for pharmacological treatment.

This review gives an overview of how physical exercise correct sarcopenia at a molecular level and how to take the benefits for the treatment of sarcopenia.

Gene set analysis of exercise that oppose sarcopenia

One of the most effective strategies to improve muscle mass and strength in adults is physical exercise [10, 11]. Resistance exercise training, more specifically for gaining fast-twitch muscles, has been claimed to reverse aging in skeletal muscle [12]. To elucidate some of these complex processes that occur in skeletal muscle during aging and to examine the effects of resistance exercise training on the skeletal muscle transcriptome, my group compared genome-wide gene expression in frail older subjects before and after resistance exercise training with that of healthy young subjects, using publicly available dataset (Fig. 1). Gene expression pattern was reversed to young in older subjects after exercise. Frailty is defined as a

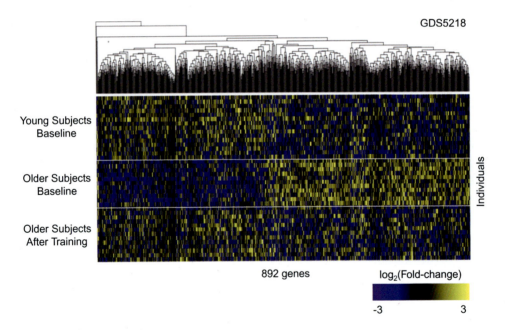

Fig. 1
Heatmap of hierarchically clustered transcriptome data in young and old human skeletal muscle after resistance exercise. Differential expression analyses were performed using a publicly available transcriptome dataset (GDS5218) containing two cohorts of young and old adults [study A: 24 year and 84 year (n = 28); study B: 25 year and 78 year (n = 36)] [13]. DEGs (differentially expressed genes) were identified by the k-means clustering algorithm (k = 50), and the expression profiles of the selected genes were depicted as a heatmap. In old skeletal muscle, 892 genes recovered to young muscle expression levels after resistance exercise from severe expression defects (mean $\log_2 FC > \pm 1$).

clinical syndrome in which the following criteria are present: weight loss, exhaustion, physical activity, walking speed, and grip strength [14]. Frailty criteria are similar to that of EWGSOP sarcopenia standard, including grip strength, walking speed, muscle performance (SPPB), and muscle mass [15], even though the cut-off ranges are somewhat different in between.

Skeletal muscle transcriptome after 24 weeks of resistance exercise showed that significantly different pathways between the frail older and young subjects were related to glucose metabolism and RNA processing [16]. Pathways related to mitochondrial function were some of the most significantly affected pathways, though the fold changes of the individual mitochondrial genes were relatively small but consistent. The genes that shift toward younger expression levels by exercise include genes related to the extracellular matrix, vascularization, glucose metabolism, and muscle contraction. Training resulted in the differential expression levels of many genes related to the connective tissue and the extracellular matrix, including collagen genes and laminin genes, suggesting significant tissue remodeling probably under the control of TGF-β signaling. Myosin heavy chain isoforms and troponin isoforms were also distinctly upregulated. Genes related to neuromuscular function are a significant group that changes after exercise. Expression of the protocadherin gamma gene cluster that may be related to muscle denervation and reinnervation was significant frailty-correlated genes and negatively correlated with exercise. Acetylcholine esterase, unc-13 homolog C (UNC13C), and MYH8 genes related to neuromuscular function, such as neurotransmitter breakdown, release, and denervation, respectively, were also expressed in correlation with frailty. Another skeletal muscle transcriptome study found genes involved in growth, cell cycle, cytokines, ubiquitin-proteasome pathway, and amino acid transport were reproducibly responses during acute exercise training [13]. Vascular endothelial growth factor A, platelet-derived growth factor A, cyclin-dependent kinase 4, eukaryotic translation initiation factor 4E, RICTOR, TWEAK receptor, FOXO1, pyruvate dehydrogenase kinase 4, and PGC1α showed increased expression, whereas IκBα, GADD45γ, and FOXO3 were decreased consistently. However, in the fast-twitch muscle fibers, young adults responded to resistance exercise with 463 genes over the cut-off value, whereas old adults responded within only 63 genes, which is somewhat disappointing in terms of aging therapeutics. In other words, this limited responsiveness in old adults is also a necessity for the development of sarcopenia therapeutics. Nonetheless, the possibility that different exercise training protocols applied to two age groups may cause the gene abundance cannot be excluded.

Exercise-induced molecular signaling in skeletal muscle

Physical exercise is the best way by which muscles can be protected against wasting. Physical exercise is generally divided into two types: aerobic (or endurance) and anaerobic (or resistance) exercise. Aerobic exercise shifts muscle fiber types toward those with increased capacity for aerobic metabolism and better ability to resist fatigue, due to a larger number of mitochondria and capillaries (types I and IIA fibers). This is typical in long-distance runners, bikers, and swimmers. These fibers contract slowly with a low peak force and generate ATP through oxidative phosphorylation of glucose and free fatty acids. The resistance exercise causes muscle hypertrophy, especially in myofibers IIX (and IIB in rodents), due to enhanced synthesis of contractile proteins with no change in the number of mitochondria, resulting in increased mass and strength. This is typical in sprinters, weight-lifters, and body-builders. These fibers generate fast contractions with a high peak force and use phosphocreatine and glucose anaerobically to generate ATP [17, 18]. Aerobic exercise induces peroxisome proliferator-activated receptor γ coactivator 1-α (PGC1-α) in humans [19] and rodents [20]. PGC1-α not only promotes mitochondrial biogenesis but also directly antagonizes protein catabolism by blocking FOXO3 [21], the master transcription factor coordinating both proteasomal and lysosomal protein degradation [22–24]. Conversely, resistance exercise stimulates mainly myofibrillar protein synthesis through increased expression of IGF-1 and activation of the PI3K/AKT pathway [25] more specifically in type IIX and IIB muscle, where mTOR-mediated protein synthesis is enhanced by activation of p70S6K and 4E-BP1 and FOXO3 is inactivated by AKT-mediated phosphorylation [22], resulting in inhibition of muscle wasting.

Systemic functions of myokines induced by exercise

Myokine, a category of cytokine, is a functional group of proteins or peptides, which are secreted from skeletal muscle cells and subsequently released into the circulation to exert endocrine or paracrine effects in other cells, tissues, or organs [26]. Acute exercise thus increases myokine concentrations in the blood [27]. The secreted myokines during exercise have been shown to act as anti-inflammatory cytokines and mediators facilitating muscle regeneration or recovery [28]. For instance, irisin, a proteolytic cleavage product from fibronectin type III domain-containing protein 5 (FNDC5), levels in blood elevated by twofold after endurance exercise of healthy adult humans and mice [29]. Apelin and IL-15 levels also increased in endurance exercised by humans and rodents [30, 31]. Many myokines have an autocrine effect on skeletal muscle such as mitochondria biogenesis, muscle fiber hypertrophy, and capillary density, thus showing the positive effects on age-related muscle atrophy. Apelin activates AMP-activated protein kinase (AMPK), thus improves insulin sensitivity via increasing glucose uptake in the skeletal muscle [32], and also promotes mitochondria biogenesis, autophagy, and anti-inflammatory pathways in myofibers [30]. Resistance exercise increased muscle strength and serum irisin levels in elderly women [33], implicating a possible application of myokine as a therapeutic strategy for the treatment of sarcopenia. The paracrine effects of myokines are on adipose tissue, liver, pancreas, endothelial, as well as bone and brain. Most exercise-induced myokines improved conditions of metabolic disorder. Irisin plays a role in the browning of white adipose tissue [29]. Irisin circulation increases after exercise and positively correlates with decreased fat mass in obese adults [34]. IL-15 has an anabolic effect resulting in adipose tissue lipolysis [35, 36]. Another example is myostatin that can inhibit activin type II receptors (ActRII), leading to skeletal muscle atrophy. Myostatin inactivation by spontaneous missense mutations or intentional genetic ablation results in hypermuscularity in mice, dogs, cows, and even in a human pedigree [37–39]. Although antagonizing myostatin with neutralizing antibodies or follistatin, another species of myokine that endogenously antagonizes myostatin, has been developed by several pharmaceuticals for treating sarcopenia, it has a drawback as a drug target because its serum levels have no correlation with age. Cathepsin B is also an exercise-induced myokine that improves memory and adult neurogenesis [40]. Exercise enhances neuronal gene expression of FNDC5, which may be involved in stimulating brain-derived neurotrophic factor (BDNF) in the hippocampus [41]. Exercise increases the expression of kynurenine aminotransferase in muscle, which converts blood levels of neurotoxic kynurenine to the neuroprotective kynurenic acid, thereby reducing depression [42]. These examples mediate muscle to brain crosstalk. Exercise induces not only myokine but also adipokine (adiponectin) or hepatokine (FGF21 and IGF-1), which are also beneficial for older adults. FGF21 and Metrln were found to be elevated in plasma after acute endurance exercise but also elevated in the plasma of diabetic individuals [43]. Further studies are needed to see whether these myokines are useful to target for the cure of metabolic disease, muscle atrophy, and cognitive diseases.

Exercise mimetics targeting AMPK and PPARβ/δ pathway

The positive effects of exercise on patients with sarcopenia have been examined in numerous studies. Given that most patients with sarcopenia have a problem with physical activity, however, there is a limit to overcome sarcopenia through exercise. Therefore, exercise mimetics (exercise pill) have become a potential therapeutic strategy for sarcopenia to make exercise effects without exercise. It was found that PPARβ/δ agonist GW1516 and exercise training synergistically increased oxidative myofibers and running endurance in adult mice [44]. Four weeks of an AMPK agonist, AICAR, treatment alone enhanced running endurance by 44% even in sedentary mice. PPARβ/δ or AMPK activates a robust gene set transcription in skeletal muscle that reprograms the metabolism. AMPK-PPARβ/δ pathway has been targeted by drug developments for the purpose of enhancing exercise benefit without real exercise in patients with sarcopenia. Metformin, a common drug for type 2 diabetes, has been known to be an AMPK agonist so that it has been examined to prevent the development of sarcopenia. The effects of metformin on muscle are still uncertain, and the exact mechanism of action is a matter of debate, although it has been reported to extend lifespan and healthspan with improving physical performance in model mice [45]. Thus, metformin has been a lot studied for pharmacological interventions for delaying aging and age-related diseases, e.g., sarcopenia.

Anabolic hormones effects on skeletal muscle

The decrease in circulating levels of several anabolic hormones with aging may contribute to the decrease in muscle mass and function in the elderly [46]. Therapies of hormonal augmentation have been studies for sarcopenia [47]. Testosterone treatment resulted in the preservation of muscle thickness in intermediate-frail and frail elderly men, while considering adverse effects, its benefits have not been clear.

Specifying the anabolic function of hormonal candidates has been carried out by decreasing the androgenic function of the chemicals. The treatment with selective androgen receptor modulator (SARM) enobosarm (also known as ostarine, MK-2866) induced a dose-dependent increase in total lean body mass with improvements in physical function in the elderly [48]. Another SARM MK-0773/PF-05314882 also increased lean body mass substantially in women with sarcopenia, without evidence of androgenization [49] (Fig. 2). The physical performance showed a tendency to increase. Despite the growing evidence, it is still earlier to decide the clinical use of anabolic hormone supplementation to manage sarcopenia [50].

Not only animal steroids such as testosterone but also plant steroids such as tomatidine and ursolic acid have anabolic effects on human skeletal muscle (Fig. 2). Ursolic acid, a pentacyclic triterpenoid enriched in apples, reduced muscle atrophy and induced muscle

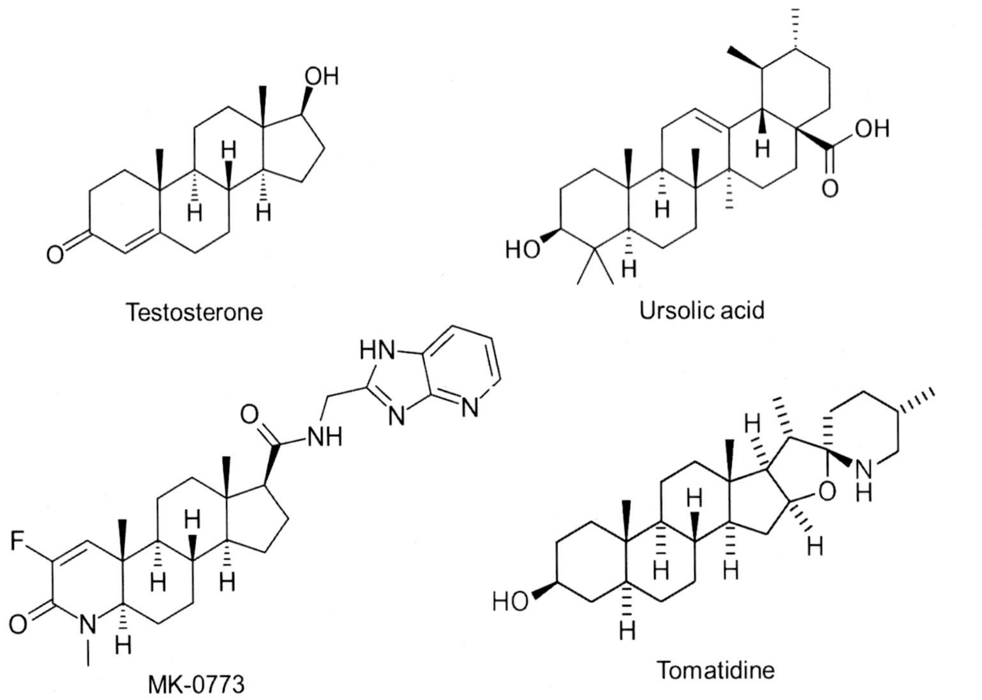

Fig. 2
Structural similarity of animal- and plant-originated steroids that are active on skeletal muscle atrophy: testosterone, SARM MK-0773, tomatidine, and ursolic acid.

hypertrophy in mice by enhancing skeletal muscle insulin/IGF-I signaling and by inhibiting atrophy-related gene expression [51]. Moreover, the effects were accompanied by reductions in adiposity with lowered blood glucose, plasma cholesterol, and triglycerides. However, the clinical trial (NCT02401113) with healthy adults was not successful. Tomatidine significantly reduced age-dependent decline in skeletal muscle mass, strength, and quality in old mice [52], accompanied by decreased adiposity [53] by stimulating mTORC1 signaling and anabolism.

Roles of autophagy pathway in skeletal muscle

With aging, dysregulation of autophagy flux inhibits lysosomal storage processes involved in muscle biogenesis. Exercise-induced autophagy activation executes in skeletal muscle regeneration and remodeling, a mechanism that enables sarcopenia intervention [54]. In the normal state of physiology, autophagy is vital for breaking down lysosomal nutrient stores to reconstruct cellular architecture using damaged cellular components, a recycling process. However, in the pathological states of muscle atrophy, such as cachexia, diabetes, and fasting, autophagy activation also enhances the loss of muscle mass via the proteolytic process. Thus, both excessive and defective autophagy is highly correlated with the loss of skeletal muscle [55].

Mechanically, in the starvation condition, AMPK phosphorylates unc-51-like kinase 1 (ULK1) at Ser317 and Ser777 and directly inhibits mTORC1 through phosphorylation of TSC1 and Raptor, thus triggering autophagy in a FOXO-dependent or -independent manner [56, 57]. In contrast, under nutrient-rich conditions, mTORC1 phosphorylates ULK1 at Ser757, resulting in inhibition of autophagy initiation. Irrespective of endurance or resistance exercise, exercise induces AMPK phosphorylation, reduces p62 accumulation while increasing expression of beclin-1, autophagy-related gene 5 (Atg5), 7 (Atg7), and 12 (Atg12), thus resulting in activation of autophagy, which likely contributes to beneficial skeletal muscle adaptation and physical performance, especially in the aged mice [58].

In addition, autophagy has been reported to contribute to satellite cell transition from quiescence to activation [59]. Appropriate autophagy is necessary for proteostasis and mitochondria biogenesis in maintaining satellite cell stemness by preventing senescence [60].

Mitochondrial function declines with aging [61]. Mitophagy plays a significant role in mitochondrial quality control in muscles, indicating that mitophagy-inducing agents may help sarcopenia [62]. Urolithin A is a benzo-coumarin compound metabolically transformed from a group of natural compounds, which increases muscle function in mice [63].

Conclusion

Practically, an exercise pill could not reproduce the multiple beneficial effects of exercise on a variety of organs in the body, because exercise not only affects too many interconnected pathways but also its effect depends on the host polymorphism and physiology. Thus, here we need patient-specific combinatorial therapeutics and precision medicine, for which necessity is a state-of-art diagnostic using multiple biomarkers [64], in sarcopenia. Nonetheless, reminding that there is no drug available at present, selective drugs based on the exercise mechanisms could be given to act on specific pathways and help at least in part patients who cannot exercise for various reasons.

The catabolic pathways outweigh the anabolic process with aging. Thus, ubiquitin-dependent proteolysis by atrogin-1 and MuRF-1 and ubiquitin-independent autophagy, as well as mTOR-dependent protein synthesis, should be considered as therapeutic interventions for sarcopenia treatment in old age by mimicking exercise.

Chemically synthesized or naturally originated small molecules and biologically synthesized nucleotides and myokines are all possible strategies for targeting exercise mechanisms that provide a variety of principles for sarcopenia therapeutics, thus leading to global healthcare of future aged society.

Acknowledgment

The author acknowledges Drs. Yong Ryoul Yang, Byungkuk Min, and Ju Yeon Kwak for statistical analyses and help.

References

[1] Cruz-Jentoft AJ, Bahat G, Bauer J, Boirie Y, Bruyere O, Cederholm T, et al. Sarcopenia: revised European consensus on definition and diagnosis. Age Ageing 2019;48(1):16–31.

[2] Chen LK, Woo J, Assantachai P, Auyeung TW, Chou MY, Iijima K, et al. Asian working Group for Sarcopenia: 2019 consensus update on sarcopenia diagnosis and treatment. J Am Med Dir Assoc 2020;21(3):300–7. e2.

[3] Jung HW, Kim SW, Kim IY, Lim JY, Park HS, Song W, et al. Protein intake recommendation for Korean older adults to prevent sarcopenia: expert consensus by the Korean geriatric society and the Korean nutrition society. Ann Geriatr Med Res 2018;22(4):167–75.

[4] Cruz-Jentoft AJ, Landi F, Schneider SM, Zuniga C, Arai H, Boirie Y, et al. Prevalence of and interventions for sarcopenia in ageing adults: a systematic review. Report of the international sarcopenia initiative (EWGSOP and IWGS). Age Ageing 2014;43(6):748–59.

[5] Kalinkovich A, Livshits G. Sarcopenia—the search for emerging biomarkers. Ageing Res Rev 2015;22:58–71.

[6] Ilich JZ, Kelly OJ, Inglis JE, Panton LB, Duque G, Ormsbee MJ. Interrelationship among muscle, fat, and bone: connecting the dots on cellular, hormonal, and whole body levels. Ageing Res Rev 2014;15:51–60.

[7] Kob R, Bollheimer LC, Bertsch T, Fellner C, Djukic M, Sieber CC, et al. Sarcopenic obesity: molecular clues to a better understanding of its pathogenesis? Biogerontology 2015;16(1):15–29.

[8] Marzetti E, Calvani R, Lorenzi M, Marini F, D'Angelo E, Martone AM, et al. Serum levels of C-terminal agrin fragment (CAF) are associated with sarcopenia in older hip fractured patients. Exp Gerontol 2014;60:79–82.

[9] Sakuma K, Aoi W, Yamaguchi A. Current understanding of sarcopenia: possible candidates modulating muscle mass. Pflugers Arch 2015;467(2):213–29.

[10] Snijders T, Verdijk LB, van Loon LJ. The impact of sarcopenia and exercise training on skeletal muscle satellite cells. Ageing Res Rev 2009;8(4):328–38.

[11] Morley JE. Editorial: sarcopenia revisited. J Gerontol A Biol Sci Med Sci 2003;58:M909–10.

[12] Melov S, Tarnopolsky MA, Beckman K, Felkey K, Hubbard A. Resistance exercise reverses aging in human skeletal muscle. PLoS One 2007;2(5), e465.

[13] Raue U, Trappe TA, Estrem ST, Qian HR, Helvering LM, Smith RC, et al. Transcriptome signature of resistance exercise adaptations: mixed muscle and fiber type specific profiles in young and old adults. J Appl Physiol (1985) 2012;112(10):1625–36.

[14] Fried LP, Tangen CM, Walston J, Newman AB, Hirsch C, Gottdiener J, et al. Frailty in older adults: evidence for a phenotype. J Gerontol A Biol Sci Med Sci 2001;56(3):M146–56.

[15] Reijnierse EM, Trappenburg MC, Blauw GJ, Verlaan S, de van der Schueren MA, Meskers CG, et al. Common ground? The concordance of sarcopenia and frailty definitions. J Am Med Dir Assoc 2016;17(4):371. e7–12.

[16] Hangelbroek RW, Fazelzadeh P, Tieland M, Boekschoten MV, Hooiveld GJ, van Duynhoven JP, et al. Expression of protocadherin gamma in skeletal muscle tissue is associated with age and muscle weakness. J Cachexia Sarcopenia Muscle 2016;7(5):604–14.

[17] Hoppeler H, Baum O, Lurman G, Mueller M. Molecular mechanisms of muscle plasticity with exercise. Compr Physiol 2011;1(3):1383–412.

[18] Hawley JA, Hargreaves M, Joyner MJ, Zierath JR. Integrative biology of exercise. Cell 2014;159(4):738–49.

[19] Pilegaard H, Saltin B, Neufer PD. Exercise induces transient transcriptional activation of the PGC-1alpha gene in human skeletal muscle. J Physiol 2003;546(Pt 3):851–8.

[20] Terada S, Goto M, Kato M, Kawanaka K, Shimokawa T, Tabata I. Effects of low-intensity prolonged exercise on PGC-1 mRNA expression in rat epitrochlearis muscle. Biochem Biophys Res Commun 2002;296(2):350–4.

[21] Sandri M, Lin J, Handschin C, Yang W, Arany ZP, Lecker SH, et al. PGC-1alpha protects skeletal muscle from atrophy by suppressing FoxO3 action and atrophy-specific gene transcription. Proc Natl Acad Sci U S A 2006;103(44):16260–5.

[22] Sandri M, Sandri C, Gilbert A, Skurk C, Calabria E, Picard A, et al. Foxo transcription factors induce the atrophy-related ubiquitin ligase atrogin-1 and cause skeletal muscle atrophy. Cell 2004;117(3):399–412.

[23] Mammucari C, Milan G, Romanello V, Masiero E, Rudolf R, Del Piccolo P, et al. FoxO3 controls autophagy in skeletal muscle in vivo. Cell Metab 2007;6(6):458–71.

[24] Zhao J, Brault JJ, Schild A, Cao P, Sandri M, Schiaffino S, et al. FoxO3 coordinately activates protein degradation by the autophagic/lysosomal and proteasomal pathways in atrophying muscle cells. Cell Metab 2007;6(6):472–83.

[25] McCall GE, Allen DL, Haddad F, Baldwin KM. Transcriptional regulation of IGF-I expression in skeletal muscle. Am J Phys Cell Phys 2003;285(4):C831–9.

[26] Pedersen BK, Febbraio MA. Muscles, exercise and obesity: skeletal muscle as a secretory organ. Nat Rev Endocrinol 2012;8(8):457–65.

[27] Christiansen T, Bruun JM, Paulsen SK, Olholm J, Overgaard K, Pedersen SB, et al. Acute exercise increases circulating inflammatory markers in overweight and obese compared with lean subjects. Eur J Appl Physiol 2013;113(6):1635–42.

[28] Ost M, Coleman V, Kasch J, Klaus S. Regulation of myokine expression: role of exercise and cellular stress. Free Radic Biol Med 2016;98:78–89.

[29] Bostrom P, Wu J, Jedrychowski MP, Korde A, Ye L, Lo JC, et al. A PGC1-alpha-dependent myokine that drives brown-fat-like development of white fat and thermogenesis. Nature 2012;481(7382):463–8.

[30] Vinel C, Lukjanenko L, Batut A, Deleruyelle S, Pradere JP, Le Gonidec S, et al. The exerkine apelin reverses age-associated sarcopenia. Nat Med 2018;24(9):1360–71.

[31] Yang H, Chang J, Chen W, Zhao L, Qu B, Tang C, et al. Treadmill exercise promotes interleukin 15 expression in skeletal muscle and interleukin 15 receptor alpha expression in adipose tissue of high-fat diet rats. Endocrine 2013;43(3):579–85.

[32] Attane C, Foussal C, Le Gonidec S, Benani A, Daviaud D, Wanecq E, et al. Apelin treatment increases complete fatty acid oxidation, mitochondrial oxidative capacity, and biogenesis in muscle of insulin-resistant mice. Diabetes 2012;61(2):310–20.

[33] Kim HJ, So B, Choi M, Kang D, Song W. Resistance exercise training increases the expression of irisin concomitant with improvement of muscle function in aging mice and humans. Exp Gerontol 2015;70:11–7.

[34] Kim HJ, Lee HJ, So B, Son JS, Yoon D, Song W. Effect of aerobic training and resistance training on circulating irisin level and their association with change of body composition in overweight/obese adults: a pilot study. Physiol Res 2016;65(2):271–9.

[35] Quinn LS, Strait-Bodey L, Anderson BG, Argiles JM, Havel PJ. Interleukin-15 stimulates adiponectin secretion by 3T3-L1 adipocytes: evidence for a skeletal muscle-to-fat signaling pathway. Cell Biol Int 2005;29(6):449–57.

[36] Pierce JR, Maples JM, Hickner RC. IL-15 concentrations in skeletal muscle and subcutaneous adipose tissue in lean and obese humans: local effects of IL-15 on adipose tissue lipolysis. Am J Physiol Endocrinol Metab 2015;308(12):E1131–9.

[37] McPherron AC, Lee SJ. Double muscling in cattle due to mutations in the myostatin gene. Proc Natl Acad Sci U S A 1997;94(23):12457–61.

[38] McPherron AC, Lawler AM, Lee SJ. Regulation of skeletal muscle mass in mice by a new TGF-beta superfamily member. Nature 1997;387(6628):83–90.

[39] Prontera P, Bernardini L, Stangoni G, Capalbo A, Rogaia D, Ardisia C, et al. 2q31.2q32.3 deletion syndrome: report of an adult patient. Am J Med Genet A 2009;149A(4):706–12.

[40] Moon HY, Becke A, Berron D, Becker B, Sah N, Benoni G, et al. Running-induced systemic cathepsin B secretion is associated with memory function. Cell Metab 2016;24(2):332–40.

[41] Wrann CD, White JP, Salogiannnis J, Laznik-Bogoslavski D, Wu J, Ma D, et al. Exercise induces hippocampal BDNF through a PGC-1alpha/FNDC5 pathway. Cell Metab 2013;18(5):649–59.

[42] Agudelo LZ, Femenia T, Orhan F, Porsmyr-Palmertz M, Goiny M, Martinez-Redondo V, et al. Skeletal muscle PGC-1alpha1 modulates kynurenine metabolism and mediates resilience to stress-induced depression. Cell 2014;159(1):33–45.

[43] Piccirillo R. Exercise-induced myokines with therapeutic potential for muscle wasting. Front Physiol 2019;10:287.

[44] Narkar VA, Downes M, Yu RT, Embler E, Wang YX, Banayo E, et al. AMPK and PPARdelta agonists are exercise mimetics. Cell 2008;134(3):405–15.

[45] Kulkarni AS, Brutsaert EF, Anghel V, Zhang K, Bloomgarden N, Pollak M, et al. Metformin regulates metabolic and nonmetabolic pathways in skeletal muscle and subcutaneous adipose tissues of older adults. Aging Cell 2018;17(2).

[46] Tenover JS. Effects of testosterone supplementation in the aging male. J Clin Endocrinol Metab 1992;75(4):1092–8.

[47] Atkinson RA, Srinivas-Shankar U, Roberts SA, Connolly MJ, Adams JE, Oldham JA, et al. Effects of testosterone on skeletal muscle architecture in intermediate-frail and frail elderly men. J Gerontol A Biol Sci Med Sci 2010;65(11):1215–9.

[48] Dalton JT, Barnette KG, Bohl CE, Hancock ML, Rodriguez D, Dodson ST, et al. The selective androgen receptor modulator GTx-024 (enobosarm) improves lean body mass and physical function in healthy elderly men and postmenopausal women: results of a double-blind, placebo-controlled phase II trial. J Cachexia Sarcopenia Muscle 2011;2(3):153–61.

[49] Papanicolaou DA, Ather SN, Zhu H, Zhou Y, Lutkiewicz J, Scott BB, et al. A phase IIA randomized, placebo-controlled clinical trial to study the efficacy and safety of the selective androgen receptor modulator (SARM), MK-0773 in female participants with sarcopenia. J Nutr Health Aging 2013;17(6):533–43.

[50] Kamel HK, Maas D, Duthie Jr EH. Role of hormones in the pathogenesis and management of sarcopenia. Drugs Aging 2002;19(11):865–77.
[51] Kunkel SD, Suneja M, Ebert SM, Bongers KS, Fox DK, Malmberg SE, et al. mRNA expression signatures of human skeletal muscle atrophy identify a natural compound that increases muscle mass. Cell Metab 2011;13(6):627–38.
[52] Ebert SM, Dyle MC, Bullard SA, Dierdorff JM, Murry DJ, Fox DK, et al. Identification and small molecule inhibition of an activating transcription factor 4 (ATF4)-dependent pathway to age-related skeletal muscle weakness and atrophy. J Biol Chem 2015;290(42):25497–511.
[53] Dyle MC, Ebert SM, Cook DP, Kunkel SD, Fox DK, Bongers KS, et al. Systems-based discovery of tomatidine as a natural small molecule inhibitor of skeletal muscle atrophy. J Biol Chem 2014;289(21):14913–24.
[54] Park SS, Seo YK, Kwon KS. Sarcopenia targeting with autophagy mechanism by exercise. BMB Rep 2019;52(1):64–9.
[55] Larsson L, Degens H, Li M, Salviati L, Lee YI, Thompson W, et al. Sarcopenia: aging-related loss of muscle mass and function. Physiol Rev 2019;99(1):427–511.
[56] Milan G, Romanello V, Pescatore F, Armani A, Paik JH, Frasson L, et al. Regulation of autophagy and the ubiquitin-proteasome system by the FoxO transcriptional network during muscle atrophy. Nat Commun 2015;6:6670.
[57] Vainshtein A, Hood DA. The regulation of autophagy during exercise in skeletal muscle. J Appl Physiol (1985) 2016;120(6):664–73.
[58] Kim YA, Kim YS, Oh SL, Kim HJ, Song W. Autophagic response to exercise training in skeletal muscle with age. J Physiol Biochem 2013;69(4):697–705.
[59] Tang AH, Rando TA. Induction of autophagy supports the bioenergetic demands of quiescent muscle stem cell activation. EMBO J 2014;33(23):2782–97.
[60] Garcia-Prat L, Martinez-Vicente M, Perdiguero E, Ortet L, Rodriguez-Ubreva J, Rebollo E, et al. Autophagy maintains stemness by preventing senescence. Nature 2016;529(7584):37–42.
[61] Short KR, Bigelow ML, Kahl J, Singh R, Coenen-Schimke J, Raghavakaimal S, et al. Decline in skeletal muscle mitochondrial function with aging in humans. Proc Natl Acad Sci U S A 2005;102(15):5618–23.
[62] Romanello V, Sandri M. Mitochondrial quality control and muscle mass maintenance. Front Physiol 2015;6:422.
[63] Ryu D, Mouchiroud L, Andreux PA, Katsyuba E, Moullan N, Nicolet-Dit-Felix AA, et al. Urolithin A induces mitophagy and prolongs lifespan in C. elegans and increases muscle function in rodents. Nat Med 2016;22(8):879–88.
[64] Kwak JY, Hwang H, Kim SK, Choi JY, Lee SM, Bang H, et al. Prediction of sarcopenia using a combination of multiple serum biomarkers. Sci Rep 2018;8(1):8574.

CHAPTER 7

Myokines: A potential key factor in development, treatment, and biomarker of sarcopenia

Wataru Aoi

Laboratory of Nutrition Science, Graduate School of Life and Environmental Sciences, Kyoto Prefectural University, Kyoto, Japan

Abstract

Skeletal muscle cells secrete various proteins/peptides, known as myokines, into the extracellular milieu. The concept of myokines could be expanded to small peptides, noncoding RNAs, and metabolites and applied to various fields including sports, health promotion, and medicine. Myokines can regulate functions such as energy metabolism, anti-inflammation, and muscle hypertrophy via autocrine, paracrine, and endocrine effects. Many myokines are secreted in response to exercise and muscle contraction, while their secretion is dysregulated in conditions such as aging and physical inactivity. Accumulating evidence suggests that several myokines regulate myogenesis and protein metabolism, which are associated with the development of sarcopenia. Some myokines may have the potential to be developed as biomarkers for sarcopenia. Understanding the role of myokines might provide insights into the mechanism and treatment of sarcopenia.

Keywords: Myokine, Skeletal muscle, Sarcopenia, Myogenesis, Protein metabolism

Introduction

It is well known that skeletal muscle functions as a supporting organ during physical activity. It also functions as a major tissue that uptakes more than 70% of blood glucose [1]. In addition, growing evidence suggests that skeletal muscle cells secrete bioactive proteins and low molecular weight peptides into the extracellular milieus and circulation. These proteins regulate the function of many organs, are anti-inflammatory, and also play a role in metabolism and muscle building, and this is referred to as the myokine theory [2]. Early studies have reported that interleukin-6 (IL-6), a typical secretory protein produced by muscle cells, was one of the first identified myokines [3–5]. Thereafter, various proteins and peptides have been identified. Furthermore, noncoding microRNAs and metabolites secreted from muscle cells have also been recognized as myokines. Such myokines can regulate the function of the muscle itself in autocrine and paracrine manners or other organs via an endocrine route and thereby contribute to physiological and pathological phenotypes such as metabolic capacity, muscle mass, bone density, hormone secretion, cognitive function, and tumorigenesis.

Exercise and muscle contraction regulate the secretion of myokines. Thus, myokines mediate exercise-induced adaptations and exert their effects on energy metabolism, nervous system, endocrine system, and immune function. Thus, the circulating level of myokines has been suggested to be involved in reduced risk of noncommunicable diseases such as type 2 diabetes, cardiovascular disease, and carcinogenesis [6–8]. Furthermore, accumulating evidence indicates that several myokines are involved in the development of age-related muscle atrophies via regulating myogenesis and protein metabolism (Fig. 1). Such myokines may also be useful as potential biomarkers for sarcopenia (Table 1). This chapter reviews the role of major myokines in myogenesis and muscle hypertrophy, as well as their potential effects on the development and treatment of sarcopenia.

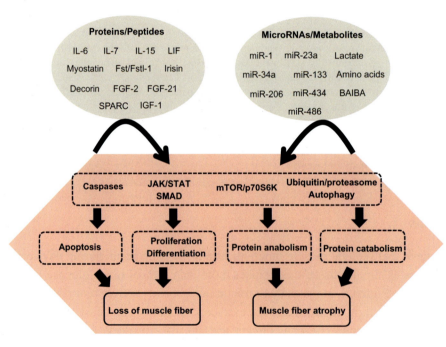

Fig. 1
The potential roles of secreted factors in the regulation of muscle mass. Skeletal muscle cells secrete several proteins and oligopeptides into the extracellular milieus and circulation. Such myokines can be involved in muscle mass maintenance by regulating myogenesis and protein metabolism via autocrine, paracrine, or paracrine routes. Further, several microRNAs and metabolites secreted from muscle cells also function as muscle mass regulators. The effect of myokines affects the development of age-related muscle atrophies. *BAIBA*, β-aminoisobutyric acid; *FGF*, fibroblast growth factor; *Fst*, follistatin; *Fstl-1*, follistatin-like-1; *IGF-1*, insulin like growth factor-1; *IL*, interleukin; *LIF*, leukemia inhibitory factor; *SPARC*, secreted protein acidic and rich in cysteine.

Table 1: Summary of myokines with potential biomarkers for sarcopenia.

Protein/peptide	Study design (age, n)	Circulating level	References
Myostatin	Cross sectional (60–92 yr, 31)	High	[9]
	Cross sectional (53–92 yr, 463)	N.D.	[10]
	Cross sectional (53–71 yr, 238)	N.D.	[11]
	Cross sectional (41–84 yr, 39)	N.D.	[12]
	Cross sectional (60– yr, 46)	N.D.	[13]
	Intervention, 8wk (55–75 yr, 31)	Decrease	[14]
	Intervention, 8wk (40–53 yr, 10)	Decrease	[15]
Fst/Fstl-1	Cross sectional (53–71 yr, 238)	N.D.	[11]
	Cross sectional (60– yr, 66)	N.D.	[13]
	Intervention, 8wk (55–75 yr, 31)	Increase	[14]
	Intervention, 8wk (40–53 yr, 10)	Increase	[15]
IGF-1	Cross sectional (60–87 yr, 3276)	Low	[16]
	Cross sectional (60– yr, 94)	Low	[17]
	Intervention, 8wk (55–75 yr, 31)	N.D.	[14]
Irisin	Cross sectional (60– yr, 153)	Low	[18]
	Cross sectional (41–84 yr, 39)	Low	[12]
	Intervention, 16wk (60–75 yr, 23)	Increase	[19]
Decorin	Cross sectional (41–84 yr, 39)	Low	[12]

The potential role of myokines as biomarkers for sarcopenia has been examined in the middle to elderly people. Cross-sectional studies showed that circulating levels of classical myokines, myostatin, and Fst/Fstl-1 are not necessarily correlated with sarcopenia, while positively changed by exercise intervention. Lower circulating levels of irisin and decorin with sarcopenia have been shown in few studies. *High*, higher in sarcopenic condition; *low*, lower in sarcopenic condition; *N.D.*, no difference between normal and sarcopenic conditions; *increase*, increase vs. baseline; *decrease*, decrease vs. baseline; *Fst*, follistatin; *Fstl-1*, follistatin-like-1; *IGF-1*, insulin like growth factor-1.

The role of myokines in myogenesis

It is well known that loss of muscle cell number is a major cause of age-related muscle atrophy [20]. Impaired myogenesis due to dysregulated differentiation of satellite cells can result in decreased cell number. Some myokines affect myogenesis positively and negatively. Growth differentiation factor 8, also known as myostatin, which belongs to the transforming growth factor-β (TGF-β) superfamily, is a typical myokine that inhibits muscle hypertrophy [21]. Indeed, an earlier study reported that circulating myostatin levels increased with aging in human beings [9]. Myostatin is secreted from the muscle cells into the blood as an inactive complex with several proteins and peptides [22]. After binding to activin type II receptors on the cell membrane, myostatin stimulates SMAD signals and decreases the levels of myogenic regulatory factors including MyoD and Pax3. As a result, it inhibits myoblast proliferation and differentiation during the process of myogenesis [21,23]. The inhibitory effect on differentiation may be partly mediated by the inactivation of the Akt/mammalian target of rapamycin (mTOR)/p70S6 pathway [24], as mentioned in the next section. Therefore, inhibiting the function of this protein can be beneficial in preventing muscle atrophy. Follistatin and its related proteins are known as inhibitors of myostatin. These proteins directly bind to myostatin and inhibit its function [21,25]. However, later studies have shown that circulating levels of myostatin and follistatin were not significantly correlated with sarcopenia conditions [10,11,13]. Thus, it is difficult to determine the effect of the myostatin-dependent pathway on age-related muscle loss and use it as a biomarker for the estimation or diagnosis of sarcopenia. In contrast, intervention by resistance training reduced myostatin and elevated follistatin levels in serum [14,15]. The level of circulating follistatin-like protein 1 (Fstl1) is also increased by a single bout of exercise in human subjects [26] and functions in an endocrine route. In animal studies, inhibition of myostatin by knockout of this gene increased muscle mass [27,28]. Although therapies targeting myostatin have been clinically investigated in human beings, further studies are required.

Decorin, a leucine-rich proteoglycan, is another secreted protein that inhibits myostatin signaling not only by direct binding but also by stimulating the expression of Mighty, a downstream factor of the myostatin cascade [29,30]. In decorin over-expressing muscle cells, the expression levels of Myod1 and follistatin were increased, whereas the levels of ubiquitin ligases, atrogin1 and MuRF1, were decreased. In addition, the old concept of sarcopenia was based on the assessment of skeletal muscle mass alone, whereas the more recent concept encompasses muscle strength and the role of physical activity. Thus, decorin secreted from muscle cells contributes to hypertrophy and prevented atrophy of the skeletal muscle. The expression of decorin is increased upon muscle contraction in human beings and mice [30]. Acute resistance exercise increased the circulating levels of decorin, which might contribute to myogenesis [30]. Inflammatory condition suppresses the expression of decorin [31]. Serum decorin level was positively correlated with skeletal muscle mass in patients with liver cirrhosis [12], suggesting that it could be a potential biomarker of sarcopenia condition with inflammatory diseases.

Several factors act through myostatin independent routes. Leukemia inhibitory factor (LIF) is a secreted protein that accelerates myogenesis. The expression of LIF is induced by intracellular Ca^{2+} level and it is released into the extracellular milieu but not into circulation [32]; thus, it acts locally in muscle tissues. LIF stimulates satellite cell proliferation mainly via activation of the JAK2-STAT3 signaling pathway and contributes to regeneration and hypertrophy [33]. Human myoblast proliferation was promoted by exogenous LIF and reduced upon knockdown of the LIF receptor [34]. The mRNA levels of LIF were markedly increased by resistance exercise in human skeletal muscle [34]. On the other hand, serum level of LIF has been reported to relatively increase with aging and diabetic conditions [11,35]. Although it exerts an endocrine effect in contrast to exercised condition, impaired signal transduction of LIF in skeletal muscle may result in aging and metabolic disorders.

A PGC-1α-dependent myokine, irisin, is released into circulation by exercise and has been shown to mediate various functions in other organs including bone, brain/nerve, and metabolic organs in an endocrine manner [36–38]. In a cross-sectional study, circulating irisin levels were significantly lower in the sarcopenic group than in the nonsarcopenic group in postmenopausal women, suggesting that irisin could be a potential biomarker of sarcopenia [18]. A study in patients with myotonic dystrophies also supports that plasma irisin levels reflect muscle mass [39]. Indeed, in an animal study, injection of irisin induced muscle hypertrophy with enhanced strength, mediated by the activation of satellite cells, thereby suggesting its function as a promyogenic factor [40]. Recently, a prospective and controlled clinical trial with elderly people showed that 16 weeks of resistance training improved muscle mass and physical performance with elevated serum irisin levels [19], suggesting that it could be a biomarker for sarcopenia itself or to determine the effect of exercise therapy.

An exercise-induced myokine, secreted protein acidic and rich in cysteine (SPARC) induces muscle differentiation. This myokine exerts several functions including improved glucose tolerance, insulin secretion, and suppression of colon tumorigenesis [41–43]. Interestingly, the expression level of SPARC in skeletal muscle was lower in aged mice than in young mice [43]. In a SPARC knockdown model, muscle atrophy was observed with upregulated SMAD3 signaling [44]. Acute exercise transiently elevates serum SPARC levels in human beings [43,45]. However, progenitor cells from aged muscle show resistance to exogenous SPARC, resulting in a differentiation shift from myogenesis to adipogenesis [46]. In contrast, the circulating levels of SPARC were considerably higher in the sarcopenic group compared to healthy individuals [17], supporting a concept of developed resistance to SPARC in aged muscle.

Furthermore, myokines have been reported to induce muscle proliferation and differentiation of satellite cells in exercise models. The levels of chitinase-3-like protein 1 are elevated in circulation and muscle tissues by exercise and activate myoblast proliferation via protease-activated receptor [47]. In addition, levels of the secreted protein, R3h domain-containing like (R3hdml), were increased during muscle cell differentiation [48]. Although muscle loss was observed in R3hdml KO mice, treatment with R3hdml stimulated satellite cell proliferation and differentiation. IL-7, detected in media from primary cultures of human myotubes differentiated from satellite cells, stimulated satellite cell migration [49]. The expression of IL-7 in skeletal muscle was elevated by resistance training [49]; therefore, IL-7 can contribute to hypertrophic adaptation via autocrine and paracrine effects. IL-6 may also stimulate exercise-induced proliferation of satellite cells during muscle regenerations [50]. However, activation of AMPK, an exercise-induced metabolic factor, reduced IL-6 expression in skeletal muscle [51], suggesting its different roles between low-grade/chronic- and moderate/transient-secretions. The extent of involvement of these myokines in age-related muscle loss is still unclear.

The role of myokines in protein anabolism and catabolism

Cross-sectional studies have reported that the circulating levels of insulin-like growth factor-1 (IGF-1) were lower in the sarcopenic group than in the nonsarcopenic group in elderly people [16,17]. There was a strong positive correlation between IGF-1 levels and muscle mass/strength, and resistance training intervention for 12 weeks resulted in higher levels of this protein [52]. IGF-I is a well-known secretory protein contributing to muscle mass [53,54]. Mice overexpressing IGF-1 exhibited hypertrophy with higher strength and accelerated muscle regeneration in both normal and dystrophic conditions [55,56]. The hypertrophic effect is mainly mediated by protein synthesis through increased Akt/mTOR/p70S6K signaling. The insulin signaling and the Akt/mTOR/p70S6K pathways play important roles in protein synthesis in muscle cells. In the anabolic cascade, the activated mTOR/p70S6K signaling causes phosphorylation of the S6-ribosomal protein and increases the translation of various proteins related to hypertrophy [57]. IGF-I overexpression can also prevent age-induced muscle atrophy in mice [58]; therefore, upregulation of IGF-I might be an appropriate strategy for inhibiting sarcopenia. In contrast, there are controversial findings regarding the effect of IGF-I administration on the elderly with respect to muscle mass and function since decreased sensitivity to IGF-I occurs in aged muscle [59].

Myostatin-induced muscle atrophy is also mediated by protein metabolism. It suppresses protein synthesis via Akt/mTOR signaling and accelerates protein degradation via the ubiquitin-proteasome pathway [60]. Deletion of myostatin can enhance Akt activity and inhibit IGF-1-induced hypertrophic effect in skeletal muscle [61]. In contrast, exposure to myostatin increases FOXO1 accumulation in the nucleus of myotubes [62]. However, intervention by resistance training reduced circulating myostatin levels with improved muscle mass in both nonsarcopenic and sarcopenic elderly men [14,15,63]. Fstl1, an inhibitor of myostatin, secreted by muscle cells upon exercise/muscle contraction, also stimulates protein synthesis via Akt/mTOR signaling [26]. Other studies showed that both insulin and IGF-1 were required for follistatin-induced muscle anabolism [64,65]. Thus, these observations suggest that the effects of myostatin and follistatin are associated with IGF-1. Recently, transcription factor IRF4 in brown adipose tissues has been shown to activate mTOR signaling in muscle, which may be mediated by the inhibitory effect of circulating myostatin [66].

Several studies have reported that irisin contributes to muscle mass preservation by improved protein metabolism in muscle cells. Application of irisin leads to activation of Akt/mTOR signaling and inhibition of ubiquitin-proteasome signaling in glucocorticoid- and denervation-induced atrophic models [67,68]. In C2C12 myotubes, exposure to irisin enhanced Akt/mTOR signaling and suppressed the expression of atrogin-1 and Murf1 [68]. FGF21 is a myokine that regulates glucose and lipid utilization in various tissues, including brown adipose tissue and skeletal muscle. It is released from skeletal muscle cells upon activation of mTORC1 [69] and Akt1 [70]. Thus, FGF21 partly mediates muscle hypertrophy-induced whole-body metabolism. However, the circulating level does not necessarily correlate with either sarcopenia status or the effect of exercise interventions. With respect to studies regarding other myokines, FGF-2 suppresses glucocorticoid-induced protein catabolism through reduced myostatin expression [71]. IL-6 and LIF can activate gp130-Akt signaling axis, which induces protein synthesis via mTORC1 independent mechanisms in cultured myotubes [72].

Recently, the importance of protein metabolism via autophagy has been suggested to be involved in age-related muscle atrophy. Some myokines such as brain-derived neurotrophic factor, myostatin, and FGF21 have been shown to regulate the autophagy [73–75] and, hence, may support the role of myokines in the modulation of protein metabolism.

MicroRNAs and metabolites as myokines

Early studies of myokines were limited to proteins and peptides. However, skeletal muscle cells have been found to secrete many kinds of nucleic acids and metabolites. Typical secreted nucleic acids are microRNAs (miRNAs) and small noncoding RNAs of approximately 19–22 nucleotides in length. A single miRNA can regulate the expression of several mRNAs and proteins by post-transcriptional regulation. Thirty percent of protein-coding genes might be regulated by miRNAs that play important roles in various physiological and pathological processes, including growth and development, cell death, adaptation, diseases, and aging. Interestingly, several miRNAs are secreted from the cells into the circulation or are taken up from the circulation into the cells [76]. miRNAs are protected against RNases by being enveloped in extracellular vesicles, such as exosomes, microvesicles, and apoptotic bodies, or by their binding with nonvesicle-associated proteins, such as lipoprotein particles [77,78]. Modulation of the function of recipient cells by circulating miRNAs (c-miRNAs) could explain the communication between skeletal muscles and other organs, along with myokine theory [79].

Since several specific miRNAs are associated with skeletal muscles, determining their circulating levels may be useful for developing biomarkers of muscle-related events, including muscle disorders and physical fitness. Serum levels of several muscle-enriched miRNAs such as miR-1, miR-133, and miR-206 are elevated in Duchenne muscular dystrophy and rhabdomyosarcoma tumors in human beings and animals [80–82]. Other candidate c-miRNAs, such as miR-378 and miR-31, have been suggested to be associated with dystrophy in human beings [83]. Furthermore, circulating levels of muscle-enriched miRNAs such as miR-1, miR-206, and miR-499 are higher in patients with chronic obstructive pulmonary disease, who often exhibit reduced muscle mass compared to normal healthy subjects [84]. In muscular atrophy, the levels of miR-23a are decreased and it is secreted into the extracellular space after being taken up by exosomes [85]. In contrast, the majority of miRNAs that are highly expressed in skeletal muscle are difficult to detect in circulation under normal physiological conditions.

Exercise changes, transiently or adaptively, the levels c-miRNAs in animals and human beings [86–88], leading to post-transcriptional regulation of proteins associated with energy metabolism and angiogenesis in adipocytes, hepatocytes, and endothelial cells. Muscle-enriched miRNAs exhibit no change in response to exercise [86,87], except for miR-486, the levels of which were decreased in response to acute and chronic exercise associated with the lower aerobic performance [89]. However, other researchers have reported that the levels of several c-miRNAs are elevated after strenuous/prolonged exercise such as running a marathon, and that, in particular, alterations in the levels of c-miR-1, c-miR-133a, c-miR-206, and c-miR-208 are closely associated with performance and muscle damage parameters [90,91]. These contradicting results may be attributed to variations in the type, intensity, and duration of exercises evaluated in different studies. Since the levels of certain miRNAs are influenced by both exercise and myopathy, it is difficult to establish the benefit of these miRNAs as reliable biomarkers for muscle diseases. This warrants the investigation of additional parameters for consideration of miRNAs as diagnostic tools.

miRNAs are also regulators of signaling pathways known to modulate muscle atrophy. Some of them can be potential biomarkers for sarcopenia. The levels of miR-21 and miR-34a are increased due to inflammation and oxidative stress and induce inhibition of myogenesis and senescence [92,93], hence supporting the relationship between inflammation and aging. Comprehensive analysis of miRNA expression in mice using miRNA-seq showed that miR-434-3p was lower in both serum and muscle of aged mice than young mice [94]. A bioinformatics analysis of c-miRNA-mRNA interactions that higher levels of circulating miR-19a-3p, miR-19b-3p, miR-20a-5p, miR-26b-5p, miR-143-3p, and miR-195-5p in younger subjects, leading to elevated protein anabolic signaling of proteins [95]. However, such response was lower in elderly subjects, which can be a cause of anabolic resistance in aging. FOXO1 activity was reduced following miR-486 overexpression in skeletal muscle cells in vitro, through decreased FOXO1 expression and increased FOXO1 phosphorylation through direct miR-486-targeting of phosphatase and tensin homolog (PTEN), a negative regulator of FOXO1-upstream kinase AKT, by miR-486 [96]. Moreover, miR-486 overexpression also reduced the induction of FOXO1 targets, MAFbx and MuRF-1 protein expression in mouse primary muscle cells following treatment with dexamethasone, a potent inducer of muscle atrophy [96]. In addition, overexpression of miR-486 protected against skeletal muscle loss in a mouse model of chronic kidney disease [96]. Furthermore, miR-486 inhibition *in vitro* slightly reduced myotube diameter, and its inhibition in vivo reduced the cross-sectional area of muscle fibers, confirming the effects of miR-486 on the regulation of skeletal muscle mass [97]. Recently, a study reported that exercise increased the baseline expression of miR-486-5p, miR-215-5p, miR-941 and decreased miR-151b expression in circulating exosomes isolated from elderly subjects [98]. The expression of exercise-regulated miRNAs was associated with IGF-1 signaling, which may contribute to exercise-induced hypertrophy [98]. However, it is unclear whether these c-miRNAs were derived from skeletal muscle cells since many of them are also expressed in other tissues. A recent study suggested that c-miRNA are likely difficult to be used as biomarkers of muscle phenotype [88].

Muscle-derived metabolites are also recognized as myokines. Lactate is well known as a typical exercise-induced metabolite secreted from contracting muscle. It is mostly released into the bloodstream from active muscle and is metabolized as a source of energy in other organs, which is referred to as the lactate shuttle [99]. For example, it is produced in fast muscle, which is low in mitochondria, and is used gradually as an energy substrate in mitochondria-rich red and cardiac muscles. It can also cross the cerebral vascular barrier and can be used as a valuable energy source in the brain. It has also been reported to act as a signaling factor and increase mitochondrial levels. In addition, many other metabolites derived from skeletal muscles have been identified by metabolome analysis. Typically, β-aminoisobutyric acid (BAIBA) is a metabolite that is secreted with skeletal muscle metabolism [100]. In addition, skeletal muscle can ameliorate symptoms of depression by metabolizing kynurenine in the bloodstream through PGC1-dependent enzymes [101]. Although the relationship between metabolites and sarcopenia in human beings is unclear, some comprehensive metabolic studies have attempted to examine this association and suggested that certain circulating metabolite profiles, including amino acids, oligopeptides, and their derivatives, were associated with muscle quality and physical fitness [102,103]. Further, a recent cross-sectional study in elderly subjects indicated that plasma proline levels independently showed a positive correlation with sarcopenia [104].

Perspective

The idea that skeletal muscle is a secretory endocrine organ has been established. Currently, more than 30 proteins and peptides, and nucleic acids and metabolites have been identified as secretory factors. Some of them are involved in skeletal muscle atrophy with aging and might have the potential to be developed as biomarkers for sarcopenia (Table 1). However, several factors secreted by muscles are yet to be identified. For example, a bioinformatics study showed that the secretome of human muscle cells includes more than 300 proteins [105]. More than 100 secretory proteins of skeletal muscle were regulated in response to exercise in human beings [106]. Furthermore, many other secretory factors, such as protein-bound molecules and contents within the extracellular vesicles, in circulation that have not been identified yet, still exist as undiscovered myokines. In the future, such unknown myokines need to be identified, which may accelerate the understanding of sarcopenia and aging.

In addition, the old concept of sarcopenia was based on the assessment of skeletal muscle mass alone, whereas the more recent concept encompasses muscle strength and the role of physical activity [107,108]. However, skeletal muscle mass does not necessarily correlate with muscle function. If the coordination of motor neurons and skeletal muscles, i.e., the excitation-contraction coupling, is impaired, it causes muscle weakness. Further study of myokines that affect this function will clarify the relationship between sarcopenia and myokines.

References

[1] Baron AD, Brechtel G, Wallace P, Edelman SV. Rates and tissue sites of non-insulin- and insulin-mediated glucose uptake in humans. Am J Physiol 1998;255:E769–74.

[2] Pedersen BK, Steensberg A, Fischer C, Keller C, Keller P, Plomgaard P, Febbraio M, Saltin B. Searching for the exercise factor: is IL-6 a candidate. J Muscle Res Cell Motil 2003;24:113–9.

[3] Pedersen BK, Febbraio M. Muscle-derived interleukin-6 – a possible link between skeletal muscle, adipose tissue, liver, and brain. Brain Behav Immun 2005;19:371–6.

[4] Pedersen BK. The anti-inflammatory effect of exercise: its role in diabetes and cardiovascular disease control. Essays Biochem 2006;42:105–17.

[5] Petersen EW, Carey AL, Sacchetti M, Steinberg GR, Macaulay SL, Febbraio MA, Pedersen BK. Acute IL-6 treatment increases fatty acid turnover in elderly humans in vivo and in tissue culture in vitro. Am J Physiol 2005;288:E155–62.

[6] Catoire M, Kersten S. The search for exercise factors in humans. FASEB J 2015;29:1615–28.

[7] Polyzos SA, Anastasilakis AD, Efstathiadou ZA, Makras P, Perakakis N, Kountouras J, Mantzoros CS. Irisin in metabolic diseases. Endocrine 2018;59:260–74.

[8] Aoi W, Sakuma K. Skeletal muscle: novel and intriguing characteristics as a secretory organ. BioDiscovery 2013;7:2 [pp. 1–9].

[9] Yarasheski KE, Bhasin S, Sinha-Hikim I, Pak-Loduca J, Gonzalez-Cadavid NF. Serum myostatin-immunoreactive protein is increased in 60–92 year old women and men with muscle wasting. J Nutr Health Aging 2002;6:343–8.

[10] Peng LN, Lee WJ, Liu LK, Lin MH, Chen LK. Healthy community-living older men differ from women in associations between myostatin levels and skeletal muscle mass. J Cachexia Sarcopenia Muscle 2018;9:635–42.

[11] Choi K, Jang HY, Ahn JM, Hwang SH, Chung JW, Choi YS, Kim JW, Jang ES, Choi GH, Jeong SH. The association of the serum levels of myostatin, follistatin, and interleukin-6 with sarcopenia, and their impacts on survival in patients with hepatocellular carcinoma. Clin Mol Hepatol 2020;26(4):492–505.

[12] Bekki M, Hashida R, Kawaguchi T, Goshima N, Yoshiyama T, Otsuka T, Koya S, Hirota K, Matsuse H, Niizeki T, Torimura T, Shiba N. The association between sarcopenia and decorin, an exercise-induced myokine, in patients with liver cirrhosis: a pilot study. J Cachexia Sarcopenia Muscle 2018;1, e00068.

[13] Ratkevicius A, Joyson A, Selmer I, Dhanani T, Grierson C, Tommasi AM, DeVries A, Rauchhaus P, Crowther D, Alesci S, Yaworsky P, Gilbert F, Redpath TW, Brady J, Fearon KC, Reid DM, Greig CA, Wackerhage H. Serum concentrations of myostatin and myostatin-interacting proteins do not differ between young and sarcopenic elderly men. J Gerontol A Biol Sci Med Sci 2011;66:620–6.

[14] Negaresh R, Ranjbar R, Baker JS, Habibi A, Mokhtarzade M, Gharibvand MM, Fokin A. Skeletal muscle hypertrophy, insulin-like growth factor 1, myostatin and follistatin in healthy and sarcopenic elderly men: the effect of whole-body resistance training. Int J Prev Med 2019;10:29.

[15] Bagheri R, Rashidlamir A, Motevalli MS, Elliott BT, Mehrabani J, Wong A. Effects of upper-body, lower-body, or combined resistance training on the ratio of follistatin and myostatin in middle-aged men. Eur J Appl Physiol 2019;119:1921–31.

[16] Bian A, Ma Y, Zhou X, Guo Y, Wang W, Zhang Y, Wang X. Association between sarcopenia and levels of growth hormone and insulin-like growth factor-1 in the elderly. BMC Musculoskelet Disord 2020;21:214.

[17] Kwak JY, Hwang H, Kim SK, Choi JY, Lee SM, Bang H, Kwon ES, Lee KP, Chung SG, Kwon KS. Prediction of sarcopenia using a combination of multiple serum biomarkers. Sci Rep 2018;8:8574.

[18] Park HS, Kim HC, Zhang D, Yeom H, Lim SK. The novel myokine irisin: clinical implications and potential role as a biomarker for sarcopenia in postmenopausal women. Endocrine 2019;64:341–8.

[19] Planella-Farrugia C, Comas F, Sabater-Masdeu M, Moreno M, Moreno-Navarrete JM, Rovira O, Ricart W, Fernández-Real JM. Circulating Irisin and myostatin as markers of muscle strength and physical condition in elderly subjects. Front Physiol 2019;10:871.

[20] Lexell J, Taylor CC, Sjöström M. What is the cause of the ageing atrophy? Total number, size and proportion of different fiber types studied in whole vastus lateralis muscle from 15- to 83-year-old men. J Neurol Sci 1988;84:275–94.

[21] Lee SJ, McPherron AC. Regulation of myostatin activity and muscle growth. Proc Natl Acad Sci U S A 2001;98:9306–11.

[22] Hill JJ, Davies MV, Pearson AA, Wang JH, Hewick RM, Wolfman NM, Qiu Y. The myostatin propeptide and the follistatin-related gene are inhibitory binding proteins of myostatin in normal serum. J Biol Chem 2002;277:40735–41.

[23] Allen DL, Unterman TG. Regulation of myostatin expression and myoblast differentiation by FoxO and SMAD transcription factors. Am J Physiol Cell Physiol 2007;292:C188–99.

[24] Trendelenburg AU, Meyer A, Rohner D, Boyle J, Hatakeyama S, Glass DJ. Myostatin reduces Akt/TORC1/p70S6K signaling, inhibiting myoblast differentiation and myotube size. Am J Physiol Cell Physiol 2009;296:C1258–70.

[25] Amthor H, Nicholas G, McKinnell I, Kemp CF, Sharma M, Kambadur R, Patel K. Follistatin complexes Myostatin and antagonises Myostatin-mediated inhibition of myogenesis. Dev Biol 2004;270:19–30.

[26] Görgens SW, Raschke S, Holven KB, Jensen J, Eckardt K, Eckel J. Regulation of follistatin-like protein 1 expression and secretion in primary human skeletal muscle cells. Arch Physiol Biochem 2013;119:75–80.

[27] Morvan F, Rondeau JM, Zou C, Minetti G, Scheufler C, Scharenberg M, Jacobi C, Brebbia P, Ritter V, Toussaint G, Koelbing C, Leber X, Schilb A, Witte F, Lehmann S, Koch E, Geisse S, Glass DJ, Lach-Trifilieff E. Blockade of activin type II receptors with a dual anti-ActRIIA/IIB antibody is critical to promote maximal skeletal muscle hypertrophy. Proc Natl Acad Sci U S A 2017;114:12448–53.

[28] McPherron AC, Lawler AM, Lee SJ. Regulation of skeletal muscle mass in mice by a new TGF-beta superfamily member. Nature 1997;387:83–90.

[29] Guiraud S, van Wittenberghe L, Georger C, Scherman D, Kichler A. Identification of decorin derived peptides with a zinc dependent anti-myostatin activity. Neuromuscul Disord 2012;22:1057–68.

[30] Kanzleiter T, Rath M, Görgens SW, Jensen J, Tangen DS, Kolnes AJ, Kolnes KJ, Lee S, Eckel J, Schürmann A, Eckardt K. The myokine decorin is regulated by contraction and involved in muscle hypertrophy. Biochem Biophys Res Commun 2014;450:1089–94.

[31] Kim S, Lee MJ, Choi JY, Park DH, Kwak HB, Moon S, Koh JW, Shin HK, Ryu JK, Park CS, Park JH, Kang JH. Roles of exosome-like vesicles released from inflammatory C2C12 myotubes: regulation of myocyte differentiation and myokine expression. Cell Physiol Biochem 2018;48:1829–42.

[32] Broholm C, Pedersen BK. Leukaemia inhibitory factor – an exercise-induced myokine. Exerc Immunol Rev 2010;16:77–85.

[33] Spangenburg EE, Booth FW. Multiple signaling pathways mediate LIF-induced skeletal muscle satellite cell proliferation. Am J Physiol Cell Physiol 2002;283:C204–11.

[34] Broholm C, Laye MJ, Brandt C, Vadalasetty R, Pilegaard H, Pedersen BK, Scheele C. LIF is a contraction-induced myokine stimulating human myocyte proliferation. J Appl Physiol (1985) 2011;111:251–9.

[35] Wang TS, Gao F, Qi QR, Qin FN, Zuo RJ, Li ZL, Liu JL, Yang ZM. Dysregulated LIF-STAT3 pathway is responsible for impaired embryo implantation in a Streptozotocin-induced diabetic mouse model. Biol Open 2015;4:893–902.

[36] Kim H, Wrann CD, Jedrychowski M, Vidoni S, Kitase Y, Nagano K, Zhou C, Chou J, Parkman VA, Novick SJ, Strutzenberg TS, Pascal BD, Le PT, Brooks DJ, Roche AM, Gerber KK, Mattheis L, Chen W, Tu H, Bouxsein ML, Griffin PR, Baron R, Rosen CJ, Bonewald LF, Spiegelman BM. Irisin mediates effects on bone and fat via αv integrin receptors. Cell 2019;178:507–8.

[37] Wang S, Pan J. Irisin ameliorates depressive-like behaviors in rats by regulating energy metabolism. Biochem Biophys Res Commun 2016;474:22–8.

[38] Boström P, Wu J, Jedrychowski MP, Korde A, Ye L, Lo JC, Rasbach KA, Boström EA, Choi JH, Long JZ, Kajimura S, Zingaretti MC, Vind BF, Tu H, Cinti S, Højlund K, Gygi SP, Spiegelman BM. A PGC1-α-dependent myokine that drives brown-fat-like development of white fat and thermogenesis. Nature 2012;481:463–8.

[39] Dozio E, Passeri E, Cardani R, Benedini S, Aresta C, Valaperta R, Corsi Romanelli M, Meola G, Sansone V, Corbetta S. Circulating Irisin is reduced in male patients with type 1 and type 2 myotonic dystrophies. Front Endocrinol 2017;8:320.

[40] Reza MM, Subramaniyam N, Sim CM, Ge X, Sathiakumar D, McFarlane C, Sharma M, Kambadur R. Irisin is a pro-myogenic factor that induces skeletal muscle hypertrophy and rescues denervation-induced atrophy. Nat Commun 2017;8:1104.

[41] Aoi W, Hirano N, Lassiter DG, Björnholm M, Chibalin AV, Sakuma K, Tanimura Y, Mizushima K, Takagi T, Naito Y, Zierath JR, Krook A. Secreted protein acidic and rich in cysteine (SPARC) improves glucose tolerance via AMP-activated protein kinase activation. FASEB J 2019;33:10551–62.

[42] Harries LW, McCulloch LJ, Holley JE, Rawling TJ, Welters HJ, Kos K. A role for SPARC in the moderation of human insulin secretion. PLoS One 2013;8:e68253.

[43] Aoi W, Naito Y, Takagi T, Tanimura Y, Takanami Y, Kawai Y, Sakuma K, Hang LP, Mizushima K, Hirai Y, Koyama R, Wada S, Higashi A, Kokura S, Ichikawa H, Yoshikawa T. A novel myokine, secreted protein acidic and rich in cysteine (SPARC), suppresses colon tumorigenesis via regular exercise. Gut 2013;62:882–9.

[44] Nakamura K, Nakano S, Miyoshi T, Yamanouchi K, Nishihara M. Loss of SPARC in mouse skeletal muscle causes myofiber atrophy. Muscle Nerve 2013;48:791–9.

[45] Matsuo K, Sato K, Suemoto K, Miyamoto-Mikami E, Fuku N, Higashida K, Tsuji K, Xu Y, Liu X, Iemitsu M, Hamaoka T, Tabata I. A mechanism underlying preventive effect of high-intensity training on colon cancer. Med Sci Sports Exerc 2017;49:1805–16.

[46] Nakamura K, Nakano S, Miyoshi T, Yamanouchi K, Matsuwaki T, Nishihara M. Age-related resistance of skeletal muscle-derived progenitor cells to SPARC may explain a shift from myogenesis to adipogenesis. Aging 2012;4:40–8.

[47] Görgens SW, Hjorth M, Eckardt K, Wichert S, Norheim F, Holen T, Lee S, Langleite T, Birkeland KI, Stadheim HK, Kolnes KJ, Tangen DS, Kolnes AJ, Jensen J, Drevon CA, Eckel J. The exercise-regulated myokine chitinase-3-like protein 1 stimulates human myocyte proliferation. Acta Physiol 2016;216:330–45.

[48] Sakamoto K, Furuichi Y, Yamamoto M, Takahashi M, Akimoto Y, Ishikawa T, Shimizu T, Fujimoto M, Takada-Watanabe A, Hayashi A, Mita Y, Manabe Y, Fujii NL, Ishibashi R, Maezawa Y, Betsholtz C, Yokote K, Takemoto M. R3hdml regulates satellite cell proliferation and differentiation. EMBO Rep 2019;20, e47957.

[49] Haugen F, Norheim F, Lian H, Wensaas AJ, Dueland S, Berg O, Funderud A, Skålhegg BS, Raastad T, Drevon CA. IL-7 is expressed and secreted by human skeletal muscle cells. Am J Physiol Cell Physiol 2010;298:C807–16.

[50] Zhang C, Li Y, Wu Y, Wang L, Wang X, Du J. Interleukin-6/signal transducer and activator of transcription 3 (STAT3) pathway is essential for macrophage infiltration and myoblast proliferation during muscle regeneration. J Biol Chem 2013;288:1489–99.

[51] Nylén C, Aoi W, Abdelmoez AM, Lassiter DG, Lundell LS, Wallberg-Henriksson H, Näslund E, Pillon NJ, Krook A. IL6 and LIF mRNA expression in skeletal muscle is regulated by AMPK and the transcription factors NFYC, ZBTB14, and SP1. Am J Physiol Endocrinol Metab 2018;315:E995–E1004.

[52] Li CW, Yu K, Shyh-Chang N, Li GX, Jiang LJ, Yu SL, Xu LY, Liu RJ, Guo ZJ, Xie HY, Li RR, Ying J, Li K, Li DJ. Circulating factors associated with sarcopenia during ageing and after intensive lifestyle intervention. J Cachexia Sarcopenia Muscle 2019;10:586–600.

[53] Adams GR. Autocrine/paracrine IGF-I and skeletal muscle adaptation. J Appl Physiol 2002;93:1159–67.

[54] Tahimic CG, Wang Y, Bikle DD. Anabolic effects of IGF-1 signaling on the skeleton. Front Endocrinol 2013;4:6.

[55] Musarò A, McCullagh K, Paul A, Houghton L, Dobtowolny G, Molinaro M, Barton ER, Sweeney HL, Rosenthal N. Localized Igf-1 transgene expression sustains hypertrophy and regeneration in senescent skeletal muscle. Nat Genet 2001;27:195–200.

[56] Barton ER, Morris L, Musarò A, Rosenthal N, Sweeney HL. Muscle-specific expression of insulin-like growth factor I counters muscle decline in mdx mice. J Cell Biol 2002;157:137–48.

[57] Bodine SC, Stitt TN, Gonzalez M, Kline WO, Stover GL, Bauerlein R, Zlotchenko E, Scrimgeour A, Lawrence JC, Glass DJ, Yancopoulos GD. Akt/mTOR pathway is a crucial regulator of skeletal muscle hypertrophy and can prevent muscle atrophy in vivo. Nat Cell Biol 2001;3:1014–9.

[58] Barton-Davis ER, Shoturma DI, Musaro A, Rosenthal N, Sweeney HL. Viral mediated expression of insulin-like growth factor I blocks the aging-related loss of skeletal muscle function. Proc Natl Acad Sci U S A 1998;95:15603–7.

[59] Li M, Li C, Parkhouse WS. Age-related differences in the des IGF-I-mediated activation of Akt-1 and p70 S6K in mouse skeletal muscle. Mech Ageing Dev 2003;124:771–8.

[60] Lokireddy S, Mouly V, Butler-Browne G, Gluckman PD, Sharma M, Kambadur R, McFarlane C. Myostatin promotes the wasting of human myoblast cultures through promoting ubiquitin-proteasome pathway-mediated loss of sarcomeric proteins. Am J Physiol Cell Physiol 2011;301:C1316–24.

[61] Morissette MR, Cook SA, Buranasombati C, Rosenberg MA, Rosenzweig A. Myostatin inhibits IGF-I-induced myotube hypertrophy through Akt. Am J Physiol Cell Physiol 2009;297:C1124–32.

[62] McFarlane C, Plummer E, Thomas M, Hennebry A, Ashby M, Ling N, Smith H, Sharma M, Kambadur R. Myostatin induces cachexia by activating the ubiquitin proteolytic system through an NF-kappaB-independent, FoxO1-dependent mechanism. J Cell Physiol 2006;209:501–14.

[63] Negaresh R, Ranjbar R, Baker JS, Habibi A, Mokhtarzade M, Gharibvand MM, Fokin A. Skeletal muscle hypertrophy, insulin-like growth factor 1, myostatin and follistatin in healthy and sarcopenic elderly men: the effect of whole-body resistance training. Int J Prev Med 2019;10:29.

[64] Kalista S, Schakman O, Gilson H, Lause P, Demeulder B, Bertrand L, Pende M, Thissen JP. The type 1 insulin-like growth factor receptor (IGF-IR) pathway is mandatory for the follistatin-induced skeletal muscle hypertrophy. Endocrinology 2012;153:241–53.

[65] Barbé C, Kalista S, Loumaye A, Ritvos O, Lause P, Ferracin B, Thissen JP. Role of IGF-I in follistatin-induced skeletal muscle hypertrophy. Am J Physiol Endocrinol Metab 2015;309:E557–67.

[66] Kong X, Yao T, Zhou P, Kazak L, Tenen D, Lyubetskaya A, Dawes BA, Tsai L, Kahn BB, Spiegelman BM, Liu T, Rosen ED. Brown adipose tissue controls skeletal muscle function via the secretion of myostatin. Cell Metab 2018;28:631–43. e3.

[67] Chang JS, Kong ID. Irisin prevents dexamethasone-induced atrophy in C2C12 myotubes. Pflugers Arch 2020;472:495–502.

[68] Reza MM, Subramaniyam N, Sim CM, Ge X, Sathiakumar D, McFarlane C, Sharma M, Kambadur R. Irisin is a pro-myogenic factor that induces skeletal muscle hypertrophy and rescues denervation-induced atrophy. Nat Commun 2017;8:1104.

[69] Guridi M, Tintignac LA, Lin S, Kupr B, Castets P, Rüegg MA. Activation of mTORC1 in skeletal muscle regulates whole-body metabolism through FGF21. Sci Signal 2015;8, ra113.

[70] Izumiya Y, Bina HA, Ouchi N, Akasaki Y, Kharitonenkov A, Walsh K. FGF21 is an Akt-regulated myokine. FEBS Lett 2008;582:3805–10.

[71] Adhikary S, Choudhary D, Tripathi AK, Karvande A, Ahmad N, Kothari P, Trivedi R. FGF-2 targets sclerostin in bone and myostatin in skeletal muscle to mitigate the deleterious effects of glucocorticoid on musculoskeletal degradation. Life Sci 2019;229:261–76.

[72] Gao S, Durstine JL, Koh HJ, Carver WE, Frizzell N, Carson JA. Acute myotube protein synthesis regulation by IL-6-related cytokines. Am J Physiol Cell Physiol 2017;313:C487–500.

[73] Yang X, Brobst D, Chan WS, Tse MCL, Herlea-Pana O, Ahuja P, Bi X, Zaw AM, Kwong ZSW, Jia WH, Zhang ZG, Zhang N, Chow SKH, Cheung WH, Louie JCY, Griffin TM, Nong W, Hui JHL, Du GH, Noh HL, Saengnipanthkul S, Chow BKC, Kim JK, Lee CW, Chan CB. Muscle-generated BDNF is a sexually dimorphic myokine that controls metabolic flexibility. Sci Signal 2019;12, eaau1468.

[74] Oost LJ, Kustermann M, Armani A, Blaauw B, Romanello V. Fibroblast growth factor 21 controls mitophagy and muscle mass. J Cachexia Sarcopenia Muscle 2019;10:630–42.

[75] Manfredi LH, Ang J, Peker N, Dagda RK, McFarlane C. G protein-coupled receptor kinase 2 regulates mitochondrial bioenergetics and impairs myostatin-mediated autophagy in muscle cells. Am J Physiol Cell Physiol 2019;317:C674–86.

[76] Mitchell PS, Parkin RK, Kroh EM, Fritz BR, Wyman SK, Pogosova-Agadjanyan EL, Peterson A, Noteboom J, O'Briant KC, Allen A, Lin DW, Urban N, Drescher CW, Knudsen BS, Stirewalt DL, Gentleman R, Vessella RL, Nelson PS, Martin DB, Tewari M. Circulating microRNAs as stable blood-based markers for cancer detection. Proc Natl Acad Sci U S A 2008;105:10513–8.

[77] Raposo G, Stoorvogel W. Extracellular vesicles: exosomes, microvesicles, and friends. J Cell Biol 2013;200:373–83.

[78] Vickers KC, Palmisano BT, Shoucri BM, Shamburek RD, Remaley AT. MicroRNAs are transported in plasma and delivered to recipient cells by high-density lipoproteins. Nat Cell Biol 2011;13:423–33.

[79] Aoi W. Frontier impact of microRNAs in skeletal muscle research: a future perspective. Front Physiol 2015;5:495.

[80] Mizuno H, Nakamura A, Aoki Y, Ito N, Kishi S, Yamamoto K, Sekiguchi M, Takeda S, Hashido K. Identification of muscle-specific microRNAs in serum of muscular dystrophy animal models: promising novel blood-based markers for muscular dystrophy. PLoS One 2011;6, e18388.

[81] Cacchiarelli D, Legnini I, Martone J, Cazzella V, D'Amico A, Bertini E, Bozzoni I. miRNAs as serum biomarkers for Duchenne muscular dystrophy. EMBO Mol Med 2011;3:258–65.

[82] Hu J, Kong M, Ye Y, Hong S, Cheng L, Jiang L. Serum miR-206 and other muscle-specific microRNAs as non-invasive biomarkers for Duchenne muscular dystrophy. J Neurochem 2014;129:877–83.

[83] Vignier N, Amor F, Fogel P, Duvallet A, Poupiot J, Charrier S, Arock M, Montus M, Nelson I, Richard I, Carrier L, Servais L, Voit T, Bonne G, Israeli D. Distinctive serum miRNA profile in mouse models of striated muscular pathologies. PLoS One 2013;8, e55281.

[84] Donaldson A, Natanek SA, Lewis A, Man WD, Hopkinson NS, Polkey MI, Kemp PR. Increased skeletal muscle-specific microRNA in the blood of patients with COPD. Thorax 2013;68:1140–9.

[85] Hudson MB, Woodworth-Hobbs ME, Zheng B, Rahnert JA, Blount MA, Gooch JL, Searles CD, Price SR. miR-23a is decreased during muscle atrophy by a mechanism that includes calcineurin signaling and exosome-mediated export. Am J Physiol Cell Physiol 2014;306:C551–8.

[86] Baggish AL, Hale A, Weiner RB, Lewis GD, Systrom D, Wang F, Wang TJ, Chan SY. Dynamic regulation of circulating microRNA during acute exhaustive exercise and sustained aerobic exercise training. J Physiol 2011;589:3983–94.

[87] Nielsen S, Åkerström T, Rinnov A, Yfanti C, Scheele C, Pedersen BK, Laye MJ. The miRNA plasma signature in response to acute aerobic exercise and endurance training. PLoS One 2014;9, e87308.

[88] D'Souza RF, Zeng N, Poppitt SD, Cameron-Smith D, Mitchell CJ. Circulatory microRNAs are not effective biomarkers of muscle size and function in middle-aged men. Am J Physiol Cell Physiol 2019;316:C293–8.

[89] Aoi W, Ichikawa H, Mune K, Tanimura Y, Mizushima K, Naito Y, Yoshikawa T. Muscle-enriched microRNA miR-486 decreases in circulation in response to exercise in young men. Front Physiol 2013;4:80.

[90] Baggish AL, Park J, Min PK, Isaacs S, Parker BA, Thompson PD, Troyanos C, D'Hemecourt P, Dyer S, Thiel M, Hale A, Chan SY. Rapid upregulation and clearance of distinct circulating microRNAs after prolonged aerobic exercise. J Appl Physiol (1985) 2014;116:522–31.

[91] Gomes CP, Oliveira-Jr GP, Madrid B, Almeida JA, Franco OL, Pereira RW. Circulating miR-1, miR-133a, and miR-206 levels are increased after a half-marathon run. Biomarkers 2014;19:585–9.

[92] Borja-Gonzalez M, Casas-Martinez JC, McDonagh B, Goljanek-Whysall K. Inflamma-miR-21 negatively regulates myogenesis during ageing. Antioxidants 2020;9:345.

[93] Fulzele S, Mendhe B, Khayrullin A, Johnson M, Kaiser H, Liu Y, Isales CM, Hamrick MW. Muscle-derived miR-34a increases with age in circulating extracellular vesicles and induces senescence of bone marrow stem cells. Aging 2019;11:1791–803.

[94] Jung HJ, Lee KP, Milholland B, Shin YJ, Kang JS, Kwon KS, Suh Y. Comprehensive miRNA profiling of skeletal muscle and serum in induced and normal mouse muscle atrophy during aging. J Gerontol A Biol Sci Med Sci 2017;72:1483–91.

[95] Margolis LM, Lessard SJ, Ezzyat Y, Fielding RA, Rivas DA. Circulating microRNA are predictive of aging and acute adaptive response to resistance exercise in men. J Gerontol A Biol Sci Med Sci 2017;72:1319–26.

[96] Xu J, Li R, Workeneh B, Dong Y, Wang X, Hu Z. Transcription factor FoxO1, the dominant mediator of muscle wasting in chronic kidney disease, is inhibited by microRNA-486. Kidney Int 2012;82:401–11.

[97] Hitachi K, Nakatani M, Tsuchida K. Myostatin signaling regulates Akt activity via the regulation of miR-486 expression. Int J Biochem Cell Biol 2014;47:93–103.

[98] Nair VD, Ge Y, Li S, Pincas H, Jain N, Seenarine N, Amper MAS, Goodpaster BH, Walsh MJ, Coen PM, Sealfon SC. Sedentary and trained older men have distinct circulating exosomal microRNA profiles at baseline and in response to acute exercise. Front Physiol 2020;11:605.

[99] Brooks GA. Lactate: glycolytic end product and oxidative substrate during sustained exercise in mammals—the "lactate shuttle". In: Gilles R, editor. Circulation, Respiration, and Metabolism. Proceedings in Life Sciences. Berlin: Springer; 1985. p. 208–18.

[100] Roberts LD, Boström P, O'Sullivan JF, Schinzel RT, Lewis GD, Dejam A, Lee YK, Palma MJ, Calhoun S, Georgiadi A, Chen MH, Ramachandran VS, Larson MG, Bouchard C, Rankinen T, Souza AL, Clish CB, Wang TJ, Estall JL, Soukas AA, Cowan CA, Spiegelman BM, Gerszten RE. β-Aminoisobutyric acid induces browning of white fat and hepatic β-oxidation and is inversely correlated with cardiometabolic risk factors. Cell Metab 2014;19:96–108.

[101] Agudelo LZ, Femenía T, Orhan F, Porsmyr-Palmertz M, Goiny M, Martinez-Redondo V, Correia JC, Izadi M, Bhat M, Schuppe-Koistinen I, Pettersson AT, Ferreira DMS, Krook A, Barres R, Zierath JR, Erhardt S, Lindskog M, Ruas JL. Skeletal muscle PGC-1α1 modulates kynurenine metabolism and mediates resilience to stress-induced depression. Cell 2014;159:33–45.

[102] Moaddel R, Fabbri E, Khadeer MA, Carlson OD, Gonzalez-Freire M, Zhang P, Semba RD, Ferrucci L. Plasma biomarkers of poor muscle quality in older men and women from the Baltimore longitudinal study of aging. J Gerontol A Biol Sci Med Sci 2016;71:1266–72.

[103] Saoi M, Li A, McGlory C, Stokes T, von Allmen MT, Phillips SM, Britz-McKibbin P. Metabolic perturbations from step reduction in older persons at risk for sarcopenia: plasma biomarkers of abrupt changes in physical activity. Metabolites 2019;9:134.

[104] Toyoshima K, Nakamura M, Adachi Y, Imaizumi A, Hakamada T, Abe Y, Kaneko E, Takahashi S, Shimokado K. Increased plasma proline concentrations are associated with sarcopenia in the elderly. PLoS One 2017;12, e0185206.

[105] Bortoluzzi S, Scannapieco P, Cestaro A, Danieli GA, Schiaffino S. Computational reconstruction of the human skeletal muscle secretome. Proteins 2006;62:776–92.

[106] Pourteymour S, Eckardt K, Holen T, Langleite T, Lee S, Jensen J, Birkeland KI, Drevon CA, Hjorth M. Global mRNA sequencing of human skeletal muscle: search for novel exercise-regulated myokines. Mol Metab 2017;6:352–65.

[107] Cruz-Jentoft AJ, Bahat G, Bauer J, Boirie Y, Bruyère O, Cederholm T, Cooper C, Landi F, Rolland Y, Sayer AA, Schneider SM, Sieber CC, Topinkova E, Vandewoude M, Visser M, Zamboni M. Writing group for the european working group on sarcopenia in older people 2 (EWGSOP2), and the Extended Group for EWGSOP2. Sarcopenia: revised European consensus on definition and diagnosis. Age Ageing 2019;48:16–31.

[108] Chen LK, Woo J, Assantachai P, Auyeung TW, Chou MY, Iijima K, Jang HC, Kang L, Kim M, Kim S, Kojima T, Kuzuya M, Lee JSW, Lee SY, Lee WJ, Lee Y, Liang CK, Lim JY, Lim WS, Peng LN, Sugimoto K, Tanaka T, Won CW, Yamada M, Zhang T, Akishita M, Arai H. Asian working group for sarcopenia: 2019 consensus update on sarcopenia diagnosis and treatment. J Am Med Dir Assoc 2020;2:300–7. e2.

CHAPTER 8

Defect of autophagy signaling in sarcopenic muscle

Kunihiro Sakuma[a], Akihiko Yamaguchi[b], and Haruyo Matsuo[c]

[a]Institute for Liberal Arts, Environment and Society, Tokyo Institute of Technology, Tokyo, Japan,
[b]Department of Physical Therapy, Health Sciences University of Hokkaido, Ishikari-Tobetsu, Hokkaido, Japan, [c]Department of Nursing, Kagoshima Medical Association Hospital, Kagoshima, Japan

Abstract

Skeletal muscle provides a fundamental basis for human function, enabling locomotion and respiration. Autophagy occurs in all eukaryotic cells and is evolutionarily conserved from yeast to human beings. The autophagy machinery is a critical pathway for cell homeostasis, but it has been insufficiently studied in skeletal muscle. Particular emphasis has been given on the role played by autophagic defects in disease pathogenesis, its involvement in atrophy, and the possible effects of exercise as a countermeasure. Recent studies indicated that the age-related defects of autophagy signaling in normal skeletal muscle, whereas denervation, unloading, and cachexia, frequently involved with aging, modulate the autophagy-dependent system. The autophagic defect in sarcopenia may be influenced by new candidates [glycogen synthase kinase (GSK)-3a, mitofusin 2, and Rubicon]. Endurance training and calorie restriction have positive effects on sarcopenia and several forms of muscle wasting by activating the autophagy system. This review describes recent research advances regarding autophagy-dependent signaling in sarcopenia.

Keywords: Sarcopenia, Aging, Autophagy, Skeletal muscle, Muscle fiber, Protein degradation

Introduction

In human beings, skeletal muscle is the most abundant tissue in the body, comprising 40%–50% of the body mass and playing vital roles in locomotion, heat production during periods of cold stress, and overall metabolism. The fact that skeletal muscle consists of the largest pool of proteins in the whole organism highlights why this specific tissue is highly sensitive to conditions that alter the balance between protein synthesis and degradation. Loss of muscle is a serious consequence of many chronic diseases and of aging itself because it leads to weakness, loss of independence, and an increased risk of death.

Previous studies using animal models demonstrated that muscle atrophy caused by various catabolic stimuli leads to similar activation of protein degradation by both the ubiquitin-proteasome system (UPS) and autophagy. Most muscle proteins, particularly myofibrillar components, are considered to be degraded by UPS. Two muscle-specific ubiquitin ligases, muscle RING finger-1 (MuRF-1) and atrophy gene-1 (atrogin-1), are markedly induced in a wide range of in vivo models of skeletal muscle atrophy, including diabetes, cancer, denervation, unweighting, and glucocorticoid treatment [1,2]. The importance of these atrophy-regulated genes in muscle wasting was confirmed through studies in knockout mice, attenuating denervation-, fasting-, and dexamethasone-induced muscle atrophy [3–5]. Interestingly, recent findings indicate that atrogin-1-knockout mice are short-lived and experience a greater loss of muscle mass during aging than control mice [6], indicating that chronic inhibition of these atrogenes should not be considered a therapeutic target to counteract sarcopenia [7,8].

Autophagy occurs in all eukaryotic cells and is evolutionarily conserved from yeast to human beings [9]. Turnover of the most long-lived proteins, macromolecules, biological membranes, and whole organelles, including mitochondria, ribosomes, the endoplasmic reticulum, and peroxisomes, is mediated by autophagy [10]. Three major mechanisms of autophagy have been described: microautophagy, in which lysosomes directly take up cytosol, inclusion bodies, and organelles for degradation; chaperone-mediated autophagy, in which soluble proteins with a particular pentapeptide motif are recognized and transported across the lysosomal membrane for degradation; macroautophagy (herein autophagy), a ubiquitous catabolic process that involves the bulk degradation of cytoplasmic components by interacting lysosomes [11,12]. This process is characterized by the engulfment of part of the cytoplasm inside double-membrane vesicles (autophagosomes). Autophagosomes subsequently fuse with lysosomes to form autophagolysosomes, in which the cytoplasmic cargo is degraded.

The autophagy machinery, a critical pathway for cell homeostasis that had been insufficiently studied in skeletal muscle, has been intensively studied in the past few years. Particular emphasis has been placed on the role played by autophagic defects in disease pathogenesis, its involvement in atrophy, and the possible effects of exercise as a countermeasure [13–15]. Indeed, the sarcopenic muscle of human beings and rodents exhibits a marked autophagic defect [16,17], leading to the inability to degrade the accumulated denatured proteins, abnormal mitochondria, and sarcoplasmic reticulum. This review aims to outline the defect of the autophagy-dependent system for sarcopenia with normal aging, with modulating factors (denervation, unloading, and cachexia frequently included in aging). In addition, we described a recent strategy for attenuating sarcopenia by autophagic activation [exercise and calorie restriction (CR)].

Autophagy-dependent signaling

Autophagy represents a refined collection of altered organelles, abnormal protein aggregates, and pathogens, similar to a selective recycling center [18] (Fig. 1). The selectivity of the autophagy process is conferred by a growing number of specific cargo receptors such as p62/SQSTM1, Nbr1, and Nix [B-cell lymphoma 2 (BCL2)/adenovirus E1B 19 kd-interacting protein (BNIP) 3L] [19]. These adaptor proteins are equipped with a cargo-binding domain,

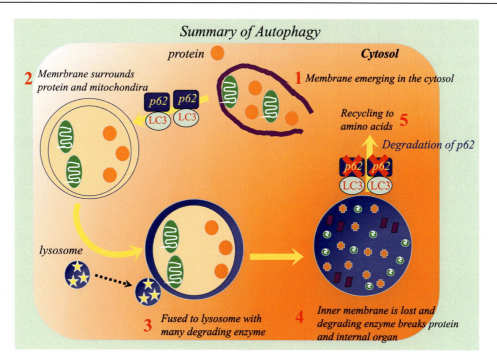

Fig. 1
Summary of autophagy. A flat vesicle called an isolate membrane appears in the cytoplasm. Subsequently, the membrane extends and surrounds denaturing proteins and unfunctional internal organelles (mitochondria) while taking in the cytoplasm (1). Its edges fusing to compose an autophagosome with the support of LC3 and p62 protein (2). The autophagosome fuses with a lysosome with many degrading enzymes (3), and then the inner membrane is lost, and degrading enzymes break inner contents (4). The amino acids gained through autodigestion are reused as nutrient sources (5). At this time, the degradation of p62 occurs.

with the ability to recognize and attach directly to molecular tags on organelles. At the same time, these adaptor proteins bind to essential autophagosome membrane proteins. Three molecular complexes mainly regulate the formation of autophagosomes: the microtubule-associated protein light chain 3 (LC3) conjugation system and the regulatory complexes governed by unc51-like kinase-1 (ULK1) and Beclin-1. The conjugation complex is composed of different proteins encoded by autophagy-related genes (Atg) [20]. The Atg12-Atg5-Atg16L1 complex, along with Atg7, plays an essential role in the conjugation of LC3 to phosphatidylethanolamine, which is required for the elongation and closure of the isolation membrane [20]. Finally, the fusion of the autophagosome with the lysosome is regulated by proteins that are largely shared with the endocytic pathway. They include the class III PI3K vacuolar protein sorting 34 (VPS34) complex II, in which Beclin-1, VPS34, and VPS154 are present, while UVRAG replaces ATG14 [21,22], which acts in cooperation with the small GTPase protein RAB7 [23], the RAB7 effector PLEKHM1, the SNARE protein syntaxin17, and the homotypic fusion and vacuole protein sorting complex (HOPS). Both autophagosome and endosome fusions with the lysosomes are negatively regulated by Rubicon, which binds to the VPS34 complex II in a mechanistic target of rapamycin (mTOR)C1-dependent manner and interferes with the activity of RAB7 and HOPS [24].

This system is under the regulation of at least two major cellular energy-sensing complexes. The ULK complex is composed of protein kinases ULK1 and ULK2, in association with the FIP200 scaffold protein and regulatory subunits ATG13 and ATG101, which are considered to activate ULK proteins by inducing conformational changes [25]. Under basal conditions, the ULK1 complex is inactivated by phosphorylation through mTORC1, whereas during autophagy induction, mTORC1 is inhibited, thus enhancing the formation of a ULK-associated complex. In addition, mTORC1 can also be negatively regulated independently of Akt by energy stress sensors such as AMP (adenosine monophosphate)-activated protein kinase (AMPK) and, in a mechanical-activity-dependent manner, through tuberous sclerosis complex 1/2. Moreover, AMPK can also directly phosphorylate ULK1 and Beclin-1 [26]. During autophagy, the ULK1 complex is localized to the isolation membrane, where it facilitates the formation of autophagosomes through interaction with the Beclin-1 complex.

Autophagic adaptation in sarcopenic muscle
Autophagic defect

Sarcopenia, the age-related loss of skeletal muscle mass, is characterized by a deterioration of muscle quantity and quality leading to a gradual slowing of movement, a decline in strength and power, increased risk of fall-related injury, and frailty [27]. von Haehling et al. [28] estimated its prevalence at 5%–13% for elderly people aged 60–70 years and 11%–50% for those aged 80 years or older. Lean muscle mass generally contributes up to ~ 50% of the total body weight in young adults, but declines with aging to 25% at 75–80 years [29].

A decline in autophagy during normal aging has been described for invertebrates and higher organisms [30]. Inefficient autophagy has been attributed a major role in the age-related accumulation of damaged cellular components, such as undegradable lysosome-bound lipofuscin, protein aggregates, and damaged mitochondria [30]. Demontis and Perrimon [31] showed that the function of the autophagy/lysosome system of protein degradation declined during aging in the skeletal muscle of *Drosophila*. This resulted in the progressive accumulation of polyubiquitin protein aggregates in senescent *Drosophila* muscle. Intriguingly, the overexpresssion of forkhead box O increases the expression of many autophagy genes, preserves the function of the autophagy pathway, and prevents the accumulation of polyubiquitin protein aggregates in the muscle of sarcopenic *Drosophila* [32]. Several investigators reported the autophagic changes in aged mammalian skeletal muscle [17,33–36]. Compared with those in young male Fischer 344 rats, amounts of Beclin-1 were significantly increased in the plantaris muscles of senescent rats [36]. Using

Western blot of fractionated homogenates and immunofluorescence microscopy, we recently demonstrated the selective induction of p62/SQSTM1 and Beclin-1 but not LC3 in the cytosol of sarcopenic muscle fibers in mice [17]. In addition, we observed significantly smaller p62/SQSTM1-positive muscle fibers in aged muscle compared with the surrounding p62/SQSTM1-negative fibers [17] (Fig. 2). In contrast, aging did not influence the amounts of Atg7 and Atg9 proteins in plantaris muscle of rat [36]. Western blot analysis by Wohlgemuth et al. [36] clearly showed a marked increase in the amount of LC3 in muscle during aging. However, they could not demonstrate an aging-related increase in the ratio of LC3-II to LC3-I, a better biochemical marker to assess ongoing autophagy. In addition, we failed to detect a marked increase in LC3-I and LC3-II (active form) proteins in aged quadriceps muscle [17]. In contrast, Wenz et al. [35] reported a significant increase in the ratio of LC3-II to LC3-I during aging (3 vs. 22 months) in the biceps femoris muscle of wild-type mice. None of the studies determining the transcript level of autophagy-linked molecules identified

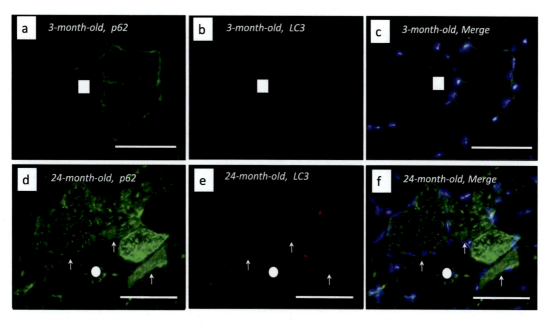

Fig. 2
Serial cryosections of the quadriceps muscle of 3- and 24-month-old mice: p62/SQSTM1 and LC3 immunoreactivity. In young quadriceps muscle, immunofluorescence labeling showed that p62/SQSTM1 was present in the membrane and at a low level in the cytosol of several muscle fibers (A). Marked increases in p62/SQSTM1 immunoreactivity were observed in the membrane and the cytosol of aged muscle fibers (D). No apparent difference in LC3 immunoreactivity was observed in the muscle between 3- and 24-month-old mice (B and E). White arrows denote the muscle fibers possessing p62/SQSTM1. Bar = 50 μm. *Data from Sakuma K, Kinoshita M, Ito Y, Aizawa M, Aoi W, Yamaguchi A. p62/SQSTM1 but not LC3 is accumulated in sarcopenic muscle of mice. J Cachexia Sarcopenia Muscle 2016;7:204–12.*

a significant increase with age [17,33,36]. Not all contributors to autophagy signaling seem to change similarly at both mRNA and protein levels in senescent skeletal muscle. Therefore, sarcopenia may include a partial defect of autophagy signaling, although a more exhaustive investigation is needed in this field. Intriguingly, a more recent study [16] using biopsy samples of young and aged human volunteers clearly showed age-dependent autophagic defects such as a decrease in the amount of Atg7 protein and the ratio of LC3-II/LC3-I protein.

Aged satellite cells are inherently more susceptible to apoptosis following cellular stress, demonstrating a shift from autophagy to apoptosis with aging [37]. Autophagy has been shown as critical for activation and proliferation by acting as a temporary energy source to fuel the initiation of proliferation [38]. A marked decline in the expression of several autophagic genes occurs in quiescent muscle satellite cells with aging [39]. The loss of autophagy results in a decline in both the number and function of satellite cells as well as muscle activity, which can be restored by autophagy re-establishment [39]. In addition, the authors, using constitutive and conditional Atg7$^{flox/flox}$ directly targeting muscle satellite cells, showed that genetic impairment of macroautophagy in young muscle satellite cells promotes entry into premature senescence by the loss of proteostasis, increased mitochondrial dysfunction, and oxidative stress [39]. Intriguingly, a reduction in autophagy and proliferation in skeletal muscle stem cells with aging was recently observed along with increased apoptosis and senescence probably due to inactivation of the AMPK/p27kip1 pathway [40]. In contrast, genetic or pharmacological activation of AMPK (AICAR) or p27kip1 signaling was effective to induce autophagy and returning the myogenic potential of aged muscle stem cells. In addition, these treatments significantly block the induction of senescence markers (p16INK4a and p21CIP1) of aged muscle stem cells [40]. Thus, autophagy may be the most prevalent pathway in muscle quiescent satellite cells.

Possible molecules modulating autophagic defect

Life-long CR alone, or combined with voluntary exercise, resulted in the mild reduction of LC3 expression and lipidation, suggesting a potential increase in autophagy flux. No significant age-related increase in autophagy-linked molecules was observed in MCK-PGC-1α (peroxisome proliferator-activated receptor γ coactivator 1α) mice [35]. PGC-1α may also enhance autophagic flux. GSK-3α was proposed as a critical regulator of aging in various organs (skeletal muscle, heart, liver, bone, etc.) via modulating mTORC1 and autophagy [41]. Intriguingly, mice with a null mutation of GSK-3α showed premature death and acceleration of age-related pathologies such as vacuolar degeneration, large tubular aggregates, sarcomere disruption, and marked sarcopenia in cardiac and skeletal muscles [41]. These GSK-3α knockout mice exhibited marked activation of mTORC1 and associated suppression of several autophagy molecules. Indeed, unrestrained activation of mTORC1 leads to marked inhibition of autophagy [42]. Therefore, it is considered that pharmacological inhibition (everolimus) of mTORC1 rescued the muscular disorder resembling sarcopenia in GSK-3α knockout mice [41]. More recently, mitofusin 2 (Mfn2) was identified as a new candidate to explain sarcopenia and impaired autophagy [43]. Mfn2 has been reported to be involved in the regulation of cell proliferation, oxidative metabolism, autophagy, mitophagy, and the unfolded protein response [44–46]. Sebastián et al. [47] demonstrated that Mfn2 deficiency in young mice resulted in marked selective atrophy of type IIB fibers and the accumulation of autophagosomes and mitophagosomes. This Mfn2-deficient young muscle exhibited significant increases in the ratio of LC3-II/I protein, p62, and BNIP3 protein accumulation very similar to those of aged muscle. Since a progressive reduction in Mfn2 occurs in mouse skeletal muscle [47], it is possible that autophagic and mitochondrial defects are regulated by Mfn2.

Rubicon negatively regulates autophagosome-lysosome fusion steps. Rubicon was originally identified as a Beclin 1-binding protein that inhibits autophagy and endocytosis [48,49]. Nakamura et al. [50] characterized the role of Rubicon in different species (aged worm, fly, and mouse) and found that its expression increased with age. Similar to the worm and fly, they [50] found that the Rubicon transcript and protein levels in kidneys and liver were higher in older mice (20 months of age) than in juvenile ones (2 months). The increase in Rubicon levels may curtail lifespan in worms and female flies and causally contributes to several age-onset phenotypes (polyQ aggregation, fibrosis, and α-synuclein accumulation) [50]. Intriguingly, Rubicon knockdown in neuronal cells extended lifespan most efficiently by activating autophagy. Rubicon systemic-knockout mice exhibit higher levels of LC3-II and reduced levels of the autophagic substrate p62. Importantly, the increase in longevity (percent survival) was completely abolished when the autophagy regulators bec-1/Beclin1, unc-51/ULK1, and atg-18/ATG18 were knocked down by RNA-I along with rub-1 [50]. Thus, the increased longevity in worms conferred by knock-down of rub-1 is dependent on autophagic activity (Beclin-1 dependent signaling). Although the functional role of Rubicon and the partner of Beclin-1 in muscle fibers should be further elucidated, the molecule's interaction may play a crucial role in the autophagic defect in sarcopenia. Fig. 3 shows a hypothesis of the functional role of Rubicon in sarcopenic muscle fibers.

Factors modulating autophagic defect in sarcopenia
Denervation

Since aged skeletal muscle exhibits the partially denervated features in neuromuscular junction (NMJ) disorganization, it is plausible that denervation affects sarcopenic symptoms. Denervation of skeletal muscle is a very popular model of atrophy because of the loss of neuromuscular activity and neurotrophic factors. Denervation induced a marked increase in

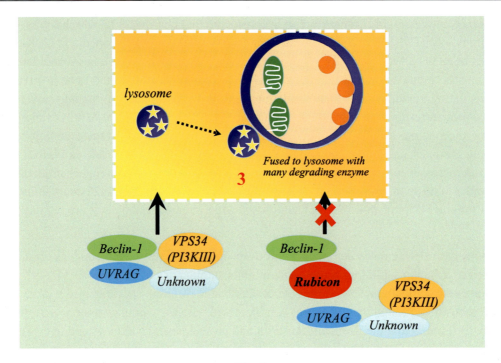

Fig. 3
The hypothesis of the functional role of Rubicon in sarcopenic muscle fibers. The autophagosome fuses with a lysosome with many degrading enzymes (Fig. 1 step 3). This response seems to be modulated by the interaction between Beclin-1 and the other Beclin-1 co-operators (VPS34, UVRAG, etc.). In contrast, the docking between Beclin-1 and Rubicon would disturb such a Beclin-1-linked co-operation and inhibit the fusion between autophagosome and lysosome, ultimately leading to an autophagic defect in sarcopenic muscle fibers.

all autophagic markers such as LC3-II, p62/SQSTM1, Beclin-1, Atg7, and ULK1 proteins [51]. The amounts of LC3-II and p62 in the mitochondria also increase, probably due to the activation of mitophagy. In contrast, Quy et al. [52] indicated that denervated muscle during the short-term (24 and 48h) exhibited autophagic suppression through the proteasome-dependent activation of mTORC1. Autophagic activating patterns may be different in early (1–2 days) and late (14 days) phases in the denervated muscle. Even though sarcopenia includes partial denervation due to the NMJ disorder, we can observe an apparent defect in autophagy-dependent signaling in aged skeletal muscle. Thus, the adaptive manner of changes in autophagic molecules after complete denervation may markedly differ from those of partial denervation occurring in sarcopenia.

Marked upregulation of the autophagy system during denervation is modulated by various upstream mediators. Denervation for 7 days upregulated the AMPKα phosphorylation status in several fast-twitch (TA, gastrocnemius) muscles and the slow-twitch soleus muscle of

C57BL/6J mice [53]. In addition, AMPKα2 deficiency led to a significant reduction in the increased ratio of LC3-II/I protein and accumulation of ubiquitin in muscle after denervation [53]. In addition to these findings, Guo et al. [53] reported that AMPKα2 is an upstream modulator of autophagy in denervated muscle. TRIM63 (MuRF-1) may also modulate the autophagic process of skeletal muscle by denervation. In 2014, Khan et al. [54] demonstrated that TRIM63, an E3 ubiquitin ligase, plays an important role in the turnover of the pentameric transmembrane protein, CHRN (cholinergic receptor, nicotinic), which is a major postsynaptic ion channel of the NMJ. In addition, most SH3GLB1 (SH3-domain GRB2-like endophilin B1) and CHRN-positive puncta were precisely overlaid with TRIM63 and accompanied by LC3 [54]. Denervation led to a marked increase of SH3GLB1 and CHRN double-positive puncta, which was almost completely blocked in TRIM63 knockout mice. TRIM63 knockout mice exhibited no significant muscle atrophy after denervation. Therefore, TRIM63 plays a crucial role in the atrophy-induced endocytic retrieval of CHRN and its subsequent autophagic processing by cooperation with SH3GLB1, LC3, and p62/SQSTM1.

Such an upstream modulator may differ between slow-twitch and fast-twitch muscle fibers. Mitochondria have been postulated to play an important role in triggering signals that contribute to muscle atrophy. PARK-2 participates in mitochondrial quality control by mitophagy. In normal mice, the denervation of slow-twitch muscle activated mitophagy by the accumulation of PARK-2 and then activated the UPS system through the translocation of nuclear factor erythroid 2-related factor 1 (NFE2L1) from the cytosol to nucleus. In contrast, PARK-2-deficient mice exhibited an atrophic delay of the soleus muscle through the inactivation of UPS by the inability to carry out nuclear translocation of NFE2L1. Autophagy deficiency in denervated soleus muscle delayed skeletal muscle atrophy, reduced mitochondrial activity, and induced oxidative stress and the accumulation of PARK2/Parkin [55].

Unloading

Since elderly individuals may frequently experience hindlimb immobilization due to osteoporosis or injury, it is plausible that unloading also affects autophagy signaling in the sarcopenic muscle. Several studies investigated the changes in autophagy-linked molecules in unloaded mammalian muscle. Recently, Smith et al. [56] demonstrated that hindlimb unweighting led to a marked increase in mRNA expressions of LC3B, Gabarapl1, and Atg4b mRNA in the quadriceps femoris muscle of mice (16–18 weeks of age) in earlier (2 days after the operation) but not later (7 days after this). Using six-month-old male mice, hindlimb unweighting for 3 but not 7 days induced the significant up-regulation of p62 mRNA in the soleus muscle, despite there being no change in Beclin-1 mRNA in both periods. Intriguingly, Cannavino et al. [57] demonstrated that a significant induction of p62 mRNA in unloaded muscle is prevented by PGC-1α overexpression but not Trolox (antioxidant treatment). Thus, the decrease in PGC-1α expression recognized in the unloaded muscle would be attributable to the increase in p62 expression. In contrast, Dupré-Aucouturier et al. [58] showed no significant change in mRNA levels of Gabarapl1, LC3B, or ULK1 in the rat soleus muscle after 2 weeks of hindlimb suspension. Although some researchers reported the mRNA induction of autophagy-related molecules after hindlimb unweighting, many researchers demonstrated no significant changes in protein levels of autophagy-linked molecules. For example, the Western blot analysis by Baehr et al. [59] demonstrated that the levels of p62, Beclin-1, and Atg7 proteins did not significantly change in the unloaded (2 weeks) soleus and tibialis anterior muscles of male F344BN rats (9 months). In addition, hindlimb unloading led to no significant change in the amount of Beclin-1 protein [60] or LC3 [61]. In contrast, some researchers reported the elevations of p62 [61] and LC3-II/I [58] at protein levels. Since the adaptive changes in autophagy-related molecules have been elucidated only in the muscle of rodents, the manner of adaptation should be investigated using human muscle samples from an unloading model. At present, it is unknown how unloading influences the defect of autophagy-dependent signaling during sarcopenia.

Cachexia

Cachexia is a complex metabolic syndrome characterized by a severe and involuntary loss of muscle mass. Cachexia is associated not only with chronic diseases, most commonly cancer, but also with other inflammatory conditions such as chronic obstructive pulmonary disease (COPD), heart failure, chronic kidney disease, AIDS, and sepsis. The overall prevalence of cachexia is approximately 1% of the global patient population, which increases to 50%–80% in patients with cancer [62]. Since patients with sarcopenia frequently show a cachexic state [63,64], we should understand the modulation of autophagy-dependent signaling by cachexia. A few general observations suggested that autophagy can be activated in the muscle of animals bearing Lewis lung carcinoma or colon 26 tumor [65]. Using three different models of cancer cachexia (colon 26, Yoshida AH-130, and Lewis lung carcinoma), Penna et al. [66] observed marked increases in the levels of Beclin-1, p62, and LC3-II (the lipidated form; a reliable marker of autophagosome formation) in the gastrocnemius muscle. OP den Kamp et al. [67] indicated that the levels of both LC3-I and -II proteins, but not LC3B mRNA, were significantly increased in the vastus lateralis muscle of patients with lung cancer cachexia. Patients with esophageal cancer also exhibit higher LC3-II/I ratios and levels of cathepsin B and L expression in muscle [68]. Since they did not detect a significant change of proteasome, calpain, or caspase 3 activity in the muscle of these patients, they consider that the autophagic-lysosomal pathway is the main proteolytic system in muscle in the presence of esophageal cancer cachexia.

The functional importance of autophagy in the pathogenesis of lung disease in COPD patients has been demonstrated [44,69]. Using lung biopsy samples, Chen et al. [44] indicated that LC3B, Beclin-1, Atg7, and Atg5 were all upregulated, and autophagosome formation was visualized using electron microscopy. In contrast, using muscle biopsy samples obtained from severe COPD patients with marked atrophy (forced expiratory volume in 1 s value of 35 ± 2% of predicted), Plant et al. [70] failed to detect significant differences in Beclin-1 and LC3 mRNA expression in the quadriceps muscle between COPD patients and control individuals. Unfortunately, they assessed the degree of muscle autophagy in COPD patients by measuring only the mRNA levels. Guo et al. [71] performed a pilot experiment and revealed significant increases in the intensity of various autophagy-linked proteins such as LC3-II in the muscle of severe COPD patients compared with that in control subjects. Although more complete elucidation of the autophagic state in the muscle of COPD patients remains to be determined, muscle in the presence of cachexia and COPD may exhibit an autophagy-activated condition. Therefore, when sarcopenia with autophagic defects leads to various cachexic symptoms, it is difficult for us to grasp the exact state (activation or inactivation?) of autophagy-dependent signaling in skeletal muscle.

Several therapeutic strategies attenuating sarcopenia due to autophagic-activation
Exercise

Various hormonal, supplemental, and pharmacological approaches may attenuate muscle atrophy by activating autophagy. This section deals with the attenuating strategy for sarcopenia by autophagic activation. The most common approach is resistance and endurance exercise. Energetic sensors, such as AMPK, sirtuin (SIRT)1, and p38-mitogen-activated protein kinase, are activated by muscle contraction. These modulators of autophagy-dependent signaling are important for acutely maintaining cellular energy homeostasis, as well as for efficient organelle and protein turnover following exercise [72]. A recent systematic review of the international sarcopenia initiative (EWGSOP and IWGS) [73] indicated that exercise interventions improve muscle strength and physical performance in sarcopenic patients. Nine weeks of resistance training prevented the loss of muscle mass and improved muscle strength in 18–20-month-old rats, accompanied by a reduced LC3-II/LC3-I ratio, reduced p62/SQSTM1 protein levels, and increased levels of autophagy regulatory proteins (Beclin-1, Atg5/12, and Atg7) [74]. In addition, endurance exercise (training) activates autophagic flux, possibly by preventing binding between BCL2 and Beclin-1 [75], although recent findings demonstrated that exercise-induced autophagy does not have an impact on physical performance, the activation of a metabolic sensor (PRKAA1), or glucose homeostasis [76]. Furthermore, Pagano et al. [77] observed that the autophagy initiator ULK1 was rapidly phosphorylated on AMPK phosphorylation residues (Ser-317 and Ser-555) in oxidative muscles during progressive endurance exercise. In contrast, mice subjected to shorter moderate to high-intensity treadmill exercise showed a general decline or no change in several autophagy-linked molecules (LC3-II, p62, and Beclin-1) [78,79].

Indeed, He et al. [75] reported that mice with BCL2 knock-in mutations, displaying intact basal autophagy but defective stress-induced autophagy, showed decreased phosphorylation and activation of AMPK and its downstream target acetyl-CoA carboxylase, probably due to the disruption of the BCL2-Beclin-1 complex. Although it is not clear whether acute exercise modulates the expression of autophagic markers, exercise (muscle contraction) activates autophagy-dependent signaling. It is reasonable that both exercises prevent sarcopenia by inhibiting autophagic defects and the denaturing and unfolding of proteins accumulation of nonfunctional mitochondria and other internal organelles. Indeed, life-long exercise (regular exercise over past 30 tears) was found to attenuate age-dependent autophagic dysfunction (a marked decrease in LC3-II and Atg7 proteins) in elderly sportsmen when compared with age-matched healthy sedentary individuals [16]. Interestingly, endurance training ameliorated several diseases with similar autophagic defects, such as in spontaneously hypersensitive rats and mutant mice with the valosin-containing protein (R155H/+) model [80] and Collagen VI [81].

Calorie restriction

CR (typically 20%–40% fewer calories) activates autophagic flux, preserves mitochondrial health, and attenuates sarcopenia in mice, rats, and rhesus monkeys [36,82,83]. CR is recognized as the most robust intervention to retard both primary aging (natural age-related deterioration) and secondary aging (accelerated aging due to disease and negative lifestyle behaviors), thereby increasing the lifespan of many species. Yang et al. [84] recently indicated that long-term CR for humans (3–15 years) also elicits the upregulation of several autophagic markers (LC3 and Beclin-1) as well as that of a molecular chaperone (heat shock protein 70). Interestingly, the effect of CR in human beings and monkeys against type II diabetes, cardiovascular disease, and sarcopenia is significant but less marked compared with that in rodents [85,86]. Recently, an attractive hypothesis was proposed suggesting that CR animals are more active than ad libitum fed animals. A recent study indicated a burst of physical activity (voluntary exercise) in CR mice just before the start of eating despite there being no significant increase in total daily activity [87]. The group hypothesized that the positive effects of CR on muscle maintenance in rodents are not merely a direct consequence of a lower energy intake, but also related to a more active behavior in a specific time frame. In contrast, a low protein diet despite ad libitum feeding also attenuates muscular atrophy of Duchenne muscular dystrophy model mice [88] and in those with type 2 diabetic nephropathy. In addition, a low protein diet containing keto acids also inhibits muscle atrophy of nephrectomized rats (one of the chronic kidney disease models) [89]. Patients with chronic kidney disease also frequently show sarcopenic symptoms. Therefore, a low protein diet despite ad libitum feeding may attenuate not only muscular atrophy but also sarcopenia, probably due to autophagic activation. More recently, CR mimetics emerged as potent compounds to activate the protective pathways of CR by promoting autophagy via a reduction in protein acetylation [90]. CR mimetics are anticipated to become part of the pharmacological armamentarium against aging and age-related cardiovascular, neurodegenerative, and malignant diseases, although the possible role of CR mimetics in attenuating sarcopenia remains to be elucidated.

Supplemental approach

Whether a supplemental approach (protein, amino acids, etc.) alleviates sarcopenia has been tested in many studies. It is widely accepted that the combination of resistance training and supplementation with amino acids has a promising role to attenuate sarcopenia [91,92]. However, supplementation of amino acids or leucine without exercise frequently failed to prevent sarcopenia [73,91], probably due to inhibiting autophagy. More recently, it was found that supplementation with dihydromyricetin, the main flavonoid component of *Ampelopsis grossedettata* (10, 50, and 100 mg/kg body weight), decreases the amount of p62/SQSTM1 proteins and increases the amount of Atg5 and Beclin-1 proteins and the ratio of LC3-II/LC3-I protein in male Sprague-Dawley rats [93]. In addition, dihydromyricetin supplementation induced the upregulation of autophagy-signaling inducers (p-AMPK/AMPK and p-ULK1/ULK1), and the downregulation of autophagy-signaling inhibitors (p-mTOR/mTOR) in both normal and autophagy-defective muscle of mice fed a high-fat diet (8 weeks). Furthermore, researchers point out the possibility of sarcopenia being attenuated by the flavanol-rich lychee extract oligonol, consisting of catechins, procyanidins, and other phenolic compounds. Supplementation with oligonol (8 weeks) of SAMP8 mice led to the elevated expression of PINK1 protein and mitochondrial biogenesis (PGC-1α and Tfam) and fusion (Mfn2 and Opa1) genes, inhibited expression of Atg13, LC3-II, p62 proteins, and decreased accumulation of autophagosomes and lysosomes in skeletal muscle [94]. Since SAMP8 mice exhibit typical features of accelerated muscle aging with a short lifespan, the authors consider that the possibility of oligonol attenuates sarcopenia. However, oligonol supplementation also inhibited the nuclear localization of NF-κB and decreased transcription of Atrogin-1 and MuRF-1 (ubiquitin-proteasome signaling), as well as autophagy-linked molecules. It should be further elucidated descriptively whether the modulation of autophagy (mitophagy)-dependent signaling following oligonol supplementation contributes to the enlargement of the muscle fiber size. Treatment with beta-hydroxy-beta-methyl butyrate (HMB) alleviates muscle atrophy caused by dexamethasone in Sprague-Dawley rats. Giron et al. [95] reported that supplementation with HMB (320 mg/kg in water) increased the grip strength and weight of the soleus and gastrocnemius muscles. Using the L6 myotube in vitro, they indirectly examined possible mechanisms of HMB in muscle fibers, demonstrating the marked autophagic inhibition of LC3-II induction and p62/SQSTM1 decrease after treatment with dexamethasone. Therefore, HMB supplementation may be a possible approach to attenuate sarcopenia [96], irrespective of the presence of an autophagic defect. In contrast, supplementation with alanine and citrulline (0.81 g/kg/d) for 14 days in mice cannot inhibit muscle atrophy under limb immobilization despite the marked increase of serum arginine in both cases and possible autophagic activation in the former [97].

Hormonal treatment

Several hormonal treatments, such as testosterone, growth hormone, and insulin-like growth factor-I, have been attempted to attenuate sarcopenia in rodents and human beings for 20 years. However, many negative and some positive findings have been obtained [91,92]. More recently, some hormonal supplementations attenuated sarcopenia by autophagic activation. In normal adult male mice, the intraperitoneal injection of T3 (20 μg/100 g BW) induced the marked activation of autophagy regarding both protein (an increase in LC3B and a decrease in p62/SQSTM1) and mRNA (LC3, p62/SQSTM1, Beclin-1, Atg5) expressions [98]. In addition, treatment with T3 further elicited the autophagy-upstream regulators, such as downregulation of the ratio of p-mTOR/mTOR and upregulation of the ratio of pAMPK/AMP and pULK1Ser555 in skeletal muscle of normal mice. Circulating thyroid hormone levels decreases with normal aging in human beings [99] and rodents [100], and treatment with T3 may attenuate sarcopenia by marked autophagic activation.

Concluding remarks

Particular emphasis has been given on the role played by autophagic defects in disease pathogenesis, including sarcopenia [16,17]. Intriguingly, the disorganization of the autophagy system may accelerate sarcopenic symptoms in rodents and human beings because of the absence of disposal of denaturing proteins and dysfunctional mitochondria, no new formation of NMJ, and/or no elegant conversion of muscle stem cells. The autophagic defects in sarcopenia may be influenced by new intriguing candidates (GSK-3α, mitofusin 2, and Rubicon). Endurance training and CR are potent countermeasures against sarcopenia that involve activating autophagy in muscle fibers.

Acknowledgments

This work was supported by a research Grant-in-Aid for Scientific Research C (No. 17K01755) from the Ministry of Education, Science, Culture, Sports, Science and Technology of Japan.

References

[1] Bodine SC, Latres E, Baumhueter S, Lai VK, Nunez L, Clarke BA, Poueymirou WT, Panaro FJ, Na E, Dharmarajan K, Pan ZQ, Valenzuela DM, DeChiara TM, Stitt TN, Yancopoulos GD, Glass DJ. Identification of ubiquitin ligases required for skeletal muscle atrophy. Science 2001;294:1704–8.

[2] Lecker SH, Jagoe RT, Gilbert A, Gomes M, Baracos V, Bailey J, Price SR, Mitch WE, Goldberg AL. Multiple types of skeletal muscle atrophy involve a common program of changes in gene expression. FASEB J 2004;18:39–51.

[3] Baehr LM, Furlow JD, Bodine SC. Muscle sparing in muscle RING finger 1 null mice: response to synthetic glucocorticoids. J Physiol 2011;589:4759–76.
[4] Cong H, Sun L, Liu C, Tien P. Inhibition of atrogin-1/MAFbx expression by adenovirus-delivered small hairpin RNAs attenuates muscle atrophy in fasting mice. Hum Gene Ther 2011;22:313–24.
[5] Drummond MJ, Dreyer HC, Pennings B, Fry C, Dhanani S, Dillon EL, Sheffield-Moore M, Volpi E, Rasmussen BB. Skeletal muscle protein anabolic response to resistance exercise and essential amino acids is delayed with aging. J Appl Physiol 2008;104:1452–61.
[6] Sandri M, Barberi L, Bijlsma AY, Blaauw B, Dyar KA, Milan G, Mammucari C, Meskers CG, Pallafacchina G, Paoli A, Pion D, Roceri M, Romanello V, Serrano AL, Toniolo L, Larsson L, Maier AB, Muñoz-Cánoves P, Musarò A, Pende M, Reggiani C, Rizzuto R, Schiaffino S. Signaling pathways regulating muscle mass in ageing skeletal muscle. The role of IGF-1-Akt-mTOR-FoxO pathway. Biogerontology 2013;14:303–23.
[7] Sakuma K, Aoi W, Yamaguchi A. Current understanding of sarcopenia: possible candidates modulating muscle mass. Pflugers Arch 2015;467:213–29.
[8] Sakuma K, Aizawa M, Aoi W, Yamaguchi A. Molecular mechanism of sarcopenia and cachexia: recent research advances. Pflugers Arch 2017;469:573–91.
[9] Levine B, Klionsky DJ. Development of self-digestion: molecular mechanisms and biological functions of autophagy. Dev Cell 2004;6:463–77.
[10] Cuervo AM. Autophagy: many paths to the same end. Mol Med 2004;9:65–76.
[11] Neel BA, Lin Y, Pessin JE. Skeletal muscle autophagy: a new metabolic regulator. Trends Endocrinol Metab 2013;24:635–43.
[12] Sandri M. New findings of lysosomal proteolysis in skeletal muscle. Curr Opin Clin Nutr Metab Care 2011;14:223–9.
[13] Ferraro E, Giammarioli AM, Chiandotto S, Spoletini I, Rosano G. Exercise-induced skeletal muscle remodeling and metabolic adaptation: redox signaling and role of autophagy. Antioxid Redox Signal 2014;21:154–76.
[14] Sanchez AM, Bernardi H, Py G, Candau RB. Autophagy is essential to support skeletal muscle plasticity in response to endurance exercise. Am J Physiol Regul Integr Comp Physiol 2014;307:R956–69.
[15] Vainshtein A, Grumati P, Sandri M, Bonaldo P. Skeletal muscle, autophagy, and physical activity: the ménage à trois of metabolic regulation in health and disease. J Mol Med 2014;92:127–37.
[16] Carnio S, LoVerso F, Baraibar MA, Longa E, Khan MM, Maffei M, Reischl M, Canepari M, Loefler S, Kern H, Blaauw B, Friguet B, Bottinelli R, Rudolf R, Sandri M. Autophagy impairment in muscle induces neuromuscular junction degeneration and precocious aging. Cell Rep 2014;8:1509–21.
[17] Sakuma K, Kinoshita M, Ito Y, Aizawa M, Aoi W, Yamaguchi A. p62/SQSTM1 but not LC3 is accumulated in sarcopenic muscle of mice. J Cachexia Sarcopenia Muscle 2016;7:204–12.
[18] Park C, Cuervo AM. Selective autophagy: talking with the UPS. Cell Biochem Biophys 2013;67:3–13.
[19] Shaid S, Brandts CH, Serve H, Dikic I. Ubiquitination and selective autophagy. Cell Death Differ 2013;20:21–30.
[20] Mizushima N, Komatsu M. Autophagy: renovation of cells and tissues. Cell 2011;147:728–41.
[21] Lamb CA, Yoshimori T, Tooze SA. The autophagosome: origins, unknown, biogenesis complex. Nat Rev Mol Cell Biol 2013;14:759–74.
[22] Levine B, Liu R, Dong X, Zhong Q. Beclin orthologs: interactive hubs of cell signaling, membrane trafficking, and physiology. Trends Cell Biol 2015;25:533–44.
[23] Amaya C, Fader CM, Colombo MI. Autophagy and proteins involved in vesicular trafficking. FEBS Lett 2015;589:3343–53.
[24] Kim YM, Jung CH, Seo M, Kim EK, Park JM, Bae SS, Kim DH. mTORC1 phosphorylates UVRAG to negatively regulate autophagosome and endosome maturation. Mol Cell 2015;57:207–18.
[25] Lin MG, Hurley JH. Structure and function of the ULK1 complex in autophagy. Curr Opin Cell Biol 2016;39:61–8.
[26] Kim J, Kim YC, Fang C, Russell RC, Kim JH, Fan W, Liu R, Zhong Q, Guan KL. Differential regulation of distinct Vps34 complexes by AMPK in nutrient stress and autophagy. Cell 2013;152:290–303.

[27] Melton 3rd LJ, Khosla S, Crowson CS, O'Connor MK, O'Fallon WM, Riggs BL. Epidemiology of sarcopenia. J Am Geriat Soc 2000;48:625–30.
[28] von Haehling S, Morley JE, Anker SD. An overview of sarcopenia: facts and numbers on prevalence and clinical impact. J Cachexia Sarcopenia Muscle 2010;1:129–33.
[29] Short KR, Vittone JL, Bigelow ML, Proctor DN, Coenen-Schimke JM, Rys P, Nair KS. Age, and aerobic exercise training effects on whole body and muscle protein metabolism. Am J Physiol Endocrinol Metab 2004;286:E92–E101.
[30] Cuervo AM, Bergamini E, Brunk UT, Dröge W, Ffrench M, Terman A. Autophagy and aging: the importance of maintaining "clean" cells. Autophagy 2005;1:131–40.
[31] Demontis F, Perrimon N. FOXO/4E-BP signaling in Drosophila muscles regulates organism-wide proteostasis during aging. Cell 2010;143:813–25.
[32] Demontis F, Perrimon N. Integration of insulin receptor/Foxo signaling and dMyc activity during muscle growth regulates body size in *Drosophila*. Development 2009;136:983–93.
[33] Gaugler M, Brown A, Merrell E, DiSanto-Rose M, Rathmacher JA, Reynolds 4th TH. PKB signaling and atrogene expression in skeletal muscle of aged mice. J Appl Physiol 2011;111:192–9.
[34] McMullen CA, Ferry AL, Gamboa JL, Andrade FH, Dupont-Versteegden EE. Age-related changes of cell death pathways in rat extraocular muscle. Exp Gerontol 2009;44:420–5.
[35] Wenz T, Rossi SG, Rotundo RL, Spiegelman BM, Moraes CT. Increased muscle PGC-1alpha expression protects from sarcopenia and metabolic disease during aging. Proc Natl Acad Sci U S A 2009;106:20405–10.
[36] Wohlgemuth SE, Seo AY, Marzetti E, Lees HA, Leeuwenburgh C. Skeletal muscle autophagy and apoptosis during aging: effects of calorie restriction and life-long exercise. Exp Gerontol 2010;45:138–48.
[37] Jejurikar SS, Henkelman EA, Cederna PS, Marcelo CL, Urbanchek MG, Kuzon Jr WM. Aging increases the susceptibility of skeletal muscle derived satellite cdells to apoptosis. Exp Gerontol 2006;41:828–36.
[38] Tang AH, Rando TA. Induction of autophagy supports the bioenergetic demands of quiescent muscle stem cell activation. EMBO J 2014;33:2782–97.
[39] Garcia-Prat L, Martinez-Vicente M, Perdiguero E, Ortet L, Rodriguez-Ubreva J, Rebollo E, Ruiz-Bonilla V, Gutarra S, Ballestar E, Serrano AL, Sandri M, Muñoz-Cánoves. Autophagy maninains stemness by preventing senescence. Nature 2016;529:37–42.
[40] White JP, Billin AN, Campbell ME, Russell AJ, Huffman KM, Kraus WE. The AMPK/p27kip1 axis regulates autophagy/apoptosis decisions in aged skeletal muscle stem cells. Stem Cell Rep 2018;11:425–39.
[41] Zhou J, Freeman TA, Ahmad F, Shang X, Mangano E, Gao E, Farber J, Wang Y, Ma XL, Woodgett J, Vagnozzi RJ, Lal H, Force T. GSK-3α is a central regulator of age-related pathologies in mice. J Clin Invest 2013;123:1821–32.
[42] Kroemer G, Marino G, Levine B. Autophagy and the integrated stress response. Mol Cell 2010;40:280–93.
[43] Sebastián D, Zorzano A. When MFN2 (mitofusin 2) met autophagy: a new age for old muscles. Autophagy 2016;12:2250–1.
[44] Chen ZH, Kim HP, Sciurba FC, Lee SJ, Feghali-Bostwick C, Stolz DB, Dhir R, Landreneau RJ, Schuchert MJ, Yousem SA, Nakahira K, Pilewski JM, Lee JS, Zhang Y, Ryter SW, Choi AM. Egr-1 regulates autophagy in cigarette smoke-induced chronic obstructive pulmonary disease. PLoS One 2008;3, e3316.
[45] Hailey DW, Rambold AS, Saptute-Krishnan P, Mitra K, Sougrat R, Kim PK, Lippincott-Schwartz J. Mitochondria supply membranes for autophagosome biogenesis during starvation. Cell 2010;141:656–67.
[46] Munoz JP, Ivanova S, Sanchez-Wandelmer J, Martinez-Cristobal P, Noguera E, Sancho A, Diaz-Ramos A, Hernandez-Alvarez MI, Sebastian D, Mauvezin C, Palacin M, Zorzano A. Mfn2 modulates the UPR and mitochondrial function via repression of PERK. EMBO J 2013;32:2348–61.
[47] Sebastián D, Sorianello E, Segalés J, Irazoki A, Ruiz-Bonilla V, Sala D, Planet E, Berenguer-Llergo A, Muñoz JP, Sánchez-Feutrie M, Plana N, Hernández-Álvarez MI, Serrano AL, Palacín M, Zorzano A. Mfn2 deficiency links age-related sarcopenia and impaired autophagy to activation of an adaptive mitophagy pathway. EMBO J 2016;35:1677–93.

[48] Matsunaga K, Saitoh T, Tabata K, Omori H, Satoh T, Kurotori N, Maejima I, Shirahama-Noda K, Ichimura T, Isobe T, Akira S, Noda T, Yoshimori T. Two Beclin 1-binding proteins, Atg14L and Rubicon, reciprocally regulate autophagy at different stages. Nat Cell Biol 2009;11:385–96.

[49] Zhong Y, Wang QJ, Li X, Yan Y, Backer JM, Chait BT, Heintz N, Yue Z. Distinct regulation of autophagic activity by Atg14L and Rubicon associated with Beclin 1-phosphatidylinositol-3-kinase complex. Nat Cell Biol 2009;11:468–76.

[50] Nakamura S, Oba M, Suzuki M, Takahashi A, Yamamuro T, Fujiwara M, Ikenaka K, Minami S, Tabata N, Yamamoto K, Kubo S, Tokumura A, Akamatsu K, Miyazaki Y, Kawabata T, Hamasaki M, Fukui K, Sango K, Watanabe Y, Kitajima TS, Okada Y, Mochizuki H, Isaka Y, Antebi A, Yoshimori T. Suppression of autophagic activity by Rubicon is a signature of aging. Nat Commun 2019;10:847.

[51] O'Leary MF, Vainshtein A, Iqbal S, Ostojic O, Hood DA. Adaptive plasticity of autophagic proteins to denervation in aging skeletal muscle. Am J Physiol Cell Physiol 2013;304:C422–30.

[52] Quy PN, Kuma A, Pierre P, Mizushima N. Proteasome-dependent activation of mammalian target of rapamycin complex 1 (mTORC1) is essential for autophagy suppression and muscle remodeling following denervation. J Biol Chem 2013;288:1125–34.

[53] Guo Y, Jin M, Tang Y, Wang T, Wei B, Feng R, Gong B, Wang H, Ji G, Lu Z. AMP-activated kinase α2 deficiency protects mice fro denervation-induced skeletal muscle atrophy. Arch Biochem Biophys 2016;600:56–60.

[54] Khan MM, Strack S, Wild F, Hanashima A, Gasch A, Brohm K, Reischl M, Carnio S, Labeit D, Sandri M, Labeit S, Rudolf R. Role of autophagy, SQSTM1, SH3GLB1, and TRIM63 in the turnover of nicotinic acetylcholine receptors. Autophagy 2014;10:123–36.

[55] Furuya N, Ikeda S, Sato S, Soma S, Ezaki J, Oliva Trejo JA, Takeda-Ezaki M, Fujimura T, Arikawa-Hirasawa E, Tada N, Komatsu M, Tanaka K, Kominami E, Hattori N, Ueno T. PARK2/Parkin -mediated mitochondrial clearance contributes to proteasome activation during slow-twitch muscle atrophy via NFE2L1 nuclear translocation. Autophagy 2014;10:631–41.

[56] Smith HK, Matthews KG, Oldham JM, Jeanplong F, Falconer SJ, Bass JJ, Senna-Salerno M, Bracegirdle JW, McMahon CD. Translational signaling, atrogenic and myogenic gene expression during unloading and reloading of skeletal muscle in myostatin-deficient mice. PLoS One 2014;9, e94356.

[57] Cannavino J, Brocca L, Sandri M, Bottinelli R, Pellegrino MA. PGC1-α over-expression prevents metabolic alterations and soleus muscle atrophy in hindlimb unloaded mice. J Physiol 2014;592(20):4575–89.

[58] Dupré-Aucouturier S, Castells J, Freyssenet D, Desplanches D. Trichostatin A, a histone deacetylase inhibitor, modulates unloaded-induced skeletal muscle atrophy. J Appl Physiol 2015;119:342–51.

[59] Baehr LM, West DW, Marcotte G, Marshall AG, De Sousa LG, Baar K, Bodine SC. Age-related deficits in skeletal muscle recovery following disuse are associated with neuromuscular junction instability and ER stress, not impaired protein synthesis. Aging 2016;8:127–46.

[60] Andrianjafiniony T, Dupré-Aucouturier S, Letexier D, Couchoux H, Desplanches D. Oxidative stress, apoptosis, and proteolysis in skeletal muscle repair after unloading. Am J Physiol Cell Physiol 2010;299:C307–15.

[61] Liu J, Peng Y, Cui Z, Wu Z, Qian A, Shang P, Qu L, Li Y, Liu J, Long J. Depressed mitochondrial biogenesis and dynamic remodeling in mouse tibialis anterior and gastrocnemius induced by 4-week hindlimb unloading. IUBMB Life 2013;64:901–10.

[62] Argilés JM, Busquets S, Stemmler B, López-Soriano FJ. Cancer cachexia: understanding the molecular basis. Nat Rev Cancer 2014;14:754–62.

[63] Yang M, Shen Y, Tan L, Li W. Prognostic value of sarcopenia in lung cancer: a systematic review and meta-analysis. Chest 2019;156:101–11.

[64] Yin J, Lu X, Qian Z, Xu W, Zhou X. New insights into the pathogenesis and treatment of sarcopenia in chronic heart failure. Theranostics 2019;9:4019–29.

[65] Asp ML, Tian M, Wendel AA, Belury MA. Evidence for the contribution of insulin resistance to the development of cachexia in tumor-bearing mice. Int J Cancer 2010;126:756–63.

[66] Penna F, Costamagna D, Pin F, Camperi A, Fanzani A, Chiarpotto EM, Cavallini G, Bonelli G, Baccino FM, Costelli P. Autophagic degradation contributes to muscle wasting in cancer cachexia. Am J Pathol 2013;182:1367–78.

[67] Op den Kamp C, Langen RC, Snepvangers FJ, de Theije CC, Schellekens JM, Laugs F, Dingemans AM, Schols AM. Nuclear transcription factor κB activation and protein turnover adaptations in skeletal muscle of patients with progressive stages of lung cancer cachexia. Am J Clin Nutr 2013;98:738–48.

[68] Tardif N, Klaude M, Lundell L, Thorell A, Rooyackers O. Autophagic-lysosomal pathway is the main proteolytic system modified in the skeletal muscle of esophageal cancer patients. Am J Clin Nutr 2013;98:1485–92.

[69] Ryter SW, Chen Z-H, Kim HP, Choi AM. Autophagy in chronic obstructive pulmonary disease. Autophagy 2009;5:235–7.

[70] Plant PJ, Brooks D, Faughnan M, Bayley T, Bain J, Singer L, Correa J, Pearce D, Binnie M, Batt J. Cellular markers of muscle atrophy in chronic pulmonary disease. Am J Respir Cell Mol Biol 2010;42:461–71.

[71] Guo Y, Gosker HR, Schols AM, Kapchinsky S, Bourbeau J, Sandri M, Jagoe RT, Debigaré R, Maltais F, Taivassalo T, Hussain SN. Autophagy in locomoter muscles of patients with chronic obstructive pulmonary disease. Am J Respir Crit Care Med 2013;188:1313–20.

[72] Liang J, Zeng Z, Zhang Y, Chen N. Regulatory role of exercise-induced autophagy for sarcopenia. Exp Gerontol 2020;130:110789 [in press].

[73] Cruz-Jentoft AJ, Landi F, Schneider SM, Zúñiga C, Arai H, Boirie Y, Chen LK, Fielding RA, Martin FC, Michel JP, Sieber C, Stout JR, Studenski SA, Vellas B, Woo J, Zamboni M, Cederholm T. Prevalence of and interventions for sarcopenia in ageing adults: a systematic review. Report of the International Sarcopenia Initiative (EQGSOP and IWGS). Age Aging 2014;43:748–59.

[74] Luo L, Lu AM, Wang Y, Hong A, Chen Y, Hu J, Li, and X., Qin, Z. H. Chronic resistance training activates autophagy and reduces apoptosis of muscle cells by modulating IGF-1 and its receptors, Akt/mTOR and Akt/FOXO3a signaling in aged rats. Exp Gerontol 2013;48:427–36.

[75] He C, Bassik MC, Moresi V, Sun K, Wei Y, Zou Z, An Z, Loh J, Fisher J, Sun Q, Korsmeyer S, Packer M, May HI, Hill JA, Virgin HW, Gilpin C, Xiao G, Bassel-Duby R, Scherer PE, Levine B. Exercise-induced BCL2-regulated autophagy is required for muscle glucose homeostasis. Nature 2012;481:511–5.

[76] Lo Verso F, Carnio S, Vainshtein A, Sandri M. Autophagy is not required to sustain exercise and PRKAA1/AMPK activity but is important to prevent mitochondrial damage during physical activity. Autophagy 2014;10:1883–94.

[77] Pagano AF, Py G, Bernadri H, Candau RB, Sanchez AM. Autophagy and protein turnover signaling in slow-twitch muscle during exercise. Med Sci Sports Exerc 2014;46:1314–25.

[78] Kim YA, Kim YS, Song W. Autophagic response to a single bout of moderate exercise in murine skeletal muscle. J Physiol Biochem 2012;68:229–35.

[79] Saleem A, Carter HN, Hood DA. p53 is necessary for the adaptive changes in cellular milieu subsequent to an acute bout of endurance exercise. Am J Physiol Cell Physiol 2014;306:C241–9.

[80] Nalbandian A, Nguyen C, Katheria V, Llewellyn KJ, Badadani M, Caiozzo V, Kimonis VE. Exercise training reverses skeletal muscle atrophy in an experimental model of VCP disease. PLoS One 2013;8, e76187.

[81] Grumati P, Coletto L, Sabatelli P, Cescon M, Angelin A, Bertaggia E, Blaauw B, Urciuolo A, Tiepolo T, Merlini L, Maraldi NM, Bernardi P, Sandri M, Bonaldo P. Autophagy is defective in collagen VI muscular dystrophies, and its reactivation rescues myofiber degeneration. Nat Med 2010;16:1313–20.

[82] McKiernan SH, Colman RJ, Lopez M, Beasley TM, Aiken JM, Anderson RM, Weindruch R. Caloric restriction delays aging-induced cellular phenotypes in rhesus monkey skeletal muscle. Exp Gerontol 2011;46:23–9.

[83] McKiernan SH, Colman RJ, Aiken E, Evans TD, Beasley TM, Aiken JM, Weindruch R, Anderson RM. Cellular adaptation contributes to calorie restriction-induced preservation of skeletal muscle in aged rhesus monkeys. Exp Gerontol 2012;47:229–36.

[84] Yang L, Licastro D, Cava E, Veronese M, Spelta F, Rizza W, Bertozzi B, Villareal DT, Hotamisligil GS, Holloszy JO. Long-term calorie restriction enhances cellular quality-control processes in human skeletal muscle. Cell Rep 2016;14:422–8.

[85] Cava E, Fontana L. Will calorie restriction work in humans? Aging 2013;5:507–14.

[86] Speakman JR, Mitchell SE. Caloric restriction. MAM 2011;32:159–221.

[87] Van Norren K, Rusli F, van Dijk M, Lute C, Nagel J, Dijk FJ, Dwarkasing J, Boekschoten MV, Luiking Y, Witkamp RF, Müller M, Steegenga WT. Behavioural changes are a major contributing factor in the reduction of sarcopenia in caloric-restricted ageing mice. J Cachexia Sarcopenia Muscle 2015;6:253–68.

[88] Madeo F, Carmona-Gutierrez D, Hofer SJ, Kroemer G. Caloric restriction mimetics against age-associated disease: targets, mechanisms, and therapeutic potential. Cell Metab 2019;29:592–610.

[89] De Palma C, Morisi F, Cheli S, Pambianco S, Cappello V, Vezzoli M, Rovere-Querini P, Moggio M, Ripolone M, Francolini M, Sandri M, Clementi E. Autophagy as a new therapeutic target in Duchenne muscular dystrophy. Cell Death Dis 2012;3, e418.

[90] Zhang YY, Huang J, Yang M, Gu LJ, Ji JY, Wang LJ, Yuan WJ. Effect of a low-protein diet supplementated with keto-acids on autophagy and inflammation in 5/6 nephrectomized rats. Biosci Rep 2015;35, e00263.

[91] Sakuma K, Yamaguchi A. Molecular mechanisms in aging and current strategies to counteract sarcopenia. Curr Aging Sci 2010;3:90–101.

[92] Sakuma K, Yamaguchi A. Sarcopenia and its intervention. In: Yu BP, editor. Nutrition, exercise and epigenetics: ageing interventions. Switzerland: Springer; 2015. p. 127–51.

[93] Shi L, Zhang T, Zhou Y, Zeng X, Ran L, Zhang Q, Zhu J, Mi M. Dihydromyricetin improves skeletal muscle insulin resistance by inducing autophagy via the AMPK signaling pathway. Mol Cell Endocrinol 2015;409:92–102.

[94] Chang YC, Chen YT, Liu HW, Chan YC, Liu MY, Hu SH, Tseng WT, Wu HL, Wang MF, Chang SJ. Oligonol alleviates sarcopenia by regulation of signaling pathways involved in protein turnover and mitochondrial quality. Mol Nutr Food Res 2019;63:1801102.

[95] Girón MD, Vílchez JD, Shreeram S, Salto R, Manzano M, Cabrera E, Campos N, Edens NK, Rueda R, López-Pedrosa JM. β-Hydroxyl-β-methylbutyrate (HMB) normalizes dexamethasone-induced autophagy-lysosomal pathway in skeletal muscle. PLoS One 2015;10:e0117520.

[96] Brioche T, Pagano AF, Py G, Chopard A. Muscle wasting and aging: experimental models, fatty infiltrations, and prevention. Mol Aspects Med 2016;50:56–87.

[97] Ham DJ, Kennedy TL, Caldow MK, Chee A, Lynch GS, Koopman R. Citrulline does not prevent skeletal muscle wasting or weakness in limb-casted mice. J Nutr 2014;145:900–6.

[98] Lesmana R, Sinha RA, Singh BK, Zhou J, Ohba K, Wu Y, Yau WW, Bay BH, Yen PM. Thyroid hormone stimulation of autophagy is essential for mitochondrial biogenesis and activity in skeletal muscle. Endocrinololgy 2016;157:23–38.

[99] Hertoghe T. The "multiple hormone deficiency" theory of aging: is human senescence caused mainly by multiple hormone deficiencies? Ann N Y Acad Sci 2005;1057:448–65.

[100] Cao L, Wang F, Yang QG, Jiang W, Wang C, Chen YP, Chen GH. Reduced thyroid hormones with increased hippocampal SNAP-25 and Munc18-1 might involve cognitive impairment during aging. Behav Brain Res 2012;229:131–7.

CHAPTER 9

Mitophagy in sarcopenic muscle and practical recommendations for exercise training

Anthony M.J. Sanchez and Robert Solsona
Laboratoire Européen Performance Santé Altitude, EA4604, University of Perpignan Via Domitia, Faculty of Sports Sciences, Font-Romeu, France

Abstract

As we grow older, we are subjected to a decline in muscle mass and strength and global alteration in cell metabolism, leading to poor physical performance. In this chapter, the modulation of mechanisms involved in skeletal muscle organelle turnover during aging, especially mitochondria, is detailed. In the last decade, studies focused on the pivotal role of several actors involved in mitophagy (i.e., the degradation of mitochondria through autophagy) such as the energy sensor AMPK, FOXO transcription factors, and the E3 ubiquitin ligases Parkin, Mul1, and Mdm2. Importantly, studies performed in sports sciences have well recognized the central role of exercise to limit alterations of mitochondrial quality control during aging. Thus, the critical role of chronic exercise in the prevention and limitation of age-related disorders is also discussed. A better understanding of the specific functions of these pathways and the effectiveness of exercise is critical to fight detrimental muscle changes that occur with aging. Finally, perspectives are provided to encourage further exploration of this topic.

Keywords: Autophagy, Mitochondria, Aging, Skeletal muscle, Parkin, AMPK, Exercise, Endurance training, Resistance training, Mitochondrial dynamics

Introduction

The maintenance of skeletal muscle is essential for the body's integrity, health, and quality of life. Disorders in skeletal muscle homeostasis are related to a loss of physiological integrity, contributing to a plethora of chronic pathologies such as diabetes, cachexia, and sarcopenia. Sarcopenia is common among aging people but can also occur earlier in life [1]. Several adverse health outcomes of sarcopenia have been reported, including a higher risk of falls, resulting in traumatisms, motor impairment, disability, and diseases leading to death [1]. Sarcopenia is associated with the outcome of many chronic diseases such as cancer, renal and heart failure, and plays an adverse role in the outcome of critically ill patients [2–5]. Of note, sarcopenia also increases the risk of developing a nosocomial infection after surgery and community-acquired pneumonia in aged people [6,7]. As the world's population grows older, thanks to progress in research and medicine, there is an increase in age-related diseases. By 2050, estimates predict that there will be a similar number of aged and young people in the world, with a large proportion over 60 years [8]. This makes a considerable economic and social challenge for the management of age-related disorders [8].

Muscle failure is associated with detrimental muscle changes accruing during the lifetime. These deleterious modifications include a decline in muscle mass and strength and a failure in cell metabolism, leading to poor physical performance [9–11]. Mitochondria are critical organelles for the maintenance of cell metabolism. They are dynamic organelles undergoing both functional and morphological (size and shape) adaptations. Aging is accompanied by enhanced production of reactive oxygen species (ROS) by mitochondria and mitoptosis (i.e., mitochondrial death), leading to cellular damages and cell death [12]. As such, mitochondrial decline during aging plays a decisive role in the alteration of muscle homeostasis, and improving mitochondrial function or removal appears as a central strategy to counteract the adverse effects of sarcopenia. Overall, approaches targeting skeletal muscle mass and mitochondrial homeostasis might be effective to preserve health or delaying diseases related to sarcopenia (Fig. 1).

Chronic exercise (or exercise training) is one of the most available strategies to enhance muscle function by improving cell metabolism and preserving or increasing cell size [13]. Physical exercise has a major impact on the whole organism and contributes to improvement

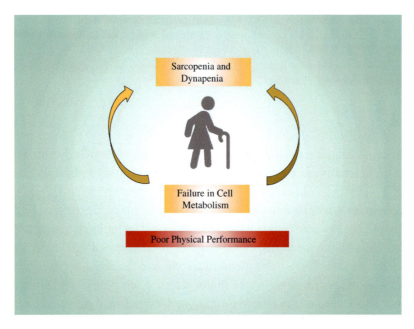

Fig. 1
Aging-related alteration in skeletal muscle.

of global homeostasis (e.g., glucose homeostasis). Chronic exercise also limits morbidity and boosts the aptitude to recover after a period of sickness. Skeletal muscle exhibits remarkable adaptive capabilities in response to exercise. Indeed, exercise affects muscle mass and metabolism through the modulation of fiber composition and size, the improvement in function of organelles and their recycling [14–16]. Among the cellular pathways involved in cell component turnover, autophagy signaling is a highly conserved eukaryotic stress and survival adaptative response that recycles cytoplasmic molecules (i.e., proteins, peptides, lipid droplets, glycogen) and organelles (e.g., mitochondria, ribosomes, peroxisomes) [17]. Importantly, the degradation of damaged mitochondria by autophagy, called "mitophagy," is critical for skeletal muscle maintenance during aging and is sensitive to exercise training. The recently identified E3 ligases Parkin (E3 ligase RING-between-RING), Mul1 (mitochondrial E3 ubiquitin-protein ligase 1), and Mdm2 (murine double minute 2) pathways were found to have a major role in muscle mitophagy and mitochondrial homeostasis, as well as exercise [13,18].

This chapter details the mechanisms underlying the age-dependent alteration of organelle turnover in skeletal muscle, especially mitophagy. Hence, the importance of mitochondrial quality control during aging and the roles of recently discovered actors such as Parkin, Mul1, and Mdm2 are highlighted. The impact of exercise training, current limitations in the literature, and further perspectives are also discussed.

Autophagy and mitochondrial dysfunction during aging
Autophagy in skeletal muscle

In skeletal muscle, there are several forms of autophagy including chaperone-mediated autophagy (CMA), microautophagy, and macroautophagy. CMA is very selective and involves the chaperone protein Hsc70/Hspa8 (heat shock cognate 71 kDa protein) that recognizes and bounds proteins with a KFERQ amino acid sequence [19]. The formed complex bounds to the lysosomal receptor LAMP-2A (lysosomal-associated membrane protein 2A), the substrate protein is then unfolded, translocated into the lumen, and degraded [20–22]. Although CMA has not been extensively studied in skeletal muscle, a recent study reported a decrease in CMA markers during aging [23]. Recent data also suggest that alteration of CMA during aging may contribute to the development of several diseases, including cancer, neurodegeneration, and other diseases [22]. On the other hand, microautophagy is mediated by the direct engulfment of portions of cytoplasm by the lysosome, but little is known about its involvement in sarcopenia. The third mechanism is the autophagosome-lysosome system, also named macroautophagy, which is usually referred to as "autophagy" (Fig. 2).

Macroautophagy is the most studied of these systems in skeletal muscle and involves the formation of a double-membrane vesicle called "autophagosome" that incorporates substrates

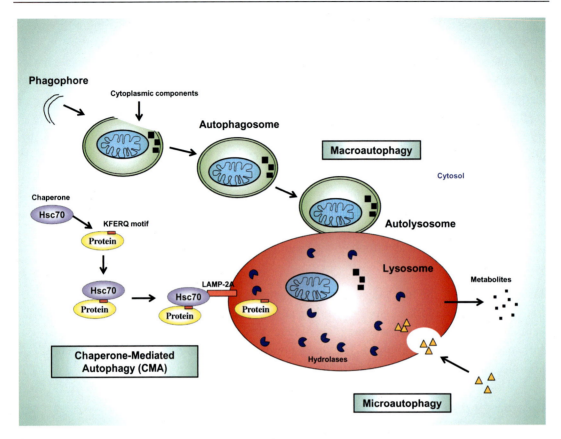

Fig. 2
Overview of three main types of autophagy: microautophagy, chaperone-mediated autophagy (CMA), and macroautophagy. Microautophagy corresponds to a two-step process: (i) invagination of lysosomal membrane and (ii) cargo breakdown in the lysosome. CMA involves the chaperone protein Hsc70/Hspa8 (heat shock cognate 71 kDa protein) that recognizes and bounds proteins with a KFERQ amino acid sequence. Then, the protein complex binds to the lysosomal receptor LAMP-2A (lysosomal-associated membrane protein 2A), and the substrate is unfolded, translocated into the lumen, and degraded. Macroautophagy involves phagophore formation, the capture of cellular components (organelles, proteins, lipids, etc.) during phagophore expansion, autophagosome completion and fusion with the lysosome. Substrates are degraded by several hydrolases within the lysosome.

such as organelles. This stage requires a protein complex that includes Unc-51-like kinase-1/2 (ULK1/2), autophagy-related proteins 13 and 100 (Atg13 and Atg100, respectively), and Fak family kinase-interacting protein of 200 kDa (FIP200). The second step corresponds to the nucleation of the autophagosomal membrane, thanks to a second protein complex that consists of Beclin-1 and phosphatidyl 3-kinase class 3/vacuole protein sorting 34 (PI3KCIII/Vps34). Of note, the microtubule-associated protein light chain 3B (LC3B) plays a critical role in the elongation and the maturation of autophagosomes. During autophagosome maturation, LC3B is lipidated and incorporated into the membrane of the autophagosome. The autophagosome subsequently fuses with the lysosome, and its contents are then degraded by several lysosomal enzymes. Selective autophagy involves autophagic receptors such as p62/SQSTM1 (sequestosome-1), OPTN (optineurin), NBR1 (neighbor of BRCA1 gene 1), NDP52 (nuclear dot protein 52 kDa), BCL2/adenovirus E1B 19 kDa protein-interacting protein 3 (BNIP3), and BNIP3-like (BNIP3L, also known as NIX) [24]. Autophagic receptors recognize cargo (i.e., misfolded and ubiquitylated proteins, damaged organelles, or intracellular pathogens) and simultaneously interact with a component of the core autophagic machinery through their LIR (LC3-interacting region) motif [25–27]. Thus, autophagic receptors bind to the LIR docking site (LDS) of LC3/GABARAP (GABA type A receptor-associated protein) family proteins to mediate the engulfment of their substrates into the forming autophagosome. The selective degradation of mitochondria by autophagy involves BNIP3 and BNIP3L located at the mitochondrial membrane. BNIP3 and BNIP3L connect to LC3 and GABARAP and thus promote autophagosome recruitment to mitochondria [28–33]. Interestingly, another mitophagy pathway involving ULK1/Rab9 (a GTP-ase)/Rip1 (receptor-interacting protein 1)/Drp1 (dynamin-related protein 1, a mitochondrial fission GTPase) complex has been identified to protect the heart against ischemia [34]. In this model, *trans*-Golgi membranes associated with Rab9 are recruited to damaged mitochondria after Rab9 phosphorylation by ULK1, leading to the association between Rab9 and Rip1 and subsequent Drp1 phosphorylation and activation by Rip1.

Several sensors have been identified to regulate autophagy and mitophagy in skeletal muscle, including the adenosine monophosphate (AMP)-activated protein kinase (AMPK) [35–38], the mechanistic/mammalian target of rapamycin complex 1 (MTORC1) [35,36,39], and the forkhead box class O (FOXO) subfamily proteins 1 and 3 (FOXO1 and FOXO3, respectively) [13,36,40]. Among actors involved in autophagy regulation, FOXO3 was first identified as a major regulator of E3 ligases, which are overexpressed in various atrophy models. Thus, FOXO3 controls MAFbx (muscle atrophy F-box)/Atrogin-1 and MuRF1 (muscle ring-finger protein 1) transcription [41,42]. Other E3 ligases, playing a central role in skeletal muscle mass regulation, have been identified, including Trim32 (tripartite motif-containing protein 32), ZNF216 (zinc finger protein 216), and the recently discovered UBR5 (ubiquitin protein ligase E3 component N-recognin 5) [43–47]. Concerning autophagy, FOXO3 controls the transcription of several autophagy genes (Atgs): Atg4B, Atg12L, Beclin, BNIP3, BNIP3L, GABARAPL1, LC3, PI3KIII, and ULK2 [28,48]. Of note, among lysosomal hydrolases, cathepsin L is an endopeptidase regulated by FOXO1 [49]. In addition to FOXO factors, AMPK is also considered as a key regulator of skeletal muscle autophagy under the condition of energy stress [17,35,36,50–52]. AMPK regulates the initiator of autophagosome formation ULK1 through phosphorylation of several residues [36,53–56]. Importantly, the AMPK-ULK1 pathway appears essential for targeting mitochondria to lysosomes after endurance exercise [38]. AMPK also regulates FOXO3 activity and stability in muscle cells [36,40,57], thereby promoting autophagy and mitophagy under the condition of energy stress. Besides these targets, it was recently shown that AMPK promotes mitochondrial fission by phosphorylating the mitochondrial fission factor (MFF, a key receptor of Drp1) enhancing mitophagy [58]. In muscle cells, AMPK activation also stimulates TBK1 (TANK-binding kinase 1) phosphorylation possibly via ULK1 [58]. TBK1 is known to contribute to efficient mitophagy via its binding with several autophagy receptors, including p62/SQSTM1, OPTN, and NDP52 [59,60]. In this way, TBK1 activation by AMPK enhances mitochondrial fission, thus facilitating autophagosome engulfment. Hence, AMPK promotes autophagy at several stages. *Per contra*, MTOR inhibits autophagy initiation through phosphorylation of ULK1 at several residues [36,53–56].

In the last decade, studies investigated skeletal muscle autophagy and mitophagy by using several approaches. Among them, autophagy is currently examined at the mRNA or protein level. The afore-described markers (i.e., Atgs) are commonly used to explore the autophagy machinery. For the interpretation of autophagy activity, the "autophagy flux assay" and "mitophagy flux assay" are specific methods to access the activity of this system. These methods are based on LC3 or p62 protein turnover and inhibitors of autophagy (NH4 Cl, bafilomycin A1, colchicine, and chloroquine) are used to suppress the fusion between autophagosomes and lysosomes or to inhibit the activity of lysosomal enzymes. To assess mitophagy flux, mitochondria are first isolated, and then, LC3 or p62 protein turnover is evaluated [61–64]. More details and other approaches (including in different cell lines and in vivo models) are reviewed in [65] (Fig. 3).

The role of autophagy in skeletal muscle has been extensively studied in the two last decades. The autophagy pathway is essential for mitochondrial and myofiber homeostasis. Autophagy deficiency in mice promotes an increase of proapoptotic markers, calpain activity, proteasomal proteases expression, and centralized nuclei [66,67]. Autophagy failure results in sarcomere disorganization, reduced force and twitch kinetics of glycolytic muscles, mitochondria impairment, and sarcoplasmic reticulum distension [66,67]. These alterations highlight the central role of this pathway in skeletal muscle homeostasis. In addition, autophagy is required for skeletal muscle adaptation to chronic exercise. Indeed, autophagy is involved in mitochondrial remodeling and fiber-type transition [68]. Of note, a study showed that cellular adaptations to endurance training are dependent on fine coordination between autophagy and mitochondrial biogenesis. Indeed, treatment with colchicine blunted the training effects on markers of muscle mitochondrial biogenesis in mice [69]. In this way, exercise is indicated as a therapeutic approach in diseases with dysfunction of autophagy and organelle turnover. Indeed, contractile activity was shown to limit autophagy suppression and reverse mitochondrial decline [63].

Mitochondrial dysfunction during aging

Mitochondria are highly plastic organelles essential for maintaining cell metabolism and their quality control has a major impact on the maintenance of skeletal muscle homeostasis [70,71]. Defective mitochondria accumulate during aging and age-related disorders.

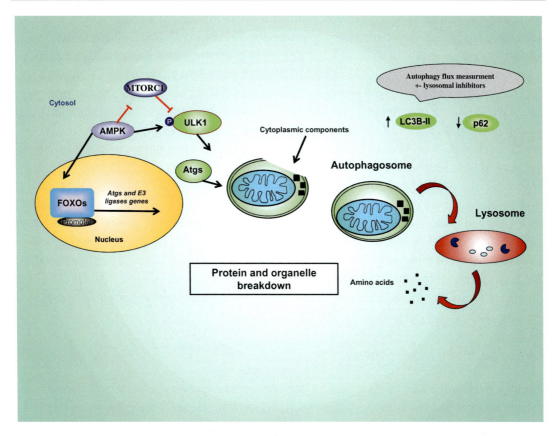

Fig. 3
Overview of autophagy and mitophagy in skeletal muscle. Upon stress that leads to AMPK (adenosine monophosphate (AMP)-activated protein kinase) and/or FOXO (forkhead box class O) activation or MTORC1 (mechanistic/mammalian target of rapamycin complex 1) inhibition, isolation membranes are generated and extend to form autophagosomes sequestering cytoplasmic components (i.e., proteins, lipids, polysaccharides, and organelles). The contents are further digested after fusion with lysosomes containing hydrolases. AMPK phosphorylates and increases FOXO3 activity, activates ULK1 (Unc-51-like kinase-1) initiating autophagosome formation, and inhibits MTORC1 under the conditions of energy stress. FOXO3 regulates the transcription of several E3 ligase genes and autophagy genes (Atgs). MTORC1 inhibits autophagosome formation by phosphorylation of ULK1. LC3B-II: microtubule-associated protein light chain 3B; p62 is also known as SQSTM1: sequestosome-1.

In addition to aerobic energy production, mitochondria coordinate important mechanisms such as cell death and signaling. Besides biogenesis and mitophagy, mitochondrial dynamics is involved in cell life and death. It refers to highly coordinated events of fusion and fission [70]. Mitochondrial fusion mediates the merging of mitochondrial membranes of two originally distinct organelles to unify their compartments, while mitochondrial fission promotes the separation of one organelle into separate mitochondria [70]. The outer mitochondrial membrane fusion proteins mitofusin 1 and 2 (Mfn1/2) mediate fusion, as well as the inner membrane fusion mediated optic atrophy 1 (OPA1) [72–76]. Mitochondrial fission allows the removal of dysfunctional mitochondria through mitophagy and is induced by Drp1 and adaptors located at mitochondrial restriction sites (e.g., the fission 1 protein, Fis1) [74,76–81]. Interestingly, a recent study examined the impact of Drp1 knockdown on adult skeletal muscle function and highlighted its critical role in muscle maintenance [82]. According to the data, Drp1 knockdown leads to severe atrophy and global impairment of muscle function. Lower ADP-stimulated respiration, impaired autophagy, enhanced oxidative stress and muscle fibrosis, denervation, and degeneration are observed [82,83]. During aging, mitochondrial dysfunctions and ubiquitination of mitochondrial proteins increase in skeletal muscle. Thus, a global decrease of mitochondrial volume, biogenesis, and reduced enzymatic activity are commonly observed during aging. Conversely, mitochondrial ROS production and mitochondrial DNA mutations are exacerbated in aged people. In addition, several studies evidenced that basal mitophagy flux is increased in skeletal muscle during aging [61,62,64]. This may contribute to explain the decline of mitochondrial content in aged muscles [18]. Altogether, these alterations in mitochondrial function may contribute to apoptosis, muscle fiber loss, and age-related sarcopenia [84–86].

Parkin pathway in sarcopenia

Recently, the involvement of E3 ligases in neurodegenerative diseases (such as Parkinson's disease) and their role in mitophagy have been investigated. Hence, Parkin (encoded by the Park2 gene) was found to play a role in Parkinson's disease but to be essential for skeletal muscle mitophagy under normal conditions and during sarcopenia. Originally, Parkin has been studied in neurons for its involvement in Parkinson's disease (hence its name) [87–89]. During Parkinson's disease, skeletal muscle dysfunctions have also been observed, such as a decrease in muscle mass and an impairment of mitochondrial respiratory chain function [90–92]. An essential regulator of Parkin is PINK1 (PTEN—induced putative kinase protein 1, PTEN being a phosphatase, and tensin homolog), which is activated by mitochondrial membrane potential depolarization. PINK1 phosphorylates Parkin on its ubiquitin-like domain, leading to its activation [89]. Phosphorylation of Parkin at Ser-65 seems essential for its mitochondrial translocation to induce mitochondrial fission and mitophagy [87,93]. Several substrates of Parkin have been identified, such as the mitochondrial outer membrane proteins Drp1, Mfn 1/2, TOMM20 (translocase of outer mitochondrial membrane 20), Fis1, VDAC (voltage-dependent anion channel), and Miro (mitochondrial Rho-GTPase) [94–99]. Their targeting results in the recruitment of the autophagy receptors LC3, p62, and NBR1 (neighbor of BRCA1 gene 1) to mitochondria [100]. Furthermore, Parkin regulates mitochondrial biogenesis by ubiquitinating the transcriptional repressor of peroxisome proliferator-γ coactivator-1α (PGC1-a), Parkin-interacting substrate (PARIS) [101]. Finally, Parkin is also involved in the production of mitochondrial-derived vesicles essential for mitochondrial quality control [102,103]. The formation of mitochondrial small vesicles that transport damaged or oxidized mitochondrial proteins or lipids to other organelles (e.g., peroxisomes or lysosomes) is stimulated by ROS before mitochondrial dysfunction [103–105]. They can also fuse with the late endosome or multivesicular body [104]. This pathway, which is independent of Drp1-related mitophagy, appears to be important for cargo delivery to lysosomes [105].

Among the multiple pathways involved in mitochondrial homeostasis and regulated by Parkin, mitophagy has been the most studied in skeletal muscle cells, including during aging. Peker and colleagues recently showed that the mitochondrial oxidative phosphorylation uncoupler CCCP (carbonyl cyanide m-chlorophenylhydrazone) induces mitophagy and atrophy in a PINK1/Parkin-dependent manner in C2C12 cells [106]. In this study, Parkin expression was not increased with CCCP treatment, but Parkin translocated to mitochondria. Importantly, Parkin ablation in myoblasts led to impaired mitochondrial turnover and accretion of dysfunctional mitochondria. Thus, Parkin appears essential for mitochondrial homeostasis in muscle cells. In vivo, the role of Parkin in skeletal muscle mitochondrial function has been confirmed using $Park2^{-/-}$ mice [107]. Parkin deficient muscles showed several dysfunctions such as a decrease of specific force production and mitochondrial respiration, and mitochondrial uncoupling. Enhanced mitochondrial fragmentation has also been suggested by the observation of an increase of Drp1 and oxidative stress markers content, as well as a decrease of Mfn2 expression. An increase in global autophagy flux (as measured using colchicine) was also found in $Park2^{-/-}$ mice. Conversely, Parkin overexpression improves mitochondrial content and quality during sepsis and prevents skeletal muscle atrophy [108]. Importantly, a study from Leduc-Gaudet and coworkers [109] highlighted that Parkin overexpression attenuates sarcopenia and improves skeletal muscle health during aging. Indeed, the authors found that Parkin overexpression attenuates the loss of muscle strength, increases mitochondrial enzymatic activity and content, and promotes hypertrophy. Parkin overexpression also limits oxidative stress, fibrosis, and apoptosis in old mice. Consistent with this, a study conducted on human beings showed that endurance exercise promotes basal Parkin expression in both young and old individuals [110]. In this study, Fis1 was also higher in active individuals compared to sedentary individuals, suggesting that fission may also contribute to exercise-related mitochondrial adaptation. Overall, Parkin appears as an important E3 ligase for skeletal muscle mass maintenance, contractile activity, and mitochondrial homeostasis during aging.

A study conducted in *Drosophila melanogaster* showed an increase of mitochondrial ubiquitination in indirect flight muscles in an age-dependent manner [111]. In this model, the authors reported that the overexpression of Parkin or PINK1 can abolish mitochondrial ubiquitination and extend lifespan. Data from this study also highlighted that Atg1 knockdown abolishes these effects, reinforcing the importance of the link between

PINK1/Parkin and mitophagy. Importantly, a series of experiments established a link between Parkin-mediated mitophagy and training-induced mitochondrial adaptations during aging. First of all, studies previously showed conflicting results on autophagy modulation during aging. Some studies found no impact of aging on the expression of several autophagy markers (i.e., ULK1, p62, Beclin-1, the ratio LC3-II/LC3-I) [112–114]. Other findings observed an increase of LC3-II and p62 protein expression and cathepsin L activity in both slow and fast muscles in aged rats, and an increase of ULK1 and Beclin level was observed in fast muscle [115]. These data suggested elevated basal autophagy in old muscles. Importantly, autophagy flux was measured by monitoring LC3 turnover with the lysosome inhibitor colchicine [115]. The authors found higher basal autophagy flux in aged muscles compared to control muscles. Recently, a study from Hood's laboratory monitored for the first time mitophagy flux on isolated mitochondria in skeletal muscles of aged rats. In this study, a higher basal mitophagy flux was found in aged muscles compared to controls, especially in inter-myofibrillar mitochondria [61,64]. Hence, mitophagy appears to be involved in the targeting of dysfunctional mitochondria during aging. This study also investigated the effect of chronic contractile activity on aged muscles. A decrease in mitophagy flux in both aged and young muscles with exercise was noted [61,64]. This result is of importance since it turns upside down the previous findings that suggested that chronic exercise stimulates basal mitophagy flux. According to these new data, chronic contractile activity does not increase basal autophagy flux. On the contrary, it decreases it, probably because exercise improves the quality of mitochondria, reducing the need to recycle these organelles. Collectively, these studies evidenced that basal mitophagy flux is increased in aged skeletal muscle and this may explain the decline of mitochondrial content observed during aging. However, exercise seems to be an effective approach to counteract age-related alteration of mitophagy and mitochondrial function (Fig. 4).

Mul1 and Mdm2 in skeletal muscle mitophagy: Perspectives in sarcopenia

Another E3 ligase, Mul1 (also known as MULAN/GIDE/MAPL/HADES), has been found to play a role in mitochondrial dynamics and signaling [116–118]. Mul1 is a RING finger and SUMO protein whose knockdown and ectopic expression both induce disturbances in mitochondrial morphology and trafficking [118]. Mul1 is located on the outer membrane of mitochondria and its RING finger motif points toward the cytoplasm. Several targets of this E3 ligase have been identified conferring a role of Mul1 in the fission machinery of mitochondria and mitophagy. Indeed, Mul1 targets and stabilizes Drp1 by SUMOylation, leading to mitochondrial fragmentation [119]. Mul1 also stabilizes ULK1 in the selenite-induced mitophagy model of HeLa cells [120] and ubiquitinates Akt in a FOXO3-dependent manner in thyroid cancer cells [121]. Recently, it was found that Mul1 regulates the hypoxia-inducible factor 1α (HIF-1α) and promotes a metabolic shift to glycolysis by modulating

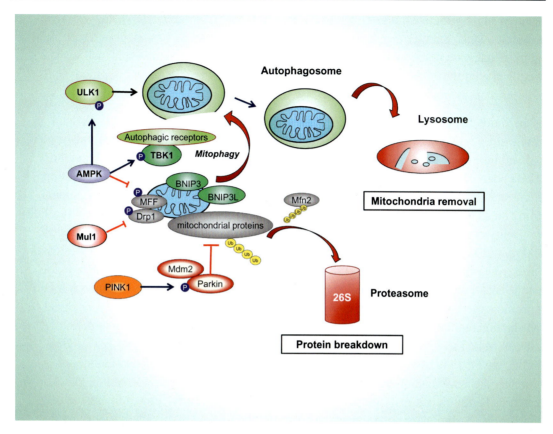

Fig. 4
Mechanisms regulating mitophagy in skeletal muscle. PINK1/Parkin (PTEN- induced putative kinase protein 1/ E3 ligase RING-between-RING), Mdm2 (murine double minute 2), and Mul1 (mitochondrial E3 ubiquitin-protein ligase 1) are involved in mitophagy through polyubiquitination of several mitochondrial proteins (such as Mfn2, mitofusin-2) that leads to their proteasomal degradation. BNIP3 (BCL2/adenovirus E1B 19 kDa protein-interacting protein 3) and BNIP3L (BNIP3L, also known as NIX) are autophagic receptors that are also involved in mitophagy. Other autophagic receptors are p62/SQSTM1 (sequestosome-1), OPTN (optineurin), NBR1 (neighbor of BRCA1 gene 1), and NDP52 (nuclear dot protein 52 kDa). AMPK (adenosine monophosphate (AMP)-activated protein kinase) promotes mitophagy through phosphorylation of MFF (mitochondrial fission factor), TBK1 (TANK-binding kinase 1), and ULK1 (Unc-51-like kinase-1).

the UBXN7 cofactor protein [122]. However, data about Mul1 in skeletal muscle, including its involvement in sarcopenia, are still limited. In primary myotubes, Mul1 was suggested to be implicated in mitophagy in an AMPK-FOXO3-dependent way [36]. It was also found that AMPK blunts the preservative effects of IGF-1 (insulin-like growth factor 1) on the contractility of sensory-innervated muscle cells via the Mul1 pathway [123]. Concerning the effects of exercise on this pathway, studies are also lacking even if it was suggested that Mul1 may play a role in adaptations to endurance exercise. Indeed, a single bout of exercise enhances Mul1 protein expression without altering its mRNA content [124], suggesting an increase of Mul1 stability during exercise. However, another study has suggested that Mul1 and mitophagy are not associated with training adaptations in type 2 diabetes mellitus [125]. Overall, even if the Mul1 pathway plays a role in mitophagy in several cellular models, its role in sarcopenia and adaptations to exercise training remains to be elucidated.

Furthermore, in the past few years, the oncoprotein Mdm2 has been involved in skeletal muscle atrophy. Mdm2 is considered as the chief E3 ligase of the transcriptional factor p53 involved in the cell cycle, autophagy, and apoptosis [126]. It was recently found that the 90 kDa heat-shock protein β isoform (Hsp90β) interacts with Mdm2, leading to alteration of p53 stability and suppression of cellular senescence [127]. Thanks to its RING domain, Mdm2 binds to the mRNAs of several cancer-related genes. Thus, Mdm2 regulates translation or stability of mRNAs encoding vascular endothelial growth factor (VEGF), the oncogene N-Myc, the X-linked inhibitor of apoptosis (XIAP), and p53 [128]. Mdm2 also participates in the proteasomal degradation of FOXO3 when FOXO3 is targeted and acetylated by the histone acetylase p300 [129]. Interestingly, the afore-described E3 ligase Parkin was found to promote the association of Mdm2 with arrestins [130] that play a critical role in signal transduction regulation at G protein-coupled receptors. Recently, the direct interaction between Mdm2 and Parkin was shown to enhance Parkin enzymatic activity [131]. This binding results in increased ubiquitination of the Parkin substrate Mfn1 and facilitates mitophagy when mitochondria lose their membrane potential. *Per contra*, Mdm2 knockdown decreases Parkin-dependent mitophagy [131]. Even if data are still limited in muscle cells, there are increasing pieces of evidence that Mdm2 plays a role in mitochondrial function. Importantly, a recent study found that Mdm2 can be imported into the mitochondria matrix independently of p53 [132]. In this way, Mdm2 suppresses the transcription of NADH-dehydrogenase 6, leading to a decrease of respiratory complex 1 activity and an enhance of ROS production. Interestingly, Mdm2 deficiency increases mitochondrial complex 1 activity and enhances skeletal muscle endurance [132]. Collectively, these data uncover previously unsuspected functions of the E3 ligases Mul1 and Mdm2 in mitochondrial function and mitophagy. These E3 ligases play critical roles in skeletal muscle homeostasis, and alteration of their function may contribute to muscle diseases. Further studies are needed to better understand the involvement of Mdm2 and Mul1 in sarcopenia and their roles in adaptations to exercise training.

Exercise modalities and practical recommendations for aging people

Exercise may improve mitochondrial function, reduce oxidative damage, and attenuate the rate of skeletal muscle mass decline. Adaptations to exercise training are related to several factors such as exercise volume and intensity, the rest between exercise bouts, recovery, nutritional considerations, genetics/epigenetics, environmental conditions, and age [13,133,134]. Responses to training, especially hypertrophy, tend to be attenuated during aging. An important mechanism involved in this mitigated response to exercise seems to be alteration of ribosome biogenesis in aged people [135]. Furthermore, as explained earlier, mitochondrial dysfunctions occur during aging and contribute to muscle failure. Resistance training may improve the physical functioning of elderly people through increases in walking endurance, leg strength, and oxidative capacity [136–138]. As frailty occurs frequently with aging, training intensity should be adjusted to protect old people from traumatic injuries. Studies on the impact of resistance training are emerging in the context of aging. Resistance training may induce several adaptations in elderly people, such as hypertrophy, the exhibition of the myonuclear domain and occasionally myonuclear accretion, augmentation of satellite cell-capillary interaction and content, and mitochondrial adaptations [139–141].

Several studies that compared the effect of resistance training at high or low intensities on elderly people found no major differences in the degree of improvement in muscle strength, fiber hypertrophy, and quality of life [142–145]. Thus, exercise intensity does not appear to be the main factor that governs adaptations to training in aged people. Regarding training volume in resistance training, little is known. However, a recent study by Hammarström and coworkers compared training with low and moderate volume with a contralateral protocol [146]. The authors found a dose-dependent relationship between the training volume and muscle adaptations. Indeed, according to this study, the moderate volume promotes higher gains in muscle mass and strength, a more pronounced type II fiber transition, and ribosome biogenesis [146,147]. Studies have to be encouraged to elucidate if manipulation of the training volume can be advised during aging and the molecular mechanism underlying the adaptations. Hypothetically, low-intensity but high-volume resistance training may stimulate mitochondrial adaptations significantly, especially in elderly individuals. Consistent with this, even if low-intensity/high-volume and high-intensity resistance training may induce similar gains in $\dot{V}O_2 peak$ (peak oxygen consumption) in old men and women, only low-intensity/high-volume leads to improvement in endurance [145]. Importantly, maximal strength training seems to promote some negative mitochondrial adaptations in aged people [148]. Furthermore, muscle strength seems to be related to mitochondrial function in adults, and dysfunction of muscle bioenergetics enhances troubles in mobility [149]. A meta-analysis also showed that Nordic walking, as a training method, promotes an increase of lower limb strength, life and sleep quality, aerobic capacity, and amelioration of body composition for elderly people [150]. Overall, these data seem to indicate that resistance training is beneficial for health in elderly people, and high-volume training should be privileged when mitochondrial adaptations are sought.

Furthermore, resistance training with eccentric actions was also suggested to generate early adaptations and higher gains in skeletal muscle strength and mass compared to other contractions modes (i.e., concentric or isometric) [151,152]. Eccentric exercises seem to promote higher effects on muscle growth and MTORC1 pathway [153]. However, effects on both hypertrophy and molecular responses (including some autophagy markers) appear relatively similar when the magnitude of the force-signal integral is normalized [154–156]. In addition, contraction mode appears less influential with prolonged high-volume resistance training, and protein and carbohydrate supplementation becomes a more critical factor to further increase muscle mass [151]. Concerning autophagy, it appears that this system is critical to preserve mitochondrial function during damaging muscle eccentric contractions [157]. However, care should be taken with eccentric exercises. Thus, only low-intensity eccentric actions should be used in aged people to minimize the occurrence of muscle damage and the risk of a traumatic injury. Otherwise, attention should be given to the possible advantages obtained by the combination of low hypoxia and eccentric endurance exercises (e.g., downhill walking sessions) on muscle function during aging since studies found advantages in rats and prediabetic people [158,159]. Further investigations have to be encouraged to better understand cellular responses on mitochondrial remodeling in response to low-intensity eccentric exercise and low hypoxia to strengthen recommendations for aged people (Fig. 5).

Conclusions and perspectives

The development of strategies to counteract the sarcopenic phenotype and its detrimental effects is critical to improve the quality of life or the capacity of aging people to recover from illness. It emphasizes the need for a better understanding of the underlying cellular mechanisms of muscle failure and the effect of chronic exercise on the subsequent dysfunctions. Thus, several pathways, including Parkin, Mul1, and Mdm2 signaling, have been shown to play a critical part in mitochondrial maintenance and mitophagy. Parkin is also required to increase the pool of functional mitochondria in muscle cells, thanks to training adaptations. The potential role of Mul1 and Mdm2 in adaptations to chronic exercise remains to be addressed during sarcopenia. Further studies on the impact of exercise and nutritional interventions on sarcopenia have to be encouraged to better understand skeletal muscle adaptations to training in elderly people. For instance, research on resistance training and mitochondrial adaptations is still limited. In addition, other forms of autophagy, including ribophagy (i.e., the degradation of ribosomes through autophagy), need further attention in the context of aging and exercise. In that matter, experiments with "ribophagy flux" measurements have to be developed to privilege correct interpretation on the modulation of this pathway.

Acknowledgments

The authors thank Prima La Casse for his advice.

Conflict of interest

The authors confirm that this article content has no conflict of interest.

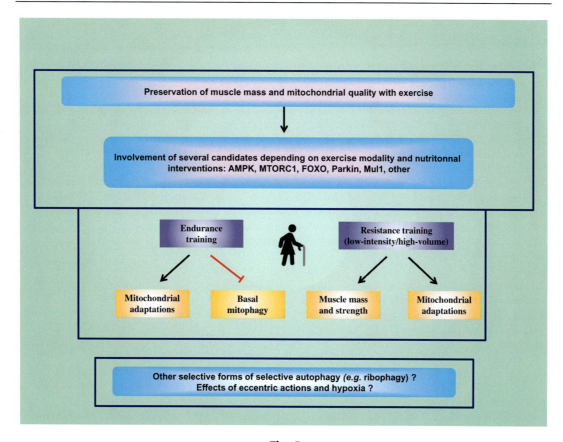

Fig. 5
Preservation of muscle mass and cell metabolism with exercise. Endurance training promotes mitochondrial adaptations and may reduce basal mitophagy flux, thanks to a higher mitochondrial quality. Resistance training (low-intensity/high-volume) may induce both improvements in muscle mass and strength, as well as mitochondrial adaptations in elderly people.

References

[1] Cruz-Jentoft AJ, Bahat G, Bauer J, et al. Sarcopenia: revised European consensus on definition and diagnosis. Age Ageing 2019;48:16–31.
[2] Baggerman MR, van Dijk DPJ, Winkens B, van Gassel RJJ, Bol ME, Schnabel RM, Bakers FC, Olde Damink SWM, van de Poll MCG. Muscle wasting associated co-morbidities, rather than sarcopenia are risk factors for hospital mortality in critical illness. J Crit Care 2020;56:31–6.
[3] Limpawattana P, Theerakulpisut D, Wirasorn K, Sookprasert A, Khuntikeo N, Chindaprasirt J. The impact of skeletal muscle mass on survival outcome in biliary tract cancer patients. PLoS ONE 2018;13, e0204985.
[4] Srikanthan P, Horwich TB, Tseng CH. Relation of muscle mass and fat mass to cardiovascular disease mortality. Am J Cardiol 2016;117:1355–60.
[5] Zhou Y, Hellberg M, Svensson P, Höglund P, Clyne N. Sarcopenia and relationships between muscle mass, measured glomerular filtration rate and physical function in patients with chronic kidney disease stages 3-5. Nephrol Dial Transplant Off Publ Eur Dial Transpl Assoc Eur Ren Assoc 2018;33:342–8.

[6] Cosquéric G, Sebag A, Ducolombier C, Thomas C, Piette F, Weill-Engerer S. Sarcopenia is predictive of nosocomial infection in care of the elderly. Br J Nutr 2006;96:895–901.
[7] Altuna-Venegas S, Aliaga-Vega R, Maguiña JL, Parodi JF, Runzer-Colmenares FM. Risk of community-acquired pneumonia in older adults with sarcopenia of a hospital from Callao, Peru 2010-2015. Arch Gerontol Geriatr 2019;82:100–5.
[8] Harper S. Economic and social implications of aging societies. Science 2014;346:587–91.
[9] Angulo J, El Assar M, Álvarez-Bustos A, Rodríguez-Mañas L. Physical activity and exercise: strategies to manage frailty. Redox Biol 2020;35, 101513.
[10] Borzuola R, Giombini A, Torre G, Campi S, Albo E, Bravi M, Borrione P, Fossati C, Macaluso A. Central and peripheral neuromuscular adaptations to ageing. J Clin Med 2020;9:741. https://doi.org/10.3390/jcm9030741.
[11] Brown LA, Guzman SD, Brooks SV. Emerging molecular mediators and targets for age-related skeletal muscle atrophy. Transl Res J Lab Clin Med 2020;221:44–57. https://doi.org/10.1016/j.trsl.2020.03.001.
[12] Skulachev VP, Longo VD. Aging as a mitochondria-mediated atavistic program: can aging be switched off? Ann N Y Acad Sci 2005;1057:145–64.
[13] Sanchez AM, Candau R, Bernardi H. Recent data on cellular component turnover: focus on adaptations to physical exercise. Cell 2019;8:542.
[14] Hood DA, Memme JM, Oliveira AN, Triolo M. Maintenance of skeletal muscle mitochondria in health, exercise, and aging. Annu Rev Physiol 2018;81:19–41. https://doi.org/10.1146/annurev-physiol-020518-114310.
[15] McGlory C, van Vliet S, Stokes T, Mittendorfer B, Phillips SM. The impact of exercise and nutrition on the regulation of skeletal muscle mass. J Physiol 2019;597(5):1251–8. https://doi.org/10.1113/JP275443.
[16] Sanchez AMJ, Bernardi H, Py G, Candau RB. Autophagy is essential to support skeletal muscle plasticity in response to endurance exercise. Am J Physiol Regul Integr Comp Physiol 2014;307:R956–69.
[17] Sanchez AMJ, Candau R, Raibon A, Bernardi H. Autophagy, a highly regulated intracellular system essential to skeletal muscle homeostasis—role in disease, exercise and altitude exposure. In: Muscle cell and tissue. IntechOpen; 2015. https://doi.org/10.5772/60698.
[18] Zhang Y, Oliveira AN, Hood DA. The intersection of exercise and aging on mitochondrial protein quality control. Exp Gerontol 2020;131:110824.
[19] Stricher F, Macri C, Ruff M, Muller S. HSPA8/HSC70 chaperone protein: structure, function, and chemical targeting. Autophagy 2013;9:1937–54.
[20] Cuervo AM. Chaperone-mediated autophagy: selectivity pays off. Trends Endocrinol Metab TEM 2010;21:142–50.
[21] Sahu R, Kaushik S, Clement CC, Cannizzo ES, Scharf B, Follenzi A, Potolicchio I, Nieves E, Cuervo AM, Santambrogio L. Microautophagy of cytosolic proteins by late endosomes. Dev Cell 2011;20:131–9.
[22] Yang Q, Wang R, Zhu L. Chaperone-mediated autophagy. In: Qin Z-H, editor. Autophagy: biology and diseases: basic science. Singapore: Springer; 2019. p. 435–52.
[23] Zhou J, Chong SY, Lim A, Singh BK, Sinha RA, Salmon AB, Yen PM. Changes in macroautophagy, chaperone-mediated autophagy, and mitochondrial metabolism in murine skeletal and cardiac muscle during aging. Aging 2017;9:583–99.
[24] Johansen T, Lamark T. Selective autophagy: ATG8 family proteins, LIR motifs and cargo receptors. J Mol Biol 2020;432:80–103.
[25] Kirkin V, Rogov VV. A diversity of selective autophagy receptors determines the specificity of the autophagy pathway. Mol Cell 2019;76:268–85.
[26] Johansen T, Lamark T. Selective autophagy mediated by autophagic adapter proteins. Autophagy 2011;7:279–96.
[27] Kim B-W, Kwon DH, Song HK. Structure biology of selective autophagy receptors. BMB Rep 2016;49:73–80.
[28] Mammucari C, Milan G, Romanello V, et al. FoxO$_3$ controls autophagy in skeletal muscle in vivo. Cell Metab 2007;6:458–71.

[29] Schweers RL, Zhang J, Randall MS, et al. NIX is required for programmed mitochondrial clearance during reticulocyte maturation. Proc Natl Acad Sci U S A 2007;104:19500–5.
[30] Zhang J, Ney PA. Role of BNIP3 and NIX in cell death, autophagy, and mitophagy. Cell Death Differ 2009;16:939–46.
[31] Zhu Y, Massen S, Terenzio M, Lang V, Chen-Lindner S, Eils R, Novak I, Dikic I, Hamacher-Brady A, Brady NR. Modulation of serines 17 and 24 in the LC3-interacting region of Bnip3 determines pro-survival mitophagy versus apoptosis. J Biol Chem 2013;288:1099–113.
[32] Novak I, Kirkin V, McEwan DG, et al. Nix is a selective autophagy receptor for mitochondrial clearance. EMBO Rep 2010;11:45–51.
[33] Hanna RA, Quinsay MN, Orogo AM, Giang K, Rikka S, Gustafsson ÅB. Microtubule-associated protein 1 light chain 3 (LC3) interacts with Bnip3 protein to selectively remove endoplasmic reticulum and mitochondria via autophagy. J Biol Chem 2012;287:19094–104.
[34] Saito T, Nah J, Oka S, et al. An alternative mitophagy pathway mediated by Rab9 protects the heart against ischemia. J Clin Invest 2019;129:802–19.
[35] Sanchez AMJ, Candau RB, Csibi A, Pagano AF, Raibon A, Bernardi H. The role of AMP-activated protein kinase in the coordination of skeletal muscle turnover and energy homeostasis. Am J Physiol Cell Physiol 2012;303:C475–85.
[36] Sanchez AMJ, Candau R, Bernardi H. AMP-activated protein kinase stabilizes FOXO3 in primary myotubes. Biochem Biophys Res Commun 2018;499(3):493–8. https://doi.org/10.1016/j.bbrc.2018.03.176.
[37] Kjøbsted R, Hingst JR, Fentz J, et al. AMPK in skeletal muscle function and metabolism. FASEB J 2018;32:1741–77.
[38] Laker RC, Drake JC, Wilson RJ, et al. Ampk phosphorylation of Ulk1 is required for targeting of mitochondria to lysosomes in exercise-induced mitophagy. Nat Commun 2017;8:548.
[39] Sanchez AMJ, Csibi A, Raibon A, Docquier A, Lagirand-Cantaloube J, Leibovitch M-P, Leibovitch SA, Bernardi H. eIF3f: a central regulator of the antagonism atrophy/hypertrophy in skeletal muscle. Int J Biochem Cell Biol 2013;45:2158–62.
[40] Sanchez AMJ, Candau RB, Bernardi H. FoxO transcription factors: their roles in the maintenance of skeletal muscle homeostasis. Cell Mol Life Sci CMLS 2014;71:1657–71.
[41] Bodine SC, Latres E, Baumhueter S, et al. Identification of ubiquitin ligases required for skeletal muscle atrophy. Science 2001;294:1704–8.
[42] Gomes MD, Lecker SH, Jagoe RT, Navon A, Goldberg AL. Atrogin-1, a muscle-specific F-box protein highly expressed during muscle atrophy. Proc Natl Acad Sci U S A 2001;98:14440–5.
[43] Cohen S, Zhai B, Gygi SP, Goldberg AL. Ubiquitylation by Trim32 causes coupled loss of desmin, Z-bands, and thin filaments in muscle atrophy. J Cell Biol 2012;198:575–89.
[44] Hishiya A, Iemura S, Natsume T, Takayama S, Ikeda K, Watanabe K. A novel ubiquitin-binding protein ZNF216 functioning in muscle atrophy. EMBO J 2006;25:554–64.
[45] Kudryashova E, Kudryashov D, Kramerova I, Spencer MJ. Trim32 is a ubiquitin ligase mutated in limb girdle muscular dystrophy type 2H that binds to skeletal muscle myosin and ubiquitinates actin. J Mol Biol 2005;354:413–24.
[46] Seaborne RA, Hughes DC, Turner DC, et al. UBR5 is a novel E3 ubiquitin ligase involved in skeletal muscle hypertrophy and recovery from atrophy. J Physiol 2019;597(14):3727–49. https://doi.org/10.1113/JP278073.
[47] Dablainville V, Sanchez AMJ. The role of the recently discovered E3 ubiquitin ligase UBR5 in skeletal muscle mass regulation. J Physiol 2019;597:4133–5.
[48] Zhao J, Brault JJ, Schild A, Cao P, Sandri M, Schiaffino S, Lecker SH, Goldberg AL. FoxO$_3$ coordinately activates protein degradation by the autophagic/lysosomal and proteasomal pathways in atrophying muscle cells. Cell Metab 2007;6:472–83.
[49] Yamazaki Y, Kamei Y, Sugita S, et al. The cathepsin L gene is a direct target of FOXO1 in skeletal muscle. Biochem J 2010;427:171–8.

[50] Sanchez AMJ, Csibi A, Raibon A, Cornille K, Gay S, Bernardi H, Candau R. AMPK promotes skeletal muscle autophagy through activation of forkhead FoxO3a and interaction with Ulk1. J Cell Biochem 2012;113:695–710.

[51] Thomson DM. The role of AMPK in the regulation of skeletal muscle size, hypertrophy, and regeneration. Int J Mol Sci 2018;19(10):3125. https://doi.org/10.3390/ijms19103125.

[52] Rocchi A, He C. Regulation of exercise-induced autophagy in skeletal muscle. Curr Pathobiol Rep 2017;5:177–86.

[53] Egan D, Kim J, Shaw RJ, Guan K-L. The autophagy initiating kinase ULK1 is regulated via opposing phosphorylation by AMPK and mTOR. Autophagy 2011;7:643–4.

[54] Goldberg AA, Nkengfac B, Sanchez AMJ, Moroz N, Qureshi ST, Koromilas AE, Wang S, Burelle Y, Hussain SN, Kristof AS. Regulation of ULK1 expression and autophagy by STAT1. J Biol Chem 2017;292:1899–909.

[55] Kim J, Guan K-L. Regulation of the autophagy initiating kinase ULK1 by nutrients: roles of mTORC1 and AMPK. Cell Cycle Georget Tex 2011;10:1337–8.

[56] Kim J, Kundu M, Viollet B, Guan K-L. AMPK and mTOR regulate autophagy through direct phosphorylation of Ulk1. Nat Cell Biol 2011;13:132–41.

[57] Sanchez AMJ. FoxO transcription factors and endurance training: a role for FoxO1 and FoxO3 in exercise-induced angiogenesis. J Physiol 2015;593:363–4.

[58] Seabright AP, Fine NHF, Barlow JP, et al. AMPK activation induces mitophagy and promotes mitochondrial fission while activating TBK1 in a PINK1-Parkin independent manner. FASEB J Off Publ Fed Am Soc Exp Biol 2020;34:6284–301.

[59] Heo J-M, Ordureau A, Paulo JA, Rinehart J, Harper JW. The PINK1-PARKIN mitochondrial ubiquitylation pathway drives a program of OPTN/NDP52 recruitment and TBK1 activation to promote mitophagy. Mol Cell 2015;60:7–20.

[60] Wild P, Farhan H, McEwan DG, et al. Phosphorylation of the autophagy receptor optineurin restricts Salmonella growth. Science 2011;333:228–33.

[61] Carter HN, Kim Y, Erlich AT, Zarrin-Khat D, Hood DA. Autophagy and mitophagy flux in young and aged skeletal muscle following chronic contractile activity. J Physiol 2018;596:3567–84.

[62] Chen CCW, Erlich AT, Hood DA. Role of Parkin and endurance training on mitochondrial turnover in skeletal muscle. Skelet Muscle 2018;8:10.

[63] Parousis A, Carter HN, Tran C, Erlich AT, Mesbah Moosavi ZS, Pauly M, Hood DA. Contractile activity attenuates autophagy suppression and reverses mitochondrial defects in skeletal muscle cells. Autophagy 2018;14:1886–97.

[64] Sanchez AMJ. Mitophagy flux in skeletal muscle during chronic contractile activity and ageing. J Physiol 2018;596:3461–2.

[65] Klionsky DJ, Abdelmohsen K, Abe A, et al. Guidelines for the use and interpretation of assays for monitoring autophagy (3rd edition). Autophagy 2016;12:1–222.

[66] Masiero E, Agatea L, Mammucari C, Blaauw B, Loro E, Komatsu M, Metzger D, Reggiani C, Schiaffino S, Sandri M. Autophagy is required to maintain muscle mass. Cell Metab 2009;10:507–15.

[67] Paré MF, Baechler BL, Fajardo VA, Earl E, Wong E, Campbell TL, Tupling AR, Quadrilatero J. Effect of acute and chronic autophagy deficiency on skeletal muscle apoptotic signaling, morphology, and function. Biochim Biophys Acta Mol Cell Res 2017;1864:708–18.

[68] Lira VA, Okutsu M, Zhang M, Greene NP, Laker RC, Breen DS, Hoehn KL, Yan Z. Autophagy is required for exercise training-induced skeletal muscle adaptation and improvement of physical performance. FASEB J Off Publ Fed Am Soc Exp Biol 2013;27:4184–93.

[69] Ju J-S, Jeon S-I, Park J-Y, Lee J-Y, Lee S-C, Cho K-J, Jeong J-M. Autophagy plays a role in skeletal muscle mitochondrial biogenesis in an endurance exercise-trained condition. J Physiol Sci JPS 2016;66:417–30.

[70] Casuso RA, Huertas JR. The emerging role of skeletal muscle mitochondrial dynamics in exercise and ageing. Ageing Res Rev 2020;58:101025.

[71] Azuma K, Ikeda K, Inoue S. Functional mechanisms of mitochondrial respiratory chain Supercomplex assembly factors and their involvement in muscle quality. Int J Mol Sci 2020;21(9):3182. https://doi.org/10.3390/ijms21093182.

[72] Eura Y, Ishihara N, Yokota S, Mihara K. Two mitofusin proteins, mammalian homologues of FZO, with distinct functions are both required for mitochondrial fusion. J Biochem (Tokyo) 2003;134:333–44.

[73] Legros F, Lombès A, Frachon P, Rojo M. Mitochondrial fusion in human cells is efficient, requires the inner membrane potential, and is mediated by mitofusins. Mol Biol Cell 2002;13:4343–54.

[74] Santel A, Fuller MT. Control of mitochondrial morphology by a human mitofusin. J Cell Sci 2001;114:867–74.

[75] Misaka T, Miyashita T, Kubo Y. Primary structure of a dynamin-related mouse mitochondrial GTPase and its distribution in brain, subcellular localization, and effect on mitochondrial morphology. J Biol Chem 2002;277:15834–42.

[76] Lee Y, Jeong S-Y, Karbowski M, Smith CL, Youle RJ. Roles of the mammalian mitochondrial fission and fusion mediators Fis1, Drp1, and Opa1 in apoptosis. Mol Biol Cell 2004;15:5001–11.

[77] Mozdy AD, McCaffery JM, Shaw JM. Dnm1p GTPase-mediated mitochondrial fission is a multi-step process requiring the novel integral membrane component Fis1p. J Cell Biol 2000;151:367–80.

[78] James DI, Parone PA, Mattenberger Y, Martinou J-C. hFis1, a novel component of the mammalian mitochondrial fission machinery. J Biol Chem 2003;278:36373–9.

[79] Frank S, Gaume B, Bergmann-Leitner ES, Leitner WW, Robert EG, Catez F, Smith CL, Youle RJ. The role of dynamin-related protein 1, a mediator of mitochondrial fission, in apoptosis. Dev Cell 2001;1:515–25.

[80] Smirnova E, Shurland DL, Ryazantsev SN, van der Bliek AM. A human dynamin-related protein controls the distribution of mitochondria. J Cell Biol 1998;143:351–8.

[81] Pitts KR, Yoon Y, Krueger EW, McNiven MA. The dynamin-like protein DLP1 is essential for normal distribution and morphology of the endoplasmic reticulum and mitochondria in mammalian cells. Mol Biol Cell 1999;10:4403–17.

[82] Dulac M, Leduc-Gaudet J-P, Reynaud O, Ayoub M-B, Guérin A, Finkelchtein M, Hussain SN, Gouspillou G. Drp1 knockdown induces severe muscle atrophy and remodelling, mitochondrial dysfunction, autophagy impairment and denervation. J Physiol 2020;598(17):3691–710. https://doi.org/10.1113/JP279802.

[83] Dablainville V, Sanchez AM. The role of Drp1 in adult skeletal muscle physiology. J Physiol 2020;598(21):4761–3. https://doi.org/10.1113/JP280423.

[84] Li H, Shen L, Hu P, et al. Aging-associated mitochondrial DNA mutations alter oxidative phosphorylation machinery and cause mitochondrial dysfunctions. Biochim Biophys Acta Mol Basis Dis 2017;1863:2266–73.

[85] Peterson CM, Johannsen DL, Ravussin E. Skeletal muscle mitochondria and aging: a review. J Aging Res 2012;2012:194821.

[86] Rezuş E, Burlui A, Cardoneanu A, Rezuş C, Codreanu C, Pârvu M, Rusu Zota G, Tamba BI. Inactivity and skeletal muscle metabolism: a vicious cycle in old age. Int J Mol Sci 2020;21(2):592. https://doi.org/10.3390/ijms21020592.

[87] Vives-Bauza C, Zhou C, Huang Y, et al. PINK1-dependent recruitment of Parkin to mitochondria in mitophagy. Proc Natl Acad Sci U S A 2010;107:378–83.

[88] Matsuda N, Sato S, Shiba K, et al. PINK1 stabilized by mitochondrial depolarization recruits Parkin to damaged mitochondria and activates latent Parkin for mitophagy. J Cell Biol 2010;189:211–21.

[89] Kondapalli C, Kazlauskaite A, Zhang N, et al. PINK1 is activated by mitochondrial membrane potential depolarization and stimulates Parkin E3 ligase activity by phosphorylating serine 65. Open Biol 2012;2:120080.

[90] Bindoff LA, Birch-Machin MA, Cartlidge NE, Parker WD, Turnbull DM. Respiratory chain abnormalities in skeletal muscle from patients with Parkinson's disease. J Neurol Sci 1991;104:203–8.

[91] Cardellach F, Martí MJ, Fernández-Solà J, Marín C, Hoek JB, Tolosa E, Urbano-Márquez A. Mitochondrial respiratory chain activity in skeletal muscle from patients with Parkinson's disease. Neurology 1993;43:2258–62.

[92] Blin O, Desnuelle C, Rascol O, Borg M, Peyro Saint Paul H, Azulay JP, Billé F, Figarella D, Coulom F, Pellissier JF. Mitochondrial respiratory failure in skeletal muscle from patients with Parkinson's disease and multiple system atrophy. J Neurol Sci 1994;125:95–101.

[93] Kim Y, Park J, Kim S, Song S, Kwon S-K, Lee S-H, Kitada T, Kim J-M, Chung J. PINK1 controls mitochondrial localization of Parkin through direct phosphorylation. Biochem Biophys Res Commun 2008;377:975–80.

[94] Tanaka A, Cleland MM, Xu S, Narendra DP, Suen D-F, Karbowski M, Youle RJ. Proteasome and p97 mediate mitophagy and degradation of mitofusins induced by Parkin. J Cell Biol 2010;191:1367–80.

[95] Chan NC, Salazar AM, Pham AH, Sweredoski MJ, Kolawa NJ, Graham RLJ, Hess S, Chan DC. Broad activation of the ubiquitin-proteasome system by Parkin is critical for mitophagy. Hum Mol Genet 2011;20:1726–37.

[96] Glauser L, Sonnay S, Stafa K, Moore DJ. Parkin promotes the ubiquitination and degradation of the mitochondrial fusion factor mitofusin 1. J Neurochem 2011;118:636–45.

[97] Wang X, Winter D, Ashrafi G, Schlehe J, Wong YL, Selkoe D, Rice S, Steen J, LaVoie MJ, Schwarz TL. PINK1 and Parkin target Miro for phosphorylation and degradation to arrest mitochondrial motility. Cell 2011;147:893–906.

[98] Sarraf SA, Raman M, Guarani-Pereira V, Sowa ME, Huttlin EL, Gygi SP, Harper JW. Landscape of the PARKIN-dependent ubiquitylome in response to mitochondrial depolarization. Nature 2013;496:372–6.

[99] Nardin A, Schrepfer E, Ziviani E. Counteracting PINK/Parkin deficiency in the activation of mitophagy: a potential therapeutic intervention for Parkinson's disease. Curr Neuropharmacol 2016;14:250–9.

[100] Heo J-M, Ordureau A, Paulo JA, Rinehart J, Harper JW. The PINK1-PARKIN mitochondrial ubiquitylation pathway drives a program of OPTN/NDP52 recruitment and TBK1 activation to promote mitophagy. Mol Cell 2015;60:7–20.

[101] Shin J-H, Ko HS, Kang H, Lee Y, Lee Y-I, Pletinkova O, Troconso JC, Dawson VL, Dawson TM. PARIS (ZNF746) repression of PGC-1α contributes to neurodegeneration in Parkinson's disease. Cell 2011;144:689–702.

[102] Bayne AN, Trempe J-F. Mechanisms of PINK1, ubiquitin and Parkin interactions in mitochondrial quality control and beyond. Cell Mol Life Sci CMLS 2019;76:4589–611.

[103] McLelland G-L, Soubannier V, Chen CX, McBride HM, Fon EA. Parkin and PINK1 function in a vesicular trafficking pathway regulating mitochondrial quality control. EMBO J 2014;33:282–95.

[104] Sugiura A, McLelland G-L, Fon EA, McBride HM. A new pathway for mitochondrial quality control: mitochondrial-derived vesicles. EMBO J 2014;33:2142–56.

[105] Soubannier V, McLelland G-L, Zunino R, Braschi E, Rippstein P, Fon EA, McBride HM. A vesicular transport pathway shuttles cargo from mitochondria to lysosomes. Curr Biol 2012;22:135–41.

[106] Peker N, Donipadi V, Sharma M, McFarlane C, Kambadur R. Loss of Parkin impairs mitochondrial function and leads to muscle atrophy. Am J Physiol Cell Physiol 2018;315(2):C164–85. https://doi.org/10.1152/ajpcell.00064.2017.

[107] Gouspillou G, Godin R, Piquereau J, et al. Protective role of Parkin in skeletal muscle contractile and mitochondrial function. J Physiol 2018;596(13):2565–79. https://doi.org/10.1113/JP275604.

[108] Leduc-Gaudet J-P, Mayaki D, Reynaud O, Broering FE, Chaffer TJ, Hussain SNA, Gouspillou G. Parkin overexpression attenuates sepsis-induced muscle wasting. Cell 2020;9(6):1454. https://doi.org/10.3390/cells9061454.

[109] Leduc-Gaudet J-P, Reynaud O, Hussain SN, Gouspillou G. Parkin overexpression protects from ageing-related loss of muscle mass and strength. J Physiol 2019;597:1975–91.

[110] Balan E, Schwalm C, Naslain D, Nielens H, Francaux M, Deldicque L. Regular endurance exercise promotes fission, Mitophagy, and oxidative phosphorylation in human skeletal muscle independently of age. Front Physiol 2019;10:1088.

[111] Si H, Ma P, Liang Q, Yin Y, Wang P, Zhang Q, Wang S, Deng H. Overexpression of pink1 or parkin in indirect flight muscles promotes mitochondrial proteostasis and extends lifespan in *Drosophila melanogaster*. PLoS ONE 2019;14, e0225214.

[112] White Z, Terrill J, White RB, McMahon C, Sheard P, Grounds MD, Shavlakadze T. Voluntary resistance wheel exercise from mid-life prevents sarcopenia and increases markers of mitochondrial function and autophagy in muscles of old male and female C57BL/6J mice. Skelet Muscle 2016;6:45.

[113] Distefano G, Standley RA, Dubé JJ, Carnero EA, Ritov VB, Stefanovic-Racic M, Toledo FGS, Piva SR, Goodpaster BH, Coen PM. Chronological age does not influence ex-vivo mitochondrial respiration and quality control in skeletal muscle. J Gerontol A Biol Sci Med Sci 2017;72:535–42.

[114] Kim Y, Triolo M, Hood DA. Impact of aging and exercise on mitochondrial quality control in skeletal muscle. Oxid Med Cell Longev 2017;2017. https://doi.org/10.1155/2017/3165396, 3165396.

[115] Baehr LM, West DWD, Marcotte G, Marshall AG, De Sousa LG, Baar K, Bodine SC. Age-related deficits in skeletal muscle recovery following disuse are associated with neuromuscular junction instability and ER stress, not impaired protein synthesis. Aging 2016;8:127–46.

[116] Peng J, Ren K-D, Yang J, Luo X-J. Mitochondrial E3 ubiquitin ligase 1: a key enzyme in regulation of mitochondrial dynamics and functions. Mitochondrion 2016;28:49–53.

[117] Neuspiel M, Schauss AC, Braschi E, Zunino R, Rippstein P, Rachubinski RA, Andrade-Navarro MA, McBride HM. Cargo-selected transport from the mitochondria to peroxisomes is mediated by vesicular carriers. Curr Biol CB 2008;18:102–8.

[118] Li W, Bengtson MH, Ulbrich A, Matsuda A, Reddy VA, Orth A, Chanda SK, Batalov S, Joazeiro CAP. Genome-wide and functional annotation of human E3 ubiquitin ligases identifies MULAN, a mitochondrial E3 that regulates the organelle's dynamics and signaling. PLoS ONE 2008;3, e1487.

[119] Braschi E, Zunino R, McBride HM. MAPL is a new mitochondrial SUMO E3 ligase that regulates mitochondrial fission. EMBO Rep 2009;10:748–54.

[120] Li J, Qi W, Chen G, et al. Mitochondrial outer-membrane E3 ligase MUL1 ubiquitinates ULK1 and regulates selenite-induced mitophagy. Autophagy 2015;11:1216–29.

[121] Kim S-Y, Kim HJ, Byeon HK, Kim DH, Kim C-H. FOXO3 induces ubiquitylation of AKT through MUL1 regulation. Oncotarget 2017;8:110474–89.

[122] Cilenti L, Di Gregorio J, Ambivero CT, Andl T, Liao R, Zervos AS. Mitochondrial MUL1 E3 ubiquitin ligase regulates hypoxia inducible factor (HIF-1α) and metabolic reprogramming by modulating the UBXN7 cofactor protein. Sci Rep 2020;10(1):1609. https://doi.org/10.1038/s41598-020-58484-8.

[123] Ding Y, Li J, Liu Z, Liu H, Li H, Li Z. IGF-1 potentiates sensory innervation signalling by modulating the mitochondrial fission/fusion balance. Sci Rep 2017;7:43949.

[124] Pagano AF, Py G, Bernardi H, Candau RB, Sanchez AMJ. Autophagy and protein turnover signaling in slow-twitch muscle during exercise. Med Sci Sports Exerc 2014;46:1314–25.

[125] Brinkmann C, Przyklenk A, Metten A, Schiffer T, Bloch W, Brixius K, Gehlert S. Influence of endurance training on skeletal muscle mitophagy regulatory proteins in type 2 diabetic men. Endocr Res 2017;42:325–30.

[126] Beyfuss K, Hood DA. A systematic review of p53 regulation of oxidative stress in skeletal muscle. Redox Rep Commun Free Radic Res 2018;23:100–17.

[127] He MY, Xu SB, Qu ZH, et al. Hsp90β interacts with MDM2 to suppress p53-dependent senescence during skeletal muscle regeneration. Aging Cell 2019;18, e13003.

[128] Fåhraeus R, Olivares-Illana V. MDM2's social network. Oncogene 2014;33:4365–76.

[129] Bertaggia E, Coletto L, Sandri M. Posttranslational modifications control FoxO3 activity during denervation. Am J Physiol Cell Physiol 2012;302:C587–96.

[130] Ahmed MR, Zhan X, Song X, Kook S, Gurevich VV, Gurevich EV. Ubiquitin ligase parkin promotes Mdm2-arrestin interaction but inhibits arrestin ubiquitination. Biochemistry 2011;50:3749–63.

[131] Kook S, Zhan X, Thibeault K, Ahmed MR, Gurevich VV, Gurevich EV. Mdm2 enhances ligase activity of parkin and facilitates mitophagy. Sci Rep 2020;10(1):5028. https://doi.org/10.1038/s41598-020-61796-4.

[132] Arena G, Cissé MY, Pyrdziak S, et al. Mitochondrial MDM2 regulates respiratory complex I activity independently of p53. Mol Cell 2018;69:594–609. e8.

[133] Figueiredo VC, de Salles BF, Trajano GS. Volume for muscle hypertrophy and health outcomes: the most effective variable in resistance training. Sports Med Auckl NZ 2018;48:499–505.

[134] Watier T, Sanchez AM. Micro-RNAs, exercise and cellular plasticity in humans: the impact of dietary factors and hypoxia. MicroRNA Shariqah United Arab Emir 2017;6:110–24.

[135] Stec MJ, Mayhew DL, Bamman MM. The effects of age and resistance loading on skeletal muscle ribosome biogenesis. J Appl Physiol (1985) 2015;119:851–7.

[136] Ades PA, Ballor DL, Ashikaga T, Utton JL, Nair KS. Weight training improves walking endurance in healthy elderly persons. Ann Intern Med 1996;124:568–72.

[137] Frontera WR, Meredith CN, O'Reilly KP, Knuttgen HG, Evans WJ. Strength conditioning in older men: skeletal muscle hypertrophy and improved function. J Appl Physiol (1985) 1988;64:1038–44.

[138] Frontera WR, Meredith CN, O'Reilly KP, Evans WJ. Strength training and determinants of VO2max in older men. J Appl Physiol (1985) 1990;68:329–33.

[139] Karlsen A, Soendenbroe C, Malmgaard-Clausen NM, et al. Preserved capacity for satellite cell proliferation, regeneration, and hypertrophy in the skeletal muscle of healthy elderly men. FASEB J Off Publ Fed Am Soc Exp Biol 2020;34(5):6418–36. https://doi.org/10.1096/fj.202000196R.

[140] Moro T, Brightwell CR, Volpi E, Rasmussen BB, Fry CS. Resistance exercise training promotes fiber type-specific myonuclear adaptations in older adults. J Appl Physiol (1985) 2020;128:795–804.

[141] Parry HA, Roberts MD, Kavazis AN. Human skeletal muscle mitochondrial adaptations following resistance exercise training. Int J Sports Med 2020;41(6):349–59. https://doi.org/10.1055/a-1121-7851.

[142] Sahin UK, Kirdi N, Bozoglu E, Meric A, Buyukturan G, Ozturk A, Doruk H. Effect of low-intensity versus high-intensity resistance training on the functioning of the institutionalized frail elderly. Int J Rehabil Res Int Z Rehabil Rev Int Rech Readaptation 2018;41:211–7.

[143] Taaffe DR, Pruitt L, Pyka G, Guido D, Marcus R. Comparative effects of high- and low-intensity resistance training on thigh muscle strength, fiber area, and tissue composition in elderly women. Clin Physiol Oxf Engl 1996;16:381–92.

[144] Hortobágyi T, Tunnel D, Moody J, Beam S, DeVita P. Low- or high-intensity strength training partially restores impaired quadriceps force accuracy and steadiness in aged adults. J Gerontol A Biol Sci Med Sci 2001;56:B38–47.

[145] Vincent KR, Braith RW, Feldman RA, Kallas HE, Lowenthal DT. Improved cardiorespiratory endurance following 6 months of resistance exercise in elderly men and women. Arch Intern Med 2002;162:673–8.

[146] Hammarström D, Øfsteng S, Koll L, Hanestadhaugen M, Hollan I, Apro W, Whist JE, Blomstrand E, Rønnestad BR, Ellefsen S. Benefits of higher resistance-training volume are related to ribosome biogenesis. J Physiol 2019;598(3):543–65. https://doi.org/10.1113/JP278455.

[147] Solsona R, Sanchez AMJ. Ribosome biogenesis and resistance training volume in human skeletal muscle. J Physiol 2020;598:1121–2.

[148] Berg OK, Kwon OS, Hureau TJ, et al. Skeletal muscle mitochondrial adaptations to maximal strength training in older adults. J Gerontol A Biol Sci Med Sci 2020;75(12):2269–77. https://doi.org/10.1093/gerona/glaa082.

[149] Zane AC, Reiter DA, Shardell M, Cameron D, Simonsick EM, Fishbein KW, Studenski SA, Spencer RG, Ferrucci L. Muscle strength mediates the relationship between mitochondrial energetics and walking performance. Aging Cell 2017;16:461–8.

[150] Bullo V, Gobbo S, Vendramin B, Duregon F, Cugusi L, Di Blasio A, Bocalini DS, Zaccaria M, Bergamin M, Ermolao A. Nordic walking can be incorporated in the exercise prescription to increase aerobic capacity, strength, and quality of life for elderly: a systematic review and meta-analysis. Rejuvenation Res 2018;21:141–61.

[151] Rahbek SK, Farup J, Møller AB, Vendelbo MH, Holm L, Jessen N, Vissing K. Effects of divergent resistance exercise contraction mode and dietary supplementation type on anabolic signalling, muscle protein synthesis and muscle hypertrophy. Amino Acids 2014;46:2377–92.

[152] Roig M, O'Brien K, Kirk G, Murray R, McKinnon P, Shadgan B, Reid WD. The effects of eccentric versus concentric resistance training on muscle strength and mass in healthy adults: a systematic review with meta-analysis. Br J Sports Med 2009;43:556–68.

[153] Norrbrand L, Fluckey JD, Pozzo M, Tesch PA. Resistance training using eccentric overload induces early adaptations in skeletal muscle size. Eur J Appl Physiol 2008;102:271–81.

[154] Ato S, Makanae Y, Kido K, Fujita S. Contraction mode itself does not determine the level of mTORC1 activity in rat skeletal muscle. Physiol Rep 2016;4(19):e12976. https://doi.org/10.14814/phy2.12976.

[155] Garma T, Kobayashi C, Haddad F, Adams GR, Bodell PW, Baldwin KM. Similar acute molecular responses to equivalent volumes of isometric, lengthening, or shortening mode resistance exercise. J Appl Physiol (1985) 2007;102:135–43.

[156] Ato S, Makanae Y, Kido K, Sase K, Yoshii N, Fujita S. The effect of different acute muscle contraction regimens on the expression of muscle proteolytic signaling proteins and genes. Physiol Rep 2017;5(15):e13364. https://doi.org/10.14814/phy2.13364.

[157] Lo Verso F, Carnio S, Vainshtein A, Sandri M. Autophagy is not required to sustain exercise and PRKAA1/AMPK activity but is important to prevent mitochondrial damage during physical activity. Autophagy 2014;10:1883–94.

[158] Rizo-Roca D, Ríos-Kristjánsson JG, Núñez-Espinosa C, Santos-Alves E, Magalhães J, Ascensão A, Pagès T, Viscor G, Torrella JR. Modulation of mitochondrial biomarkers by intermittent hypobaric hypoxia and aerobic exercise after eccentric exercise in trained rats. Appl Physiol Nutr Metab Physiol Appl Nutr Metab 2017;42:683–93.

[159] Klarod K, Philippe M, Gatterer H, Burtscher M. Different training responses to eccentric endurance exercise at low and moderate altitudes in pre-diabetic men: a pilot study. Sport Sci Health 2017;13:615–23.

CHAPTER 10

Underlying mechanisms of sarcopenic obesity

Melanie Rauen, Leo Cornelius Bollheimer, and Mahtab Nourbakhsh
Geriatric Medicine (Medical Clinic VI), RWTH Aachen University Hospital, Aachen, Germany

Abstract
Sarcopenic obesity is a multifactorial syndrome that is characterized by the co-occurrence of obesity and sarcopenia. The pathogenic mechanisms of sarcopenia and obesity seem to be synergistically connected and increase the risk of all-cause mortality in aging populations. With the increasing trend of obesity in our globally growing aging population, sarcopenic obesity will become a major public health issue over the next few decades. Thus, capturing the underlying mechanisms of sarcopenic obesity has strong potential in the development of preventive strategies, which may reduce the future burden of morbidity and mortality. This chapter focuses on the current definitions, diagnostic criteria, and knowledge of dysregulated pathways and the common molecular mechanisms of sarcopenia and obesity that are possibly involved in the pathogenesis of sarcopenic obesity.

Keywords: Fatty acids, Inflammation, Insulin resistance, Lipids, Metabolism, Myokines, Obesity, Sarcopenia, Satellite cells, Skeletal muscle

Introduction

Sarcopenia is mostly known as progressive loss of skeletal muscle mass and function by aging. Patients suffering from sarcopenia are likely to have higher risks of frailty and falls and even increased mortality [1–3]. Its prevalence is estimated to range from 9.9% up to 40.4% [4]. It is difficult to determine a more specific number, as cut-offs in diagnosis appear to differ for populations worldwide [5]. However, aging is not the only condition that has been linked to sarcopenia. The European working group on sarcopenia in older people (EWGSOP) proposed the concept of primary sarcopenia (age-related) and secondary sarcopenia (disease-related, malnutrition-related, and inactivity-related) [6,7]. Diabetes type 2 [8], osteoarthritis [9], chronic kidney disease [10], cardiovascular disease [11,12], chronic liver disease [13], and chronic obstructive lung disease [14] are a few conditions that have been associated with sarcopenia. In particular, obesity synergistically interacts with sarcopenia, deteriorating health status beyond either condition separately [15,16]. Both the onset and severity of sarcopenia are impaired by physical inactivity and fat-rich diets, resulting in increased body fat mass relative to muscle mass, a condition designated as "sarcopenic obesity" [17]. With the rising rates of obese individuals [18] in the elderly population [19], sarcopenic obesity may become a major health threat not only to the elderly population. There is increasing evidence that sarcopenic obesity also occurs in younger populations depending on the applied diagnostic [20]. Moreover, a consensus on sarcopenic obesity definition and diagnostic criteria has not yet been established [21,22], and the estimated sarcopenic obesity prevalence in different studies may be obscured by inconsistencies of applied diagnostic tools for obesity, sarcopenia, and sarcopenic obesity [23]. Nevertheless, several clinical studies have suggested that insulin resistance, inflammation, and high levels of circulating free fatty acids may play an important role in the development of sarcopenic obesity [24]. Moreover, in vitro studies could implicate distinct signaling pathways, potentially linking obesity with pathological muscle impairments.

Diagnostic criteria
Obesity

Obesity is a complex disease involving an excessive amount and/or abnormal distribution of body fat. The international diagnosis of obesity includes body mass index, waist circumference, waist-to-hip ratio, and body fat rate [17,25]. Initially, body mass index has been commonly used as the most convenient tool for the diagnosis of obesity in sarcopenic individuals [23,26,27]. However, the sufficiency of body mass index to determine obesity in adults has been questioned in the past [23,28,29]. The fat mass may start declining with aging. However, the loss of lean body mass that starts in middle age is typically continued by an increase in fat mass [30]. As a result, the total body weight may remain stable or increase slightly, although the body fat increases while lean body mass decreases. Moreover, it was shown that individuals with normal body mass index and body fat rate can have a high degree of metabolic dysregulation [31]. This phenomenon, defined as normal weight obesity, was associated with a significantly higher risk of cardiometabolic dysfunction and with higher mortality [31]. Especially at older ages, visceral fat and relative loss of fat-free mass may become relatively more important than body mass index [32,33]. Not only muscle mass but also overall fat-free mass declines with aging [34]. Currently, the term lean mass is commonly used to describe the fat-free mass in the body. A recent study identified a link between falls and higher body mass index [35]. In line with this observation, various studies emphasized the importance of body composition analysis using imaging techniques, such as dual-energy X-ray absorptiometry, computed tomography, magnetic resonance imaging, ultrasound, and elemental partition analysis [23,25,27,29,36,37]. However, a few drawbacks of these methods have to be considered. The operation of imaging devices is often expensive and technically challenging. Some of the technical equipment requires additional adjustments for highly obese patients. Therefore, most reported studies on obesity tried to find a compromise toward a feasible diagnostic standard individually.

Sarcopenia

A wide variety of tests and tools have been established for the characterization of sarcopenia in practice and research [38]. The latest consensus on the diagnosis of sarcopenia recommends a selection of tools depending on the patient's disability or morbidity, access to technical resources, or the purpose of testing, such as monitoring of disease progression or rehabilitation and recovery. In clinical practice, a basic 5-item questionnaire has been established as a primary screen for sarcopenia risk [39]. This tool and its variants are inexpensive and convenient, but they have low-to-moderate sensitivity, mostly detecting severe cases of low muscle strength [40]. More sensitive tools for the diagnosis of sarcopenia include assessment of physical performance and measurement of skeletal muscle mass using three main imaging techniques, dual-energy X-ray absorptiometry; bioelectrical impedance analysis; computed tomography, magnetic resonance spectroscopy, or magnetic resonance imaging [26,41–43].

Sarcopenic obesity

Different definitions of sarcopenic obesity exist, and its diagnostic and exclusion criteria are not commonly established. Therefore, the prevalence rate of sarcopenic obesity can vary significantly within different studies depending on the applied diagnostics [22,44,45]. The diagnostic criteria for sarcopenic obesity certainly rely on the most current consensus of the definition and diagnosis for sarcopenia and obesity, bearing modifications and adjustments during the last two decades (Table 1). Initially, sarcopenic obesity was diagnosed as a body fat rate exceeding the population level by 60%, and the dual-energy X-ray absorptiometry or bioelectrical impedance analysis estimated that muscle mass was lower than the population level by 60% [46,47]. Since the revision of the European consensus for the definition of sarcopenia, sarcopenic obesity diagnoses progressively include a comprehensive evaluation of muscle strength and muscle function, and the association of sarcopenic obesity with increased waist circumference and impaired muscle mass and strength is well documented in the quadriceps [48,49]. Moreover, the diagnosis of sarcopenia can be obscured by advanced obesity [23,38]. Among the most convenient diagnostic criteria for sarcopenia in adults and the elderly, body fat rate seems to be more reliable and indicative in the detection of sarcopenic obesity than body mass index methods in these studies [44,45]. It was recently reported that the grip-to-body mass index ratio can serve as a diagnostic tool for sarcopenic obesity in children aged between 6 and 10 years [50]. However, the gold standard in sarcopenic obesity diagnosis includes body composition imaging using abdominal magnetic resonance (MR) and the simultaneous quantification of muscle mass and subcutaneous and visceral fat [51].

A systematic review was recently performed to summarize the available literature on the definitions and the diagnostic criteria for sarcopenic obesity, which were proposed or applied in human studies [52]. In general, the majority of the reports on sarcopenic obesity

Table 1: Most frequently used parameters for the diagnosis of sarcopenia, obesity, or sarcopenic obesity.

Sarcopenia	Sarcopenic obesity	Obesity
	60% lower skeletal muscle mass and 60% higher body fat than the population mean level	
Fat-free mass index	→ ←	Fat mass index
Appendicular skeletal mass	→ ←	Visceral fat mass
Appendicular skeletal mass/hight^2	→ ←	Waist circumference
Appendicular skeletal mass/body weight	→ ←	Body fat mass
Appendicular skeletal mass/hight^2 and gait speed or handgrip strength	→ ←	Body mass index

were cross-sectional studies, which applied different tools or cut-offs for the diagnosis of sarcopenic obesity in six different fields of interest, including the definition of relevant biological factors, comorbidities, impaired physical action, musculoskeletal disorders, mental health, and hospitalization. Thus, the results could not allow for consensus on the definition and diagnostic criteria of sarcopenic obesity with wide clinical applicability and consistent cut-off values.

Pathogenesis of sarcopenic obesity

Several different factors are known to increase the complexity of sarcopenic obesity pathogenesis. They include age-related decline of physical activities, changes in body composition and fat metabolism, low-grade inflammation, and insulin resistance [53]. Therefore, it is important to take these factors and their molecular pathways into account while addressing the underlying mechanisms of sarcopenic obesity.

Aging results in a progressive decline of skeletal muscle mass and physical activity [54,55]. Obesity is the main cause of systemic low-grade inflammation. Proinflammatory cells such as macrophages accumulate in aged adipose tissue, creating an inflammatory milieu, which induces insulin resistance. Thus, obesity and aging induce substantial changes in fat metabolism, which lead to increased fat deposits in nonadipose tissue, such as skeletal muscles. In turn, the intramuscular lipids induce local inflammation in skeletal muscle, which

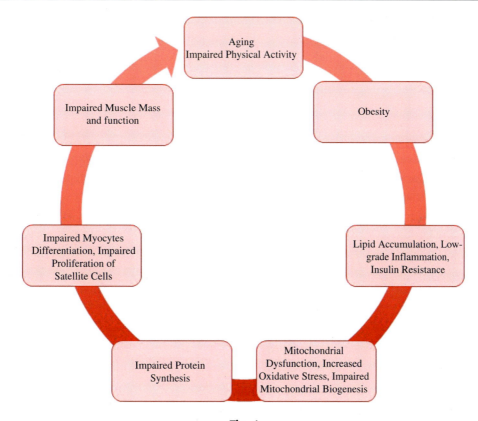

Fig. 1
Pathogenic cycle of sarcopenic obesity.

leads to impaired physical activity, and is the main trigger of sarcopenic obesity [56]. Obesity and sarcopenia result in a pathological cycle by interaction and influencing each other by involving multiple signaling pathways at systemic and cellular levels (Fig. 1).

Metabolism

Lipid accumulation

Lipids are a group of fat-soluble tissue compounds classified as fats or phospholipids. Fats are the fatty acid esters of glycerol, present as monoglycerides, diglycerides, or triglycerides, and compose the primary energy depot. Fatty acids are organic acids largely defined by the length and saturation of the aliphatic side chain attached to a carboxylic acid. In mammals, these side chains normally contain an even number of carbon atoms, and fatty acids are grouped into short chain (2–6 carbon atoms), medium chain (8–12 carbon atoms), long chain (14–18 carbon atoms), and longer chain (20–26 carbon atoms). The major types of fatty acids in the circulation and the tissues of mammals are the long-chain and longer-chain fatty acids with varying degrees of saturation. These include palmitic acid (C16:0), palmitoleic acid (C16:1), stearic acid (C:18:0), oleic acid (C18:1n-9), linoleic acid (C18:2n-6), and, particularly in smaller mammals, arachidonic acid (20:4n-6) and docosahexaenoic acid (22:6n-3). While C16–C18 fatty acids can act as signaling molecules, such as diacylglycerols (DAGs) or ceramides, C20–C22 unsaturated fatty acids can also serve as basic structures for the synthesis of signaling molecules, such as prostaglandins and leukotrienes [57].

In young adults, up to 50% of the bodyweight comprises the lean muscle mass, which declines progressively to approximately 25% with aging. Concomitantly, body fat deposits increase, particularly in visceral adipose tissue [58,59]. Excessive body fat deposits, as in obesity, are associated with elevated plasma triglycerides levels, high low-density lipoprotein (LDL)-Chol, and low high-density lipoprotein (HDL)-Chol contents [38,39]. Triglycerides are transported in the form of VLDL in the bloodstream. The excess of circulating triglycerides is not only stored in visceral adipose tissue, but also accumulate in the liver, heart, pancreas, or skeletal muscle (Fig. 2) [60–62]. Hence, obesity has been shown to increase fat deposits at intracellular levels in adipocytes and nonadipogenic cells, such as skeletal muscle cells and adipose tissue-resident macrophages (ATMs) via VLDL receptor (VLDLR), which is an important target for diet-induced obesity and inflammation [40,41].

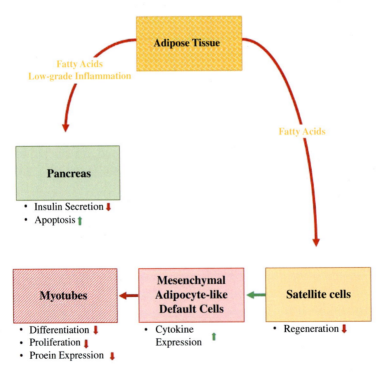

Fig. 2
Relevant pathways in sarcopenic obesity.

In skeletal muscle tissue, increased fatty acid deposits were shown to induce lipotoxicity, inhibit the regeneration of satellite cells, and promote their differentiation into mesenchymal adipocyte-like default cells. The accumulation of mesenchymal adipocyte-like default cells in muscle tissue reduces the regenerative capacity of muscle tissue [63].

In adipose tissue, adipose tissue macrophages (ATMs) uptake lipids primarily from circulating free fatty acids and necrotic adipocytes [64]. Muscle and adipose tissue are the main sources of free fatty acids, where triglyceride lipoproteins are hydrolyzed by lipoprotein lipase. Distinct genetic mutations in lipoprotein lipase have been shown to reduce lipid storage in macrophages and increase circulating free fatty acid levels [19]. The high level of circulating lipids deposits as a triacylglycerol or its derivatives, such as diacylglycerol, long-chain acyl CoA, and ceramide, in skeletal muscle cells [65,66]. Several previous reports established the association of intra-myocellular diacylglycerol, long-chain acyl CoA, and ceramide with decreased insulin sensitivity [67]. It was shown that these molecules interact with different targets in the insulin signaling pathway [68]. In pancreatic islet cells, accumulation of saturated palmitic acid was reported to inhibit cell proliferation and lead to decreased insulin production and secretion [61,69]. Based on the established links between excessive lipid storage in obesity and insulin resistance in muscle, the role of fatty acids should be considered not only as an alternative energy substrate to glucose.

Mitochondrial dysfunction

Adequate energy supply and sufficient protein synthesis are the most relevant prerequisites for muscle health and function. Mitochondria play a crucial role in the oxidative production of energy, including oxidative phosphorylation to produce cellular adenosine triphosphate. They also play important roles in ion homeostasis, several metabolic pathways, apoptosis and programmed cell death, and reactive oxygen species production and consumption. All of these functions are significant in aging. Mitochondrial dysfunction has been implicated in aging and aging-associated diseases involving inadequate adenosine triphosphate synthesis, Ca^{2+} homeostasis, central metabolic pathways, or radical production. However, the mechanisms and regulation of reactive oxygen species formation by mitochondria remain poorly understood. Aging may lead to the accumulation of dysfunctional components in mitochondria caused directly by radicals or mutation of nuclear or mitochondrial DNA [70,71]. These effects may be further aggravated by the degradation of protective mechanisms against mitochondrial destruction [72]. The biogenesis of mitochondria is in turn regulated by the peroxisome proliferator-activated receptor-gamma coactivator 1-alpha [73–75]. For instance, exercise has been shown to activate this coactivator and to improve the low mitochondrial biogenesis in aging [76]. Excessive deposit of intra-myocellular lipids results in mitochondrial dysfunction, which elevates the production of reactive oxygen species and decreases new protein synthesis [77,78]. The most consequential result of this is a successive decline of fatty acid oxidation, which triggers the onset of insulin resistance [79]. Previous reports have suggested that reactive oxygen species can establish a destructive positive feedback loop via different pathways by insulin resistance, which in turn further increases reactive oxygen species production [80]. Further studies have shown that insulin resistance also impacts the size of mitochondria and the expression of mitochondrial genes [81]. Although the complex link between mitochondrial function in the pathogenesis of insulin resistance is well recognized, the underlying pathways remain to be identified.

Insulin resistance

Insulin regulates cell growth and promotes energy storage. Dysregulation of its pathway causes different metabolic disorders. Insulin acts at the cellular level by binding to the insulin receptor, which is then internalized by clathrin-mediated endocytosis. The mechanism and regulation of clathrin-mediated endocytosis of insulin receptors are still not known. After the binding of multiple insulin molecules, the insulin receptor acts as an autophosphorylating tyrosine kinase by suppressing its autoinhibitory conformation [82,83]. Activated insulin receptor kinase cascade recruits and activates two major signaling pathways, the phosphatidylinositol 3-kinase (PI3K)/AKT pathway and the MAPK pathway. The PI3K-PKB/AKT pathway is primarily responsible for controlling metabolism. The dysregulation of the insulin-mediated activation of the MAPK pathway has been shown to contribute to the development of insulin resistance [84,85]. Insulin insensitivity is characterized by suboptimal insulin-stimulated uptake of glucose into muscle and adipose tissue. In turn, this causes weight gain, wherein adipose tissue expands and accommodates lipids [86].

Inflammation

Obesity is often caused by a chronic imbalance between energy expenditure and energy intake. The expansion and hypertrophy of adipose tissue contribute to the chronic, low-grade inflammatory state. In particular, visceral fat secretes a variety of cytokines, such as C-reactive protein, interleukin-6, and tumor necrosis factor-α. Chronic accumulation of inflammatory cytokines during aging leads to a redox imbalance that plays an important role in age-related diseases [87]. According to the latest research, C-reactive protein, interleukin-6, and tumor necrosis factor-α are considered to be the most related cytokines of sarcopenia [87]. However, there is no clearly defined link between any cytokine and sarcopenic obesity. Only a few studies have reported elevated levels of these inflammatory cytokines in distinctly defined sarcopenic obesity groups.

Analysis of the changes of C-reactive protein levels in an aging population revealed three subpopulations: sarcopenic patients with the highest C-reactive protein levels, sarcopenic obesity patients and nonsarcopenic obese patients with high C-reactive protein levels, and patients with normal body composition with the lowest C-reactive protein levels. A cross-sectional study including 237,838 South Korean participants demonstrated that a high level of C-reactive protein was associated with sarcopenic obesity independent of sex or age [88]. However, a stronger association was reported in female and younger (< 60 years) subjects. Another cross-sectional study of 1370 obese bariatric surgery candidates aged ≥ 18 revealed that age is also an independent predictor of sarcopenic obesity in obese female subjects aged > 60 years [89].

A previous community-based study of 378 men and 493 women (> 65 years) showed that sarcopenic obesity diagnosed based on grip strength and body mass index was associated with elevated levels of interleukin-6 and C-reactive protein after adjusting for age, sex, education, smoking history, and physical activity [90]. A recent study of sarcopenic obesity prevalence in 64 obese elderly women (> 68 years) revealed that sarcopenic obesity diagnosed based on body fat rate and dual-energy X-ray absorptiometry was significantly associated with interleukin-6 [91].

A possible implication of tumor necrosis factor-α in sarcopenic obesity pathogenesis was first suggested by the association between − 308 G/A tumor necrosis factor-α gene polymorphism, which increases tumor necrosis factor-α expression, and appendicular skeletal muscle mass [92]. In this study, tumor necrosis factor-α expression was associated with sarcopenic obesity diagnosed based on body mass index and dual-energy X-ray absorptiometry.

Muscle atrophy

Aging is accompanied by an imbalance between regeneration and degradation of muscle tissue, which leads to a progressive decline of skeletal muscle mass [93]. It has been well established that increasing fat deposits and declining muscle mass are the major modifications in skeletal muscle tissue observed during aging [94]. Increasing fat deposits and intra-myocellular fat exacerbates muscle mass decline by interfering with mitochondrial function and by the activation of proinflammatory pathways as mentioned earlier. Additionally, skeletal muscle expresses a variety of endocrine factors, called myokines, that exert effects in autocrine, paracrine, or endocrine manner to regulate regenerative and degenerative processes in skeletal muscle and other tissues (Table 2) [56,95,98–109,111–113]. The best-studied myokines, thus far, are musclin, LIF, interleukin-4, interleukin-6, interleukin-7, interleukin-15, and myostatin, the latter of which negatively regulates myogenesis in an autocrine manner [101,114]. Myostatin is a member of the transforming growth factor-β superfamily and has been shown to activate Smad 2 and 3, which regulate genes involved in the differentiation of muscle stem cells, called satellite cells, protein synthesis, and degradation in myofibers [115,116]. In addition, myostatin can inhibit the proliferation of satellite cells through paired-box-protein 7 [110]. Previous studies have suggested that blocking of myostatin enhances skeletal muscle growth, which was associated with increased protein synthesis and signaling of mammalian target of rapamycin complex-1 [117]. Mammalian target of rapamycin complex-1 activates protein synthesis and cell growth by adequate energy resources, nutrient availability, oxygen abundance, and proper growth factors. Therefore, all processes that are required for protein synthesis affect the mammalian target of rapamycin complex-1 activation.

Table 2: Regulatory factors involved in skeletal muscle biogenesis and fat metabolism.

Factor	Mechanisms
Angiopoietin-like 4	Induced by exercise, involved in lipid metabolism [95–97]
Apelin	Decreased by aging, regulates water and food intake, induces satellite cells proliferation [98]
Brain-derived neurotrophic factor	Expressed in satellite cells and enhances fat oxidation [99]
Beta-aminoisobutyric acid	Expressed in skeletal muscle, inhibits obesity-induced inflammation, and insulin resistance [100]
Decorin	Promotes muscle hypertrophy, inhibits myostatin
Fibroblast growth factor-21	Regulates mitophagy and muscle mass [101]
Interleukin-6	Induced by exercise [102,103]
Interleukin-15	Induced in skeletal muscle by inflammation, promotes myositis via CD^{8+} T cells [104]
Insulin-like growth factor-1	Induces muscle growth via mammalian target of rapamycin [105]
Insulin	Stimulates protein synthesis in skeletal muscle [106]
Leukemia inhibitory factor	Induced by exercise, stimulates muscle regeneration [107]
Meteorin-like protein	Regulates insulin sensitivity, facilitates skeletal muscle repair [108]
Musclin	Regulates glucose metabolism, contributes to obesity and insulin resistance [109]
Myostatin	Produced and secreted by myocytes, inhibits muscle cell growth and differentiation [98,103,110]

Growth hormones

Endocrine factors influence body composition, and testosterone is one of the best-studied factors involved in the augmentation of skeletal muscle mass and increased protein synthesis in muscle cells [118]. Levels of this hormone decline with age and are individually affected by nutrition and physical activity [119–121]. Several studies have reported that short-term testosterone administration to elderly men elevates skeletal muscle strength and protein synthesis [120–123]. Similar results were obtained with growth hormones [120,124,125]. Interestingly, low levels of testosterone together with a decline in insulin-like growth factor-I were shown to increase the risk of frailty in an aging population [126]. In contrast, 6 months' supplementation of testosterone in healthy elderly men with low endogenous testosterone levels could not enhance their functional mobility or muscle strength [127]. Although testosterone, growth, or insulin-like growth hormones play key roles in maintaining muscle health, their possible improving effects on muscle function in aging remain elusive.

Intervention strategies in sarcopenic obesity

Recent clinical studies on sarcopenia and obesity highlighted effective outcomes from nonpharmacological interventions via an adequate nutrition regime and exercise. However, there are no studies explicitly addressing sarcopenic obesity in an aging population combined with exercise and nutritional interventions, including specific weight loss targets. Although the current evidence on successful interventions in sarcopenic obesity is limited, combined exercise and nutrition interventions, exercise interventions, and nutritional interventions for sarcopenic obesity should be addressed. Skeletal muscle is activated most strongly by exercise, which dramatically increases the uptake and utilization of oxygen and energy substrates. These changes occur within a very short time, highlighting the ability of the skeletal muscle to respond rapidly and effectively to physical stress. However, long-term exercise induces an adaptive response, which elevates oxidative capacity, mitochondrial density, and insulin sensitivity in skeletal muscle [128,129].

In a study of obese aging and frail older adults, positive effects on body weight and physical performance were achieved using a complex intervention combining a weight loss diet and exercise [76]. The exercise program consisted of strength and endurance, balance, and flexibility exercises. The diet intervention involved an energy deficit of 500–750 kcal/d and protein supplementation of 1 g/kg body weight/d. The best effects on function were found in the combined weight loss diet and exercise group compared to the separate interventions or no intervention groups. Although interventions with weight loss are not favorable for sarcopenic patients, there is evidence of complex interventions combining exercise and nutritional supplementation in sarcopenia [130]. Resistance training together with protein or amino acid was reported to provide beneficial effects on muscle function and/or muscle size. In several studies, supplementation of vitamin D was addressed to attenuate the progressive loss of muscle mass in sarcopenic adults [131,132]. However, the results were not conclusive based on suboptimal inclusion criteria and the diverging results regarding balance, gait, muscle strength, and function [96,133]. Similarly, a meta-analysis found no effect of vitamin D supplementation in older adults [97]. The vast variations in the characteristics of different study populations, the unknown level of vitamin D deficiency at the study initiation, and vitamin D doses do not currently allow reliable conclusions [134].

Conclusion

Current research shows that a complex interacting network of inflammatory and metabolic pathways underlies the pathogenesis of sarcopenic obesity. Although some pieces of this puzzle seem to be identified as discussed here, further extensive studies under standard clinical definitions and procedures are required to capture the whole picture. A widely accepted definition and diagnostic cut-off criteria are essential prerequisites for advancing the clinical research on underlying mechanisms of sarcopenic obesity. Until then, solid guidelines for successful intervention strategies cannot be established. According to our most current knowledge from clinical studies, the most promising approach is an individually developed combination of exercise programs comprising strength and aerobic exercise and a dietary regime that can ensure supervised moderate weight loss and protein supplementation. This strategy may have some detectable positive effects on the function and quality of muscle tissue in sarcopenic obese elderly people. From a public health perspective, any stage of improvement will be clinically relevant and an important achievement, considering the high vulnerability of frail sarcopenic older adults.

References

[1] Kamijo Y, Kanda E, Ishibashi Y, Yoshida M. Sarcopenia and frailty in PD: impact on mortality, malnutrition, and inflammation. Perit Dial Int 2018;38(6):447–54.

[2] Schneider DA, Trence DL. Possible role of nutrition in prevention of sarcopenia and falls. Endocr Pract 2019;25(11):1184–90.

[3] Zhang X, Huang P, Dou Q, Wang C, Zhang W, Yang Y, et al. Falls among older adults with sarcopenia dwelling in nursing home or community: a meta-analysis. Clin Nutr 2020;39(1):33–9.

[4] Mayhew AJ, Amog K, Phillips S, Parise G, McNicholas PD, de Souza RJ, et al. The prevalence of sarcopenia in community-dwelling older adults, an exploration of differences between studies and within definitions: a systematic review and meta-analyses. Age Ageing 2019;48(1):48–56.

[5] Moreira VG, Perez M, Lourenço RA. Prevalence of sarcopenia and its associated factors: the impact of muscle mass, gait speed, and handgrip strength reference values on reported frequencies. Clinics (Sao Paulo) 2019;74:e477.

[6] Cruz-Jentoft AJ, Baeyens JP, Bauer JM, Boirie Y, Cederholm T, Landi F, et al. Sarcopenia: European consensus on definition and diagnosis: report of the European Working Group on Sarcopenia in Older People. Age Ageing 2010;39(4):412–23.

[7] Cruz-Jentoft AJ, Bahat G, Bauer J, Boirie Y, Bruyère O, Cederholm T, et al. Sarcopenia: revised European consensus on definition and diagnosis. Age Ageing 2019;48(1):16–31.

[8] Mesinovic J, Zengin A, De Courten B, Ebeling PR, Scott D. Sarcopenia and type 2 diabetes mellitus: a bidirectional relationship. Diabetes Metab Syndr Obes 2019;12:1057–72.

[9] Kemmler W, Teschler M, Goisser S, Bebenek M, von Stengel S, Bollheimer LC, et al. Prevalence of sarcopenia in Germany and the corresponding effect of osteoarthritis in females 70 years and older living in the community: results of the FORMoSA study. Clin Interv Aging 2015;10:1565–73.

[10] Watanabe H, Enoki Y, Maruyama T. Sarcopenia in chronic kidney disease: factors, mechanisms, and therapeutic interventions. Biol Pharm Bull 2019;42(9):1437–45.

[11] von Haehling S. Muscle wasting and sarcopenia in heart failure: a brief overview of the current literature. ESC Heart Fail 2018;5(6):1074–82.

[12] Bellanti F, Romano AD, Lo Buglio A, Castriotta V, Guglielmi G, Greco A, et al. Oxidative stress is increased in sarcopenia and associated with cardiovascular disease risk in sarcopenic obesity. Maturitas 2018;109:6–12.

[13] Hsu C-S, Kao J-H. Sarcopenia and chronic liver diseases. Expert Rev Gastroenterol Hepatol 2018;12(12):1229–44.

[14] Benz E, Trajanoska K, Lahousse L, Schoufour JD, Terzikhan N, De Roos E, et al. Sarcopenia in COPD: a systematic review and meta-analysis. Eur Respir Rev 2019;28(154):190049.

[15] Parr EB, Coffey VG, Hawley JA. 'Sarcobesity': a metabolic conundrum. Maturitas 2013;74(2):109–13.

[16] Distefano G, Standley RA, Zhang X, Carnero EA, Yi F, Cornnell HH, et al. Physical activity unveils the relationship between mitochondrial energetics, muscle quality, and physical function in older adults. J Cachexia Sarcopenia Muscle 2018;9(2):279–94.

[17] Heber D, Ingles S, Ashley JM, Maxwell MH, Lyons RF, Elashoff RM. Clinical detection of sarcopenic obesity by bioelectrical impedance analysis. Am J Clin Nutr 1996;64(3 Suppl):472S–7S.

[18] Blüher M. Obesity: global epidemiology and pathogenesis. Nat Rev Endocrinol 2019;15(5):288–98.

[19] Lechleitner M. Obesity in elderly. Wien Med Wochenschr 2016;166(3–4):143–6.

[20] Stefanaki C, Peppa M, Boschiero D, Chrousos GP. Healthy overweight/obese youth: early osteosarcopenic obesity features. Eur J Clin Invest 2016;46(9):767–78.

[21] Nezameddin R, Itani L, Kreidieh D, El Masri D, Tannir H, El Ghoch M. Understanding sarcopenic obesity in terms of definition and health consequences: a clinical review. Curr Diabetes Rev 2020;16(9):957–61. https://doi.org/10.2174/1573399816666200109091449.
[22] Donini LM, Busetto L, Bauer JM, Bischoff S, Boirie Y, Cederholm T, et al. Critical appraisal of definitions and diagnostic criteria for sarcopenic obesity based on a systematic review. Clin Nutr 2019;39(8):2368–88.
[23] Johnson Stoklossa CA, Sharma AM, Forhan M, Siervo M, Padwal RS, Prado CM. Prevalence of sarcopenic obesity in adults with class II/III obesity using different diagnostic criteria. J Nutr Metab 2017;2017, 7307618.
[24] Stenholm S, Harris TB, Rantanen T, Visser M, Kritchevsky SB, Ferrucci L. Sarcopenic obesity: definition, cause and consequences. Curr Opin Clin Nutr Metab Care 2008;11(6):693–700.
[25] Ponti F, Santoro A, Mercatelli D, Gasperini C, Conte M, Martucci M, et al. Aging and imaging assessment of body composition: from fat to facts. Front Endocrinol (Lausanne) 2020;10:861.
[26] De Stefano F, Zambon S, Giacometti L, Sergi G, Corti MC, Manzato E, et al. Obesity, muscular strength, muscle composition and physical performance in an elderly population. J Nutr Health Aging 2015;19(7):785–91.
[27] Kelly OJ, Gilman JC, Boschiero D, Ilich JZ. Osteosarcopenic obesity: current knowledge, revised identification criteria and treatment principles. Nutrients 2019;11(4):747.
[28] Romero-Corral A, Somers VK, Sierra-Johnson J, Thomas RJ, Collazo-Clavell ML, Korinek J, et al. Accuracy of body mass index in diagnosing obesity in the adult general population. Int J Obes (Lond) 2008;32(6):959–66.
[29] Donini LM, Pinto A, Giusti AM, Lenzi A, Poggiogalle E. Obesity or BMI paradox? Beneath the tip of the iceberg. Front Nutr 2020;7:53.
[30] Kalyani RR, Corriere M, Ferrucci L. Age-related and disease-related muscle loss: the effect of diabetes, obesity, and other diseases. Lancet Diabetes Endocrinol 2014;2(10):819–29.
[31] Oliveros E, Somers VK, Sochor O, Goel K, Lopez-Jimenez F. The concept of normal weight obesity. Prog Cardiovasc Dis 2014;56(4):426–33.
[32] Bosello O, Vanzo A. Obesity paradox and aging. Eat Weight Disord 2019;26(1):27–35. https://doi.org/10.1007/s40519-019-00815-4.
[33] Hunter GR, Gower BA, Kane BL. Age related shift in visceral fat. Int J Body Compos Res 2010;8(3):103–8.
[34] Strugnell C, Dunstan DW, Magliano DJ, Zimmet PZ, Shaw JE, Daly RM. Influence of age and gender on fat mass, fat-free mass and skeletal muscle mass among Australian adults: the Australian diabetes, obesity and lifestyle study (AusDiab). J Nutr Health Aging 2014;18(5):540–6.
[35] Kioh SH, Mat S, Kamaruzzaman SB, Ibrahim F, Mokhtar MS, Hairi NN, et al. Does lower lean body mass mediate the relationship between falls and higher body mass index in Asian older persons? J Aging Phys Act 2019;1–8.
[36] Ribeiro SML, Kehayias JJ. Sarcopenia and the analysis of body composition. Adv Nutr 2014;5(3):260–7.
[37] Donini LM, Rosano A, Di Lazzaro L, Lubrano C, Carbonelli M, Pinto A, et al. Impact of disability, psychological status, and comorbidity on health-related quality of life perceived by subjects with obesity. Obes Facts 2020;13(2):191–200.
[38] Cruz-Jentoft AJ, Bahat G, Bauer J, Boirie Y, Bruyere O, Cederholm T, et al. Sarcopenia: revised European consensus on definition and diagnosis. Age Ageing 2019.
[39] Gade J, Quick AA, Beck AM, Ronholt F, Vinther A. SARC-F in hospitalized, geriatric medical patients – feasibility, prevalence of risk of sarcopenia, and characteristics of the risk group, including one-year follow-up. Clin Nutr ESPEN 2020;37:80–6.
[40] Krzyminska-Siemaszko R, Deskur-Smielecka E, Kaluzniak-Szymanowska A, Lewandowicz M, Wieczorowska-Tobis K. Comparison of diagnostic performance of SARC-F and its two modified versions (SARC-CalF and SARC-F+EBM) in community-dwelling older adults from Poland. Clin Interv Aging 2020;15:583–94.
[41] Schweitzer L, Geisler C, Pourhassan M, Braun W, Gluer CC, Bosy-Westphal A, et al. What is the best reference site for a single MRI slice to assess whole-body skeletal muscle and adipose tissue volumes in healthy adults? Am J Clin Nutr 2015;102(1):58–65.

[42] Sergi G, De Rui M, Stubbs B, Veronese N, Manzato E. Measurement of lean body mass using bioelectrical impedance analysis: a consideration of the pros and cons. Aging Clin Exp Res 2017;29(4):591–7.

[43] Grimm A, Meyer H, Nickel MD, Nittka M, Raithel E, Chaudry O, et al. Evaluation of 2-point, 3-point, and 6-point Dixon magnetic resonance imaging with flexible echo timing for muscle fat quantification. Eur J Radiol 2018;103:57–64.

[44] Kemmler W, Teschler M, Weissenfels A, Sieber C, Freiberger E, von Stengel S. Prevalence of sarcopenia and sarcopenic obesity in older German men using recognized definitions: high accordance but low overlap! Osteoporos Int 2017;28(6):1881–91.

[45] Oliveira TM, Roriz AKC, Barreto-Medeiros JM, Ferreira AJF, Ramos L. Sarcopenic obesity in community-dwelling older women, determined by different diagnostic methods. Nutr Hosp 2019;36(6):1267–72.

[46] Wannamethee SG, Atkins JL. Muscle loss and obesity: the health implications of sarcopenia and sarcopenic obesity. Proc Nutr Soc 2015;74(4):405–12.

[47] Chung JY, Kang HT, Lee DC, Lee HR, Lee YJ. Body composition and its association with cardiometabolic risk factors in the elderly: a focus on sarcopenic obesity. Arch Gerontol Geriatr 2013;56(1):270–8.

[48] Wada O, Kurita N, Kamitani T, Mizuno K. Implications of evaluating leg muscle mass and fat mass separately for quadriceps strength in knee osteoarthritis: the SPSS-OK study. Clin Rheumatol 2019;39(5):1655–61. https://doi.org/10.1007/s10067-019-04879-6.

[49] Johnson Stoklossa CA, Ghosh SS, Forhan M, Sharma AM, Terada T, Siervo M, et al. Poor physical function as a marker of sarcopenia in adults with class II/III obesity. Curr Dev Nutr 2017;2(3). nzx008-nzx.

[50] Gontarev S, Jakimovski M, Georgiev G. Using relative handgrip strength to identify children at risk of sarcopenic obesity. Nutr Hosp 2020;34(3):490–6.

[51] Kim S, Kim TH, Jeong CW, Lee C, Noh S, Kim JE, et al. Development of quantification software for evaluating body composition contents and its clinical application in sarcopenic obesity. Sci Rep 2020;10(1):10452.

[52] Di Lorenzo L, Pipoli A, Manghisi NM, Clodoveo ML, Corbo F, De Pergola G, et al. Nutritional hazard analysis and critical control points at work (NACCPW): interdisciplinary assessment of subjective and metabolic work-related risk of the workers and their prevention. Int J Food Sci Nutr 2020;1–7.

[53] Lynch GM, Murphy CH, Castro EDM, Roche HM. Inflammation and metabolism – the role of adiposity in Sarcopenic obesity. Proc Nutr Soc 2020;1–27.

[54] Murton AJ. Muscle protein turnover in the elderly and its potential contribution to the development of sarcopenia. Proc Nutr Soc 2015;74(4):387–96.

[55] Murton AJ, Marimuthu K, Mallinson JE, Selby AL, Smith K, Rennie MJ, et al. Obesity appears to be associated with altered muscle protein synthetic and breakdown responses to increased nutrient delivery in older men, but not reduced muscle mass or contractile function. Diabetes 2015;64(9):3160–71.

[56] Kalinkovich A, Livshits G. Sarcopenic obesity or obese sarcopenia: a cross talk between age-associated adipose tissue and skeletal muscle inflammation as a main mechanism of the pathogenesis. Ageing Res Rev 2017;35:200–21.

[57] Kruger MC, Coetzee M, Haag M, Weiler H. Long-chain polyunsaturated fatty acids: selected mechanisms of action on bone. Prog Lipid Res 2010;49(4):438–49.

[58] Sakuma K, Yamaguchi A. Sarcopenic obesity and endocrinal adaptation with age. Int J Endocrinol 2013;2013:204164.

[59] Sakuma T, Yamashita K, Miyakoshi T, Shimodaira M, Yokota N, Sato Y, et al. Postchallenge hyperglycemia in subjects with low body weight: implication for small glucose volume. Am J Physiol Endocrinol Metab 2017;313(6):E748–56.

[60] Summers SA. Ceramides in insulin resistance and lipotoxicity. Prog Lipid Res 2006;45(1):42–72.

[61] Garris DR. Cytochemical analysis of pancreatic islet lipoapoptosis: hyperlipidemia-induced cytoinvolution following expression of the diabetes (db/db) mutation. Pathobiology 2005;72(3):124–32.

[62] Wei W, Qi X, Reed J, Ceci J, Wang HQ, Wang G, et al. Effect of chronic hyperghrelinemia on ingestive action of ghrelin. Am J Physiol Regul Integr Comp Physiol 2006;290(3):R803–8.

[63] Lee EJ, Jan AT, Baig MH, Ahmad K, Malik A, Rabbani G, et al. Fibromodulin and regulation of the intricate balance between myoblast differentiation to myocytes or adipocyte-like cells. FASEB J 2018;32(2):768–81.

[64] Shapiro H, Pecht T, Shaco-Levy R, Harman-Boehm I, Kirshtein B, Kuperman Y, et al. Adipose tissue foam cells are present in human obesity. J Clin Endocrinol Metab 2013;98(3):1173–81.

[65] Watt MJ, Dzamko N, Thomas WG, Rose-John S, Ernst M, Carling D, et al. CNTF reverses obesity-induced insulin resistance by activating skeletal muscle AMPK. Nat Med 2006;12(5):541–8.

[66] Adams 2nd JM, Pratipanawatr T, Berria R, Wang E, DeFronzo RA, Sullards MC, et al. Ceramide content is increased in skeletal muscle from obese insulin-resistant humans. Diabetes 2004;53(1):25–31.

[67] Kob R, Bollheimer LC, Bertsch T, Fellner C, Djukic M, Sieber CC, et al. Sarcopenic obesity: molecular clues to a better understanding of its pathogenesis? Biogerontology 2015;16(1):15–29.

[68] Consitt LA, Bell JA, Houmard JA. Intramuscular lipid metabolism, insulin action, and obesity. IUBMB Life 2009;61(1):47–55.

[69] van Herpen NA, Schrauwen-Hinderling VB. Lipid accumulation in non-adipose tissue and lipotoxicity. Physiol Behav 2008;94(2):231–41.

[70] Balaban RS, Nemoto S, Finkel T. Mitochondria, oxidants, and aging. Cell 2005;120(4):483–95.

[71] Larsson NG. Somatic mitochondrial DNA mutations in mammalian aging. Annu Rev Biochem 2010;79:683–706.

[72] Baker BM, Haynes CM. Mitochondrial protein quality control during biogenesis and aging. Trends Biochem Sci 2011;36(5):254–61.

[73] Summermatter S, Troxler H, Santos G, Handschin C. Coordinated balancing of muscle oxidative metabolism through PGC-1alpha increases metabolic flexibility and preserves insulin sensitivity. Biochem Biophys Res Commun 2011;408(1):180–5.

[74] Summermatter S, Thurnheer R, Santos G, Mosca B, Baum O, Treves S, et al. Remodeling of calcium handling in skeletal muscle through PGC-1alpha: impact on force, fatigability, and fiber type. Am J Physiol Cell Physiol 2012;302(1):C88–99.

[75] Summermatter S, Baum O, Santos G, Hoppeler H, Handschin C. Peroxisome proliferator-activated receptor {gamma} coactivator 1{alpha} (PGC-1{alpha}) promotes skeletal muscle lipid refueling in vivo by activating de novo lipogenesis and the pentose phosphate pathway. J Biol Chem 2010;285(43):32793–800.

[76] Derbre F, Gomez-Cabrera MC, Nascimento AL, Sanchis-Gomar F, Martinez-Bello VE, Tresguerres JA, et al. Age associated low mitochondrial biogenesis may be explained by lack of response of PGC-1alpha to exercise training. Age (Dordr) 2012;34(3):669–79.

[77] Aon MA, Bhatt N, Cortassa SC. Mitochondrial and cellular mechanisms for managing lipid excess. Front Physiol 2014;5:282.

[78] Lipina C, Hundal HS. Lipid modulation of skeletal muscle mass and function. J Cachexia Sarcopenia Muscle 2017;8(2):190–201.

[79] Pagel-Langenickel I, Bao J, Pang L, Sack MN. The role of mitochondria in the pathophysiology of skeletal muscle insulin resistance. Endocr Rev 2010;31(1):25–51.

[80] Di Meo S, Iossa S, Venditti P. Skeletal muscle insulin resistance: role of mitochondria and other ROS sources. J Endocrinol 2017;233(1):R15–42.

[81] Cade WT. The manifold role of the mitochondria in skeletal muscle insulin resistance. Curr Opin Clin Nutr Metab Care 2018;21(4):267–72.

[82] Scapin G, Dandey VP, Zhang Z, Prosise W, Hruza A, Kelly T, et al. Structure of the insulin receptor-insulin complex by single-particle cryo-EM analysis. Nature 2018;556(7699):122–5.

[83] Scapin G, Potter CS, Carragher B. Cryo-EM for small molecules discovery, design, understanding, and application. Cell Chem Biol 2018;25(11):1318–25.

[84] Banks AS, McAllister FE, Camporez JP, Zushin PJ, Jurczak MJ, Laznik-Bogoslavski D, et al. An ERK/Cdk5 axis controls the diabetogenic actions of PPARgamma. Nature 2015;517(7534):391–5.

[85] Gehart H, Kumpf S, Ittner A, Ricci R. MAPK signalling in cellular metabolism: stress or wellness? EMBO Rep 2010;11(11):834–40.

[86] Abdullahi A, Amini-Nik S, Jeschke MG. Animal models in burn research. Cell Mol Life Sci 2014;71(17):3241–55.
[87] Chung HY, Cesari M, Anton S, Marzetti E, Giovannini S, Seo AY, et al. Molecular inflammation: underpinnings of aging and age-related diseases. Ageing Res Rev 2009;8(1):18–30.
[88] Park CH, Do JG, Lee YT, Yoon KJ. Sarcopenic obesity associated with high-sensitivity C-reactive protein in age and sex comparison: a two-center study in South Korea. BMJ Open 2018;8(9), e021232.
[89] Molero J, Moize V, Flores L, De Hollanda A, Jimenez A, Vidal J. The impact of age on the prevalence of Sarcopenic obesity in bariatric surgery candidates. Obes Surg 2020;30(6):2158–64.
[90] Schrager MA, Metter EJ, Simonsick E, Ble A, Bandinelli S, Lauretani F, et al. Sarcopenic obesity and inflammation in the InCHIANTI study. J Appl Physiol 2007;102(3):919–25.
[91] Nascimento DDC, Oliveira SDC, Vieira DCL, Funghetto SS, Silva AO, Valduga R, et al. The impact of sarcopenic obesity on inflammation, lean body mass, and muscle strength in elderly women. Int J Gen Med 2018;11:443–9.
[92] Di Renzo L, Sarlo F, Petramala L, Iacopino L, Monteleone G, Colica C, et al. Association between -308 G/A TNF-alpha polymorphism and appendicular skeletal muscle mass index as a marker of sarcopenia in normal weight obese syndrome. Dis Markers 2013;35(6):615–23.
[93] Henze H, Jung MJ, Ahrens HE, Steiner S, von Maltzahn J. Skeletal muscle aging – stem cells in the spotlight. Mech Ageing Dev 2020;189:111283.
[94] Stenholm S, Rantanen T, Heliovaara M, Koskinen S. The mediating role of C-reactive protein and handgrip strength between obesity and walking limitation. J Am Geriatr Soc 2008;56(3):462–9.
[95] Ogborn DI, Gardiner PF. Effects of exercise and muscle type on BDNF, NT-4/5, and TrKB expression in skeletal muscle. Muscle Nerve 2010;41(3):385–91.
[96] Annweiler C, Allali G, Allain P, Bridenbaugh S, Schott AM, Kressig RW, et al. Vitamin D and cognitive performance in adults: a systematic review. Eur J Neurol 2009;16(10):1083–9.
[97] Muir SW, Montero-Odasso M. Effect of vitamin D supplementation on muscle strength, gait and balance in older adults: a systematic review and meta-analysis. J Am Geriatr Soc 2011;59(12):2291–300.
[98] Rosales-Soto G, Diaz-Vegas A, Casas M, Contreras-Ferrat A, Jaimovich E. Fibroblast growth factor-21 potentiates glucose transport in skeletal muscle fibers. J Mol Endocrinol 2020.
[99] Mathers JL, Farnfield MM, Garnham AP, Caldow MK, Cameron-Smith D, Peake JM. Early inflammatory and myogenic responses to resistance exercise in the elderly. Muscle Nerve 2012;46(3):407–12.
[100] Guo A, Li K, Xiao Q. Sarcopenic obesity: myokines as potential diagnostic biomarkers and therapeutic targets? Exp Gerontol 2020;139:111022.
[101] Das DK, Graham ZA, Cardozo CP. Myokines in skeletal muscle physiology and metabolism: recent advances and future perspectives. Acta Physiol (Oxf) 2020;228(2), e13367.
[102] Besse-Patin A, Montastier E, Vinel C, Castan-Laurell I, Louche K, Dray C, et al. Effect of endurance training on skeletal muscle myokine expression in obese men: identification of apelin as a novel myokine. Int J Obes (Lond) 2014;38(5):707–13.
[103] Carol A, Witkamp RF, Wichers HJ, Mensink M. Bovine colostrum supplementation's lack of effect on immune variables during short-term intense exercise in well-trained athletes. Int J Sport Nutr Exerc Metab 2011;21(2):135–45.
[104] Hou X, Li Z, Higashi Y, Delafontaine P, Sukhanov S. Insulin-like growth factor I prevents cellular aging via activation of mitophagy. J Aging Res 2020;2020:4939310.
[105] Klymenko O, Brecklinghaus T, Dille M, Springer C, de Wendt C, Altenhofen D, et al. Histone deacetylase 5 regulates interleukin 6 secretion and insulin action in skeletal muscle. Mol Metab 2020;42, 101062.
[106] Scheler M, Irmler M, Lehr S, Hartwig S, Staiger H, Al-Hasani H, et al. Cytokine response of primary human myotubes in an in vitro exercise model. Am J Physiol Cell Physiol 2013;305(8):C877–86.
[107] Eaton M, Granata C, Barry J, Safdar A, Bishop D, Little JP. Impact of a single bout of high-intensity interval exercise and short-term interval training on interleukin-6, FNDC5, and METRNL mRNA expression in human skeletal muscle. J Sport Health Sci 2018;7(2):191–6.
[108] Subbotina E, Sierra A, Zhu Z, Gao Z, Koganti SR, Reyes S, et al. Musclin is an activity-stimulated myokine that enhances physical endurance. Proc Natl Acad Sci U S A 2015;112(52):16042–7.

[109] Fujimoto T, Sugimoto K, Takahashi T, Yasunobe Y, Xie K, Tanaka M, et al. Overexpression of Interleukin-15 exhibits improved glucose tolerance and promotes GLUT4 translocation via AMP-activated protein kinase pathway in skeletal muscle. Biochem Biophys Res Commun 2019;509(4):994–1000.

[110] McFarlane C, Hennebry A, Thomas M, Plummer E, Ling N, Sharma M, et al. Myostatin signals through Pax7 to regulate satellite cell self-renewal. Exp Cell Res 2008;314(2):317–29.

[111] Nelke C, Dziewas R, Minnerup J, Meuth SG, Ruck T. Skeletal muscle as potential central link between sarcopenia and immune senescence. EBioMedicine 2019;49:381–8.

[112] Pillon NJ, Bilan PJ, Fink LN, Klip A. Cross-talk between skeletal muscle and immune cells: muscle-derived mediators and metabolic implications. Am J Physiol Endocrinol Metab 2013;304(5):E453–65.

[113] Nylen C, Aoi W, Abdelmoez AM, Lassiter DG, Lundell LS, Wallberg-Henriksson H, et al. IL6 and LIF mRNA expression in skeletal muscle is regulated by AMPK and the transcription factors NFYC, ZBTB14, and SP1. Am J Physiol Endocrinol Metab 2018;315(5):E995–E1004.

[114] Severinsen MCK, Pedersen BK. Muscle-organ crosstalk: the emerging roles of myokines. Endocr Rev 2020;41(4):594–609.

[115] Lessard SJ, MacDonald TL, Pathak P, Han MS, Coffey VG, Edge J, et al. JNK regulates muscle remodeling via myostatin/SMAD inhibition. Nat Commun 2018;9(1):3030.

[116] Biglari S, Afousi AG, Mafi F, Shabkhiz F. High-intensity interval training-induced hypertrophy in gastrocnemius muscle via improved IGF-I/Akt/FoxO and myostatin/Smad signaling pathways in rats. Physiol Int 2020;107. https://doi.org/10.1556/2060.2020.00020.

[117] Welle SL. Myostatin and muscle fiber size. Focus on "Smad2 and 3 transcription factors control muscle mass in adulthood" and "Myostatin reduces Akt/TORC1/p70S6K signaling, inhibiting myoblast differentiation and myotube size". Am J Physiol Cell Physiol 2009;296(6):C1245–7.

[118] De Toni L, Agoulnik AI, Sandri M, Foresta C, Ferlin A. INSL3 in the muscolo-skeletal system. Mol Cell Endocrinol 2019;487:12–7.

[119] Hilbert-Walter A, Buttner R, Sieber C, Bollheimer C. Testosterone in old age: an up-date. Dtsch Med Wochenschr 2012;137(41):2117–22.

[120] Ipsa E, Cruzat VF, Kagize JN, Yovich JL, Keane KN. Growth hormone and insulin-like growth factor action in reproductive tissues. Front Endocrinol (Lausanne) 2019;10:777.

[121] Jager R, Mohr AE, Carpenter KC, Kerksick CM, Purpura M, Moussa A, et al. International society of sports nutrition position stand: probiotics. J Int Soc Sports Nutr 2019;16(1):62.

[122] Urban RJ, Bodenburg YH, Gilkison C, Foxworth J, Coggan AR, Wolfe RR, et al. Testosterone administration to elderly men increases skeletal muscle strength and protein synthesis. Am J Physiol 1995;269(5 Pt 1):E820–6.

[123] Altarawneh MM, Hanson ED, Betik AC, Petersen AC, Hayes A, McKenna MJ. Effects of testosterone suppression, hindlimb immobilization, and recovery on [(3)H]ouabain binding site content and Na(+), K(+)-ATPase isoforms in rat soleus muscle. J Appl Physiol (1985) 2020;128(3):501–13.

[124] Halmos T, Suba I. The physiological role of growth hormone and insulin-like growth factors. Orv Hetil 2019;160(45):1774–83.

[125] Forrest L, Sedmak C, Sikder S, Grewal S, Harman SM, Blackman MR, et al. Effects of growth hormone on hepatic insulin sensitivity and glucose effectiveness in healthy older adults. Endocrine 2019;63(3):497–506.

[126] Yeap BB, Chubb SA, Flicker L, McCaul KA, Ebeling PR, Hankey GJ, et al. Associations of total osteocalcin with all-cause and cardiovascular mortality in older men. The health in men study. Osteoporos Int 2012;23(2):599–606.

[127] Emmelot-Vonk MH, Verhaar HJ, Nakhai Pour HR, Aleman A, Lock TM, Bosch JL, et al. Effect of testosterone supplementation on functional mobility, cognition, and other parameters in older men: a randomized controlled trial. JAMA 2008;299(1):39–52.

[128] Lira VA, Benton CR, Yan Z, Bonen A. PGC-1alpha regulation by exercise training and its influences on muscle function and insulin sensitivity. Am J Physiol Endocrinol Metab 2010;299(2):E145–61.

[129] Friedrichsen M, Mortensen B, Pehmoller C, Birk JB, Wojtaszewski JF. Exercise-induced AMPK activity in skeletal muscle: role in glucose uptake and insulin sensitivity. Mol Cell Endocrinol 2013;366(2):204–14.

[130] Goisser S, Kemmler W, Porzel S, Volkert D, Sieber CC, Bollheimer LC, et al. Sarcopenic obesity and complex interventions with nutrition and exercise in community-dwelling older persons – a narrative review. Clin Interv Aging 2015;10:1267–82.
[131] Annweiler C, Schott-Petelaz AM, Berrut G, Kressig RW, Bridenbaugh S, Herrmann FR, et al. Vitamin D deficiency-related quadriceps weakness: results of the Epidemiologie De l'Osteoporose cohort. J Am Geriatr Soc 2009;57(2):368–9.
[132] Annweiler C, Bridenbaugh S, Schott AM, Berrut G, Kressig RW, Beauchet O. Vitamin D and muscle function: new prospects? Biofactors 2009;35(1):3–4.
[133] Annweiler C, Schott AM, Berrut G, Fantino B, Beauchet O. Vitamin D-related changes in physical performance: a systematic review. J Nutr Health Aging 2009;13(10):893–8.
[134] Cipriani C, Pepe J, Piemonte S, Colangelo L, Cilli M, Minisola S. Vitamin d and its relationship with obesity and muscle. Int J Endocrinol 2014;2014:841248.

CHAPTER 11

Vascular aging and sarcopenia: Interactions with physiological functions during exercise

Naoyuki Hayashi
Faculty of Sport Sciences, Waseda University, Saitama, Japan

Abstract
Sarcopenia includes reductions in the skeletal muscle mass, which could be related to the circulatory responses to exercise that support the degree of exertion associated with movements, the blood flow supporting the activities of neurons in the central and peripheral nervous systems, and the regulation of temperature, as well as supporting digestion and absorption. Reduced blood flow could be related to the pathological pathways of sarcopenia. Studies have shown that the age-related decline in blood flow reduces the exchange of oxygen, energy sources, metabolites, and heat between blood and cells, thereby aggravating the trophic state in cells. This chapter addresses vascular aging, focusing on the roles of the functions of skeletal muscle and cerebral, ocular, splanchnic, and skin vessels on locomotion and exercise. Sarcopenia could be bidirectionally related to marked impairments in the cardiovascular system resulting from reduced muscle activity.

Keywords: Blood flow, Exercise, Skeletal muscle, Cerebral vessels, Ocular vessels, Internal organs, Skin vessels

Introduction

Sarcopenia is prevalent in the elderly population and is strongly associated with disability [1,2]. In addition, sarcopenic obesity was found to be moderately associated with an increased risk of cardiovascular disease via sarcopenia, with obesity alone being insufficient to explain this increased risk [3].

The skeletal muscle mass decreases with aging. A longitudinal study involving 71-year-old (mean age) subjects with a 9-year follow-up found a 5.7% reduction in the cross-sectional area of the total anterior muscle without changes in body weight, body mass index, or physical activity [4]. Moreover, the age-related decline in muscle mass was found to be greater in females, while the quality of muscles decreased in both sexes [5]. Various other studies have also focused on muscle mass [6–8].

Leg muscles are more affected by aging than arm muscles in human beings [9], while hindlimb muscles are also more severely affected than the forelimbs in quadruped mammals [10,11]. This is particularly significant, given that lower-limb function has a stronger impact on the quality of life than upper-limb function in humans, and dysfunction therein can result in falls [12]. It is, therefore, necessary to understand the physiological functions supporting exercise to understand the effect of sarcopenia on locomotion.

Reductions in skeletal muscle mass can be related to neural and circulatory responses to exercise. Disuse atrophy exaggerated the blood-pressure responses to passive stretching of triceps surae muscles in rats, which simulates mechanical change of muscle contraction [13]. This pressor response originates from mechano- and metabosensitive receptors in skeletal muscles [14]. The primary pathway of the exercise pressor reflex arc includes group-III and group-IV afferent fibers, and so an exaggerated pressor response is related to neural input from skeletal muscles and the pathway of the exercise pressor reflex. Aging and the reduction in muscle mass induced by sarcopenia can alter neural and circulatory responses.

The blood flow supports the exertion associated with relatively long-duration movements, whereas the neuromuscular system directly affects both the short- and long-term strengths during exercise. Blood flow also supports the activities of neurons in the central and peripheral nervous systems, and the regulation of temperature, as well as digestion and the absorption of nutrients in internal organs that are required to support muscle movements.

Reduced blood flow could be related to the pathological pathways of sarcopenia. Many studies have found that aging results in declines of the central and peripheral blood flows and the functioning of the associated vessels. Such declines reduce the exchange of oxygen, energy sources, metabolites, and heat between blood and cells, aggravating the trophic state in cells. For example, glial cells could affect the development of sarcopenia via glial regulation in blood vessels [15]. Thus, vascular aging could be related to the aging of neural systems and impairment of locomotive functions that result in sarcopenia, and vice versa. This chapter addresses the bidirectional relationship between vascular aging and sarcopenia.

Role of peripheral blood flow during exercise

Blood flow has diverse roles, including (1) providing oxygen and nutrients such as glucose, amino acids, and fatty acids; (2) removing metabolites such as carbon dioxide and lactic acid; (3) maintaining optimal ion concentrations, such as by removing hydrogen ions; (4) transporting hormones [16]; (5) maintaining the shapes of different tissues, including the brain and penis; and (6) regulating the core temperature. Most of these roles are related to exercise or locomotion, and they are dependent on maintaining—but not exceeding—the appropriate blood flow.

The blood flow is generally greater for a tissue that has greater metabolic needs. For example, blood flow to the active muscles increases substantially during exercise, while blood flow to the kidney and some other internal organs decreases [17]. The blood flows to cerebral and ocular organs that have important roles in maintaining the central nervous and visual systems increase or at least remain stable during exercise. Cycling exercise increases blood flow in the internal carotid artery (ICA), which supplies blood to the brain, while ICA blood flow was found to return to near resting levels during high-intensity exercises [18]. Static knee extension at 30% of the maximal voluntary contraction was also reported to increase blood flow in the ICA [19]. Maintaining vision requires the ocular blood flow (OBF) to remain stable, which comprises the retinal and choroidal circulations. The retinal circulation exists in the inner part of the retina and is characterized by a low blood supply, whereas the choroidal circulation exists on the outside of the retina, and has a very high blood supply [20]. Dynamic exercise at a heart rate of 100–140 bpm increases the choroidal flow by up to 30% of the resting baseline, depending upon the intensity, but does not alter the retinal flow [21,22]. Meanwhile, the choroidal flow did not change from the resting baseline value during exhaustive exercise, and the retinal flow decreased only slightly (by 13%) [22].

The competition in blood flow between exercising muscles and nonexercising organs results in the decrease of splanchnic blood flow during exercise [23]. Pulsed Doppler ultrasonography has revealed that long-duration exercise is associated with reductions in the blood flow in splanchnic regions by 30% to 50% [24–26]. In addition, the renal blood flow decreased in response to a handgrip exercise [27]. Blood flow in the portal vein decreased by 80% relative to the resting baseline immediately after 60 min of exercise [28]. Blood flow responses to exercise in healthy humans are mainly related to the vasodilation response to metabolites in active muscles and sympathetic vasoconstriction in inactive organs. For example, the role of sympathetic activation in the vasoconstriction of nonexercising organs has been demonstrated by comparing blood flow responses in the portal vein and femoral artery during arm cranking between normal subjects and subjects with a spinal cord lesion [29].

Increases in the skin blood flow are particularly marked during high-intensity exercise at high temperatures and humidities. The blood flow in nonglabrous skin areas gradually increases with the body temperature during exercise to dissipate heat from the skin [30,31]. These responses make substantial contributions to the maintenance of thermoregulatory homeostasis [32]. The importance of arteriovenous anastomoses on heat dissipation has also been reported, since the main physiological role of these direct connections between small arteries and small veins is the transport of heat from the body core to surface areas [33].

Loss of vascular functions relevant to sarcopenia

Vascular aging is associated with changes in the mechanical and structural properties of the vascular wall, which leads to the loss of arterial elasticity [34].

Peripheral arterial disease (PAD) was shown to be accompanied by reductions in the mass, strength, and physical performance of skeletal muscle, that is, sarcopenia. A systematic review demonstrated that sarcopenia and lower-limb PAD have musculoskeletal consequences, with both sarcopenia and PAD being accompanied by oxidative stress, skeletal muscle mitochondrial impairments, inflammation, and inhibition of specific pathways regulating muscle synthesis and protection [35].

Later we discuss vascular aging in several organs and their effects on exercise.

Skeletal-muscle vessels

It is well established that the blood flow in exercising skeletal muscles is closely related to their metabolic and oxygen demands [17,36,37]. Blood is needed to support the metabolism associated with exercise, and so, any insufficiency in the blood flow will directly restrict the exercise and locomotion abilities. Exercise intolerance is caused by inadequate blood flow to skeletal muscle. Vascular alterations due to aging decrease the exercise performance by impairing the blood flow [38], and decreased capillary density [39], and thickening of vascular walls [40] are well-known changes related to aging.

The relationship between capillarization and muscle size was shown in a comparative study involving groups of 22- and 74-year-old subjects [41]. The capillary supply to muscle fibers was related to the fiber size, regardless of age and sex. The distributions of capillaries in skeletal muscles were found to be similar in healthy active older and young people. The age-related capillary rarefaction maintains the coupling between the fiber size of skeletal muscle and capillarization. To the author's knowledge, a direct relationship between a reduced blood flow to skeletal muscle and changes in skeletal muscle mass and/or function has not been reported. However, considering the important role of capillaries in oxygen and nutrition delivery [42,43], the muscle blood flow contributes to maintaining the function of skeletal muscles.

In addition to the possible effects of a reduced blood flow to skeletal muscle aggravating trophic states in muscle cells, the effects on satellite cells should also be noted. The mechanisms contributing to sarcopenia include reduced satellite-cell function. Nutritional interventions might be an effective therapeutic strategy for improving satellite-cell function in aging muscles [44].

Cerebral vessels

We cannot overlook the role of the cerebral flow in terms of sarcopenia being caused by nerves. A proposed neurological model of sarcopenia suggests that the pathology of sarcopenia is gliogenic, implying that aging and disuse atrophy of Schwann cells may be major contributors to the complex etiology of sarcopenia [45]. Aging, Alzheimer's disease (AD), and leukoaraiosis are associated with decreased vascular density, and cerebrovascular dysfunction precedes and accompanies cognitive dysfunction and neurodegeneration. A decline in cerebrovascular angiogenesis may inhibit the recovery from hypoxia-induced capillary loss [46].

The brain constitutes about 2% of the body mass while its metabolic rate can be up to 20% of that of the whole body, and so a steady and sufficient cerebral blood flow (CBF) is important to maintaining brain function. Age-related declines in cardiovascular function may impair CBF regulation, leading to the disruption of neuronal homeostasis [47].

CBF is related to cognitive function. A higher blood velocity in the middle cerebral artery (MCAv), which supplies nutrients to large areas of the brain, was found to be correlated with faster response times in the Stroop test, which tests executive function and cognition [48]. Response times on the Stroop test were found to be slower in old than in young subjects, and a higher MCAv was correlated with faster response times on the Stroop test.

The CBF decreases with aging. A longitudinal study involving a follow-up lasting more than 6 years found that the regional cerebral blood flow (rCBF), as measured using positron-emission tomography, decreased in both 14 normotensive patients and 14 treated hypertensive participants, but with different patterns of change in these two groups [49]. Cross-sectional studies have also shown that older subjects have lower CBFs. Transcranial Doppler flowmetry revealed age-related declines in the MCAv in 307 healthy males aged 18–79 years [50]. Studies using other techniques, including color duplex sonography for measuring the extracranial cerebral arteries [51] and phase-contrast magnetic resonance imaging for measuring the total CBF [52], have revealed global age-related decreases in the CBF in healthy adults. Studies applying various techniques to various target areas have also found decreases in CBF in older subjects.

Lower CBFs in various parts of the brain compared with the normal aged population have been reported in AD patients and patients with mild cognitive impairment (MCI). A longitudinal study showed that the CBF in the posterior cingulate gyrus was lower in MCI and AD patients than in control subjects, while MCI patients had higher CBFs in the left hippocampus, right amygdala, and rostral head of the right caudate nucleus, the ventral putamen, and the globus pallidus [53]. A cross-sectional study found lower rCBFs in AD patients than in cognitively normal subjects in the right inferior parietal cortex extending to the bilateral posterior cingulate gyri, bilateral superior and middle frontal gyri, and left inferior parietal lobe, while the MCI patients also showed a trend for a lower CBF in the right inferior parietal lobe [54]. In a retrospective cohort study, subjects who converted to AD over a 3-year follow-up showed lower CBFs in the bilateral parahippocampal gyri, precunei, posterior cingulate cortices, bilateral parietal association areas, and the right middle temporal gyrus, while those who did not convert also showed lower CBFs in the posterior cingulated cortices and the right caudate nucleus compared with controls before the follow-up [55]. A study with a 6-year follow-up found that cerebral atrophy increased as CBF declined after the age of 60. An excessive decrease in CBF, gray and white matter hypodensities, and cerebral atrophy were found to be related to cognitive decline [56]. These findings together indicate that a decline in CBF is related to the impairment of cognitive function.

Impaired cognitive function is related to an impaired ability to perform the activities of daily living (ADL). The ADL are the basic self-maintenance activities that are essential to life, such as eating, changing clothes, moving around, toileting, dressing, and bathing. The instrumental ADL (IADL) are more-complex everyday tasks, such as preparing a meal or managing finances [57], as well as higher functions of daily living that are not included as ADLs, such as telephone use, shopping, housework, transportation, going out, and managing medications and money. A systematic review found that IADL deficits were present in patients with MCI in 35 of 37 studies [58]. Reduced abilities to perform the ADL and IADL aggravate sarcopenia.

Ocular vessels

Vision is essential for locomotion ability, and a continuous supply of blood to the retina is essential for vision since the visual system has a high oxygen demand and oxygen is not stored in the retina or surrounding tissues [59]. The OBF to the retina is as small as 2 mL/s, and it plays a fundamental role in vision [20]. Changing the arterial partial pressure of carbon dioxide by manipulating respiration showed that changes in OBF are associated with changes in visual acuity [60]. An increase in the choroidal blood flow was associated with improved contrast sensitivity in healthy humans after sildenafil administration [61], while no effect on ocular hemodynamics was detected using color Doppler ultrasonography in patients with erectile dysfunction [62]. Many types of blindness are due to abnormalities of the fundus circulation, and so improving the OBF could help to prevent eye diseases and myopia.

Aging results in structural and functional impairments in ocular vascular networks [63] and consequently increases the risk of vision impairment in older people [64]. Eye diseases such as diabetic retinopathy, glaucoma, and age-related macular degeneration are relatively common. A review of United States data on the prevalence rates of visual impairment, blindness, and selected eye conditions—both self-reported and medically diagnosed—in 31,000 adults found that the prevalence of visual impairment was 9.3%, including 0.3% with blindness [65]. The prevalence of poor vision was as high as 1% in more than 6000 urban Chinese, and this was related to aging [66]. Myopic retinopathy is present in roughly 40% of highly myopic eyes and is a common cause of visual impairment [67]. Preventing ocular vascular dysfunction can help to maintain vision and consequently also the locomotion ability.

The elasticity of ocular vessels has been reported to increase with age. One variable, called the blow-out time (BOT), reflects for how long a large blood flow is maintained during a single heartbeat. A larger BOT indicates greater nutrition being supplied to the periphery, and its values in various areas of the ocular circulation decrease with aging regardless of the type of ocular vasculature [68,69].

Exercise is beneficial to patients with diseases of the visual system [70,71]. People who engage in physical activity have lower rates of glaucomatous vision loss [72]. Another correlational study that analyzed the data of more than 8000 children in Ireland revealed that refractive errors and vision problems were significantly associated with increased sedentary behavior and decreased physical activity [71].

The mechanisms that could be triggered to benefit vision remain unclear. Considering the importance of vision to many human activities, including locomotion, further studies are needed to identify mechanisms underlying improvements in vision. It is feasible that ocular diseases related to the impairment of ocular vessels will one day be found to benefit from exercise [70].

Splanchnic vessels

The splanchnic circulation supplies nutrients to the body via digestion and absorption mainly at rest, and it restricts the blood flow to secure the blood flow to active muscles during exercise. Blood in organs from the stomach to the large intestine, including the liver, pancreas, and spleen, is supplied from part of the splanchnic circulation. The splanchnic circulation accounts for 25% of the cardiac output at rest [17], and it consists of the celiac artery (CA), superior mesenteric artery (SMA), and inferior mesenteric artery (IMA). The CA supplies blood to the stomach, liver, and spleen; the SMA supplies the duodenum, jejunum, ileum, ascending colon, transverse colon, and pancreas; the IMA supplies blood to the descending colon, sigmoid colon, and upper rectum. This circulation is essential to maintaining digestion and absorption in the alimentary tract.

The splanchnic blood flow decreases during exercise so that blood can be distributed preferentially to muscles and maintain the blood pressure in the presence of a substantial decrease in vessel resistance associated with vasodilation in active muscles.

Unfortunately, little is known about age-related changes in splanchnic circulation. Postprandial hypotension is reportedly common in elderly patients and is a cause of syncope [73]. Symptomatic hypotension tends to occur more often and sooner after meal ingestion than before meal ingestion [74]. After meal ingestion and orthostatic head-up tilt testing, 22% of functionally independent elderly people were found to exhibit symptomatic hypotension, while 12% experienced this during preprandial testing. While the underlying mechanism is not fully understood, it might be secondary to a blunted sympathetic response to a meal. Hypotension can lead to a fear of going out, lack of exercise, and orthostatic hypotension.

Several research groups have measured the splanchnic blood flow and oxygen uptake before and after consuming a meal in groups of young and middle-aged normal volunteers [75–78]. However, to the author's knowledge, no comparison has been performed between young and aged groups, and so further studies are needed on the effects of aging on splanchnic circulation.

Skin vessels

Climate changes associated with global warming will have serious impacts on human beings. The ICCP (Intergovernmental Panel on Climate Change) reported that warming of the climate system is unequivocal and projected that the global average surface temperature is likely to increase by the end of the century by between 0.3°C and 4.8°C [79]. The climate change projected to occur by the middle of this century will impact human health, mainly by exacerbating health problems that already exist. Throughout the 21st century, climate change is expected to lead to increases in ill-health in many regions, and especially in developing countries with low incomes, as compared to a baseline without climate change. The risks that global warming present to human health include an increase in heat-related deaths during periods of hot weather. An epidemiological survey of heat-related deaths in Japan from 1968 to 1994 showed that even a small increase in the atmospheric temperature can lead to a considerable increase in heat-related mortality and found that half of the increased deaths occurred in children (4 years and below) and the elderly (70 years and above) regardless of sex [80]. This situation will make temperature regulation by the skin vasculature increasingly important for allowing elderly people to exercise, including jogging and walking outside.

The main mechanism for coping with heat exposure includes the distribution of the cardiac output to the skin and skin vasodilation. This mechanism is weaker in the elderly people, with the skin blood flow at a given core temperature being lower in this population due to a greater vessel resistance. This age-related attenuation was found to be due to both axon-reflex-mediated and nitric-oxide-mediated vasodilation [81].

Heat dissipation from the skin during exercise is more important than at rest due to the additional heat produced by skeletal muscle activities, and this dissipation is reduced in elderly people. The cardiac output when exercising in a hot environment was reported to be reduced in older people [82], and the distribution of the cardiac output to the skin was also less efficient [83]. These factors together result in less heat dissipation from the skin.

Environmental heat stress and exercise increase physiological strain, which is manifested by increases in the core temperature and cardiovascular strain and results in reduced aerobic performance [84]. An increase in the cardiovascular strain in a hot environment—including a depressed cardiac output and mean arterial pressure—was associated with reductions in the sustainable and maximal power outputs during prolonged, intense self-paced exercise [85]. Exercising in a hot environment is associated with a thermoregulatory burden that is associated with cardiovascular challenges and influences cerebral function, all of which potentially contribute to fatigue and impair the ability to sustain power output during exercise [86]. Thus, the reduction in skin blood flow associated with aging decreases exercise and locomotion abilities.

Veins

Veins serve as blood reservoirs since they contain more than 60% of the circulating blood. Venous constriction can maintain arterial blood pressure when blood loss occurs.

Venous thrombosis and ulcers have been extensively studied since these conditions can be life-threatening [87]. Epidemiological studies have shown that age is a risk factor for thrombosis in veins and arteries [88]. Venous thromboembolism is the most common vascular disease after acute myocardial infarction and stroke. Changes in blood coagulation, inflammation, and immune response may be interdependently linked to induce thrombosis [89]. Hemmeryckx et al. [90] reported that venous valves become more fragile in association with a procoagulant and inflammatory blood phenotype in aged mice.

Less attention has been paid to the effects of healthy aging on the functioning of the central and peripheral venous systems than on the central and peripheral arteries.

Other factors resulting in circulatory impairments related to aging

Central arteries

The blood is driven from the heart and transported to the peripheral organs via the central arteries. The central arteries are highly extensible, and so their arterial walls are stretched during systole. During diastole, the stretched arterial wall returns to its original dimensions due to its elasticity, which results in the stored blood being sent to the periphery (Windkessel model).

Age-related changes in the diameters of the thoracic and abdominal aortas have been studied extensively, and it is now generally accepted that their diameters increase with age. The aorta also stiffens with age [91–93], and its effective diameter in the proximal region is reduced [94], a process known as arteriosclerosis. The greatest difference in aortic stiffness is observed in the abdominal region, whereas the greatest difference in diameter is in the ascending aorta [95].

These changes lead to an increase in the pulse pressure, which places an additional strain on the aorta and limits its buffering capacity, which appears to affect the endurance capacity. Vaitkevicius et al. [93] found that indices of arterial stiffness were inversely related to the maximal oxygen uptake. However, age-related increases in the central arterial stiffness were not observed in females who remained highly physically active [92]. The function of the central arteries contributes to the working capacity.

Baroreflex

The baroreflex is important for the ability of human beings to stand in an upright position. Information about the pressure that is sensed in the carotid and aortic arch attached to the arteries is processed in the brainstem to modulate the activity of the autonomic nervous system to the vasculature and heart. A fall in blood pressure instantaneously induces vasoconstriction and increases the heart rate and stroke volume. Impairment of the baroreflex function severely impairs the standing posture and locomotion.

Reduced baroreflex sensitivity is one of the first alterations in autonomic functions related to aging in human beings. The ability of the carotid baroreflex to defend against a hypotensive stimulus is reduced in older subjects both at rest and during exercise [96,97]. The most obvious problem associated with an impaired baroreflex is syncope, which is a common condition that reduces the working capacity or can even be life-threatening in severe cases.

Blood volume

An increase in the plasma volume (PV) or circulating blood volume (BV) improves thermoregulation during exercise to protect human beings against heat. Both responses are physiologically important for optimal human performance. A PV or BV with an adequate oxygen-carrying capacity is critical to ensuring that sufficient oxygen is provided to active tissues.

The PV and BV appear to be lower in older people, including in the older males when expressed relative to the body weight, body surface area, or estimated fat-free mass [98]. Aging was associated with a decrease in BV due to reductions in both the PV and erythrocyte-cell volume in healthy females, whereas the PV and BV were maintained with age in physically active females [99].

However, Koons et al. [100] reported the contradictory finding that the BV did not differ between older and younger males and females. Those authors explained that the conflicting results could be due to studies including subjects with different age ranges and initial aerobic capacities. While the effects of aging on the PV and BV remain controversial, an increased PV or BV is related to an increase in working capacity, as demonstrated in a study of the effects of acute PV expansion on thermoregulation in young subjects due to an acute increase in the cardiac filling pressure induced by saline infusion [101].

Possible counteractions to vessel aging

A regular exercise habit and proper nutrition can be effective in preventing or treating sarcopenia with few side effects [102,103], while taking appropriate drugs and stopping smoking have also been reported as effective treatments [34]. Promoting muscle protein anabolism by consuming an adequate amount of high-quality protein at each meal in combination with physical activity may be a promising strategy to preventing or delaying the onset of sarcopenia [104]. A large amount of moderate-to-vigorous-intensity physical activity seems to delay the onset of sarcopenia [105].

It is difficult to describe the effects of nutrition and exercise on the function, especially at each vascular site. While many vessels show similar trends in their adaptations, site differences are also known to exist. For example, exercise habits have been shown to improve vascular stiffness in many parts of the body [106], whereas their effects on improving vascular stiffness can vary between individuals and parts of the body [107]. Later, we discuss some typical effects of exercise on the vasculature.

Exercise training is well known to improve cardiovascular function and increase the vascular transport capacity of skeletal muscle. Performing exercise for as short as 4 weeks was reported to increase the muscle blood-flow response to vasodilation stimuli in both the young and elderly people [108]. Aging-induced reductions and training-induced enhancements of endothelial vasodilation were demonstrated in rats, with both occurring via the nitric oxide vasodilation mechanisms in highly oxidative skeletal muscle [109]. A review proposed two mechanisms for explaining the training-induced increases in muscle blood flow: (1) structural remodeling of the vascular tree and (2) altered vasomotor reactivity of arteries and arterioles. In addition, the fiber composition of muscles exerts powerful influences on the vascular structure and function [110].

It is also well known that regular exercise increases cerebral flow and cognitive function in elderly people. Murrell et al. [111] found that the cerebrovascular reactivity to carbon dioxide and vasodilation stimuli was elevated after 12 weeks of training both at rest and during exercise, regardless of age. Cardiovascular fitness was shown to be associated with the sparing of brain tissue and cognitive function in older people [112]. Thus, exercise habits can induce favorable changes in cerebral vessels.

Training interventions are also well known to improve central arterial elasticity. Regular aerobic exercise attenuates age-related reductions in central arterial elasticity and restores the elasticity in previously sedentary healthy middle-aged and older males [113]. The improvements in central arterial elasticity induced by aerobic exercise training were influenced by the total energy expenditure of the training rather than its intensity in postmenopausal females [114].

Okazaki et al. [115] reported on the effects of combining exercise and nutrition interventions. After 8 weeks of training with the postexercise consumption of protein and carbohydrate, the increases in core temperature were attenuated more than with a normal training regimen and associated with enhanced cutaneous vasodilation and sweating in both young and elderly subjects.

Summary

Sarcopenia not only reduces the function and structure of muscles but also causes marked impairments of the cardiovascular system as a result of reduced muscle activity.

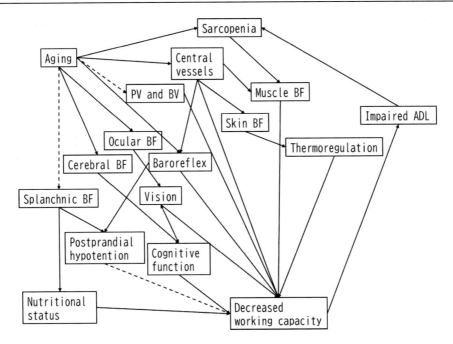

Fig. 1
Possible interrelationships among sarcopenia, vessel aging, and exercise. Sarcopenia can be related to impairments in the function and structure of muscles and the cardiovascular system that result from reduced muscle activity. Impairment of the cardiovascular system restricts muscle activity, and this, in turn, worsens sarcopenia further. Speculative connections are indicated using dashed lines. *ADL*, activities of daily living; *BF*, blood flow; *PV*, plasma volume; *BV*, blood volume.

This impairment of the cardiovascular system, in turn, restricts muscle activity and, hence, also the exercise and locomotion abilities, which worsen sarcopenia further. These complex interrelations are shown in Fig. 1, in which some of the connections are still speculative.

Some of the connections in Fig. 1 are related to declines in functioning (e.g., cognition and thermoregulation) and cannot be explained by vascular aging alone. At present, we can only show the connections, but these associations can be viewed positively. Future research should attempt to improve our understanding of these complex processes.

References

[1] Baumgartner RN. Body composition in healthy aging. Ann N Y Acad Sci 2000;904:437–48.
[2] Baumgartner RN, Koehler KM, Gallagher D, Romero L, Heymsfield SB, Ross RR, et al. Epidemiology of sarcopenia among the elderly in New Mexico. Am J Epidemiol 1998;147:755–63.
[3] Stephen WC, Janssen I. Sarcopenic-obesity and cardiovascular disease risk in the elderly. J Nutr Heal Aging 2009;13:460–6.
[4] Frontera WR, Reid KF, Phillips EM, Krivickas LS, Hughes VA, Roubenoff R, et al. Muscle fiber size and function in elderly humans: a longitudinal study. J Appl Physiol 2008;105:637–42.

[5] Shimokata H, Ando F, Yuki A, Otsuka R. Age-related changes in skeletal muscle mass among community-dwelling Japanese: a 12-year longitudinal study. Geriatr Gerontol Int 2014;14(Suppl1):85–92.
[6] Clark BC, Manini TM. Sarcopenia ≠Dynapenia. 2008;63:829–34.
[7] Janssen I. Evolution of sarcopenia research. Appl Physiol Nutr Metab 2010;35:707–12.
[8] Visser M, Schaap LA. Consequences of sarcopenia. Clin Geriatr Med 2011;27:387–99.
[9] Oertel G. Changes in human skeletal muscles due to ageing. Acta Neuropathol 1986;69:309–13.
[10] Stalberg E, Fawcett PR. Macro EMG in healthy subjects of different ages. J Neurol Neurosurg Psychiatry 1982;45:870–8.
[11] McDonagh MJ. Mechanical properties of muscles from *Xenopus borealis* following maintenance in organ culture. Comp Biochem Physiol Part A Physiol 1984;77:377–82.
[12] Larsson L, Degens H, Li M, Salviati L, Lee YL, Thompson W, et al. Sarcopenia: aging-related loss of muscle mass and function. Physiol Rev 2019;99:427–511.
[13] Hayashi N, Koba S, Yoshida T. Disuse atrophy increases the muscle mechanoreflex in rats. J Appl Physiol 2005;99:1442–5.
[14] Kaufman MP, Forster HV. Reflexes controlling circulatory, ventilator and airway responses to exercise. In: Handbook of physiology. Exercise: regulation and integration of multiple systems. Bethesda, MD: Am. Physiol. Soc.; 1996. p. 381–447. sect. 12, chapt. 10.
[15] Haydon PG, Carmignoto G. Astrocyte control of synaptic transmission and neurovascular coupling. Physiol Rev 2006;86:1009–31.
[16] Hall JE. Guyton and Hall textbook of medical physiology. Saunders; 2015.
[17] Rowell LB. Human cardiovascular control. Oxford University Press; 1993.
[18] Sato K, Ogoh S, Hirasawa A, Oue A, Sadamoto T. The distribution of blood flow in the carotid and vertebral arteries during dynamic exercise in humans. J Physiol 2011;589:2847–56.
[19] Hirasawa A, Sato K, Yoneya M, Sadamoto T, Bailey DM, Ogoh S. Heterogeneous regulation of brain blood flow during low-intensity resistance exercise. Med Sci Sport Exerc 2016;48:1829–34.
[20] Delaey C, van de Voorde J. Regulatory mechanisms in the retinal and choroidal circulation. Ophthalmic Res 2000;32:249–56.
[21] Hayashi N, Ikemura T, Someya N. Effects of dynamic exercise and its intensity on ocular blood flow in humans. Eur J Appl Physiol 2011;111:2601–6.
[22] Ikemura T, Hayashi N. Ocular circulatory responses to exhaustive exercise in humans. Eur J Appl Physiol 2012;112:3313–8.
[23] Hayashi N, Yamaoka-Endo M, Someya N, Fukuba Y. Blood flow in non-muscle tissues and organs during exercise: nature of splanchnic and ocular circulation. J Phys Fit Sport Med 2012;1:281–6.
[24] Bergeron R, Kjar M, Simonsen L, Low JB, Skovgaard D, Howlett K, et al. Splanchnic blood flow and hepatic glucose production in exercising humans: role of renin-angiotensin system. Am J Physiol Regul Integr Comp Physiol 2001;281:1854–61.
[25] Perko MJ, Nielsen HB, Skak C, Clemmesen JO, Schroeder TV, Secher NH. Mesenteric, coeliac and splanchnic blood flow in humans during exercise. J Physiol 1998;513:907–13.
[26] Qamar MI, Read AE. Effects of exercise on mesenteric blood flow in man. Gut 1987;28:583–7.
[27] Momen A, Bower D, Leuenberger UA, Boehmer J, Lerner S, Alfrey EJ, et al. Renal vascular response to static handgrip exercise: sympathetic vs. autoregulatory control. Am J Physiol Hear Circ Physiol 2005;289:1770–6.
[28] Rehrer NJ, Smets A, Reynaert H, Goes E, DE Meirleir K. Effect of exercise on portal vein blood flow in man. Med Sci Sport Exerc 2001;33:1533–7.
[29] Thijssen DHJ, Steendijk S, Hopman MTE. Blood redistribution during exercise in subjects with spinal cord injury and controls. Med Sci Sport Exerc 2009;41:1249–54.
[30] Rasch W, Cabanac M. Vasomotor response of the human face: laser-Doppler measurements during mild hypo- and hyperthermia. Acta Physiol Scand 1993;147:431–6.
[31] White MD, Cabanac M. Physical dilatation of the nostrils lowers the thermal strain of exercising humans. Eur J Appl Physiol Occup Physiol 1995;70:200–6.

[32] González-Alonso J, Crandall CG, Johnson JM. The cardiovascular challenge of exercising in the heat. J Physiol 2008;586:45–53.
[33] Walløe L. Arterio-venous anastomoses in the human skin and their role in temperature control. Temperature 2016;3:92–103.
[34] Jani B, Rajkumar C. Ageing and vascular ageing. Postgrad Med J 2006;82:357–62.
[35] Pizzimenti M, Meyer A, Charles AL, Giannini M, Chakfé N, Lejay A, et al. Sarcopenia and peripheral arterial disease: a systematic review. J Cachexia Sarcopenia Muscle 2020;11:866–86.
[36] Andersen P, Saltin B. Maximal perfusion of skeletal muscle in man. J Physiol 1985;366:233–49.
[37] Fadel PJ. Reflex control of the circulation during exercise. Scand J Med Sci Sport 2015;25:74–82.
[38] Borisov AB, Huang SK, Carlson BM. Remodeling of the vascular bed and progressive loss of capillaries in denervated skeletal muscle. Anat Rec 2000;258:292–304.
[39] Coggan AR, Spina RJ, King DS, Rogers MA, Rogers MA, Brown M, et al. Histochemical and enzymatic comparison of the gastrocnemius muscle of young and elderly men and women. J Gerontol 1992;47:B71–6.
[40] Moreau P, D'Uscio LV, Lüscher TF. Structure and reactivity of small arteries in aging. Cardiovasc Res 1998;37:247–53.
[41] Barnouin Y, McPhee JS, Butler-Browne G, Bosutti A, De Vito G, Jones DA, et al. Coupling between skeletal muscle fiber size and capillarization is maintained during healthy aging. J Cachexia Sarcopenia Muscle 2017;8:647–59.
[42] Hudlicka O, Brown M, Egginton S. Angiogenesis in skeletal and cardiac muscle. Physiol Rev 1992;72:369–417.
[43] Degens H, Turek Z, Hoofd LJ, Van't Hof MA, Binkhorst RA. The relationship between capillarisation and fibre types during compensatory hypertrophy of the plantaris muscle in the rat. J Anat 1992;180:455–63.
[44] Alway SE, Myers MJ, Mohamed JS. Regulation of satellite cell function in sarcopenia. Front Aging Neurosci 2014;6:1–15.
[45] Kwan P. Sarcopenia: the gliogenic perspective. Mech Ageing Dev 2013;134:349–55.
[46] Brown WR, Thore CT. Review: cerebral microvascular pathology in ageing and neurodegeneration. Neuropathol Appl Neurobiol 2011;37:56–74.
[47] Tarumi T, Zhang R. Cerebral blood flow in normal aging adults: cardiovascular determinants, clinical implications, and aerobic fitness. J Neurochem 2018;144:595–608.
[48] Lucas SJE, Ainslie PN, Murrell CJ, Thomas KN, Franz EA, Cotter JD. Effect of age on exercise-induced alterations in cognitive executive function: relationship to cerebral perfusion. Exp Gerontol 2012;47:541–51.
[49] Beason-Held LL, Moghekar A, Zonderman AB, Kraut MA, Resnick SM. Longitudinal changes in cerebral blood flow in the older hypertensive brain. Stroke 2007;38:1766–73.
[50] Ainslie PN, Cotter JD, George KP, Lucas S, Murrell C, Shave R, et al. Elevation in cerebral blood flow velocity with aerobic fitness throughout healthy human ageing. J Physiol 2008;586:4005–10.
[51] Scheel P, Ruge C, Petruch UR, Schöning M. Color duplex measurement of cerebral blood flow volume in healthy adults. Stroke 2000;31:147–50.
[52] Stoquart-ElSankari S, Balédent O, Gondry-Jouet C, Makki M, Godefroy O, Meyer ME. Aging effects on cerebral blood and cerebrospinal fluid flows. J Cereb Blood Flow Metab 2007;27:1563–72.
[53] Dai W, Lopez OL, Carmichael OT, Becker JT, Kuller LH, Gach HM. Mild cognitive impairment and alzheimer disease: patterns of altered cerebral blood flow at MR imaging. Radiology 2009;250:856–66.
[54] Johnson NA, Jahng GH, Weiner MW, Miller BL, Chui HC, Jagust WJ, et al. Pattern of cerebral hypoperfusion in Alzheimer's disease and mild cognitive impairment measured with arterial spin-labeling MR imaging: initial experience. Int Congr Ser 2006;1290:108–22.
[55] Hirao K, Ohnishi T, Hirata Y, Yamashita F, Mori T, Moriguchi Y, et al. The prediction of rapid conversion to Alzheimer's disease in mild cognitive impairment using regional cerebral blood flow SPECT. Neuroimage 2005;28:1014–21.
[56] Meyer JS, Rauch G, Rauch RA, Haque A. Risk factors for cerebral hypoperfusion, mild cognitive impairment, and dementia. Neurobiol Aging 2000;21:161–9.

[57] Lawton MP, Brody EM. Assessment of older people: self-maintaining and instrumental activities of daily living. Gerontologist 1969;9:179–86.
[58] Jekel K, Damian M, Wattmo C, Hausner L, Bullock R, Connelly PJ, et al. Mild cognitive impairment and deficits in instrumental activities of daily living: a systematic review. Alzheimer's Res Ther 2015;7:17.
[59] Wangsa-Wirawan ND. Retinal oxygen. Arch Ophthalmol 2003;121:547.
[60] Hayashi N, Ikemura T, Someya N. Changes in ocular flow induced by hypo- and hypercapnia relate to static visual acuity in humans. Eye Rep 2011;1:e8.
[61] Sponsel WE, Paris G, Sandoval SS, Sanford DK, Harrison JM, Elliott WR, et al. Sildenafil and ocular perfusion. N Engl J Med 2000;342:1680.
[62] Kurtulan E, Gulcu A, Secil M, Celebi I, Aslan G, Esen AA. Effects of sildenafil on ocular perfusion demonstrated by color Doppler ultrasonography. Int J Impot Res 2004;16:244–8.
[63] Wen SW, Wong CHY. Aging- and vascular-related pathologies. Microcirculation 2019;26, e12463.
[64] World Health Organization. Universal eye health: a global action plan 2014–2019. Spain: WHO Press; 2013. p. 1–19.
[65] Ryskulova A, Turczyn K, Makuc DM, Cotch MF, Klein RJ, Janiszewski R. Self-reported age-related eye diseases and visual impairment in the United States: results of the 2002 National Health Interview Survey. Am J Public Health 2008;98:454–61.
[66] Liang YB, Friedman DS, Wong TY, Zhan SY, Sun LP, Wang JJ, Duan XR, Yang XH, Wang FH, Zhou Q, Wang NL, Handan Eye Study Group. Prevalence and causes of low vision and blindness in a rural Chinese adult population: the Handan Eye Study. Ophthalmology 2008;115:1965–72.
[67] Buch H, Vinding T, la Cour M, Appleyard M, Jensen GB, Vesti NN. Prevalence and causes of visual impairment and blindness among 9980 Scandinavian adults. Ophthalmology 2004;111:53–61.
[68] Miyaji A, Ikemura T, Hayashi N. Effect of aging on the blowout time in various ocular vessels. J Aging Sci 2016;4:148.
[69] Kobayashi T, Shiba T, Kinoshita A, Matsumoto T, Hori Y. The influences of gender and aging on optic nerve head microcirculation in healthy adults. Sci Rep 2019;9:15636.
[70] Anderson AJ. Exercise and glaucoma: positive steps toward finding another modifiable risk factor to prevent vision loss. Ophthalmology 2019;126:965–6.
[71] Quigley C, Zgaga L, Vartsakis G, Fahy G. Refractive error and vision problems in children: association with increased sedentary behavior and reduced exercise in 9-year-old children in Ireland. JAAPOS 2019;23:159e1–6.
[72] Lee MJ, Wang J, Friedman DS, Boland MV, De Moraes CG, Ramulu PY. Greater physical activity is associated with slower visual field loss in glaucoma. Ophthalmology 2019;126:958–64.
[73] Luciano GL, Brennan MJ, Rothberg MB. Postprandial hypotension. Am J Med 2010;123:281.e1–6.
[74] Maurer M, Karmally W, Rivadeneira H, Parides M, Bloomfield D. Upright posture and postprandial hypotension in elderly persons. Ann Intern Med 2000;133:533.
[75] Hamada Y, Miyaji A, Hayashi N. Effect of postprandial gum chewing on diet-induced thermogenesis. Obesity 2016;24:878–85.
[76] Kashima H, Eguchi K, Miyamoto K, Fujimoto M, Endo MY, Aso-Someya N, et al. Suppression of oral sweet taste sensation with *Gymnema sylvestre* affects postprandial gastrointestinal blood flow and gastric emptying in humans. Chem Senses 2017;42:295–302.
[77] Madsen JL, Søndergaard SB, Møller S. Meal-induced changes in splanchnic blood flow and oxygen uptake in middle-aged healthy humans. Scand J Gastroenterol 2006;41:87–92.
[78] Someya N, Endo MY, Fukuba Y, Hayashi N. Blood flow responses in celiac and superior mesenteric arteries in the initial phase of digestion. Am J Physiol Regul Integr Comp Physiol 2008;294:R1790–6.
[79] IPCC. Fifth assessment report; 2014.
[80] Nakai S, Itoh T, Morimoto T. Deaths from heat-stroke in Japan: 1968–1994. Int J Biometeorol 1999;43:124–7.
[81] Minson CT, Holowatz LA, Wong BJ, Kenney WL, Wilkins BW. Decreased nitric oxide- and axon reflex-mediated cutaneous vasodilation with age during local heating. J Appl Physiol 2002;93:1644–9.

[82] Kenney WL, Morgan AL, Farquhar WB, Brooks EM, Pierzga JM, Derr JA. Decreased active vasodilator sensitivity in aged skin. Am J Physiol Circ Physiol 1997;272:H1609–14.

[83] Kenney WL, Zappe DH. Effect of age on renal blood flow during exercise. Aging Clin Exp Res 1994;6:293–302.

[84] Nybo L, Rasmussen P, Sawka MN. Performance in the heat-physiological factors of importance for hyperthermia-induced fatigue. In: Comprehensive physiology. Hoboken, NJ, USA: John Wiley & Sons; 2014. p. 657–89.

[85] Périard JD, Cramer MN, Chapman PG, Caillaud C, Thompson MW. Cardiovascular strain impairs prolonged self-paced exercise in the heat. Exp Physiol 2011;96:134–44.

[86] Périard JD, Racinais S, Sawka MN. Adaptations and mechanisms of human heat acclimation: applications for competitive athletes and sports. Scand J Med Sci Sport 2015;25(S1):20–38.

[87] Siccama RN, Janssen KJM, Verheijden NAF, Oudega R, Bax L, van Delden JJM, et al. Systematic review: diagnostic accuracy of clinical decision rules for venous thromboembolism in elderly. Ageing Res Rev 2011;10:304–13.

[88] Wilkerson WR, Sane DC. Aging and thrombosis. Semin Thromb Hemost 2002;28:555–68.

[89] Previtali E, Bucciarelli P, Passamonti SM, Martinelli I. Risk factors for venous and arterial thrombosis. Blood Transfus 2011;9:120–38.

[90] Hemmeryckx B, Emmerechts J, Bovill EG, Hoylaerts MF, Lijnen HR. Effect of ageing on the murine venous circulation. Histochem Cell Biol 2012;137:537–46.

[91] McEniery CM, Yasmin HIR, Qasem A, Wilkinson IB, Cockcroft JR. Normal vascular aging: differential effects on wave reflection and aortic pulse wave velocity – the Anglo-Cardiff Collaborative Trial (ACCT). J Am Coll Cardiol 2005;46:1753–60.

[92] Tanaka H, DeSouza CA, Seals DR. Absence of age-related increase in central arterial stiffness in physically active women. Arterioscler Thromb Vasc Biol 1998;18:127–32.

[93] Vaitkevicius PV, Fleg JL, Engel JH, O'Connor FC, Wright JG, Lakatta LE, et al. Effects of age and aerobic capacity on arterial stiffness in healthy adults. Circulation 1993;88:1456–62.

[94] Mitchell GF, Lacourcière Y, Ouellet JP, Izzo JL, Neutel J, Kerwin LJ, et al. Determinants of elevated pulse pressure in middle-aged and older subjects with uncomplicated systolic hypertension: the role of proximal aortic diameter and the aortic, pressure-flow relationship. Circulation 2003;108:1592–8.

[95] Hickson SS, Butlin M, Graves M, Taviani V, Avolio AP, McEniery CM, et al. The relationship of age with regional aortic stiffness and diameter. JACC Cardiovasc Imaging 2010;3:1247–55.

[96] Credeur DP, Holwerda SW, Boyle LJ, Vianna LC, Jensen AK, Fadel PJ. Effect of aging on carotid baroreflex control of blood pressure and leg vascular conductance in women. Am J Physiol Circ Physiol 2014;306:H1417–25.

[97] Fisher JP, Kim A, Young CN, Fadel PJ. Carotid baroreflex control of arterial blood pressure at rest and during dynamic exercise in aging humans. Am J Physiol Integr Comp Physiol 2010;299:R1241–7.

[98] Davy KP, Seals DR. Total blood volume in healthy young and older men. J Appl Physiol 1994;76:2059–62.

[99] Jones PP, Davy KP, DeSouza CA, van Pelt RE, Seals DR. Absence of age-related decline in total blood volume in physically active females. Am J Physiol Circ Physiol 1997;272:H2534–40.

[100] Koons NJ, Suresh MR, Schlotman TE, Convertino VA. Interrelationship between sex, age, blood volume, and VO$_2$max. Aerosp Med Hum Perform 2019;90:362–8.

[101] Nose H, Mack GW, Shi XR, Morimoto K, Nadel ER. Effect of saline infusion during exercise on thermal and circulatory regulations. J Appl Physiol 1990;69:609–16.

[102] Sanchis-Gomar F, Gómez-Cabrera MC, Viña J. The loss of muscle mass and sarcopenia: non hormonal intervention. Exp Gerontol 2011;46:967–9.

[103] Volkert D. The role of nutrition in the prevention of sarcopenia. Wiener Medizinische Wochenschrift 2011;161:409–15.

[104] Bosaeus I, Rothenberg E. Nutrition and physical activity for the prevention and treatment of age-related sarcopenia. Proc Nutr Soc 2016;75:174–80.

[105] Mijnarends DM, Koster A, Schols JMGA, Meijers JMM, Halfens RJG, Gudnason V, et al. Physical activity and incidence of sarcopenia: the population-based AGES—Reykjavik study. Age Ageing 2016;45:614–20.

[106] Green DJ. Exercise training as vascular medicine. Exerc Sport Sci Rev 2009;37:196–202.
[107] Santos-Parker JR, LaRocca TJ, Seals DR. Aerobic exercise and other healthy lifestyle factors that influence vascular aging. Adv Physiol Educ 2014;38:296–307.
[108] Green DJ, Cable NT, Fox C, Rankin JM, Taylor RR. Modification of forearm resistance vessels by exercise training in young men. J Appl Physiol 1994;77:1829–33.
[109] Spier SA, Delp MD, Meininger CJ, Donato AJ, Ramsey MW, Muller-Delp JM. Effects of ageing and exercise training on endothelium-dependent vasodilation and structure of rat skeletal muscle arterioles. J Physiol 2004;556:947–58.
[110] Laughlin MH, Roseguini B. Mechanisms for exercise training-induced increases in skeletal muscle blood flow capacity: differences with interval sprint training versus aerobic endurance training. J Physiol Pharmacol 2008;59(Suppl 7):71–88.
[111] Murrell CJ, Cotter JD, Thomas KN, Lucas SJE, Williams MJA, Ainslie PN. Cerebral blood flow and cerebrovascular reactivity at rest and during sub-maximal exercise: effect of age and 12-week exercise training. Age (Omaha) 2013;35:905–20.
[112] Colcombe SJ, Erickson KI, Scalf PE, Kim JS, Prakash R, McAuley E, et al. Aerobic exercise training increases brain volume in aging humans. J Gerontol Ser A Biol Sci Med Sci 2006;61:1166–70.
[113] Tanaka H, Dinenno FA, Monahan KD, Clevenger CM, DeSouza CA, Seals DR. Aging, habitual exercise, and dynamic arterial compliance. Circulation 2000;102:1270–5.
[114] Sugawara J, Inoue H, Hayashi K, Yokoi T, Kono I. Effect of low-intensity aerobic exercise training on arterial compliance in postmenopausal women. Hypertens Res 2004;27:897–901.
[115] Okazaki K, Goto M, Nose H. Protein and carbohydrate supplementation increases aerobic and thermoregulatory capacities. J Physiol 2009;587:5585–90.

CHAPTER 12

Dysphagia of cachexia and sarcopenia

Haruyo Matsuo[a] and Kunihiro Sakuma[b]

[a]*Department of Nursing, Kagoshima Medical Association Hospital, Kagoshima, Japan,* [b]*Institute for Liberal Arts, Environment and Society, Tokyo Institute of Technology, Tokyo, Japan*

Abstract

Cachexia is defined as a complex metabolic syndrome characterized by the loss of body weight. Inflammatory cytokines are closely linked to losses of appetite and skeletal muscle mass, shortening survival, and worsening the quality of life. Since dysphagia is frequently observed in the elderly, there is no evidence that cachexia directly induces dysphagia. Sarcopenia may be attributed to changes in the central nervous system, muscle fibers, hormonal balance, nutritional status, and lifestyle. Disorders of skeletal muscle are induced by neuromuscular disease, stroke, and head and neck carcinoma. Almost all these studies revealed associations between dysphagia and sarcopenia. Dysphagia is an important clinical problem causing malnutrition, dehydration, suffocation, aspiration pneumonia, and death. This review focuses on assessment tools, prevalence, and outcomes of cachexia, sarcopenia, and dysphagia associated with major diseases.

Keywords: Cachexia, Sarcopenia, Dysphagia, Anorexia, Malnutrition, Swallowing assessment

Introduction

Cachexia is defined as a complex metabolic syndrome characterized by the loss of body weight. The overall prevalence of cachexia is approximately 11% [1] of the global patient population, it affects more than 50% of cancer patients, and is responsible for approximately 30% [1–3] of the total deaths. The incidence of this syndrome among cancer patients is very high, with the distribution varying by tumor type. The underlying mechanisms that cause cachexia are not well-understood. Cachexia is associated with not only cancers, but also with other inflammatory conditions such as COPD, liver and heart failure, AIDS, and sepsis. Muscle loss is a serious consequence of many chronic diseases and of the aging process itself because it leads to weakness, loss of independence, and an increased risk of death [4]. Cachexia in cancer patients is a prognostic factor indicating decreased resistance to chemotherapy and radiation therapy, reduced effectiveness of anticancer drugs, and an increased risk of postoperative complications [5]. In COPD, repeated exacerbations lead to the progression of the primary disease and an increased rate of cachexia complications [6]. Patients with cardiac cachexia exhibit a progressive involuntary weight loss [7]. Early interventions are important because the nutritional status and oral physical function rapidly decline with the progression of cachexia. Early skeletal muscle loss in cachexia occurs due to metabolic abnormalities and decreased oral intake due to anorexia. Cachexic weight loss and decreased oral intake can lead to dysphagia. Although dysphagia is frequently observed in the elderly, there is no evidence that cachexia directly induces dysphagia. Unlike stroke and head and neck disease, which are frequently associated with dysphagia, few studies of dysphagia in patients with COPD and CHF have been conducted. As for the relationship between cancer cachexia and dysphagia, Lees [8] reported only that patients with head and neck cancer show weight loss and dysphagia at the start of treatment.

Sarcopenia is an age-related condition characterized by the gradual decline of muscle mass and strength. It leads to a reduction in physical performance and represents a risk condition for several negative health-related outcomes [9]. Sarcopenia is essentially a result of aging, but it can occur at any age if it includes cachexia, malnutrition, or disuse syndrome. A systemic review demonstrated that sarcopenia is associated with poor survival in cancer patients [10]. Loss of muscle mass and muscle strength can be greater in patients with moderate-to-severe COPD [11, 12] or during acute COPD exacerbations [13], especially loss of muscle from the lower libs [11, 14, 15]. In advanced stages of CHF, a loss of skeletal muscle mass is commonly observed, which contributes to reduced exercise capacity and frailty [16–18]. Older patients with sarcopenia are more prone to reductions in physical activity, oral intake, and quality of life. A generalized loss of skeletal muscle mass and strength also affects muscles of the head and neck. Recent studies suggest that malnutrition and sarcopenia may contribute to the development of dysphagia.

Dysphagia in sarcopenia is defined as that resulting from the presence of sarcopenia in both the whole body and swallowing-related muscles [19]. A flow chart is used to diagnose dysphagia in sarcopenia; a definitive diagnosis is made based on five diagnostic criteria, but these cannot be implemented for all patients in clinical practice from a practical standpoint. In contrast with the well-defined diagnostic criteria for sarcopenia, including the reference of muscle mass and physical function or muscle strength, the diagnostic criteria for sarcopenic dysphagia have not yet been standardized [9, 20]. Since dysphagia is an important clinical problem causing malnutrition, dehydration, suffocation, aspiration pneumonia, and death, it is necessary to accurately understand the degree of dysphagia as well as the treatment of the disease. This review focuses on assessment tools, prevalence, and outcomes of cachexia, sarcopenia, and dysphagia associated with major diseases. In addition, after clarifying the focus of previous swallowing evaluations, future directions of research in this area are discussed.

Cachexia
Definition of cachexia

Cachexia is defined as a complex metabolic syndrome characterized by the loss of body weight, which negatively affects mortality, morbidity, and quality of life. Cachexia is associated not only with cancers but also with other inflammatory conditions such as COPD, liver and heart failure, AIDS, and sepsis. The overall prevalence of cachexia is approximately

11% [1] of the global patient population, it affects more than 50% of cancer patients, it is responsible for approximately 30% [1–3] of death. The incidence of the syndrome among cancer patients is very high, with the distribution varying by tumor type; in patients with gastric or pancreatic cancer, the incidence is more than 80%, whereas approximately 50% of patients with lung, prostate, and colon cancers are affected, and around 40% of patients with breast tumors or some leukemia develops the syndrome [21, 22]. However, the underlying mechanisms that cause cachexia are not well understood. Approximately 10 years have passed since the definition of cachexia was published by Evans et al. [23]. In 2011, the definition of cachexia was published: "Cancer cachexia is multifactorial defined by an ongoing loss of skeletal muscle mass (with or without loss of fat mass) that cannot be fully reversed by conventional nutritional support and leads to progressive functional impairment" [24]. This definition is used worldwide in conjunction with stage classification [25] to consider cancer cachexia.

Condition of cachexia

Cachexia occurs in cancer as well as in a variety of chronic debilitating diseases. Chronic inflammation leads to decreased muscle mass and weakness, which worsens physical function and quality of life [26]. Metabolic abnormalities, anorexia, and other conditions increase catabolism, resulting in decreased energy intake and a treatment-resistant malnutrition state [23, 27]. Cachexia is viewed as a systemic inflammatory condition mediated by various cytokines [26]. Cachexia, one of the possible factors for sarcopenia, induces early loss of skeletal muscle. Early multimodal interventions are important because nutritional status and physical function rapidly decline according to the progression of cachexia. Skeletal muscle plays a central role in metabolism that influences energy, protein metabolism, body temperature regulation, and insulin sensitivity [28]. Decreased muscle mass due to chronic debilitating diseases and aging can lead to a number of pathological conditions, including dynapenia, malaise, decreased immune strength, susceptibility to infection, glucose intolerance, dyslipidemia, osteoporosis, falls, and fractures, as well as reduced muscle strength and physical function, resulting in poorer QOL and prognosis [28].

The anorexia, the hallmark symptom of cachexia, leads to decreased oral intake and progressive malnutrition, which greatly affects prognosis. Anorexia and metabolic abnormalities are associated with activation of proinflammatory cytokines (TNF-α, IL-1, IL-6) in cachexia. The inflammatory cytokines impair the appetite by stimulating the secretion of neuropeptide Y (NPY) and corticotropin-releasing hormone (CRH), leading to anorexia [29]. In addition to the numerous molecular mediators of cachexia, mechanical and digestive factors have been identified [30, 31]. Tumor burden or chemotherapy may lead to nausea, dysphagia, mucositis, pancreatic insufficiency, and malabsorption [32], resulting in reduced food intake and subsequently weight loss [33]. The aforementioned consensus-definition for cachexia has been validated [34]. The decreased oral intake is caused by anorexia, impaired

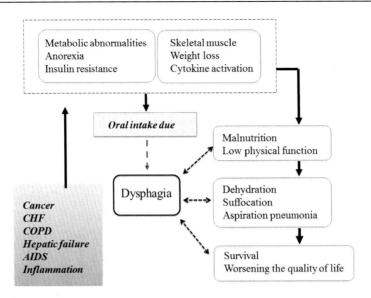

Fig. 1
Association between cachexia and dysphagia Cachexia occurs with a chronic wasting disease. Metabolic abnormalities, anorexia, weight loss, and skeletal muscle loss are associated with malnutrition. These symptoms may result in the decreased oral intake and have a major effect on dysphagia. Dysphagia is likely to be associated with dehydration, asphyxia, aspiration pneumonia, life-threatening illness, and poor quality of life.

gastrointestinal transit, and adverse effects of cancer treatment (surgery, chemotherapy, radiation therapy). Decreased body weight and oral intake due to cachexia and anorexia may affect dysphagia and malnutrition. There is no evidence at this time that cachexia is the direct inducer for dysphagia. Although it is widely accepted that dysphagia could be primary caused by aging, stroke, or head-and-neck diseases, we have often encountered dysphagia without such diseases in patients with cachexia in daily clinical practice (Fig. 1).

Sarcopenia
Definition of sarcopenia

Sarcopenia results from a progressive and systemic loss of skeletal muscle and is associated with reduced physical function, falls, fractures, disability, hospitalization, muscle weakness, and a poor quality of life [9]. The prevalence of sarcopenia has been estimated to range between 1% and 33%. However, these figures depend on the adopted operational definitions, place where research is conducted, and frailty status of the studied individuals [35, 36]. The term sarcopenia was first proposed in 1988 by Rosenberg [37]. Its etymological origins are two Greek words "sarx" and "penia," which translates into "flesh" and "reduced or deficiency." Originally, sarcopenia was considered to lead to impaired physical performance and poor subsistence, noncancer populations and to be characterized by a loss of skeletal muscle mass, skeletal muscle strength, and physical performance [9, 38, 39]. Later, sarcopenia was also found to impair survival in a variety of clinical conditions (e.g., cancer) [40]. By the early 2000s, various causes of age-related sarcopenia were recognized, including systemic inflammation, oxidative stress, a decline in anabolic hormones, reduced physical function, and anorexia. At present, both primary sarcopenia (age-related) and secondary sarcopenia (disease-related) are recognized.

Based on previous epidemiological studies, multiple operational definitions have been proposed to estimate (or determine) sarcopenia. In 2010, the European Working Group on Sarcopenia for Older Persons (EWGSOP) [9] proposed a new operational definition of sarcopenia of aging and diagnostic criteria. These groups used different reference values to define sarcopenia of aging, highlighting the fact that different reference values are necessary for different ethnic groups [41]. In 2014, the Asian Working Group for Sarcopenia (AWGS) proposed diagnostic criteria based on the characteristics of Asian populations [41]. In 2018, the EWGSOP2 added low muscle strength as a key characteristic of low muscle quality and the presence of low muscle quantity to confirm the diagnosis. Furthermore, the EWGSOP2 recommended the use of the SARC-F and speedup screening, which indicates that muscle strength, such as handgrip strength, should be measured and an accurate diagnosis of the skeletal muscle mass should be made. One was an update by the EWGSOP2 [42], and the other was on the management of sarcopenia of aging by the International Clinical Practice Guidelines for Sarcopenia (ICFSR) [43]. In addition, in 2019, AWGS released a new algorithm and recommended strategies for the early identification of those at risk of sarcopenia in primary care settings, even without a diagnostic device. Although the diagnostic criteria vary between different study groups, it is common for the criteria to comprise "skeletal muscle mass," "physical function," and "muscle strength" [44].

Condition of sarcopenia

Sarcopenia is an age-related condition characterized by the gradual decline of muscle mass and strength. It leads to a reduction in physical performance and represents a risk condition for several negative health-related outcomes [9]. Sarcopenia can be classified as either primary (age) or secondary (activities, nutrition, and diseases). Primary sarcopenia is an aging-associated loss of muscle mass. Secondary sarcopenia predominantly involves a loss of muscle mass without emphasis placed on muscle function. Activity-related sarcopenia can be caused by prolonged bed rest, a sedentary lifestyle, deconditioning, or zero-gravity conditions. Nutrition-related sarcopenia occurs when there is inadequate dietary intake of energy and protein, malabsorption, gastrointestinal problems, or medications that result in anorexia. Disease-related sarcopenia is associated with inflammatory disease, malignancy, endocrine disease, and advanced organ failure [39].

A person loses 1% of their muscle mass with each year of age, and aging is the most important factor in sarcopenia. Rogers et al. [38] showed that muscle mass decreases with aging, even with continued exercise. Daily bed rest reduces muscle mass by 0.5% [45]. Malnutrition and intake of low protein and amino acid can trigger sarcopenia. Matone et al. [46] showed that approximately 15% of acute care hospital admissions developed sarcopenia and that long-term bed rest and poor nutrition were risks for accelerating sarcopenia. Roubenoff et al. [47] reported that sarcopenia may be attributed to changes in the central nervous system, muscle fibers, hormonal balance, nutritional status, and lifestyle. Loss of muscle mass can result in functional impairments associated with muscle weakness, such as respiratory dysfunction, which can affect mortality. Sarcopenia is essentially a result of aging, but it can occur at any age if the underlying disease is cachexia, malnutrition, or disuse syndrome (Fig. 2).

The decline of a skeletal muscle occurring with aging is systemic and exerts detrimental effects beyond impairing the mobility function. Disorders of skeletal muscle are induced by neuromuscular disease, stroke, and head and neck carcinoma [48]. Such disorders are commonly associated with dysphagia, which is caused by an abnormality in the movement of either fluid or food into the mouth and stomach via the pharynx and esophagus. Dysphagia is an important clinical problem causing malnutrition, dehydration, and aspiration pneumonia. Grelot et al. [49] showed that swallowing muscles were active even during time periods

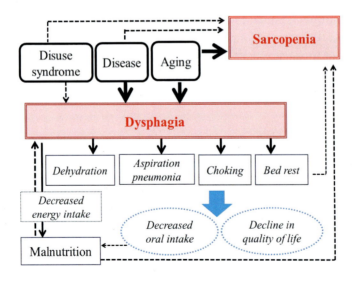

Fig. 2
Possible relationship between dysphagia and sarcopenia development Dysphagia is essentially caused by age and disease. Dysphagia is likely to be associated with dehydration, aspiration pneumonia, choking, and bed rest. Sarcopenia is essentially a result of aging, but it can occur at any age if the underlying disease, malnutrition, bed rest, or disuse syndrome.

without any swallowing activity, are regulated by the respiratory center in the brainstem, and show activities that are mainly synchronized with expiration. Interestingly the swallowing muscles are considered to be striated muscles, but their embryological characteristics are different from those of somatic muscle, the skeletal muscles of the extremities, and it is considered that disuse muscle atrophy is less likely than in general somatic muscle [50]. Therefore, when evaluating the pathogenesis of sarcopenia, it is necessary to consider the differences between it and generalized somatic muscle. Malnutrition is one possible cause of sarcopenia, and the two often overlap. Sánchez-Rodríguez et al. [51] reported that sarcopenia was present in 76% of hospitalized patients aged 70 years or older who presented with malnutrition. Malnutrition is a common cause of dysphagia [52, 53] and also secondary sarcopenia. However, there is no report of basic research showing that malnutrition is a direct cause of swallowing muscle atrophy. Many of the swallowing muscles are composed of slow muscle fibers and may be prone to be affected by malnutrition [52, 53]. Furthermore, dysphagia can lead to reduced energy intake, resulting in nutritional deficiencies. In summary, dysphagia may lead to malnutrition and sarcopenia. Older patients with sarcopenia are more prone to reductions in physical activity, oral intake, and quality of life. A generalized loss of skeletal muscle mass and strength also affects muscles of the head and neck. Recent studies suggest that malnutrition and sarcopenia may contribute to the development of dysphagia. In 1996, Veldee and Peth [54] proposed a hypothesis whereby malnutrition may cause dysphagia. In 2012, Kuroda and Kuroda [55] reported an association between arm circumference and swallowing function using the term "sarcopenic dysphagia" in a review article and presented it as a new concept of dysphagia. In 2015, Clave and Shaker [56], a worldwide leading researcher in dysphagia, used the term "sarcopenic dysphagia" in a review article. Sporns et al. [57] showed that muscle mass loss in swallowing-related muscles was associated with dysphagia in patients with acute stroke, and muscle mass showed a greater decrease with more advanced age. Also, several clinical studies reported associations with tongue thickness and muscle mass [58], tongue pressure and dysphagia [59], handgrip strength [60], and nutritional status [61]. Interestingly, systemic muscle mass loss and sarcopenia have been shown to contribute to the development of dysphagia. Maeda et al. [62] showed that skeletal muscle mass is a predictor of dysphagia development in older adults. Yoshimura et al. [63] reported an association between systemic sarcopenia and dysphagia in rehabilitated older adults. These reports suggest the possibility of dysphagia being associated with sarcopenia.

In 2019, a position paper on sarcopenia and dysphagia was presented. Dysphagia in sarcopenia is defined as dysphagia resulting from the presence of sarcopenia in both the whole body and swallowing-related muscles [19]. A flow chart is used to diagnose dysphagia in sarcopenia; a definitive diagnosis is made based on five diagnostic criteria, but these cannot be implemented for all patients in clinical practice from a practical standpoint. Furthermore, there are no criteria for direct assessment of swallowing strength or for defining swallowing muscle mass loss. In addition, few clinical studies have been reported using this flowchart and it is not well established in clinical practice. In contrast with the well-defined diagnostic criteria for sarcopenia, including the reference of muscle mass and physical function or muscle strength, the diagnostic criteria for sarcopenic dysphagia have not yet been standardized [9, 20]. The risk factors of sarcopenia include age, history of clinical disease, and physical frailty, including reduced activities of daily living. Almost all these studies revealed the associations between dysphagia and sarcopenia. The prevalence and mechanism of dysphagia in sarcopenia, as well as effective interventions, are still unclear and require further investigation.

Dysphagia
Definition of dysphagia

Swallowing is the movement of fluids and food from the outside into the mouth and then through the pharynx and esophagus into the stomach. Dysphagia occurs from abnormalities in either of these processes. The process of swallowing can be divided into four consecutive stages: (1) oral preparatory stage, (2) oropharyngeal stage, (3) pharyngeal stage, and (4) esophageal stage. The first two steps correspond to pharyngeal and bolus formation and delivery to the pharynx. The pharyngeal phase requires precise coordination of respiration and swallowing for airway defense during the swallowing reflex phase. During the esophageal stage, the bolus is transported to the stomach by esophageal peristalsis. Seven cranial nerves and more than 25 muscles are involved, and any neurological or structural defect affects swallowing. Swallowing should be understood as a series of movements and should be evaluated at each stage.

Cancer

The progression of cancer cachexia involves the activation of tumor-released proteolysis-inducing factor (PIF), lipid mobilizing factor [27], and other proinflammatory cytokines. Anorexia is common in patients with cancer and is a major component of cancer cachexia. Large amounts of proinflammatory cytokines (TNF-α, IL-1β, IL-6) are released from macrophages, mononuclear leukocytes, and lymphocytes [64]. The inflammatory cytokines not only act on skeletal muscle but also increase leptin receptors in the hypothalamus, causing leptin-like effects and decreasing appetite. There are numerous factors leading to anorexia in patients with cachexia. The primary cause is an increase in proinflammatory cytokines and tumorigenic factors, but dysphagia caused by the tumor is also a possibility. Inflammatory cytokines and tumorigenic factors influence anorexia, hypermetabolism, and the decreased muscle and fat mass. Although the dominant cause of weight and muscle mass loss is cachexia, dysphagia or obstruction of the gastrointestinal tract by a tumor may also be causative [65]. Cachexia in cancer patients is a prognostic factor indicating decreased resistance to chemotherapy and radiation therapy, reduced the effectiveness of anticancer drugs, and an increased risk of postoperative complications [5]. A number of symptoms and complications of advanced cancer, anticancer treatment, or medical comorbidities can adversely affect patients who have retained their appetite and ability to eat or digest food [66, 67]. Insufficient dietary intake and decreased appetite are major factors leading to loss of muscle mass.

Weight loss of cancer cachexia is caused by a variable degree of reduced food intake and deranged metabolism. Cancer cachexia is modulated by a variety of tumor and treatment-related symptoms. Indeed, a number of symptoms of advanced tumor and anticancer treatment can influence patients' appetite and ability to eat. These are referred to as nutritional impact symptoms (NIS) and include symptoms such as anorexia, pain, and fatigue. The decreased weight loss affects the NIS: stomatitis, dysphagia, nausea, emesis, constipation, and taste disorder [68]. The ESPEN guidelines of 2009 suggest that around 50% of patients with weight loss are hypermetabolic [69]. The metabolic change would be accompanied by anorexia, fatigue, and nausea, which, in turn, exacerbate weight loss. It is estimated that 25%–57% of patients with tumors of the head and neck already have a markedly impaired nutrition status at the time of diagnosis and before beginning treatment [70, 71]. Weight loss due to inadequate dietary intake as a result of dysphagia frequently occurs in head and neck cancer patients [72–74]. Many cancer patients experience eating difficulty and weight loss during the course of anticancer treatment. Lees [8] suggested that 57% of patients with head and neck cancer experience weight loss at the start of radiation therapy. Based on a questionnaire survey, more than 33% of patients with cancer cachexia showed dysphagia (swallowing problems). In another cross-sectional study, Omlin et al. [68] used a checklist to assess the frequency of NIS in a mixed cancer population. They indicated that dysphagia is one of the frequent symptoms in this population (11.5%). Studies of dysphagia in patients with cancer have involved only limited assessments of dysphagia as they have used only questionnaires and checklists, with no detailed survey or analysis being defined. The gold standard for evaluation of swallowing is a videofluoroscopic examination of swallowing (VF) and videoendoscopic examination of swallowing (VE). VF can be evaluated morphologically and functionally to accurately assess the presence and severity of dysphagia and risk of aspiration. On the other hand, VE diagnosis evaluates structural abnormalities during the pharyngeal phase but cannot assess the oral phase of swallowing; thus, VE alone is a very limited tool for swallowing evaluation (Table 1). Questionnaires used to subjectively assess dysphagia in patients with cancer are personal measures of patients or clinicians and inaccurate for assessing dysphagia. There is a discrepancy in the literature with respect to the correlation between subjective and objective swallowing evaluations. Pauloski et al. [75] reported an excellent correlation between the swallowing function assessed by VF and patient-reported dysphagia. In contrast, Jensen et al. [76] found little concordance between dysphagia-related complaints and objective parameters. An objective evaluation may underestimate the severity of dysphagia in patients. We believe that a combination of clinical and objective methods is essential for defining the swallowing function and in diagnosing dysphagia accurately. At present, insufficient evidence suggests

Table 1: Comparison of clinical advantages of VF, VE, and checklist.

Apply	VF	VE	Checklist
Initial evaluation	○		○
Oral function	○		○
Pharyngeal and laryngeal functions	○	○	○
Esophageal function	○		○
Dynamic evaluation	○	○	
Secretion evaluation		○	
Anatomic deviations		○	
Biofeedback		○	
Simplicity		○	○
Exposure		○	
Time constraint		○	○

possible cachectic dysphagia in patients with cancer. Assessment of the swallowing function is not common in diagnostic testing of cachexia. However, patients with cancer may have dysphagia associated with cachexia, and dysphagia would be more severe in the presence of cachexia, anorexia, and muscle atrophy. Dysphagic impairment is a clinically relevant acute and long-term complication in patients with cancer. Dysphagia is common in patients with cancer. Most studies on this complication have been focused on patients with head and neck cancers, but swallowing disorders may also be present in patients with other malignancies. Dysphagia in cancer patients is often caused by a malignant tumor in the head and neck region. The frequency and severity of dysphagia depend on the cancer stage and location of the tumor, as the tumor may affect the motility associated with swallowing [77–81]. Several studies showed significant rates of pretreatment dysphagia. Pauloski et al. [78] found dysphagia in 28.2% of patients with stage T2 or more oral cancers, 50.9% of pharyngeal cancer, and 28.9% of laryngeal cancer. In another retrospective study, Nguyen et al. [81] reported dysphagia in 5% of patients with all tumor stages of oral, 33% of pharyngeal, 29% of laryngeal, and 52% of hypopharyngeal cancers. In addition, Stenson et al. [79] categorized dysphagia severity in the presence of stage III or more oral cancer: 28% mild impairment, 34% mild-moderate impairment, and 4% moderate-severe impairment. Furthermore, in addition to dysphagia caused by the tumor, increased age would also be associated with increased baseline swallowing dysfunction. Garcia-Peris et al. [82] reported dysphagia in 50.6% of patients with head and neck cancer treated with surgery and radiotherapy or chemotherapy. Surgical interventions for head and neck cancer result in anatomic or neurologic disorders [83]. Combinations of chemotherapy may increase acute toxicity and dysphagia, but this has not been elucidated [84]. Complications such as cancer or chemotherapy interfere with normal swallowing function. It is necessary to recognize that side effects of cancer and chemotherapy can lead to decreased swallowing function and further progression of cachexia. Therefore, evaluation and management of dysphagia should be incorporated into the diagnosis and treatment plan for cachexia.

Sarcopenia in patients with cancer is an important problem that has an impact on shortening survival. The prevalence of sarcopenia in patients with cancer ranges between 27.3% and 66.7% [85]. A systemic review demonstrated that sarcopenia is associated with poor survival in patients with cancer [10]. Pamoukdjian et al. [86] found that 39% of patients with cancer had pretreatment sarcopenia, and pretreatment sarcopenia resulted in postoperative complications, chemotherapy toxicity, and poor survival. Multiple clinical studies reported that sarcopenia in gastrointestinal cancer surgery is a risk factor for postoperative complications. Hodari et al. [87], in a large study, showed that patients with severe sarcopenia who underwent esophagectomy had significantly higher rates of postoperative cardiovascular complications and mortality. Reisinger et al. [88] reported that greater muscle mass loss during preoperative chemoradiotherapy (CRT) in patients with esophageal cancer in cases of stage III or higher induced a significantly higher incidence of fatal postoperative complications. Huang et al. [89] showed that sarcopenia in elderly patients undergoing radical gastrectomy for gastric cancer was an independent predictor of 1-year mortality. Sarcopenia was assessed by muscle mass, handgrip strength, and walking speed, and the receiver operating characteristic (ROC) curve demonstrated an increased predictive power for 1-year mortality with the inclusion of sarcopenia. In multivariate analysis, decreased skeletal muscle mass was not predictive of 1-year mortality, and the measurement of muscle function is important as a preoperative assessment criterion for sarcopenia. Lieffers et al. [90] found that 39% of colorectal cancer surgery cases had sarcopenia, and the sarcopenia group had a significantly longer postoperative hospital stay compared with the nonsarcopenia group, with sarcopenia shown to be an independent risk factor for the development of postoperative infectious complications. Reisinger et al. [91] reported that the presence of sarcopenia in colorectal cancer cases was significantly correlated with in-hospital mortality. In addition, patients with reduced skeletal muscle mass after chemotherapy treatment were shown to develop a high rate of grade III or higher toxicity and have a lower survival rate [92, 93]. Surgical techniques and chemotherapy that consider sarcopenia in all patients with cancer, even before treatment, may be effective in improving the quality of life and survival.

Malnutrition is a factor in the development of sarcopenia and is found in many patients with cancer. Approximately 35 to 60% of patients with head and neck cancer present with malnutrition and more than 10% weight loss [94]. In addition, patients with head and neck cancer experience weight loss, gastrointestinal distress, anorexia, and sarcopenia before, during, and after their oncological treatment [95]. Radiation therapy plays a pivotal role in most patients with head and neck cancer and is associated with many toxicities, like xerostomia, oral mucositis, and dysphagia, resulting in further deterioration of the nutritional status [96–99]. Many patients present with symptomatic tumors that lead to decreased oral intake before the initiation of treatment, with most patients experiencing a loss of more than 5% of pretreatment [100–102]. Concurrent chemotherapy and radiation result in significant systemic toxicities, including nausea, vomiting, anorexia, and dysphagia [100–102].

Rankher et al. [103] reported that in patients with oral cancer, surgery and chemoradiotherapy can easily cause dysphagia. These reductions in oral intake may also affect weight and skeletal muscle mass loss.

Dysphagia is frequently observed in patients with esophageal and head and neck cancers. However, the relationship between sarcopenia and dysphagia in the gastrointestinal region has rarely been tested. van Maria Rijn-Dekker [104] reported an association between sarcopenia and dysphagia in patients with head and neck cancer treated with radiation therapy. In this study, late radiation-induced toxicity endpoints were patient- and physician-rated xerostomia and physician-rated dysphagia, 6 and 12 months after treatment. Patient-rated xerostomia was assessed using European Organization for Research Treatment of Cancer EORTC QLQ-H&N35 questionnaires [105], and physician-rated xerostomia and dysphagia were assessed using the Common Terminology Criteria for Adverse Events (CTCAE, v.4, 03) [106], respectively. In multivariable analysis, patients with sarcopenia were associated with physician-rated xerostomia and dysphagia 6 and 12 months after treatment. In a report on sarcopenia before and after oral cancer surgery, postoperative chemoradiotherapy is a risk factor for weight loss, decreased skeletal muscle mass, and dysphagia at discharge [107]. In addition, Mekhail et al. [108] reported that acute reactions to chemoradiotherapy at 1 month occurred in 80% of patients and dysphagia in 90% of patients. The mucositis and nausea associated with postoperative chemotherapy can make oral intake difficult, leading to less challenging dietary patterns and tube feeding management, and further reducing the swallowing function. Langendijk et al. [109] showed that xerostomia and dysphagia can affect the quality of life. In addition, increased radiation-induced toxicity in patients with sarcopenia has also been shown to affect the quality of life. Previous studies showed that surgery and chemoradiation can affect postoperative weight loss and swallowing function, but it is unclear whether cancer affects dysphagia in sarcopenia. No clear link has been found between patients with cancer and dysphagia in sarcopenia, so future high-quality intervention studies are needed.

Chronic obstructive pulmonary disease

Cachexia is a serious clinical problem of many chronic diseases. The World Health Organization predicts that it will become the third leading cause of mortality worldwide in 2020 [110]. Chronic obstructive pulmonary disease (COPD) is a chronic inflammatory disorder of the lung and whole body caused mainly by tobacco smoking. Inflammatory metabolic abnormalities are thought to cause weight loss and sarcopenia [111]. Increased levels of inflammatory cytokines such as tumor necrosis factor-alpha (TNF-α), interleukin-6 (IL-6), and C-reactive protein (CRP) induce decreased lean body mass and exercise tolerance in patients with COPD [112–114]. NF-κB activation occurs in the skeletal muscle of COPD patients with low body weight [115]. Patients with cachexia were suggested to have prominent systemic inflammation and anorexia [7]. COPD patients have increased anorectic leptin secretion [116].

COPD is characterized by chronic airflow limitation leading to pathologic alterations in the lungs with consequent extrapulmonary effects. It is not a completely reversible disease, generating systemic complications and comorbidities that contribute to the worsening of the disease and that can lead to death [117, 118]. In COPD, the primary disease progresses by repeated exacerbation, and the complication rate of cachexia increases [6]. Wagner et al. [119] found that in approximately 25% of patients with COPD developing cachexia, coexisting cachexia increases mortality in COPD patients. Since exacerbations inevitably leads to a worsening of lung function [120] and an increased risk of mortality [121], decreasing the number of exacerbations is important. A literature review of the relationship between dysphagia and exacerbations in COPD suggests that the presence of dysphagia exacerbates the COPD, especially when the incoordination of the swallowing reflex occurs with consequent laryngeal aspiration [122, 123]. O'Kane et al. [124], in a systematic review, six of the seven studies surveyed documented some kind of alteration in the swallowing process of patients with COPD. Unstable dysphagia with aspiration may be a predictor of COPD exacerbation. At present, insufficient evidence suggests the association between dysphagia and COPD of cachexia. Dysphagia would have a cause of exacerbation, but its effects on COPD patients with cachexia are not well recognized. Good-Fratturelli et al. [125] reported that the incidence of dysphagia associated with COPD was 85%, with laryngeal penetration and aspiration observed in 28% and 42% of subjects, respectively. Furthermore, complications secondary to swallowing impairments, such as aspiration pneumonia, dehydration, and airway obstruction, have been shown to contribute to disease exacerbations [126]. Recent research focuses on the correlation between COPD and dysphagia and on the relationship between dysphagia and increased exacerbations [123, 127]. In addition, in their hospital-based case-control study, some authors found a higher prevalence of dysphagia in individuals with COPD than in controls [128, 129]. Stein et al. [128] and Mokhlesi et al. [129] reported 84% and 20% of the COPD patients with moderate to severe disease, respectively. Terada et al. [130] reported that an abnormal swallowing reflex exacerbates the COPD more frequently.

In addition, two recent studies suggest that the duration of the events of the pharyngeal phase of swallowing is longer in COPD patients than in healthy controls when assessed through VF [131, 132]. Cvejic et al. [133], in a case-control study using VF, demonstrated that patients with stable and moderate COPD were more likely to have laryngeal penetration of contents and aspiration of large fluid volumes of swallowing. VF or VE are reliable methods for detecting dysphagia, but from a practical viewpoint, VF or VE cannot be adopted for all patients. In addition, there is no validated dysphagia screening for COPD patients. The evaluation method used in the study may lead to an underestimation of dysphagia.

Dysphagia is known to have devastating effects on nutritional status. Garand et al. [134] found that oropharyngeal swallowing impairment was observed in all COPD patients. Interestingly, patients with COPD have no specific neurological or structural etiology known to account for dysphagia. Maltais et al. [135] reported that it is related, at least in part, to poor nutrition and reduced exercise tolerance with generalized weakness present in the COPD patients. In addition, Jones et al. [136] reported that the prevalence of sarcopenia was 14.5% in the stable COPD patients. Dysphagia is associated with an increased risk of aspiration and malnutrition and may affect the swallowing muscles. The clinical consequences of cachexia are dependent on both weight loss and systemic inflammation, which accompany cachexia development [137, 138]. Skeletal muscle wasting is an important component of cachexia; in addition, it can be easily assumed that muscle wasting leads to the impairment of swallowing function. However, when considering the limited number of studies and the absence of randomized controlled trials, it is evident that more research is needed to study the relationship between the COPD and dysphagia. Further studies are needed to assess the association between cachexia and dysphagia in COPD, because of differences in selection criteria, definitions, and evaluation methods.

COPD is a condition characterized by chronic inflammation and extrapulmonary changes that negatively affect physical functions (e.g., lower levels of physical activity and reductions in muscle mass strength) [139–144]. The presence of such factors is also closely related to the presence of sarcopenia. In COPD patients, prevalence estimates range from 15% to 55% [140, 145]. Loss of muscle mass and muscle strength can be greater in patients with moderate-to-severe COPD [11, 12] or during acute COPD exacerbations [13], especially loss of muscle from the lower limbs [11, 14, 15]. Lee et al. [146] showed that COPD occurs mainly in middle-aged and older people and that sarcopenia in COPD can occur irrespective of age. While the prevalence of sarcopenia increases notably with aging, the higher prevalence in COPD patients is unlikely to be explained by age alone. There are biological mechanisms whereby respiratory impairment contributes to muscle deterioration [11], and patients with more severe emphysema have a lower muscle mass [12]. A systemic review indicated that sarcopenia is prevalent in a significant proportion of patients with COPD and negatively impacts important clinical outcomes [47]. Various meta-analyses showed that those with sarcopenia had, on average, poorer FEV1% predicted and performance than those without sarcopenia [147]. Although sarcopenia has also been shown to contribute to a poorer prognosis in patients with COPD, no studies have been reported on mortality. Sarcopenia is a clinically important condition that is prevalent within a large proportion of patients with COPD. Early detection of sarcopenia is extremely important as it may be useful in the rehabilitation of COPD patients and treatment of respiratory failure management.

Dysphagia may be present in COPD patients and is associated with malnutrition and aspiration pneumonia, which can cause COPD exacerbations. Few studies have been reported on COPD patients and dysphagia. Good-Fratturelli et al. [118] found that 65% of COPD patients experienced difficulty in swallowing and 49% had dysphagia. Mokhlesi et al. [148] noted that COPD-induced pulmonary hyperinflation can make swallowing difficult, leading to inadequate laryngeal elevation. COPD is associated with secondary sarcopenia caused by decreased physical activity due to dysphagia on exertion, systemic inflammation, and malnutrition. These may be associated with dysphagia, but there are no reports of dysphagia in patients with COPD and sarcopenia. Sarcopenia is a frequent extrapulmonary condition in COPD patients. Sarcopenia is an important factor in considering dysphagia, but there are no methods or diagnostic criteria for assessing sarcopenic dysphagia, and future research findings are awaited.

Chronic heart failure

Chronic heart failure (CHF) is a recurrent and progressive syndrome. CHF affects up to 2% of the population in the developed countries and is therefore considered to be a massive socioeconomic health burden [7]. The prevalence of cachexia in CHF ranges from 5% to 15% [149–151]. The progress of CHF leads to high five-year mortality rates of 50% or more [152–154]. Cachexia in the context of CHF has been termed cardiac cachexia and presents a progressive involuntary weight loss [7]. Tian et al. [155] suggested that muscle mass loss due to cachexia was found not only in skeletal muscle but also in heart muscle. Malnutrition and cachexia occur in many patients with CHF, leading to decreased quality of life and increased mortality. CHF is the most common admission diagnosis [156], and cachexia has been associated with a higher readmission rate [157]. Cardiac cachexia is thought to affect between 8% and 42% of patients with CHF [158]. Sundaram and Fang [159] found a mortality rate in cachexic CHF patients being as high as 20%–30% at 1 year.

Levine et al. [160] found an increased the blood level of TNF-α with cardiac cachexia. The increased TNF-α, IL-6, and TNF-α receptor in CHF patients is a poor prognostic factor [161, 162]. Langhans and Hrupka [163] reported that TNF-α and IL-1 act directly on the brain to reduce appetite. The inflammatory cytokines may be closely modulated to the pathogenesis of CHF. Cardiac cachexia is one of the factors that worse nutritional status. The major nutritional dysfunction in CHF patients is represented by malnutrition. Various clinical studies have found that patients with CHF are in a prevalent malnutrition state from 54% to 69% [164, 165]. Matsuo et al. [166] reported that the prevalence of malnutrition was approximately 56% in patients undergoing cardiac rehabilitation after CHF. Malnutrition is more commonly encountered in patients with CHF, at times progressing to overt cardiac cachexia, which is characterized by protein-calorie malnutrition with muscle wasting and peripheral edema. Poehlman et al. [167] reported an increased resting energy expenditure with cardiac cachexia. Anker and Coats [168] found that anorexia was present in 10%–20% of patients with CHF. The nutritional status would deteriorate if the energy intake is not sufficiently secured. CHF patients have anorexia for a variety of reasons. Symptoms of CHF, such as dyspnea and malaise, lead to reduced activity, decreased activity of life, and loss of muscle mass. As a result, the decrease of oral intake would worsen the nutritional status. Decreased skeletal muscle strength with impairment of daily function is considered characteristic of malnutrition that it has been incorporated into its definition [169, 170]. Few studies have focused on the combination of nutrition and exercise therapy among CHF patients. Pineda-Juarez et al. [171] found that the combination of branched-chain amino acid (BCAA) supplementation and resistance exercise can significantly ameliorate sarcopenia and cachexia in CHF patients. The authors found that clinical and physical improvements were caused by the resistance exercise independently from BCAA supplementation. In general, there is consensus that sarcopenia requires appropriate physical therapy and nutrition management in addition to treatment for the primary disease [172]. A more recent systematic review indicated the effectiveness of nutrition and exercise therapy for the elderly in sarcopenia [173, 174].

However, little is known about the relationship between dysphagia and cardiovascular disease, including CHF. Ferraris et al. [175] showed preoperative heart failure was at increased risk of dysphagia. Altman et al. [176] reported that dysphagia was associated with congestive heart failure and increases the length of hospital stay 1.8 times in patients with CHF. Dysphagia is suspected to have a significant impact on clinical outcomes in patients with CHF. Although it is widely accepted that dysphagia could be primarily caused by stroke or head-and-neck diseases, we have often encountered dysphagia without such diseases in older patients with CHF in daily clinical practice. However, there is little evidence regarding the prevalence of dysphagia in these patients. It is necessary to identify dysphagia as well as an assessment of CHF and cardiac cachexia. Decreased swallowing function is ascribed by aging and impaired intestinal absorption and reduced intake of energy and protein, leading to the incidence or exacerbation of dysphagia [177, 178]. Future studies should determine whether dysphagia contributes to poor nutritional status in patients with CHF.

CHF is an important clinical problem causing declines in physical function, quality of life, and clinical outcomes [179–183]. The prevalence of sarcopenia increases in patients suffering from CHF. Fulster et al. [183] reported that 20% of patients with CHF had sarcopenia and significantly reduced handgrip strength, quadriceps muscle strength, and exercise tolerance. In advanced stages of CHF, a loss of skeletal muscle mass is commonly observed, which contributes to a reduced exercise capacity and frailty [16–18]. Interestingly, CHF patients with a preserved ejection fraction demonstrate a high prevalence of sarcopenic obesity [184–186]. Another contributing factor to sarcopenia is a variable degree of malnutrition that may be caused by inflammatory cytokines [179, 180]. Undernutrition is common among patients with CHF [181], and it increases the risks of mortality and rehospitalization [182, 183]. Among older CHF patients, undernutrition-related outcomes include sarcopenia, which is associated with a further decline in the physical function and activities of daily living (ADLs) [187].

Important clinical outcomes among patients with CHF include a decreased physical function, dysphagia, and mortality. However, there is insufficient evidence for dysphagia in CHF patients, especially in older patients. Furthermore, there is no direct report of dysphagia in CHF and sarcopenia patients. Particularly, hospitalized older adults are often malnourished and those with undernutrition and sarcopenia tend to have poor short-term outcomes, including the inability to perform independent ADLs and dysphagia [63]. Dysphagia is associated with a reduced physical function after acute care [188, 189] and is highly prevalent in community-dwelling frail older patients [190]. In addition, Matsuo et al. [191] showed that the incidence of dysphagia during hospital admission is negatively associated with functional recovery and 1-year survival rates in CHF patients. A decreased swallowing function can result from both aging and impaired intestinal absorption and reduced intake of energy and protein, and this leads to the development or exacerbation of dysphagia [192, 193]. Swallowing management of hospitalized CHF patients is essential for improving the nutritional status, physical function, and life expectancy. It is easy to predict that dysphagia can lead to reduced energy intake, consequently resulting in undernutrition, and nutritional and exercise therapies during hospitalization are conversely necessary to improve dysphagia. Validation is required to determine whether improvements in undernutrition and sarcopenia lead to the prevention of dysphagia in patients with CHF.

Conclusions

Cachexic and sarcopenic weight loss and decreased oral intake can lead to dysphagia. Clinical evaluation of swallowing should be performed routinely. There is little evidence regarding the prevalence of dysphagia in COPD and CHF. Since there is considerable variation among studies determining dysphagia, it is probable that the evaluation methods used in these study may elicit an underestimation of dysphagia. Dysphagia is an important clinical problem causing malnutrition, dehydration, suffocation, aspiration pneumonia, and death. We should accurately understand the degree of dysphagia and the treatment of the disease. Therefore, evaluation and management of dysphagia should be incorporated into the diagnosis and treatment plan for cachexia and sarcopenia. Further studies are needed to evaluate the association between cachexia and dysphagia in sarcopenia.

References

[1] Argilés JM, Busquest S, Stemmler B, Lopez-Soriano FJ. Cancer cachexia: understanding the molecular basis. Nat Rev Cancer 2014;14:754–62.
[2] von Haehling S, Anker SD. Prevalence, incidence and clinical impact of cachexia: facts and numbers—update 2014. J Cachexia Sarcopenia Muscle 2014;1:129–33.
[3] Tisdale MJ. Cachexia in cancer patients. Nat Rev Cancer 2002;2:862–71.
[4] Sakuma K, Aoi W, Yamaguchi A. Molecular mechanism of sarcopenia and cachexia: recent research advances. Pflugers Arch 2017;469:573–91.
[5] Murphy KT, Lynch GS. Update on emerging drugs for cancer cachexia. Expert Opin Emerg Drugs 2009;14:619–32.
[6] Schols AM, Broekhuizen R, Weling-Scheepers CA, Wouters EF. Body composition and mortality in chronic obstructive pulmonary disease. Am J Clin Nutr 2005;82:53–9.
[7] Fornaro A, Olivotto I, Rigacci L, Ciaccheri M, Tomberli B, Ferrantini C, Coppini R, Girolami F, Mazzarotto F, Chiostri M, et al. Comparison of long-term outcome in anthracycline-related versus idiopathic dilated cardiomyopathy: a single centre experience. Eur J Heart Fail 2018;20:898–906.

[8] Lees J. Incidence of weight loss in head and neck cancer patients on commencing radiotherapy treatment at a regional oncology centre. Eur J Cancer Care 1999;8:133–6.

[9] Cruz-Jentoft AJ, Baeyens JP, Bauer JM, Boirie Y, Cederholm T, Landi F, Martin FC, Michel JP, Rolland Y, Schneider SM, et al. Sarcopenia: European consensus on definition and diagnosis: report of the European Working Group on Sarcopenia in Older People. Age Ageing 2010;39:412–23.

[10] Shachar SS, Williams GR, Muss HB, Nishijima TF. Prognostic value of sarcopenia in adults with solid tumours: a meta-analysis and systematic review. Eur J Cancer 2016;57:58–67.

[11] Maltais F, Decramer M, Casaburi R, Barreiro E, Burelle Y, Richard Debigare PN, Dekhuizen R, Franssen F, Gayan-Ramirez G, et al. An official American Thoracic Society/European Respiratory Society statement: update on limb muscle dysfunction in chronic obstructive pulmonary disease. Am J Respir Crit Care Med 2014;189:e15–62.

[12] Celli BR, Locantore N, Tal-Singer R, Riley J, Miller B, Vestbo J, HYates JC, Silverman EK, Owen CA, Miguel D, Pinto-Plata V, EFM W, Rosa F, Agusti A, ECLIPSE Study Investigators. Emphysema and extrapulmonary tissue loss in COPD: a multi-organ loss of tissue phenotype. Eur Respir J 2018;51:1702146.

[13] Spruit MA, Gosselink R, Troosters T, Kasran A, Gayan-Ramirez G, Bogaerts P, Bouillon R, Decramer M. Muscle force during an acute exacerbation in hospitalised patients with COPD and its relationship with CXCL8 and IGF-I. Thorax 2003;58:752–6.

[14] Rabe KF, Watz H. Chronic obstructive pulmonary disease. Lancet 2017;389:1931–40.

[15] Abdulai RM, Jensen TJ, Patel NR, Polkey MI, Jansson P, Celli BR, Rennard SI. Deterioration of limb muscle function during acute exacerbation of chronic obstructive pulmonary disease. Am J Respir Crit Care Med 2018;197:433–49.

[16] Uchmanowicz I, Loboz-Rudnicka M, Szelag P, Jankowska-Polanska B, Loboz-Grudzien K. Frailty in heart failure. Curr Heart Fail Rep 2014;11:266–73.

[17] Kato A. Muscle wasting is associated with reduced exercise capacity and advanced disease in patients with chronic heart failure. Future Cardiol 2013;9:767–70.

[18] Szulc P, Feyt C, Chapurlat R. High risk of fall, poor physical function, and low grip strength in men with fracture—the STRAMBO study. J Cachexia Sarcopenia Muscle 2016;7:299–311.

[19] Fujishima I, Fujiu-Kurachi M, Arai H, Hyodo M, Kagaya H, Maeda K, Mori T, Nishioka S, Oshima F, Ogawa S, et al. Sarcopenia and dysphagia: position paper by four professional organizations. Geriatr Gerontol Int 2019;19:91–7.

[20] Chen LK, Lee WJ, Peng LN, Liu LK, Arai H, Akishita M, Asian Working Group for Sarcopenia. Recent advances in Sarcopenia Research in Asia: 2016 update from the Asian Working Group for Sarcopenia. J Am Med Dir Assoc 2016;17, 767.e1–7.

[21] Dewys WD, Begg C, Lavin PT, Band PR, Bennett JM, Bertino JR, Cohen MH, Douglass Jr HO, Engstrom PF, Ezdinli EZ, et al. Prognostic effect of weight loss prior to chemotherapy in cancer patients. Eastern Cooperative Oncology Group. Am J Med 1980;69:391–497.

[22] Teunissen SC, Wesker W, Kruitwagen C, de Haes HC, Voest EE, de Graeff A. Symptom prevalence in patients with incurable cancer: a systematic review. J Pain Symptom Manage 2007;34:94–104.

[23] Evans WJ, Morley JE, Argiles J, Bales C, Baracos V, Guttridge D, Jatoi A, Kalantar-Zadeh K, Lochs H, Mantovani G, et al. Cachexia: a new definition. Clin Nutr 2008;27:793–9.

[24] Fearon K, Strasser F, Anker SD, Bosaeus I, Bruera E, Fainsinger RL, Jatoi A, Loprinzi C, MacDonald N, Mantovani G, et al. Definition and classification of cancer cachexia: an international consensus. Lancet Oncol 2011;12:489–95.

[25] Radbruch L, Elsner F, Trottenberg P, Strasser F, Fearon K. Clinical practice guidelines on cancer cachexia in advanced cancer patients with a focus on refractory cachexia. European Palliative Care Research Collaborative: Aachen 2010.

[26] Muscaritoli M, Anker SD, Argiles J, Aversa Z, Bauer JM, Biolo G, Boirie Y, Bosaeus I, Cederholm T, Costelli P, et al. Consensus definition of sarcopenia, cachexia and pre-cachexia: joint document elaborated by Special Interest Groups (SIG) "cachexia-anorexia in chronic wasting diseases" and "nutrition in geriatrics". Clin Nutr 2010;29:154–9.

[27] Tisdale MJ. Mechanisms of cancer cachexia. Physiol Rev 2009;89:381–410.
[28] Biolo G, Cederholm T, Muscaritoli M. Muscle contractile and metabolic dysfunction is a common feature of sarcopenia of aging and chronic diseases: from sarcopenic obesity to cachexia. Clin Nutr 2014;33:737–48.
[29] Esper DH, Hard WA. The cancer cachexia syndrome: a review of metabolic and clinical manifestations. Nutr Clin Pract 2005;20:369–76.
[30] Fearon K, Arends J, Baracos V. Understanding the mechanisms and treatment options in cancer cachexia. Nat Rev Clin Oncol 2013;10:90–9.
[31] Tuca A, Jimenez-Fonseca P, Gascon P. Clinical evaluation and optimal management of cancer cachexia. Crit Rev Oncol Hematol 2013;88:625–36.
[32] Deutsch J, Kolhouse JF. Assessment of gastrointestinal function and response to megesterol acetate in subjects with gastrointestinal cancers and weight loss. Support Care Cancer 2004;12:503–10.
[33] Wigmore SJ, Plester CE, Ross JA, Fearon KC. Contribution of anorexia and hypermetabolism to weight loss in anicteric patients with pancreatic cancer. Br J Surg 1997;84:196–7.
[34] Blum D, Stene GB, Solheim TS, Fayers P, Hjermstad MJ, Baracos VE, Fearon K, Strasser F, Kaasa S, Euro-Impact. Validation of the consensus-definition for cancer cachexia and evaluation of a classification model—a study based on data from an international multicentre project (EPCRC-CSA). Ann Oncol 2014;25:1635–42.
[35] Cruz-Jentoft AJ, Landi F, Schneider SM, Zuniga C, Arai H, Boirie Y, Chen LK, Fielding RA, Martin FC, Michel JP, et al. Prevalence of and interventions for sarcopenia in ageing adults: a systematic review. Report of the International Sarcopenia Initiative (EWGSOP and IWGS). Age Ageing 2014;43:748–59.
[36] Buckinx F, Reginster J-Y, Brunois LC, Beaudart C, Croisier J-L, Petermans J, Bruyere O. Prevalence of sarcopenia in a population of nursing home residents according to their frailty status: results of the SENIOR cohort. J Musculoskelet Neuronal Interact 2017;17:209–17.
[37] Rosenberg IH. Summary comments: epidemiologic and methodologic problems in determining nutritional status of older persons. Am J Clin Nutr 1989;50:1231–3.
[38] Baumgartner RN, Koehler KM, Gallagher D, Romero L, Heymsfield SB, Ross RR, Garry PJ, Lindeman RD. Epidemiology of sarcopenia among the elderly in New Mexico. Am J Epidemiol 1998;147:755–63.
[39] Janssen I, Heymsfield SB, Ross R. Low relative skeletal mass (sarcopenia) in older persons is associated with functional impairment and physical disability. J Am Geriatr Soc 2002;50:889–96.
[40] Prado CM, Lieffers JR, McCargar LI, Reiman T, Sawyer MB, Martin L, Baracos VE. Prevalence and clinical implications of sarcopenia obesity in patients with solid tumours of the respiratory and gastrointestinal tracts: a population-based study. Lancet Oncol 2008;9:629–35.
[41] Chen LK, Liu LK, Woo J, Assantachai P, Auyeung TW, Bahyah KS, Chou MY, Chen LY, Hsu PS, Krairit O, Lee JS, Lee WJ, Lee Y, Liang CK, Limpawattana P, Lin CS, Peng LN, Satake S, Suzuki T, Won Wu CH, Wu CH, Wu SN, Zhang T, Zeng P, Akishita M, Arai H. Sarcopenia in Asia: consensus report of the Asian Working Group for Sarcopenia. J Am Med Dir Assoc 2014;15:95–101.
[42] Cruz-Jentoft AJ, Bahat G, Bauer J, Boirie Y, Bruyere O, Cederholm T, Cyrus C, Francesco L, Yves R, Sayer AA, Schneider SM, Sieber CC, Topinkova E, Vandewoude M, Visser M, Zamboni M, Writing Group for the European Working Group on Sarcopenia in Older People (EWGSOP2), and the Extended Group for EWGSOP2. Sarcopenia: revised European consensus on definition and diagnosis. Age Ageing 2019;48:16–31.
[43] Dent E, Morley JE, Cruz-Jentoft AJ, Arai H, Kritchevsky SB, Guralnik J, Bauer JM, Pahor M, Clark BC, Cesari M, Ruiz J, Sieber CC, Aubertion-Leheudre M, Waters DL, Visvanathan R, Landi F, Villareal DT, Fielding R, Won CW, Theou O, et al. International Clinical Practice Guidelines for Sarcopenia (ICFSR): screening, diagnosis and management. J Nutr Health Aging 2018;22:1148–61.
[44] Chen L-K, Woo J, Assantachai P, Auyeng T-W, Chou M-Y, Iijima K, Jang HC, Lin K, Kim M, Kim S, Kojima T, Kuzuya M, Lee JSW, Lee SY, Lee W-J, Lee Y, Liang C-K, Lim J-Y, Lim WS, Peng K-N, Sugimoto K, Tanaka T, Won CW, Yamada M, Zhang T, Akishita M, Arai H. Asian Working Group for Sarcopenia: 2019 consensus update on sarcopenia diagnosis and treatment. J Am Med Dir Assoc 2020;21:300–307.e2. https://doi.org/10.1016/j.jamda.2019.12.012 [Epub 2020 Feb 4].

[45] Biolo G, Pisot R, Mazzucco S, Di Girolamo FG, Roberta S, Lazzer S, Bruno G, Reggiani C, Passaro A, Rittweger J, Gasparini M, Simunic B, Narici M. Anabolic resistance assessed by oral stable isotope ingestion following bed rest in young and older adult volunteers: relationships with changes in muscle mass. Clin Nutr 2017;36:1420–6.

[46] Martone AM, Bianchi L, Abete P, Bellelli G, Bo M, Cherubini A, Corica F, Bari MD, Maggio M, Mance GM, Mazetti E, Rizzo MR, Rossi A, Volpato S, Landi F. The incidence of sarcopenia among hospitalized older patients: results from the Glisten study. J Cachexia Sarcopenia Muscle 2017;8:907–14.

[47] Roubenoff R, Hughes VA. Sarcopenia: current concepts. J Gerontol A Biol Sci Med Sci 2000;55:M716–24.

[48] Dellis S, Papadopoulou S, Krikonis K, Zigras F. Sarcopenic dysphagia. A narrative review. J Frailty Sarcopenia Falls 2018;3:1–7.

[49] Grelot L, Barillot JC, Bianchi AL. Pharyngeal motoneurones: respiratory-related activity and responses to laryngeal afferents in the decerebrate cat. Exp Brain Res 1989;78:336–44.

[50] Sokoloff AJ, Douglas M, Rahnert JA, Burkholder T, Easley KA, Luo Q. Absence of morphological and molecular correlates of sarcopenia in the macaque tongue muscle styloglossus. Exp Gerontol 2016;84:40–8.

[51] Sánchez-Rodríguez D, Ester M, Natalia R-N, Ramon M, Vazquez-Ibar O, Escalada F, Muniesa JM. Prevalence of malnutrition and sarcopenia in a post-acute care geriatric unit: applying the new ESPEN definition and EWGSOP criteria. Clin Nutr 2017;36:1339–44.

[52] Veldee MS, Peth CD. Can protein-calorie malnutrition cause dysphagia? Dysphagia 1992;7:86–101.

[53] Hudson HM, Daubert CR, Mills RH. The interdependency of protein-energy malnutrition, aging, and dysphagia. Dysphagia 2000;15:31–8.

[54] Veldee MS, Peth LD. Can protein-calorie malnutrition cause dysphagia? Dysphagia 1992;7:86–101.

[55] Kuroda Y, Kuroda R. Relationship between thinness and swallowing function in Japanese older adults: implications dysphagia. J Am Geriatr Soc 2012;60:1785–6.

[56] Clave P, Shaker R. Dysphagia: current reality and scope of the problem. Nat Rev Gastroenterol Hepatol 2015;12:259–70.

[57] Sporns PB, Muhle P, Hanning U, Suntrup-Krueger S, Schwindt W, Eversmann J, Warnecke T, Wirth R, Zimmer S, Dziewas R. Atrophy of swallowing muscles is associated with severity of and age in patients with acute stroke. J Am Med Dir Assoc 2017;18:635.e631–7.

[58] Tamura F, Kikutani T, Tohara T, Yoshida M, Yaegaki K. Tongue thickness relates to nutritional status in the elderly. Dysphagia 2012;27:556–61.

[59] Robbins J, Humpal NS, Banaszynski K, Hind J, Rogus-Pulia N. Age-related differences in pressures generated during isometric presses and swallows by healthy adults. Dysphagia 2016;31:90–6.

[60] Buehring B, Hind J, Fidler E, Krueger D, Binkley N, Robbins J. Tongue strength is associated with jumping mechanography performance and handgrip strength but not with classic functional tests in older adults. J Am Geriatr Soc 2013;61:418–22.

[61] Sakai K, Nakayama E, Tohara H, Maeda T, Sugimoto M, Takehisa T, Takehisa Y, Ueda K. Tongue strength is associated with grip strength and nutritional status in older adult inpatients of a rehabilitation hospital. Dysphagia 2017;32:241–9.

[62] Maeda K, Takaki M, Akagi J. Decreased skeletal muscle mass and risk factors of sarcopenic dysphagia: a prospective observational cohort study. J Gerontol A Biol Sci Med Sci 2017;72:1290–4.

[63] Yoshimura Y, Wakabayashi H, Bise T, Nagano F, Shimazu S, Shiraishi A, Yamaga M, Koga H. Sarcopenia is associated with worse recovery of physical function and dysphagia, and a lower rate of home discharge in Japanese hospitalized adults undergoing convalescent rehabilitation. Nutrition 2019;61:111–8.

[64] Bonetto A, Aydogdu T, Kunzeritzky N, Guttridge DC, Khuri S, Koniaris LG, Zimmers TA. STAT3 activation in skeletal muscle links muscle wasting and the acute phase response in cancer cachexia. PLoS One 2011;6, e22538.

[65] Aapro M, Arends J, Bozzetti F, Fearon K, Grunberg SM, Herrstedt J, Hoplinson J, Jacquelin-Ravel N, Jatoi A, Koasa S, Strasser F. Early recognition of malnutrition and cachexia in the cancer patients: a position paper of a European School of Oncology Task Force. Ann Oncol 2014;25:1492–9.

[66] Grosvenor M, Bulcavage L, Chlebowski RT. Symptom potentially influencing weight loss in a cancer population. Correlations with primary site, nutritional status, and chemotherapy administration. Cancer 1989;63:330–4.

[67] Blum D, Omlin A, Baracos VE, Solheim TS, Tan BH, Stone P, Kaasa S, Feearon K, Strasser F, European Palliative Care Research Collaborative. Cancer cachexia: a systematic literature review of items and domains associated with involuntary weight loss in cancer. Crit Rev Oncol Hematol 2011;80:114–44.

[68] Omlin A, Blum D, Wierecky J, Haile SR, Ottery FD, Strasser F. Nutrition impact symptoms in advanced cancer patients: frequency and specific interventions, a case-control study. J Cachexia Sarcopenia Muscle 2013;4:55–61.

[69] Bozzetti F, Arends J, Lundholm K, Micklewright A, Zurcher G, Muscaritoli M, ESPEN. ESPEN guidelines on parenteral nutrition: non-surgical oncology. Clin Nutr 2009;28:445–54.

[70] Tisdale MJ. Cancer cachexia metabolic alterations and clinical manifestations. Nutrition 1997;13:1–7.

[71] Westin T, Jansson A, Zenckert C, Hallstrom T, Edstrom S. Mental depression is associated with malnutrition in patients with head and neck cancer. Arch Otolaryngol Head Neck Surg 1988;114:1449–53.

[72] Beaver MS, Matheny KE, Roberts DB, Myers JN. Predictors of weight loss during radiation therapy. Otolaryngol Head Neck Surg 2001;125:645–8.

[73] Schattner M. Enteral nutritional support of the patient with cancer: route and role. J Clin Gastroenterol 2003;36:297–302.

[74] Newman LA, Vieira F, Schwiezer V, Samant S, Murry T, Woodson G, Kumar P, Robbins KT. Eating and weight changes following chemoradiation therapy for advanced head and neck cancer. Arch Otolaryngol Head Neck Surg 1998;124:589–92.

[75] Pauloski BR, Rademaker AW, Logmann JA, Lazarus CL, Newman L, Hamner L, MacCracken E, Gaziano J, Stachowiak L. Swallow function and perception of dysphagia in patients with head and neck cancer. Head Neck 2002;24:555–65.

[76] Jensen K, Bonde Jensen A, Grau C. The relationship between observer-based toxicity scoring and patient assessed symptom severity after treatment for head and neck cancer. A correlative cross sectional study of the DAHANCA toxicity scoring system and the EORTC quality of life questionnaires. Radiother Oncol 2006;78:298–305.

[77] Logemann JA, Rademaker AW, Paulowski BR, Lazarus CL, Mittal BB, Brockstein B, MacCracken E, Haraf DJ, Vokes EE, Newman LA, et al. Site of disease and treatment protocol as correlates of swallow function in patients with head and neck cancer treated with chemoradiation. Head Neck 2006;28:64–73.

[78] Pauloski BR, Rademaker AW, Logemann JA, Stein D, Beery Q, Newman L, Hanchett C, Tusant S, MacCracken E. Pretreatment swallowing function in patients with head and neck cancer. Head Neck 2000;22:474–82.

[79] Stenson KM, MacCracken E, List M, Haraf DJ, Brockstein B, Weichselbaum R, Vokes EE. Swallowing function in patients with head and neck cancer prior to treatment. Arch Otolaryngol Head Neck Surg 2000;126:371–7.

[80] Nguyen NP, Moltz CC, Frank C, Vos P, Smith HJ, Karisson U, Dutta S, Midyett FA, Barloon J, Sallah S. Dysphagia following chemoradiation for locally advanced head and neck cancer. Ann Oncol 2004;15:303–88.

[81] Nguyen NP, Vos P, Moltz CC, Frank C, Millar C, Smith HJ, Dutta S, Alfieri A, Lee H, Martinez T, et al. Analysis of the factors influencing dysphagia severity diagnosis of head and neck cancer. Br J Radiol 2008;81:706–10.

[82] Garcia-Peris P, Paron L, Velasco C, de la Cuerda C, Cambior M, Breton I, Herencia H, Verdaguer J, Navarro C, Clave P. Long-term prevalence of oropharyngeal dysphagia in head and neck cancer patients: impact on quality of life. Clin Nutr 2007;26:710–7.

[83] Kronenberger MB, Meijers AD. Dysphagia following head and neck surgery. Dysphagia 1994;9:236–44.

[84] Dysphagia Section, Oral Care Study Group, Multinational Association of Supportive Care in Cancer (MASCC)/International Society of Oral Oncology (ISOO), Raber-Durlacher JE, Brennan MT, Verdonck-de Leeuw IM, Gibson RJ, Eilers JG, Waltimo T, Bots CP, Michelet M, Sollecito TP, Rouleau TS, et al. Swallowing dysfunction in cancer patients. Support Care Cancer 2012;20:433–43.

[85] Gibson DJ, Burden ST, Strauss BJ, Todd C, Lal S. The role of computed tomography in evaluating body composition and the influence of reduced muscle mass on clinical outcome in abdominal malignancy: a systematic review. Eur J Clin Nutr 2015;69:1079–86.

[86] Pamoukdjian F, Bouilet T, Levy V, Soussan M, Zelek L, Paillaud E. Prevalence and predictive value of pre-therapeutic sarcopenia in cancer patients: a systematic review. Clin Nutr 2017;37:1101–13. pii, S0261-5614(17) 30249-2.

[87] Hodari A, Hammond ZT, Borgi JF, Tsiouris A, Rubinfeld I. Assessment of morbidity and mortality after esophagectomy using a modified frailty index. Ann Thorac Surg 2013;96:1240–5.

[88] Reisinger KW, Bosmans JW, Uittenbogaart M, Alsoumali A, Poeze M, Sosef MN, Derikx JP. Loss of skeletal muscle mass during neoadjuvant chemoradiotherapy predicts postoperative mortality in esophageal cancer surgery. Ann Surg Oncol 2015;22:4445–52.

[89] Huang DD, Chen XX, Chen XY, Chen XY, Wang SL, Shen X, Chen XL, Yu Z, Zhuang CL. Sarcopenia predicts 1-year mortality in elderly patients undergoing curative gastrectomy for gastric cancer: a prospective study. J Cancer Res Clin Oncol 2016;142:2347–56.

[90] Lieffers JR, Bathe OF, Fassbender K, Winget M, Baracos VE. Sarcopenia is associated with postoperative infection and delayed recovery from colorectal cancer resection surgery. Br J Cancer 2012;107:931–6.

[91] Reisinger KW, van Vugt JL, Tegels JJ, Snijders C, Hulsewe KW, Hoofwilk AG, Stoot JH, Meyenfeldt MF, Beets GL, Derikx JP, Poeze M. Functional compromise reflected by sarcopenia, frailty, and nutritional depletion predicts adverse postoperative outcome after colorectal cancer surgery. Ann Surg 2015;261:345–52.

[92] Jung HW, Kim JW, Kim JY, Kim SW, Yang HK, Lee JW, Lee KW, Kim DW, Kang SB, Kim KL, Kim CH, Kim JH. Effect of muscle mass on toxicity and survival in patients with colon cancer undergoing adjuvant chemotherapy. Support Care Cancer 2015;23:687–94.

[93] Miyamoto Y, Baba Y, Sakamoto Y, Ohuchi M, Tokunaga R, Kurashige J, Hiyoshi Y, Iwagami S, Yoshida N, Watanabe M, Baba H. Negative impact of skeletal muscle loss after systemic chemotherapy in patients with unresectable colorectal cancer. PLoS One 2015;10, e0129742.

[94] Alshadwi A, Nadershah M, Carlson ER, Young LS, Burke PA, Daley BJ. Nutritional considerations for head and neck cancer patients: a review of the literature. J Oral Maxillofac Surg 2013;71:1853–60 [Internet].

[95] Garg M, Kabarriti R, Bontempo A, Romano M, Ohri N, Viswanathan S, et al. The impact of dietary regimen compliance on outcomes for head and neck cancer patients treated with definitive radiation therapy. J Clin Oncol 2015;33:3307–13. Available from [Internet].

[96] García-Peris P, Lozano MA, Velasco C, de La Cuerda C, Iriondo T, Bretón I, Camblor M, Navarro C. Prospective study of resting energy expenditure changes in head and neck cancer patients treated with chemoradiotherapy measured by indirect calorimetry. Nutrition 2005;21:1107–12. https://doi.org/10.1016/j.nut.2005.03.006.

[97] Lonbro S, Petersen GB, Andersen JR, Johansen J. Prediction of critical weight loss during radiation treatment in head and neck cancer patients is dependent on BMI. Support Care Cancer 2016;24:2101–9. https://doi.org/10.1007/s00520-015-2999-8.

[98] Mick R, Vokes EE, Weichselbaum RR, Panje WR. Prognostic factors in advanced head and neck cancer patients undergoing multimodality therapy. Otolaryngol Head Neck Surg 1991;105:62–73.

[99] Ghadjar P, Hayoz S, Zimmermann F, Bodis S, Kaul D, Badakhshi H, Bernier J, Studer G, Plasswilm L, Budach V, Aebersold DM, Swiss Group for Clinical Researech (SAKK). Impact of weight loss on survival after chemoradiation for locally advanced head and neck cancer: secondary results of randomized phase III trial (SAKK 10/94). Radiat Oncol 2015;10:21.

[100] Adelstein D, Li Y, Adams G, Wagner H, Kish J, Ensley J, Schuller DE, Forastiere AA. An intergroup phase III comparison of standard radiation therapy and two schedules of concurrent chemoradiotherapy in patients with unresectable squamous cell head and neck cancer. J Clin Oncol 2003;21:92–8.

[101] Forastiere A, Goepfert H, Maor M, Pajak T, Weber R, Morrison W, Glisson B, Trotti A, Ridge JA, Chao C, Peters G, Lee DJ, et al. Concurrent chemotherapy and radiotherapy for organ preservation in advanced laryngeal cancer. N Engl J Med 2003;349:2091–8. https://doi.org/10.1056/NEJMoa031317.

[102] List MA, Siston A, Haraf D, Schumm P, Kies M, Stenson K, Vokes E. Quality of life and performance in advanced head and neck cancer patients on concomitant chemoradiotherapy: a prospective examination. J Clin Oncol 1999;17:1020.

[103] Rankher A, Russo L, Schattner M, Schwartz L, Scott B, Shike M. Enteral nutrition support of head and neck cancer patients. Nutr Clin Pract 2007;22:68–73.

[104] van Maria Rijn-Dekker I, van den Bosch L, van den Hoek JGM, Bijl HP, van Evert Aken SM, van der Hoorn A, Oosting SF, Halmos GB, Witjes MJH, van der Hans Laan P, Langendijk JA, Steenbakkers RJHM. Impact of sarcopenia on survival and late toxicity in head and neck cancer patients treated with radiotherapy. Radiother Oncol 2020;147:103–10.

[105] Bjordal K, De Graeff A, Fayers PM, Hammerlid E, Van Pottelsberghe C, Curran D, Ahiner-Elmqvist M, Maher EJ, Meyza JW, Bredart A, Soderholm AL, Arraras JJ, Feine JS, Abendstein H, Morton RP, Pignon T, Huguenin P, Bottomly A, Kaasa S. A 12 country field study of the EORTC QLQ-C30 (version 3.0) and the head and neck cancer specific module (EORTC QLQ-H and N35) in head and neck patients. Eur J Cancer 2000;36:1796–807.

[106] National Cancer Institute, Cancer Therapy Evaluation Program (CTEP). Common toxicity criteria for adverse events v4.03 (CTCAE). 2009. Available from http://ctep.cancer.gov/protocolDevelopment/electronic_applications/docs/ctcaev3.pdf; 2009.

[107] Kagifuku Y, Tohara H, Wakasugi Y, Susa C, Nakane A, Toyoshima M, Nakakuki K, Kabasawa Y, Harada H, Minakuchi S. What factors affect changes in body composition and swallowing function in patients hospitalized for oral cancer surgery? Clin Interv Aging 2020;15:1–7.

[108] Makhail TM, Adelstein DJ, Rybicki LA, Larto MA, Saxton JP, Lavertu P. Enteral nutrition during the treatment of head and neck carcinoma: is a percutaneous endoscopic gastrostomy tube preferable to a nasogastric tube? Cancer 2001;91:1785–90.

[109] Langendijk JA, Doornaert P, Verdonck-de Leeuw IM, Leemans CR, Aaronson NK, Slotman BJ. Impact of late treatment-related toxicity on quality of life among patients with head and neck cancer treated with radiotherapy. J Clin Oncol 2008;26:3770–6.

[110] Masayuki I, Takao T, Kenji N, Hiroyuki N, Kazutetsu A. Undernutrition in patients with COPD and its treatment. Nutrients 2013;5:1316–35.

[111] Barnes PJ, Celli BR. Systemic manifestations and comorbidities of COPD. Eur Respir J 1999;58:321–8.

[112] Di Francia M, Barbier D, Mega JL, Orehek L. Tumor necrosis factor-alpha levels and weight loss in chronic obstructive pulmonary disease. Am J Respir Crit Care Med 1994;150:1453–5.

[113] Eid AA, Ionescu AA, Nixon LS, Lewis-Jenkins V, Marrhews SB, Griffiths TL, Shale DJ. Inflammatory response and body composition in chronic obstructive pulmonary disease. Am J Respir Crit Care Med 2001;15:1414–8.

[114] Brokhuizen R, Wouters EF, Creutzberg EC, Schols AM. Raised CRP levels mark metabolic and functional impairment in advanced COPD. Thorax 2006;61:17–22.

[115] Agusti A, Morla M, Sauleda J, Saus C, Busquets X. NF-κB activation and iNOS upregulation in skeletal muscle of patients with COPD and low body weight. Thorax 2004;59:483–7.

[116] Kumor-Kisielewska A, Kiersznieska-Stepien D, Pietras T, Kroczynska-Bednarek J, Kurmanowska Z, Antczak A, Gorski P. Assessment of leptin and resistin levels in patients with chronic obstructive pulmonary disease. Pol Arch Med Wewn 2013;123:215–20.

[117] Ferrari R, Tanni SE, Faganello MM, Caram LM, Lucheta PA, Godoy I. Three-year follow-up study of respiratory and systemic manifestations of chronic obstructive pulmonary disease. Braz J Med Biol Res 2011;44:46–52.

[118] Fabbri LM, Luppi F, Beghe B, Rabe KF. Update in chronic obstructive pulmonary disease 2005. Am J Respir Crit Care Med 2006;173:1056–65.

[119] Wagner PD. Possible mechanisms underlying the development of cachexia in COPD. Eur Respir J 2008;31:492–501.

[120] Decramer M, Janssens W, Miravitlles M. Chronic obstructive pulmonary disease. Lancet 2012;379:1341–51.

[121] Soler-Cataluna JJ, Martinez-Garcia MA, Roman Sanchez P, Salcedo E, Navarro M, Ochando R. Severe acute exacerbations and mortality in patients with chronic obstructive pulmonary disease. Thorax 2005;60:925–31.

[122] Kobayashi S, Kubo H, Yanai M. Impairment of the swallowing reflex in exacerbations of COPD. Thorax 2007;62:1017.

[123] Gross RD, Atwood Jr CW, Ross SB, Olszewski JW, Eichhorn KA. The coordination of breathing and swallowing in chronic obstructive pulmonary disease. Am J Respir Crit Care Med 2009;179:559–65.

[124] O'Kane L, Groher M. Dysphagia and obstructive pulmonary disease: a systematic review. Rev CEFAC 2009;11:499–506.

[125] Good-Fratturelli MD, Curlee RF, Holle JL. Prevalence and nature of dysphagia in VA patients with COPD referred for videofluoroscopic swallow examination. J Commun Disord 2000;33:93–110.

[126] Steidl E, Ribeiro CS, Goncalves BF, Fernandes N, Antunes V, Mancopes R. Relationship between dysphagia and exacerbations in chronic obstructive pulmonary disease: a literature review. Int Arch Otorhinolaryngol 2015;19:74–9.

[127] Ghannouchi I, Speyer R, Doma K, Cordier R, Verin E. Swallowing function and chronic respiratory disease: systematic review. Respir Med 2016;117:54–64.

[128] Stein M, Williams AJ, Grossman F, Weinberg AS, Zuckerbraun L. Cricopharyngeal dysfunction in chronic obstructive pulmonary disease. Chest 1990;97:347–52.

[129] Mokhlesi B, Morris AL, Huang CF, Curcio AJ, Barrett TA, Kamp DW. Increased prevalence of gastroesophageal reflux symptoms in patients with COPD. Chest 2001;119:1043–8.

[130] Terada K, Muro S, Ohara T, Kudo M, Ogawa E, Hoshino Y, Hirai T, Niimi A, Chin K, Mishima M. Abnormal swallowing reflex and COPD exacerbations. Chest 2010;137:326–32.

[131] de Deus Chaves R, Chiarion Sassi F, Davison Mangilli L, Jayanthi SK, Cukier A, Zilberstein B, Furquim de Andrade CR. Swallowing transit times and valleculae residue in stable chronic obstructive pulmonary disease. BMC Pulm Med 2014;14:62.

[132] Cassiani RA, Santos CM, Baddini-Martinez J, Dantas RO. Oral and pharyngeal bolus transit in patients with chronic obstructive pulmonary disease. Int J Chron Obstruct Pulmon Dis 2015;10:489–96.

[133] Cvejic L, Harding R, Churchward T, Turton A, Finlay P, Massey D, Bardin PG, Guy P. Laryngeal penetration and aspiration in individuals with stable COPD. Respirology 2011;16:269–75.

[134] Garand KL, Strange C, Paoletti L, Hopkins-Rossabi T, Martin-Harris B. Oropharyngeal swallowing physiology and swallowing-related quality of life in underweight patients with concomitant advanced chronic obstructive pulmonary disease. Int J Chron Obstruct Pulmon Dis 2018;29:2663–71.

[135] Maltais F, Decramer M, Casaburi R, Barreiro E, Burelle Y, Debigare R, Dekhujizen PN, Franssen F, Gayan-Ramirez G, Gea J, et al. An official American Thoracic Society/European Respiratory Society statement: update on limb muscle dysfunction in chronic obstructive pulmonary disease. Am J Respir Crit Care Med 2014;189:e15–62.

[136] Jones SE, Maddocks M, Kon SS, Canavan JL, Nolan CM, Clark AL, Polkey MI, Man WD. Sarcopenia in COPD: prevalence, clinical correlates and response to pulmonary rehabilitation. Thorax 2015;70:213–8.

[137] Rahman A, Jafry S, Jeejeebhoy K, Nagpal AD, Pisani B, Agarwala R. Malnutrition and cachexia in heart failure. JPEN J Parenter Enteral Nutr 2016;40:475–86.

[138] Saitoh M, Ishida J, Doehner W, von Haehling S, Anker MS, Coats AJS, Anker SD, Springer J. Sarcopenia, cachexia, and muscle performance in heart failure: review update 2016. Int J Cardiol 2017;238:5–11.

[139] Byun MK, Cho EN, Chang J, Ahn CM, Kim HJ. Sarcopenia correlates with systemic inflammation in COPD. Int J Chron Obstruct Pulmon Dis 2017;12:669–75.

[140] Jones SE, Maddocks M, Kon SSC, Canavan JL, Nolan CM, Clark AL, Polkey MI, Man WD. Sarcopenia in COPD: prevalence, clinical correlates and response to pulmonary rehabilitation. Thorax 2015;70:213–8.

[141] da Rocha Lemos Costa TM, Costa FM, Moreira CA, Rabelo LM, Boguszewski CL, Borba VZC. Sarcopenia in COPD: relationship with COPD severity and prognosis. J Bras Pneumol 2015;41:415–21.

[142] Rolland Y, Czerwinski S, Abellan Van Kan G, Morley JE, Cesari M, Onder G, Woo J, Baumgarter R, Boirie Y, Chumlea WMC. Sarcopenia: its assessment, etiology, pathogenesis, consequences and future perspectives. J Nutr Health Aging 2011;12:433–50.

[143] Annegarn J, Meijer K, Passos VL, Stute K, Wiechert J, Savelberg HHCM, Schols AMW, Wouters EFW, Spruit MA. Problematic activities of daily life are weakly associated with clinical characteristics in COPD. J Am Med Dir Assoc 2012;13:284–90.

[144] Weldam SWM, Schuurmans MJ, Liu R, Lammers J-WJ. Evaluation of quality of life instruments for use in COPD care and research: a systematic review. Int J Nurs Stud 2013;50:688–707.

[145] Cebron Lipovec N, Schols AM, Van den Borst B, Beijers RJ, Kosten T, Omersa D, Lainscak M. Sarcopenia in advanced COPD affects cardiometabolic risk reduction by short-term high-intensity pulmonary rehabilitation. J Am Med Dir Assoc 2016;17:814–20.

[146] Lee LW, Lin CM, Li HC, Hsiao PL, Chung AC, Hsieh CJ, Wu PC, Hsu SF. Body composition changes in male patients with chronic obstructive pulmonary disease: aging or disease process? PLoS One 2017;12, e0180928.

[147] Sepulneda-Loyola W, Osadmnik C, Phu S, Morita AA, Duque G, Probst VS. Diagnosis, prevalence, and clinical impact of sarcopenia in COPD: a systematic review and meta-analysis. J Cachexia Sarcopenia Muscle 2020. https://doi.org/10.1002/jcsm.12600.

[148] Mokhlesi B, Logemann JA, Rademaker AW, Stangl CA, Corbridge TC. Oropharyngeal deglutition in stable COPD. Chest 2002;121:361–9.

[149] Von Haeling S, Anker SD. Prevalence, incidence and clinical impact of cachexia: facts and numbers—update 2014. J Cachexia Sarcopenia Muscle 2014;5:261–3.

[150] Christensen HM, Kistorp C, Schou M, Keller N, Zerahn B, Frystyk J, Schwarz P, Faber J. Prevalence of cachexia in chronic heart failure and characteristics of body composition and metabolic status. Endocrine 2013;43:626–34.

[151] Okoshi MP, Capalbo RV, Romeiro FG, Okoshi K. Cardiac cachexia: perspectives for prevention and treatment. Arq Bras Cardiol 2017;108:74–80.

[152] Cohen-Solal A, Jacobson AF, Piña IL. Beta blocker dose and markers of sympathetic activation in heart failure patients: interrelationships and prognostic significance. ESC Heart Fail 2017;4:499–506.

[153] Yoshihisa A, Watanabe S, Yokokawa T, Misaka T, Sato T, Suzuki S, Oikawa M, Kobayashi A, Takeishi Y. Associations between acylcarnitine to free carnitine ratio and adverse prognosis in heart failure patients with reduced or preserved ejection fraction. ESC Heart Fail 2017;4:360–4. 71.

[154] Fornaro A, Olivotto I, Rigacci L, Ciaccheri M, Tomberli B, Ferrantini C, Coppini R, Girolami F, Mazzarotto F, Chiostri M, et al. Comparison of long-term outcome in anthracycline-related versus idiopathic dilated cardiomyopathy: a single centre experience. Eur J Heart Fail 2018;20:898–906.

[155] Tian M, Nishijima Y, Asp ML, Srout MB, Reiser PJ, Bekury MA. Cardiac alterations in cancer-induced cachexia in mice. Int J Oncol 2010;37:347–53.

[156] Pfuntner A. Statistical brief #148: most frequent conditions in U.S. Hospitals, 2010. Rockville, MD: Agency for Healthcare Research and Quality; 2012. p. 1–11.

[157] Aziz EF, Javed F, Pratap B, Musat D, Nader A, Pilimi S, Alivar CL, Herzog E, Kukin ML. Malnutrition as assessed by nutritional risk index is associated with worse outcome in patients admitted with acute decompensated heart failure: an ACAP-HF data analysis. Heart Int 2011;6, e2.

[158] Okoshi MP, Capalbo RV, Romeiro FG, Okoshi K. Cardiac cachexia: perspectives for prevention and treatment. Arq Bras Cardiol 2017;108:74–80.

[159] Sundaram V, Fang JC. Gastrointestinal and liver issues in heart failure. Circulation 2016;133:1696–703.

[160] Levine B, Kalman J, Mayer L, Fillit HM, Packer M. Elevated circulating levels of tumor necrosis factor in severe chronic heart failure. N Engl J Med 1990;323:236–41.

[161] Rauchhaus M, Doehner W, Francis DP, Davos C, Kemp M, Liebenthal C, Niebauer J, Hooper J, Volk HD, Coats AJ, Anker SD. Plasma cytokine parameters and mortality in patients with chronic heart failure. Circulation 2000;102:3060–7.

[162] Ferrari R, Bachetti T, Confortini R, Opasich C, Febo O, Corti A, Cassani G, Visioli O. Tumor necrosis factor soluble receptors in patients with various degrees of congestive heart failure. Circulation 1995;92:1479–86.

[163] Langhans W, Hrupka B. Interleukins and tumor necrosis factor as inhibitors of food intake. Neuropeptides 1999;33:415–24.

[164] Aquilani R, Opasich C, Verri M, Boschi F, Febo O, Pasini E, Pastoris O. Is nutritional intake adequate in chronic heart failure patients? J Am Coll Cardiol 2003;42:1218–23.

[165] Narumi T, Arimoto T, Funayama A, Kadowaki S, Otaki Y, Nishiyama S, Takahashi H, Shishido T, Miyashita T, Miyamoto T, et al. Prognostic importance of objective nutritional indexes in patients with chronic heart failure. J Cardiol 2013;62:307–13.

[166] Matsuo H, Yoshimura Y, Fujita S, Maeno Y. Risk of malnutrition is associated with poor physical function in patients undergoing cardiac rehabilitation following heart failure. Nutr Diet 2019;76:82–8.

[167] Poehlman ET, Scheffers J, Gottlieb SS, Fisher ML, Vaitekevicius P. Increased resting metabolic rate in patients with congestive heart failure. Ann Intern Med 1994;121:860–2.

[168] Anker SD, Coats AJ. Cardiac cachexia: a syndrome with impaired survival and immune and neuroendocrine activation. Chest 1999;115:836–47.

[169] White JV, Guenter P, Jensen G, Malone A, Schofield M, Academy Malnutrition Work Group, A.S.P.E.N. Malnutrition Task Force, A.S.P.E.N. Board of Directors. Consensus statement: Academy of Nutrition and Dietetics and American Society for Parenteral and Enteral Nutrition: characteristics recommended for the identification and documentation of adult malnutrition (undernutrition). JPEN J Parenter Enteral Nutr 2012;36:275–83.

[170] Jensen GL, Compher C, Sullivan DH, Mullin GE. Recognizing malnutrition in adults: definitions and characteristics, screening, assessment, and team approach. JPEN J Parenter Enteral Nutr 2013;37:802–7.

[171] Pineda-Juarez JA, Sanchez-Ortiz NA, Castillo-Martínez L, Orea-Tejeda A, Cervantes-Gaytan R, Keirns-Davis C, Perez-Ocampo C, Quiroz-Bautista K, Tenorio-Dupont M, Ronquillo-Martinez A. Changes in body composition in heart failure patients after a resistance exercise program and branched chain amino acid supplementation. Clin Nutr 2015. https://doi.org/10.1016/j.clnu.2015.02.004 [Epub ahead of print].

[172] Wakabayashi H, Sakuma K. Rehabilitation nutrition for sarcopenia with disability: a combination of both rehabilitation and nutrition care management. J Cachexia Sarcopenia Muscle 2014;5:269–77.

[173] Malafarina V, Uria-Otano F, Iniesta R, Gil-Guerrero L. Effectiveness of nutritional supplementation on muscle mass in treatment of sarcopenia in old age: a systematic review. J Am Med Dir Assoc 2013;14:10–7.

[174] Yoshimura Y, Wakabayashi H, Yamada M, Kim H, Harada A, Arai H. Interventions for treating sarcopenia: a systematic review and meta-analysis of randomized controlled studies. J Am Med Dir Assoc 2017;18:553. e1–553.e16.

[175] Ferraris VA, Ferraris SP, Moritz DM, Welch S. Oropharyngeal dysphagia after cardiac operations. Ann Thorac Surg 2011;71:1792–5.

[176] Altman KW, Yu GP, Schaefer SD. Consequence of dysphagia in the hospitalized patient: impact on prognosis and hospital resources. Arch Otolaryngol Head Neck Surg 2010;136:784–9.

[177] Hudson HM, Daubert CR, Mills RH. The interdependency of protein-energy malnutrition, aging, and dysphagia. Dysphagia 2011;15:31–8.

[178] Metra M, Mentz RJ, Chiswell K, Bloomfield DM, Cleland JG, Cotter G, Davison BA, Dittrich HC, Fiuzat M, Givertz MM, et al. Acute heart failure in elderly patients: worse outcomes and differential utility of standard prognostic variables. Insights from the PROTECT trial. Eur J Heart Fail 2015;17:109–18.

[179] Quinones PA, Seidl H, Holle R, Kuch B, Meisinger C, Hunger M, Kirchberger I. New potential determinants of disability in aged persons with myocardial infarction: results from the KORINNA-study. BMC Geriatr 2014;14:34.

[180] García-Olmos L, Batlle M, Aguilar R, Porro C, Carmona M, Alberquilla A, Sanchez-Gomez LM, Mouge E, Lopez-Rodriguez AB, Benito L, Barios N, Somon A, Martinez-Alvarez M, Lique EM, Garcia-Benito C. Disability and quality of life in heart failure patients: a cross-sectional study. Fam Pract 2019;38:693–8.

[181] Chen C, Lim JT, Chia NC, Wang L, Tysinger B, Zissimopoulos J, Chong MZ, Wang Z, Koh GC, Yuan JM, Tan KB, Chia KS, Cook AR, Malhotra R, Chan A, Ma S, Ng TP, Koh WP, Goldman DP, Yoong J. The long-term impact of functional disability on hospitalization spending in Singapore. J Econ Ageing 2019;14:100193.

[182] Wu L-W, Chen W-L, Peng T-C, Chiang S-T, Yang H-F, Sun Y-S, Chan J-Y, Kao T-W. All-cause mortality risk in elderly individuals with disabilities: a retrospective observational study. BMJ Open 2016;6, e011164.

[183] Fulster S, Tacke M, Sandek A, Ebner N, Tsxhope C, Doehner W, Anker SD, von Haehling S. Muscle wasting in patients with chronic heart failure: results from the studies investigating co-morbidities aggravating heart failure (SICA-HF). Eur Heart J 2013;34:512–9.

[184] Sengul Aycicek G, Sumer F, Canbaz B, Kara O, Ulger Z. Sarcopenia evaluated by fat-free mass index in patients with chronic heart failure. Eur J Intern Med 2015;26, e34.

[185] Bekfani T, Pellicori P, Morris DA, Ebner N, Valentova M, Steinbeck L, Wachter R, Elsner S, Sliziuk V, Schefold JC, Sandek A, Doehner W, Cleland JG, Lainscak M, Anker SD, von Haehling S. Sarcopenia in patients with heart failure with preserved ejection fraction: impact on muscle strength, exercise capacity and quality of life. Int J Cardiol 2016;222:41–6.

[186] Narumi T, Watanabe T, Kadowaki S, Takahashi T, Yokoyama M, Kinoshita D, Honda Y, Funayama A, Nishiyama S, Takahashi H, Arimoto T, Shishido T, Miyamoto T, Kubota I. Sarcopenia evaluated by fat-free mass index is an important prognostic factor in patients with chronic heart failure. Eur J Intern Med 2015;26:118–22.

[187] Yoshimura Y, Wakabayashi H, Bise T, Tanoue M. Prevalence of sarcopenia and its association with activities of daily living and dysphagia in convalescent rehabilitation ward inpatients. Clin Nutr 2018;37:2022–8.

[188] Matsuo H, Yoshimura Y, Ishizaki N, Ueno T. Dysphagia is associated with functional decline during acute-care hospitalization of older patients. Geriatr Gerontol Int 2017;17:1610–6.

[189] Carrion S, Cabre M, Monteis R, Roca M, Palomera E, Serra-Prat M, Rofes L, Clave P. Oropharyngeal dysphagia is a prevalent risk factor for malnutrition in a cohort of older patients admitted with an acute disease to a general hospital. Clin Nutr 2015;34:436–42.

[190] Furuta M, Komiya-Nonaka M, Akifusa S, Shimazaki Y, Adachi M, Kinoshita T, Kikutani T, Yamashita Y. Interrelationship of oral health status, swallowing function, nutritional status, and cognitive ability with activities of daily living in Japanese elderly people receiving home care services due to physical disabilities. Community Dent Oral Epidemiol 2013;41:173–81.

[191] Matsuo H, Yoshimura Y, Fujita S, Maeno Y. Incidence of dysphagia and its association with functional recovery and 1-year mortality in hospitalized older patients with heart failure: a prospective cohort study. JPEN J Parenter Enteral Nutr 2020. https://doi.org/10.1002/jpwn.1845 [Epub ahead of print].

[192] Hudson HM, Daubert CR, Mills RH. The interdependency of protein-energy malnutrition, aging, and dysphagia. Dysphagia 2000;15:31–8.

[193] Metra M, Mentz RJ, Chiswell K, Bloomfield DM, Cleland JG, Cotter G, Davison BA, Dittrich HD, Fiuzat M, Givertz MM, et al. Acute heart failure in elderly patients: worse outcomes and differential utility of standard prognostic variables. Insights from the PROTECT trial. Eur J Heart Fail 2015;7:109–18.

CHAPTER 13

Mechanisms of decline in muscle quality in sarcopenia

Takashi Yamada
School of Health Sciences, Sapporo Medical University, Sapporo, Japan

Abstract
Sarcopenia is a geriatric syndrome that was originally defined as the loss of muscle mass, whereas loss of muscle strength and function come to the forefront in the revised guidelines of sarcopenia (the European Working Group on Sarcopenia in Older People 2, 2018). Accordingly, a decline in muscle quality is increasingly being considered as an important feature in sarcopenia; muscle quality has generally been used to describe the loss of force per cross-sectional area (i.e., specific force). In this chapter, the mechanisms underlying reduced specific force production will be discussed using the data from aged human beings and animals, especially focusing on the intrinsic contractile properties in skeletal muscle fibers. The loss of specific force can be due to decreased Ca^{2+} release from the sarcoplasmic reticulum, reduced myofibrillar Ca^{2+} sensitivity, and/or decreased ability of the cross-bridges to generate force.
Keywords: Muscle weakness, Muscle quality, Specific force, Excitation-contraction coupling, Cross-bridge, Reactive oxygen/nitrogen species (ROS/RNS)

Introduction

In 2010, the original definition of sarcopenia by the European Working Group on Sarcopenia in Older People (EWGSOP) added muscle function to former definitions based only on detection of low muscle mass [1]. In its 2018 definition, EWGSOP2 uses low muscle strength as the primary parameter of sarcopenia, as it is recognized that strength is better than mass in predicting adverse outcomes [2]. Indeed, it has been shown that the elderly with weak muscles are more susceptible to fall-related injuries than age-matched controls with stronger muscles [3–5]. Because of the significant correlation between muscle size and strength in normal subjects [6], it has been assumed that decreased muscular strength is simply due to decreased muscle mass, that is, muscle wasting. However, in many conditions, including sarcopenia, muscle weakness is observed despite normal muscle mass or the decrease in muscle mass cannot explain the reduction in force production, suggesting a decline in muscle quality [7,8]. The term "muscle quality" has generally been applied to muscle function delivered per unit of muscle mass [9,10]. Multiple factors can affect muscle quality including muscle composition, metabolism, fat infiltration, fibrosis, and neural activation [7,10,11]. Alternatively, skeletal muscle weakness can be caused by intrinsic contractile defects in the muscle fibers. In this chapter, we will discuss decreased force production in sarcopenia, especially focusing on the mechanisms intrinsic to skeletal muscle fibers.

A decline in muscle quality in sarcopenia

Although the loss of muscle mass is associated with the reduction in strength in older adults, this strength decline is much more rapid than the concomitant loss of muscle mass [8]. Theoretically, muscle force production is proportional to the muscle cross-sectional area (CSA) in the normal subjects [6]. However, loss of force per CSA (i.e., specific force) has been repeatedly observed in skeletal muscle from aged human beings and animals (Tables 1 and 2). This loss of specific force has also been observed in the inactivated muscles (e.g., bed rest, casting, and spaceflight) (Tables 3 and 4). Fig. 1 shows the relationship

Table 1: Quantifications of muscle wasting and weakness in aged human beings.

Study	Subject (year)	Muscle	Preparation	Fiber type	Muscle mass change (%)	Specific force change (%)
[12]	Male (68 vs 28)	Vastus lateralis	In vivo		− 24% (CSA)	− 27%
		Biceps brachii	In vivo		− 20%: NS (CSA)	− 14%
[13]	Male (73–81 vs 25–31)	Quadriceps	Skinned fiber	Type I	+ 10%: NS (CSA)	− 5%: NS
				Type IIa	− 28% (CSA)	− 28%
[14]	Male (74 vs 37)	Vastus lateralis	Skinned fiber	Type I	− 6% (CSA)	− 28%
				Type IIa	+ 4% (CSA)	− 31%
[15]	Male (73 vs 30)	Vastus lateralis	Skinned fiber	Type I	− 22% (CSA)	− 22%
				Type IIa	− 12% (CSA)	− 16%
[16]	Male (74 vs 25)	Plantar flexor	In vivo		− 17% (CSA)	− 30%
[17]	Male (66 vs 32)	Vastus lateralis	Skinned fiber	Type I	+ 12%: NS (CSA)	− 25%
				Type IIa	+ 6%: NS (CSA)	− 33%
[18]	Male (67 vs 24)	Knee extensor	In vivo		− 17% (CSA)	− 31%
[19]	Male (80 vs 23)	Vastus lateralis	Skinned fiber		− 25%: NS (CSA)	− 43%
[20]	Male (71 vs 23)	Vastus lateralis	In vivo		− 31% (CSA)	− 16%: NS
			Skinned fiber	Type I	− 16% (CSA)	− 10%
				Type IIa	− 15%: NS (CSA)	− 26%
[21]	Female (72 vs 22)	Knee extensor	In vivo		− 25% (CSA)	− 17%
[22]	Male and female (79 vs 26)	Vastus lateralis	Skinned fiber	Type I	+ 7%: NS (CSA)	+ 13%: NS
				Type IIa	− 10%: NS (CSA)	− 13%: NS

NS, not significant.

Table 2: Quantifications of muscle wasting and weakness in aged animals.

Study	Subject (month)	Muscle	Condition	Fiber type	Muscle mass change (%)	Specific force change (%)
[23]	Male mouse (26–27 vs 9–10)	Soleus	Whole muscle		− 12%: NS (CSA)	− 15%: NS
		EDL	Whole muscle		− 6%: NS (CSA)	− 22%: NS
[24]	Rat (30 vs 12)	Soleus	Skinned fiber	Type I	+ 5%: NS (Diameter)	− 14%
[25]	Male rat (24 vs 12)	Soleus	Skinned fiber	Type I	− 8%: NS (CSA)	− 20%
	Male rat (30 vs 12)	Soleus	Skinned fiber	Type I	+ 11%: NS (CSA)	− 22%
	Male rat (36 vs 12)	Soleus	Skinned fiber	Type I	− 36% (CSA)	− 31%
	Male rat (37 vs 12)	Soleus	Skinned fiber	Type I	− 22% (CSA)	− 47%
[26]	Mouse (20–24 vs 2–6)	Soleus	Intact fiber		− 27% (CSA)	− 19%
		EDL	Intact fiber		3%: NS (CSA)	− 26%
[27]	Male rat (32–36 vs 8–12)	Semimembranosus	Skinned fiber	Type IIB	− 10%: NS (CSA)	− 27%
[28]	Male rat (27–29 vs 3)	EDL	Whole muscle		− 8%: NS (CSA)	− 28%
[29]	Mouse (26–28 vs 10–12)	EDL	Whole muscle		− 8%: NS (CSA)	− 26%
[30]	Male rat (34–40 vs 6–23)	Soleus	Skinned fiber	Type I	− 15% (Diameter)	− 21%
[31]	Male mouse (12–22 vs 2–6)	EDL	Whole muscle		+ 21% (CSA)	− 13%

NS, not significant.

Table 3: Quantifications of muscle wasting and weakness in inactivated human beings.

Study	Subject (year)	Condition	Muscle	Preparation	Fiber type	Muscle mass change (%)	Specific force change (%)
[32]	Male (28)	Bed rest (6 wk)	Vastus lateralis	In vivo		−14% (CSA)	−13%
[33]	Male (43)	Bed rest (17 d)	Soleus	Skinned fiber	Type I	−10% (CSA)	−1%: NS
[34]	Male	Spaceflight (17 d)	Soleus	Skinned fiber	Type I	−15% (CSA)	−4%
[35]	Female (26)	Suspension (12 d)	Soleus	Skinned fiber	Type I	−14% (CSA)	−5%
			Gastrocnemius	Skinned fiber	Type I	−3%: NS (CSA)	−9%
[15]	Male (73)	Bed rest (3.5 mo)	Vastus lateralis	Skinned fiber	Type I	−51% (CSA)	−55%
					Type IIa	−26% (CSA)	−42%
					Type IIx	−24% (CSA)	−37%
[36]	Male (32)	Bed rest (84 d)	Vastus lateralis	Skinned fiber	Type I	−28% (CSA)	−28%
[18]	Male (24)	Casting (2 wk)	Knee extensor	In vivo		−9% (CSA)	−23%
	Male (67)	Casting (2 wk)	Knee extensor	In vivo		−5% (CSA)	−17%
[37]	Male and Female (22)	Suspension (23 d)	Vastus lateralis	Skinned fiber	Type I	−9% (CSA)	−9%: NS
					Type II	−23% (CSA)	−23%

NS, not significant.

Table 4: Quantifications of muscle wasting and weakness in inactivated animals.

Study	Subject	Condition	Muscle	Preparation	Fiber type	Muscle mass change (%)	Specific force change (%)
[38]	Male SD rat (275–300 g)	Suspension (2 wk)	Soleus	Skinned fiber	Type I	−64% (CSA)	−28%
			Gastrocnemius	Skinned fiber	Type I	−57% (CSA)	−20%
					Type II	−31% (CSA)	13%: NS
[39]	Male SD rat (−)	Suspension (2 wk)	Soleus	Skinned fiber	Type I	−42% (CSA)	−19%
[33]	Male SD rat (−)	Suspension (2 wk)	Soleus	Skinned fiber	Type I	−51% (CSA)	−12%
[40]	F344 rats (30 mo)	Suspension (7 d)	Soleus	Skinned fiber	Type I	−17% (CSA)	−30%
			Gastrocnemius	Skinned fiber	Type I	−27% (CSA)	−24%
					Type II	−13%: NS (CSA)	−29%
[24]	F344 rats (12 mo)	Suspension (7 d)	Soleus	Skinned fiber	Type I	−12% (CSA)	−15%
	F344 rats (30 mo)	Suspension (7 d)	Soleus	Skinned fiber	Type I	−20% (CSA)	−30%
[41]	Male C57BL/6 mice (8–12 wk)	Suspension (7 d)	Soleus	Skinned fiber	Type I	−33% (CSA)	−15%
					Type IIa	−33% (CSA)	−20%
					Type IIx/b	−16% (CSA)	−17%
	Male ICR mice (8–12 wk)	Suspension (7 d)	Soleus	Skinned fiber	Type I	−39% (CSA)	−13%
					Type IIa	−21% (CSA)	−13%
	Male CBA/J mice (8–12 wk)	Suspension (7 d)	Soleus	Skinned fiber	Type I	−34% (CSA)	−11%
[42]	Male SD rat (275–300 g)	Suspension (2 wk)	Soleus	Skinned fiber	Type IIa	−36% (CSA)	−12%
			Adductor longus	Skinned fiber	Type I	−59% (CSA)	−17%
					Type I	−60% (CSA)	6%: NS
[43]	F344 rats (−)	Suspension (2 wk)	Semimembranosus	Skinned fiber	Type IIB	−42% (CSA)	−38%
					Type IIx/b	−49% (CSA)	−18%

SD, Sprague-Dawley; HS, hindlimb suspension; F344, Fisher 344 Brown Norway F1 hybrid; NS, not significant.

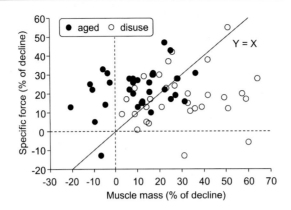

Fig. 1
Relationship between the degree of reduction in muscle mass and specific force in aged and inactivated subjects. The plotted data include the findings in Tables 1–4, except the studies using in vivo voluntary contractions where age-related alterations in the nervous system, such as the loss of motor neurons and the remodeling of motor units, could affect the force production.

between the degree of reduction in muscle mass and specific force in aged and inactivated subjects. The plotted data include the findings in Tables 1–4, except the studies using in vivo voluntary contractions where age-related alterations in the nervous system, such as the loss of motor neuron and the remodeling of motor units, could affect the force production [7,11]. Interestingly, the degree of reduction in specific force appears to be higher than that in muscle mass in aged subjects, indicating that decline in muscle quality is an important feature in sarcopenia.

Ideally, one experimental approach for understanding the age-related muscle contractile dysfunction is to use isolated whole muscles, stimulated and perfused in a muscle bath. Indeed, several studies have reported a significant reduction in specific force production in fast- and slow-twitch skeletal muscles from aged animals [23,28,31]. However, an increased noncontractile extracellular component, including connective [44] and adipose tissues [45,46], was observed in aged subjects, which could cause a reduced specific force in whole muscle level [47]. Moreover, skeletal muscles are generally composed of a mixture of fiber types with markedly different cellular functional properties, which then can be differently affected in age-related muscle weakness. Thus, with this approach, it is difficult to explore cellular mechanisms. Many of the issues associated with studying mechanisms behind weakness in whole muscles are overcome by using single muscle fibers [48]. The application of the single fiber technique to the intrinsic contractile dysfunction in muscle fibers from aged subjects was first published by Larsson et al. [13], and since then this technique has significantly contributed to improving our understanding of the cellular mechanisms of sarcopenia. Cross-sectional studies using single muscle fibers obtained from aged human beings and animals show a reduction in muscle fiber specific force in both slow-twitch type I and fast-twitch type II fibers (Tables 1 and 2).

Age-related alterations in intracellular activation-contraction pathway in skeletal muscle fibers

As depicted in Fig. 2, skeletal muscle contraction is elicited by the chain of events in muscle fibers. Acetylcholine released from the end terminals of α-motor neurons binding to its receptor in the sarcolemma activates voltage-dependent Na^+ channels and an action potential is generated. An action potential is conducted into the transverse tubules (t-tubules) and activates the t-tubular voltage sensor, the dihydropyridine receptor (DHPR), which is localized in close connection to the Ca^{2+} release channel of the sarcoplasmic reticulum (SR), the ryanodine receptor 1 (RyR1). Conformational coupling links the DHPR and the RyR1 in skeletal muscle, and Ca^{2+} is released from the SR into the myoplasm in skeletal muscle [49]. Ca^{2+} then binds to troponin (Tn)-C, relieving the inhibitory binding of Tn-I to tropomyosin (Tm) and actin. Tm moves over the surface of actin, exposing the myosin-binding sites on actin. The myosin heads can then bind to actin and cross-bridge cycling starts to generate force. Ca^{2+} is continuously pumped back into the SR by the

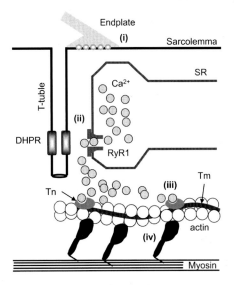

Fig. 2
Diagram of the chain of events leading to muscle force production. Acetylcholine released from the end terminals of α-motor excites the muscle (i). The action potential is conducted into the transverse tubules (t-tubules) and activates the t-tubular voltage sensor, the dihydropyridine receptor (DHPR), which is localized in close connection to the Ca^{2+} release channel of the sarcoplasmic reticulum (SR), the ryanodine receptor 1 (RyR1). Conformational coupling links the DHPR and the RyR1 in skeletal muscle and Ca^{2+} is released from the SR into the myoplasm in skeletal muscle (ii). Ca^{2+} then binds to troponin (Tn)-C, relieving the inhibitory binding of Tn-I to tropomyosin (Tm) and actin. Tm moves over the surface of actin, exposing the myosin-binding sites on actin. The myosin heads can then bind to actin and cross-bridge cycling starts to generate force.

SR Ca^{2+} pump (SERCA) during contraction. When SR Ca^{2+} release is stopped, the free myoplasmic Ca^{2+} concentration decreases and the muscle fiber relaxes. Loss of specific force can result from dysfunction of any of the events described earlier. We will discuss how defective functions of specific processes can cause a reduction in specific force in aged muscles.

Decreased Ca^{2+} release from the sarcoplasmic reticulum in skeletal muscle fiber from aged subjects

In 1995, Delbono and colleagues have demonstrated using fast-twitch single fibers from human vastus lateralis muscle that the peak Ca^{2+} transient studied with Ca^{2+} selective fluorescent indicator mag-fura-2 was significantly lower in aged human beings than in young ones [50]. In later studies, they confirmed the reduction in depolarization-evoked SR Ca^{2+} release in the fast-twitch single muscle fibers from senescent mice [51–53]. The lower peak Ca^{2+} transient was associated with a reduction in DHPR charge movement and reduction in the number of DHPR α1 subunits without changes in the number of RyR1 in aged muscles [53–55]. They suggested, therefore, that DHPR-unlinked RYR1 is increased with age, and thus, the reduction in voltage-gated SR Ca^{2+} release is due in part to the DHPR-RyR1 uncoupling in aged skeletal muscle fibers. Using transmission electron microscopy, Boncompagni et al. [56] have demonstrated significant modifications of Ca^{2+} release unit (CRU), formed by the T-tubules and the SR terminal, and a drastic reduction in CRU frequency in aging human beings, suggesting disrupted communication between the DHPR and the RyR1. However, there are conflicting data showing no major changes in the relative abundance of the DHPR α1 subunits in aged rats [57] and human beings [58]. Although the reason for these discrepancies is uncertain, further studies with genetic overexpression of DHPR α1 would more directly clarify the importance of DHPR-RyR1 coupling in aged muscles.

Russ et al. [59] reported that the SR Ca^{2+} release rate measured in SR vesicles is reduced with aging in rat fast-twitch gastrocnemius muscles, indicating an impaired RyR1 function. The impairment in SR Ca^{2+} release is not due to a reduction in RYR1 expression but appears to be related to a loss of calstabin1 (FK506-binding protein 12, FKBP12) expression and interaction of this protein with RYR1. Indeed, weakened molecular interaction between RYR1 and calstabin1 has been associated with impaired Ca^{2+} release in myocardial infarction [60]. Alternatively, decreased SR Ca^{2+} release could result simply from there being less Ca^{2+} stored in the SR in muscle fibers of aged subjects [61]. It has been reported that in both type I and type II fibers, both the endogenous and maximal releasable SR Ca^{2+} content are ~15% lower in the muscle of aged human beings compared with young ones [62]. In line with this, SR Ca^{2+} release induced by caffeine, a well-studied agonist of the RyR1, is reduced in muscle fibers from aged mice [63]. Previous studies suggest that the reduced SR Ca^{2+} content and concomitant decreases in SR Ca^{2+} release in skeletal muscle fibers with aging could arise from dysfunction of the RyR1 in the SR. Andersson et al. [64] have shown that RyR1 in fast-twitch extensor digitorum longus (EDL) muscles from aged mice undergoes nitrosative post-translational modifications (PTMs) and dissociation of calstabin1, resulting in "leaky" channels with increased open probability. This leads to intracellular Ca^{2+} leak, which in turn reduces SR Ca^{2+} content and tetanic Ca^{2+} in aged muscle fibers.

Reduced myofibrillar Ca^{2+} sensitivity in skeletal muscle fiber from aged subjects

The mechanism underlying skeletal muscle weakness has extensively been explored using skinned muscle fibers, that is, muscle fibers with their surface membrane removed either chemically or mechanically. Skinned fibers can be activated by increasing the free Ca^{2+} concentration ($[Ca^{2+}]$) in the bath. The isometric force produced at each $[Ca^{2+}]$ was expressed as a percentage of the corresponding maximum force and analyzed by fitting a Hill curve to ascertain the pCa at half-maximum force (pCa$_{50}$), which is traditionally used as an indicator of the myofibrillar Ca^{2+} sensitivity. Only a few studies, however, have examined the effect of aging on the myofibrillar Ca^{2+} sensitivity of single muscle fibers in human beings. Straight et al. [65] have reported a decreased myofibrillar Ca^{2+} sensitivity in all fiber types examined (I, I/IIa, IIa, IIa/x) from vastus lateralis muscle in aged human beings compared to young ones, with the largest effect on type I fibers (pCa$_{50}$ decreased ~ 0.14 pCa units). Lamboley et al. [62] have demonstrated that in type II fibers, but not in type I fibers, from vastus lateralis muscle in aged human beings had a reduced specific force and Ca^{2+} sensitivity (pCa$_{50}$ decreased ~ 0.05 pCa units) relative to that in young ones. Two other studies from the same research group reported similar results, with the mean pCa$_{50}$ in the type II fibers being 0.08 and 0.09 pCa units lower in the aged human beings relative to the young ones [66,67], although this differences did not reach the significance level in those studies.

The molecular basis of reduced myofibrillar Ca^{2+} sensitivity occurring with age is uncertain. One possibility is that it is due to oxidative PTMs of contractile apparatus. Reactive oxygen and nitrogen species (ROS/RNS) are generated in skeletal muscle during contraction and in pathological conditions [68,69] (see Section "Mechanisms behind intrinsic contractile dysfunction in skeletal muscle fiber from aged subjects: Role of reactive oxygen/nitrogen species (ROS/RNS)"). There is a substantial amount of evidence of increased oxidative PTMs in myofibrillar proteins with age [27,70]. S-glutathionylation of fast troponin I (TnI$_f$) has Ca^{2+}-sensitizing effect, which is regarded as an important mechanism helping delay the onset of muscle fatigue during exercise [71]. It has been shown that S-glutathionylation of TnI$_f$ by treating skinned type II fibers with reduced glutathione markedly increased Ca^{2+} sensitivity, but the increase was significantly smaller in aged human beings, suggesting a decreased ability of S-glutathionylation of TnI$_f$ to counter the fatiguing effects of metabolites on Ca^{2+}

sensitivity [62]. Massive oxidative treatment of skinned type II fibers irreversibly blocks the Ca^{2+}-sensitizing effect of S-glutathionylation [72], presumably causing irreversible oxidative PTMs of the critical cysteine on TnI_f. These findings raise the possibility that the type II fibers in the aged subjects had undergone a certain level of irreversible oxidative PTMs, which is known to cause irreversible decreases in Ca^{2+} sensitivity and specific force in isolated fibers and muscles.

Decreased ability of the cross-bridges to generate force in skeletal muscle fiber from aged subjects

A number of previous studies, using chemically or mechanically skinned fibers, have reported that the maximal Ca^{2+}-activated force (F_{max}) is lower in either or both type I and type II fibers in aged subjects compared to young subjects (see Tables 1 and 2). In principle, the decrease in F_{max} in skinned fiber can be due to a decreased number of force producing cross-bridge and/or impaired cross-bridge function with decreased force per cross-bridge. To understand age-related muscle weakness mediated by alterations in cross-bridge events, it is important to review the steps involved in cross-bridge cycling and force generation. In brief, when myosin initially binds to actin, the actomyosin is in a weak binding state (Fig. 3). With the subsequent release of inorganic phosphate (P_i), the cross-bridge transforms into a strong binding state and goes through the power stroke, generating force. ADP is then released, returning the cross-bridge to the rigor complex [73]. The strong binding high-force states are thought to be the dominant form during a maximal isometric contraction.

Myosin is the most abundant protein and comprises about 30% of total muscle proteins. Each myosin molecule is composed of two myosin heavy chains (MyHCs) and four myosin light chains (MLCs). D'Antona et al. [15] have demonstrated that MyHC concentration decreases in type I and IIa fibers in vastus lateralis muscles from sedentary aged human beings and is linearly related to the specific force of corresponding fiber types from the same subjects. In line with this, reduction in MyHC, but not in actin, content has been found in semimembranosus muscles from aged rats [74]. Several studies have reported a lower synthesis rate of MyHC in aged subjects [75,76], which appears to be regulated by transcriptional level [77]. These changes result in a reduced myosin-to-actin ratio, which may decrease the number of active cross-bridges contributing to force generation, providing one of the mechanisms for age-related decline in specific force. Several studies, however, reported no difference in MyHC content between muscles from younger and older individuals, despite an age-related decline in specific force, suggesting mechanisms other than loss of myosin can be involved in the deleterious changes in myofibrillar function in aged muscles [20,78].

There is growing evidence to suggest that PTMs of myosin can compromise muscle function. Skeletal muscle myosin contains 40 cysteines [79], including two highly reactive cysteines in myosin subfragment 1 (i.e., Cys 697 and 707). Oxidation of these two cysteines has

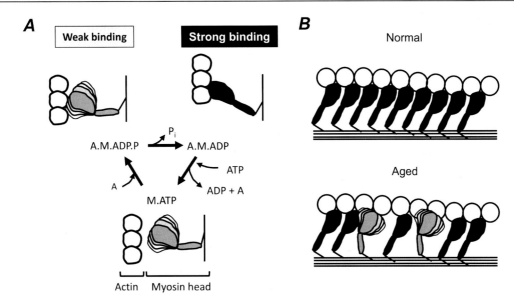

Fig. 3

Age-related changes in myosin content and structure in skeletal muscle. (A) Model for the molecular mechanisms of force generation, based on electron paramagnetic resonance (EPR) results. EPR resolves two distinct myosin structural states, and force is generated in a transition from one of these (weak binding, characterized by dynamic disorder and a bent shape, gray) to the other (strong binding, characterized by rigid order and a straight shape, black). *A*, actin; *M*, myosin. (B) The amount of myosin and the steady-state fraction of myosin heads in the strong-binding (force-generating) structural state during a maximal isometric contraction are reduced in fibers from aged subjects. *(A) Adapted from Lowe DA, Surek JT, Thomas DD, Thompson LV. Electron paramagnetic resonance reveals age-related myosin structural changes in rat skeletal muscle fibers. Am J Physiol 2001;280:C540–7.*

been shown to have dramatic effects on the functional properties of myosin, particularly in interactions with actin, resulting in significant deterioration of cross-bridge [80,81]. The nitric oxide (NO•) donor sodium nitroprusside inhibited myofibrillar function caused by reversible oxidation of myosin in rabbit muscle fibers [82].

Importantly, Thompson and colleagues demonstrated that PTMs in the catalytic domain of myosin provide a molecular explanation for myofibrillar dysfunction with aging [27,83,84]. Permeabilized semimembranosus fibers were spin-labeled, specifically at myosin Cys707, and were used to resolve and quantify the structural states of the myosin head by electron paramagnetic resonance (EPR) spectroscopy to determine the fraction of myosin head in the strong-binding (force-generating) states during a maximal isometric contraction. They showed that the fraction of myosin heads in the strong-binding structural states is 30% lower in type II fibers from aged rats, which is comparable to the 27% age-related decline in specific force [27] (Fig. 3). They also indicated that the age-related PTMs in myosin can be due to protein oxidation, as indicated by a decrease in the number of free cysteine residues.

Consistent with this finding, the number of reactive cysteines in catalytically active myosin fragment, heavy meromyosin, significantly decreased with age [85]. To sum up, it might well be that degenerative alterations in myosin molecules are likely to contribute to both a decreased number of force producing cross-bridge and impaired cross-bridge functions with decreased force per cross-bridge in age-related myofibrillar dysfunction. Of note, PTMs in other myofibrillar proteins may also play a role in the impairment of individual muscle fiber function. By using proteome analysis, Brocca et al. [20] found the phosphorylation of several proteins, including MLC-2 slow and TnT as well as the carbonylation of MyHC in aged human beings. Phosphorylation of TnT results in a decrease in the maximal actomyosin ATPase activity and a reduction in its sensitivity to Ca^{2+} [20].

In addition to the ability to generate force, maximum unloaded shortening velocity (V_0) is altered by age. It has been demonstrated, although with some differential effects depending on the study, that V_0 was reduced with age in both fast- and slow-twitch fiber types [13,17,19,20,86]. In most cases, reduction in V_0 was accompanied by weaker specific force in aged subjects. This may suggest that muscle fibers from aged subjects have impaired cross-bridge kinetics and therefore a lower capacity to generate force per area of contractile apparatus [19].

Ochala et al. [17] have shown in human single fibers that aging induces alterations in fiber elasticity in both type I and type IIa fibers. A greater instantaneous stiffness per force unit was observed in activated fibers from aged human beings. They suggest that the increased stiffness can be due to an increase in the number and proportion of weak binding low-force state cross-bridges. On the other hand, Lim et al. [22] have reported that passive force is greater in both type I and IIa fibers of aged human beings. These cellular alterations may not directly influence contractile dysfunction but may explain the muscle-tendon stiffness found in aged human beings [87].

Mechanisms behind intrinsic contractile dysfunction in skeletal muscle fiber from aged subjects: Role of disuse

Skeletal muscle strength declines with age even when maintaining an active lifestyle [88]. "Primary sarcopenia" refers to sarcopenia that has no other specific cause than aging, while "secondary sarcopenia" refers to sarcopenia that has causal factors other than (or in addition to) aging [2]. Physical inactivity contributes to the development of secondary sarcopenia, whether due to a sedentary lifestyle or to disease-related immobility [89]. It has been demonstrated, using electromyogram (EMG) activity, that the mean amplitude of each EMG burst during normal use (i.e., daily living) was less than 20% of maximum voluntary contraction (MVC) in leg muscles from healthy young human beings [90]. Based on the size principle, slow-twitch type I fibers are predominantly recruited in daily living, and hence, this type of fibers are susceptible to inactivation-induced muscle wasting and weakness. If this is also the case in aging, the confounding impact of disuse should be observed in type I fibers in aged subjects. In support of this notion, Bottinelli and colleagues have shown that the degree of reduction in specific force in type I fibers from sedentary aged human beings (− 22%) [15] is greater than that from physically active aged human beings (− 10%) [20]. However, the decline in the specific force of type I fiber with aging is observed even in world-class masters athletes [19], suggesting the existence of factors other than inactivity to induce age-related intrinsic contractile dysfunction in type I fibers.

A reduction in size and the number of fast-twitch type II fibers is a typical feature of sarcopenia [12,91–94]. The use of heavy load results in the recruitment of type II fibers, and hence, high-intensity resistance training (i.e., > 70% of 1 repetition maximum) is generally recommended to maximize muscle hypertrophy and strength gain [95]. However, as mentioned earlier, the loading intensity during normal daily living is not high enough to regularly recruit the type II fibers, and thus, this type of fibers are not frequently used over the years and decades unless one performs strength training during senescence. In other words, the fast-twitch fiber-specific inactivation would play an important role, even in primary sarcopenia.

The qualitative adaptations of contractile proteins appear to play a larger role than quantitative adaptations in primary sarcopenia. In healthy young human beings, disuse has been shown to cause a lower specific force of muscle fibers with lower myosin concentration [96,97]. In line with this, reduction in specific force was associated with loss of myosin in sedentary aged human beings [15]. On the other hand, in active aged human beings, intrinsic contractile dysfunction of muscle fibers was not accompanied by loss of myosin but was related to the PTMs of contractile proteins [20]. Thus, these findings imply that impaired cross-bridge function with decreased force per cross-bridge (e.g., PTMs of myosin) rather than a decreased number of force producing cross-bridge (e.g., loss of myosin) may contribute to the mechanisms underlying decline in specific force in primary sarcopenia.

Mechanisms behind intrinsic contractile dysfunction in skeletal muscle fiber from aged subjects: Role of reactive oxygen/nitrogen species (ROS/RNS)

The molecular basis of intrinsic contractile dysfunction occurring with age is uncertain. One possibility is that it is due to ROS- and/or RNS-induced PTMs in skeletal muscle proteins (see Sections "Decreased Ca^{2+} release from the sarcoplasmic reticulum in skeletal muscle fiber from aged subjects", "Reduced myofibrillar Ca^{2+} sensitivity in skeletal muscle fiber from aged subjects", "Decreased ability of the cross-bridges to generate force in skeletal muscle fiber from aged subjects", and "Mechanisms behind intrinsic contractile dysfunction in skeletal muscle fiber from aged subjects: Role of disuse"). $NO^{\bullet}$ and its derivative peroxynitrite anion ($ONOO^{\bullet-}$) depresses force production in skeletal muscle [82,98]. ROS

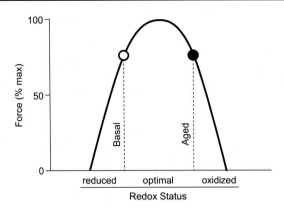

Fig. 4

Redox modulation of force production in skeletal muscle. The *curve* depicts a biphasic response of force as cellular redox status is altered. The *open circle* is the proposed status of healthy adult muscle fibers under basal conditions. The *closed circle* is the proposed status of aged muscle fibers. Model adapted from Reid MB. Redox modulation of skeletal muscle contraction: what we know and what we don't. J Appl Physiol 2001;90:724–31 and Reid MB, Durham WJ. Generation of reactive oxygen and nitrogen species in contracting skeletal muscle: potential impact on aging. Ann N Y Acad Sci 2002;959:108–16.

promotes skeletal muscle force under basal conditions but inhibits force in conditions where ROS production is exaggerated [99–102]. Reid and Durham [103] have modeled these biphasic effects as a bell-shaped continuum of contractile function across a range of redox statuses (Fig. 4). A growing body of evidence indicates that aging exaggerates the effects of muscle-derived ROS. The redox status of aged muscle appears to be shifted rightward. This age-related alteration may reflect the combined effects of accelerated ROS production and increased susceptibility of regulatory proteins to oxidative modification [103–105].

Accelerated reactive oxygen/nitrogen species (ROS/RNS) in skeletal muscle fiber from aged subjects

The superoxide anion ($O_2^{\bullet-}$) and $NO^{\bullet}$ are the primary free radicals and converted to secondary ROS and RNS. $O_2^{\bullet-}$ is dismuted by $O_2^{\bullet-}$ dismutase (SOD) to hydrogen peroxide (H_2O_2) or react with $NO^{\bullet}$ to form $ONOO^{\bullet-}$. Further, H_2O_2 can be decomposed by antioxidative enzymes, including catalase and glutathione (GSH) peroxidase to H_2O and O_2 [68]. H_2O_2 also reacts with free transition metals, such as Fe^{2+}, and converted to hydroxyl radical ($OH^{\bullet}$) (Fenton reaction). Moreover, both H_2O_2 and $OH^{\bullet}$ can react with GSH to generate thiyl radicals ($GS^{\bullet}$). ROS/RNS are involved in both cellular adaptive and maladaptive processes [106]. The biological effects of ROS/RNS depend on a combination of factors, including the type and concentration of ROS/RNS and its production site [107].

Mitochondrial respiration has been considered a major source of $O_2^{\bullet-}$ production in skeletal muscle. Complexes I and III are the two major sites of $O_2^{\bullet-}$ production in mitochondria

[108]. Although early reports suggested that 2%–5% of the total oxygen consumed by mitochondria is reduced to $O_2^{\bullet-}$ [109,110], more recent studies indicate that only ~ 0.1%–0.2% of oxygen consumed by the mitochondria forms $O_2^{\bullet-}$ [108,111,112]. With aging, ROS production is likely to be accelerated in skeletal muscle due to an age-dependent decline in mitochondrial function characterized by increased electron displacement from the transport chain [113–115]. Moreover, in human beings, a significant reduction in the number of large motorneurons, which tend to innervate type II fibers, occurs with aging, indicating some denervated muscle fibers in aged muscles [116,117]. Experimental denervation was shown to result in a large sustained increase in muscle mitochondrial ROS production [114]. Thus, denervation of individual muscle fibers may lead to a fiber-specific increase in mitochondrial ROS generation [105].

$O_2^{\bullet-}$ is also generated by enzymes such as NADPH oxidase (NOX) [118], phospholipase A_2 [119], xanthine oxidase [120], and uncoupled $NO^{\bullet}$ synthase (NOS) [121]. Of these enzymes, NOX2 is proposed to be a major contributor to $O_2^{\bullet-}$ production in skeletal muscle both at rest and during contraction [122]. The activation of NOX2 requires the interaction of cytosolic subunits p47^{phox}, p67^{phox}, and Rac1 with membrane-bound subunits gp91^{phox} and p22^{phox} [123]. In striated muscles, Ward et al. [124] have revealed that the microtubule network acts as the mechanotransducer to activate NOX2-dependent ROS generation, a pathway termed X-ROS signaling, during contractile activity and stretch. NOX2 is preferentially localized to the plasma membrane [125], SR [126], and the T-tubular membrane [127,128]. These sites are close to ion channels and pumps, which are essential for excitation-contraction coupling. Moreover, the SR and T-tubules are located around the myofibrils where the cross-bridges generate force. It is therefore assumed that the major excitation-contraction coupling proteins would be exposed readily to the $O_2^{\bullet-}$-derived radicals. Age-related alterations in NOX2 expression vary across studies, with some showing increases [129] and others showing no changes or even decreases [105,130,131]. Thus, the biological importance of NOX2 has not been established in aged skeletal muscle.

Xanthine oxidase has been demonstrated to contribute to oxidative stress in skeletal muscle from aged rodents [120,132], although this age-related increase in xanthine oxidase activity is not observed universally [133]. Xanthine oxidase-induced ROS production has shown to be increased during exhaustive exercise. Ryan et al. [134] showed that inhibition of xanthine oxidase by allopurinol, a structural isomer of hypoxanthine, reduces ROS production and improved skeletal muscle function in response to isometric contractions in aged mice. These data suggest that xanthine oxidase contributes at least partially to oxidant production during contractions.

$NO^{\bullet}$ is synthesized from L-arginine and O_2 by NOS. Mammalian skeletal and cardiac muscle fiber constitutively expresses neuronal- and endothelial-NOS (nNOS and eNOS, respectively), whereas inducible NOS (iNOS) is upregulated in response to inflammatory insults. In the physiological context, nNOS is the principal source of NO• in skeletal muscle. It is mostly compartmentalized to the sarcolemma submembrane scaffold, as a peripheral member of the dystrophin-glycoprotein complex (DGC) [135]. A small fraction of nNOS protein is also detectable in the SR and mitochondria [136]. Recent studies demonstrated a colocalization of RyR1 with nNOS in isolated mouse cardiomyocytes [137] and skeletal muscle from healthy human subjects [138]. The rate of NO• production was shown to be increased during repeated tetani in isolated mouse skeletal muscle fibers [139]. nNOS is activated by Ca^{2+} and calmodulin and the K_m of Ca^{2+} for the activation of nNOS is ~ 200 nM [140]. Thus, the Ca^{2+} transient during tetanus, which reaches 1–2 μM and even higher close to the RyR1, sufficiently activates nNOS and generates NO• in muscle fibers. Since NO• is highly diffusible and considered to have a wide range of effects exceeding 100 μm [141], most subcellular proteins can be targeted by their biological actions. Most studies have demonstrated that nNOS expression declines with age and NO• production appears to decrease in skeletal muscle [142,143]. Conversely, Capanni et al. [144] have reported that, in aged rats, the nNOS amount in skeletal muscle increases both in the soluble and microsomal fractions and that additional cytoplasmic localization appears. Notably, it has been demonstrated that dislocated nNOS from membrane to cytoplasm leads to the production of NO• and activates protein degradation pathway in 2 models of disuse-induced muscle atrophy, tail suspension, and denervation [145]. Given that some denervation of muscle fibers occurs with age [116], these denervated fibers may account for the NO• production in aged muscles. Thus, although existing findings predict that NO• signaling may play a lesser role in the muscles of aged subjects, a clear consensus is yet to be obtained.

$ONOO^{•-}$ is produced by the reaction of NO• and $O_2^{•-}$ and is a potent oxidizing and nitrating agent able to react with a wide range of biomolecules. The rates of $ONOO^{•-}$ production in vivo have been estimated to be as high as 50–100 μM per min [146]. Despite the short half-life at physiological conditions (~ 10 ms), it could influence cellular targets within ~ 5–20 μm [147]. The formation of $ONOO^{•-}$ from NO• and $O_2^{•-}$ can occur about six times faster than the rate at which SOD can convert $O_2^{•-}$ to H_2O_2 [148]. Thus, when NO• is produced at a high rate, it will rapidly react with $O_2^{•-}$ to produce $ONOO^{•-}$ even in the presence of the physiological amount of SOD. $ONOO^{•-}$ reacts with amino acid side chains such as tyrosine, forming 3-nitrotyrosine (3-NT). Substantial studies have revealed that 3-NT is increased in skeletal muscle from aged mice [149–151]. Murakami et al. [149] showed that mitochondrial proteins are more prone to nitration during aging. Nuss et al. [152] reported that 3-NT modified creatine kinase is found in aged muscle, which may account for its reduction in function. Schöneich et al. [153] demonstrated that $ONOO^{•-}$ selectively nitrates the tyrosine residues of the type 2a SERCA isoform and disrupts its enzymatic function in skeletal muscles from aged rats. These findings imply that accelerated production of $ONOO^{•-}$ may play an important role in functional deficits seen in aged muscles.

Increased susceptibility of regulatory proteins to oxidative modification in skeletal muscle fiber

According to the evidence of increased oxidative damage in muscle from aged subjects [70,154], one would expect a general decline of cellular antioxidative capacity in aged muscles. However, available data suggest that aging is associated with increased activity of antioxidative enzymes, including SOD, catalase, and glutathione peroxidase (GPX), glutathione S-transferase (GST), and glutathione reductase (GR) [155–157]. Age-related adaptation of antioxidative enzymes appears to be muscle fiber-type specific, with the most prominent increase found in slow-twitch type I fibers [157,158]. The mechanism responsible for the upregulation of major antioxidative enzyme activities in aged muscles is not clear, but one possibility is that increased production of ROS by mitochondria from aged muscles may stimulate antioxidative enzyme activities. Oh-Ishi et al. [158] reported that the activity and content of CuZn SOD in soleus muscles are significantly higher in old rats than in young rats, whereas no significant change is found in the expression levels of CuZn SOD mRNA levels. In line with this, the lower expression level of Mn SOD mRNA has been observed in aged rat muscles, despite a significant increase in Mn SOD activity [159]. Thus, these data suggest that an age-related increase in SOD activity is not induced by enhanced gene expression, but rather, translational and/or posttranslational mechanisms [160].

Reduced GSH is the most abundant nonprotein thiol source in muscle cells present in millimolar concentrations and is the most important antioxidant. GSH not only serves as a substrate for GPX and GST to reduce H_2O_2, but GSH also scavenges $OH^{\bullet}$ [161]. GSH can be recycled by GR that catalyzes the reduction of glutathione disulfide (GSSG) to the reduced GSH. As reviewed by Ji et al. [156], GSH regulation is not compromised in aged skeletal muscles. It has been shown that aging causes no significant alteration of GSH content or GSH/GSSG ratio in rat fast-twitch vastus lateralis muscles, whereas there is an increase in GSH content in slow-twitch soleus muscle from old rats [157].

Given that the antioxidative capacities do not decrease with aging, it is conceivable that intrinsic contractile dysfunction in aged muscles may relate to an increased susceptibility of cellular membranes and proteins to damage induced by oxidant challenge. In support of this notion, it has been demonstrated that the oxidant challenge induced by the xanthine oxidase system depresses the maximum tetanic tension of fatigued diaphragm muscle from aged rats, but not from young rats [162]. Incubation of rat EDL muscle with $NO^{\bullet}$ donor, S-nitrosocysteine, resulted in a more severe muscle injury in aged animals compared to the young animals [163]. Additionally, muscles from old mice appear to be more susceptible to oxidative injury caused by eccentric contraction (lengthening contraction) [164].

Within proteins, the modifications of thiol moiety (−SH) in cysteine residues are most firmly implicated as a mechanism for the regulation of muscle contractility [165]. ROS/RNS oxidizes thiols reversibly to form disulfide bonds in several E-C coupling proteins, including myosin, actin, tropomyosin, troponin, RyR1, SR Ca^{2+}-ATPase, and Na^+-K^+-ATPase [165]. Among these, myofibrillar proteins are relatively susceptible to redox modifications because exposure to ROS/RNS affected mainly the myofibrillar function [99,166,167], although PTMs of Ca^{2+} handling proteins such as RyR1 also contribute to muscle dysfunction in aged muscle [64]. It is likely that proteins in aged skeletal muscles are more susceptible to oxidative modification, rendering muscle fibers more sensitive to oxidant effects.

Interventions to counteract the age-related loss of muscle quality

Strength training is among the most effective interventions for loss of muscle mass and strength in aged muscles [12,168–171]. An acute bout of exercise provoked higher levels of ROS generation in aged muscles than young muscles working at a comparable intensity [172]. In young subjects, exercise-induced ROS production evokes adaptive responses in skeletal muscle fibers. These include an increase in antioxidative enzymes and heat shock proteins, which render the muscle more resistant to oxidative stress [104,173,174]. Although several studies reported a reduced cytoprotective adaptation to exercise in aged muscles [157,175], it seems that aged skeletal muscles do not necessarily lose adaptability to exercise [156]. Ji et al. [176] showed that chronic training increases GPX, but not SOD and catalase, activity in vastus lateralis muscle in aged rats to a level higher than that seen in young sedentary rats. In line with this, Hammeren et al. [177] demonstrated a significant increase in GPX activity with chronic training in the soleus and red gastrocnemius muscles. Importantly, chronic training resulted in lower levels of malondialdehyde, a lipid peroxidative intermediate, in vastus lateralis and soleus muscles from aged rats [157]. These data suggest that chronic training increases the resistance of aged muscles to oxidative damage, and hence, the muscle quality is preserved in aged subjects.

It has been suggested that the combination of aging and inactivity induces a reduction in the concentration of myosin in skeletal muscle fibers, resulting in lower specific force production due to fewer cross-bridges per muscle fiber area [15] (see Section "Decreased ability of the cross-bridges to generate force in skeletal muscle fiber from aged subjects"). Given that inactivity is commonly present in the aged population, prevention of loss of myosin is important to reverse age-related decline in muscle fiber quality. A reduction in mechanical stimuli appears to be a dominant factor triggering the proteolysis of myosin in skeletal muscle [178–181]. Importantly, although myosin synthesis has been reported to decline with age [75], resistance training can shift the balance between protein synthesis and degradation toward synthesis in elderly subjects, thereby counteracting the age-induced loss of myosin [77,182–184]. Moreover, resistance training in combination with amino acid-containing nutrition would have a synergistic effect on muscle protein synthesis [185,186]. Esmarck et al. [187] has demonstrated that over a 12 week resistance training period, the CSA of quadriceps femoris muscle is significantly increased when protein is ingested immediately after exercise. On the other hand, some studies have not found benefits from protein supplementation in aged subjects [188,189].

Concluding remarks

In this chapter, we have summarized various cellular mechanisms that can induce a decline in muscle quality in aged muscles. Experimental results obtained mostly from single muscle fibers show that intrinsic contractile properties are affected in skeletal muscle fibers from aged subjects. This includes decreased Ca^{2+} release from the SR, reduced myofibrillar Ca^{2+} sensitivity, and/or decreased ability of the cross-bridges to generate force. Dysregulation of muscle contractility is likely mediated, at least in part, by an age-related increase in ROS/RNS production, which leads to harmful PTMs of several key muscle proteins. Moreover, ROS/RNS-induced irreversible modifications of cellular proteins accelerate their rate of degradation by calpain [190] and the ubiquitin-proteasome pathway [191,192]. Although antioxidative adaptations to oxidative stress may decline with aging, aged human beings can still benefit from regular exercise to preserve muscle quality by upregulating muscle antioxidative capacities. Further studies are needed to determine the nature of the link between intrinsic contractile dysfunction and molecular maladaptations in aged muscle fibers. A better understanding of the loss of muscle cellular quality may be instrumental in leading to the discovery and use of therapeutic interventions to prevent or improve primary and/or secondary sarcopenia.

References

[1] Cruz-Jentoft AJ, Baeyens JP, Bauer JM, Boirie Y, Cederholm T, Landi F, Martin FC, Michel JP, Rolland Y, Schneider SM, Topinkova E, Vandewoude M, Zamboni M. Sarcopenia: European consensus on definition and diagnosis: report of the European Working Group on Sarcopenia in Older People. Age Ageing 2010;39:412–23.

[2] Cruz-Jentoft AJ, Bahat G, Bauer J, Boirie Y, Bruyere O, Cederholm T, Cooper C, Landi F, Rolland Y, Sayer AA, Schneider SM, Sieber CC, Topinkova E, Vandewoude M, Visser M, Zamboni M. Sarcopenia: revised European consensus on definition and diagnosis. Age Ageing 2019;48:16–31.

[3] Bischoff-Ferrari HA, Orav JE, Kanis JA, Rizzoli R, Schl Gl M, Staehelin HB, Willett WC, Dawson-Hughes B. Comparative performance of current definitions of sarcopenia against the prospective incidence of falls among community-dwelling seniors age 65 and older. Osteoporos Int 2015;26:2793–802.

[4] Gehlsen GM, Whaley MH. Falls in the elderly: part II, balance, strength, and flexibility. Arch Phys Med Rehabil 1990;71:739–41.

[5] Schaap LA, Van Schoor NM, Lips P, Visser M. Associations of sarcopenia definitions, and their components, with the incidence of recurrent falling and fractures: the longitudinal aging study Amsterdam. J Gerontol A Biol Sci Med Sci 2018;73:1199–204.

[6] Maughan RJ, Watson JS, Weir J. Strength and cross-sectional area of human skeletal muscle. J Physiol 1983;338:37–49.

[7] Clark BC, Manini TM. Sarcopenia =/= dynapenia. J Gerontol A Biol Sci Med Sci 2008;63:829–34.

[8] Goodpaster BH, Park SW, Harris TB, Kritchevsky SB, Nevitt M, Schwartz AV, Simonsick EM, Tylavsky FA, Visser M, Newman AB. The loss of skeletal muscle strength, mass, and quality in older adults: the health, aging and body composition study. J Gerontol A Biol Sci Med Sci 2006;61:1059–64.

[9] Barbat-Artigas S, Rolland Y, Zamboni M, Aubertin-Leheudre M. How to assess functional status: a new muscle quality index. J Nutr Health Aging 2012;16:67–77.

[10] McGregor RA, Cameron-Smith D, Poppitt SD. It is not just muscle mass: a review of muscle quality, composition and metabolism during ageing as determinants of muscle function and mobility in later life. Longev Healthspan 2014;3:9.

[11] Clark BC, Manini TM. What is dynapenia? Nutrition 2012;28:495–503.

[12] Klitgaard H, Mantoni M, Schiaffino S, Ausoni S, Gorza L, Laurent-Winter C, Schnohr P, Saltin B. Function, morphology and protein expression of ageing skeletal muscle: a cross-sectional study of elderly men with different training backgrounds. Acta Physiol Scand 1990;140:41–54.

[13] Larsson L, Li X, Frontera WR. Effects of aging on shortening velocity and myosin isoform composition in single human skeletal muscle cells. Am J Physiol 1997;272:C638–49.

[14] Frontera WR, Suh D, Krivickas LS, Hughes VA, Goldstein R, Roubenoff R. Skeletal muscle fiber quality in older men and women. Am J Physiol 2000;279:C611–8.

[15] D'Antona G, Pellegrino MA, Adami R, Rossi R, Carlizzi CN, Canepari M, Saltin B, Bottinelli R. The effect of ageing and immobilization on structure and function of human skeletal muscle fibres. J Physiol 2003;552:499–511.

[16] Morse CI, Thom JM, Mian OS, Muirhead A, Birch KM, Narici MV. Muscle strength, volume and activation following 12-month resistance training in 70-year-old males. Eur J Appl Physiol 2005;95:197–204.

[17] Ochala J, Frontera WR, Dorer DJ, Hoecke JV, Krivickas LS. Single skeletal muscle fiber elastic and contractile characteristics in young and older men. J Gerontol A Biol Sci Med Sci 2007;62:375–81.

[18] Suetta C, Hvid LG, Justesen L, Christensen U, Neergaard K, Simonsen L, Ortenblad N, Magnusson SP, Kjaer M, Aagaard P. Effects of aging on human skeletal muscle after immobilization and retraining. J Appl Physiol 2009;107:1172–80.

[19] Power GA, Minozzo FC, Spendiff S, Filion ME, Konokhova Y, Purves-Smith MF, Pion C, Aubertin-Leheudre M, Morais JA, Herzog W, Hepple RT, Taivassalo T, Rassier DE. Reduction in single muscle fiber rate of force development with aging is not attenuated in world class older masters athletes. Am J Physiol Cell Physiol 2016;310:C318–27.

[20] Brocca L, Mcphee JS, Longa E, Canepari M, Seynnes O, de Vito G, Pellegrino MA, Narici M, Bottinelli R. Structure and function of human muscle fibres and muscle proteome in physically active older men. J Physiol 2017;595:4823–44.

[21] McPhee JS, Cameron J, Maden-Wilkinson T, Piasecki M, Yap MH, Jones DA, Degens H. The contributions of fiber atrophy, fiber loss, in situ specific force, and voluntary activation to weakness in sarcopenia. J Gerontol A Biol Sci Med Sci 2018;73:1287–94.

[22] Lim JY, Choi SJ, Widrick JJ, Phillips EM, Frontera WR. Passive force and viscoelastic properties of single fibers in human aging muscles. Eur J Appl Physiol 2019;119:2339–48.

[23] Brooks SV, Faulkner JA. Contractile properties of skeletal muscles from young, adult and aged mice. J Physiol 1988;404:71–82.

[24] Thompson LV, Johnson SA, Shoeman JA. Single soleus muscle fiber function after hindlimb unweighting in adult and aged rats. J Appl Physiol 1998;84:1937–42.

[25] Thompson LV, Brown M. Age-related changes in contractile properties of single skeletal fibers from the soleus muscle. J Appl Physiol 1999;86:881–6.

[26] González E, Messi ML, Delbono O. The specific force of single intact extensor digitorum longus and soleus mouse muscle fibers declines with aging. J Membr Biol 2000;178:175–83.

[27] Lowe DA, Surek JT, Thomas DD, Thompson LV. Electron paramagnetic resonance reveals age-related myosin structural changes in rat skeletal muscle fibers. Am J Physiol 2001;280:C540–7.

[28] Urbanchek MG, Picken EB, Kalliainen LK, Kuzon Jr WM. Specific force deficit in skeletal muscles of old rats is partially explained by the existence of denervated muscle fibers. J Gerontol A Biol Sci Med Sci 2001;56:B191–7.

[29] McArdle A, Dillmann WH, Mestril R, Faulkner JA, Jackson MJ. Overexpression of HSP70 in mouse skeletal muscle protects against muscle damage and age-related muscle dysfunction. FASEB J 2004;18:355–7.

[30] Husom AD, Ferrington DA, Thompson LV. Age-related differences in the adaptive potential of type I skeletal muscle fibers. Exp Gerontol 2005;40:227–35.

[31] Chan S, Head SI. Age- and gender-related changes in contractile properties of non-atrophied EDL muscle. PLoS One 2010;5, e12345.

[32] Berg HE, Larsson L, Tesch PA. Lower limb skeletal muscle function after 6 wk of bed rest. J Appl Physiol 1997;82:182–8.

[33] Widrick JJ, Fitts RH. Peak force and maximal shortening velocity of soleus fibers after non-weight-bearing and resistance exercise. J Appl Physiol 1997;82:189–95.

[34] Widrick JJ, Knuth ST, Norenberg KM, Romatowski JG, Bain JL, Riley DA, Karhanek M, Trappe SW, Trappe TA, Costill DL, Fitts RH. Effect of a 17 day spaceflight on contractile properties of human soleus muscle fibres. J Physiol 1999;516:915–30.

[35] Widrick JJ. Effect of P(i) on unloaded shortening velocity of slow and fast mammalian muscle fibers. Am J Physiol Cell Physiol 2002;282:C647–53.

[36] Trappe S, Trappe T, Gallagher P, Harber M, Alkner B, Tesch P. Human single muscle fibre function with 84 day bed-rest and resistance exercise. J Physiol 2004;557:501–13.

[37] Lamboley CR, Wyckelsma VL, Perry BD, Mckenna MJ, Lamb GD. Effect of 23-day muscle disuse on sarcoplasmic reticulum Ca2+ properties and contractility in human type I and type II skeletal muscle fibers. J Appl Physiol (1985) 2016;121:483–92.

[38] Gardetto PR, Schluter JM, Fitts RH. Contractile function of single muscle fibers after hindlimb suspension. J Appl Physiol 1989;66:2739–49.

[39] Bangart JJ, Widrick JJ, Fitts RH. Effect of intermittent weight bearing on soleus fiber force-velocity-power and force-pCa relationships. J Appl Physiol 1997;82:1905–10.

[40] Thompson LV, Shoeman JA. Contractile function of single muscle fibers after hindlimb unweighting in aged rats. J Appl Physiol 1998;84:229–35.

[41] Stelzer JE, Widrick JJ. Effect of hindlimb suspension on the functional properties of slow and fast soleus fibers from three strains of mice. J Appl Physiol 2003;95:2425–33.

[42] Riley DA, Bain JL, Romatowski JG, Fitts RH. Skeletal muscle fiber atrophy: altered thin filament density changes slow fiber force and shortening velocity. Am J Physiol Cell Physiol 2005;288:C360–5.

[43] Kim JH, Thompson LV. Non-weight bearing-induced muscle weakness: the role of myosin quantity and quality in MHC type II fibers. Am J Physiol Cell Physiol 2014;307:C190–4.

[44] Alnaqeeb MA, Zaid NSA, Goldspink G. Connective tissue changes and physical properties of developing and ageing skeletal muscle. J Anat 1984;139:677–89.

[45] Goodpaster BH, Carlson CL, Visser M, Kelley DE, Scherzinger A, Harris TB, Stamm E, Newman AB. Attenuation of skeletal muscle and strength in the elderly: the Health ABC Study. J Appl Physiol 2001;90:2157–65.

[46] Visser M, Goodpaster BH, Kritchevsky SB, Newman AB, Nevitt M, Rubin SM, Simonsick EM, Harris TB. Muscle mass, muscle strength, and muscle fat infiltration as predictors of incident mobility limitations in well-functioning older persons. J Gerontol A Biol Sci Med Sci 2005;60:324–33.

[47] Payne AM, Dodd SL, Leeuwenburgh C. Life-long calorie restriction in Fischer 344 rats attenuates age-related loss in skeletal muscle-specific force and reduces extracellular space. J Appl Physiol 2003;95:2554–62.

[48] Frontera WR, Zayas AR, Rodriguez N. Aging of human muscle: understanding sarcopenia at the single muscle cell level. Phys Med Rehabil Clin N Am 2012;23:201–7. xiii.

[49] Dulhunty AF. Excitation-contraction coupling from the 1950s into the new millennium. Clin Exp Pharmacol Physiol 2006;33:763–72.

[50] Delbono O, O'Rourke KS, Ettinger WH. Excitation-calcium release uncoupling in aged single human skeletal muscle fibers. J Membr Biol 1995;148:211–22.

[51] González E, Messi ML, Zheng Z, Delbono O. Insulin-like growth factor-1 prevents age-related decrease in specific force and intracellular Ca2+ in single intact muscle fibres from transgenic mice. J Physiol 2003;552:833–44.

[52] Jiménez-Moreno R, Wang ZM, Gerring RC, Delbono O. Sarcoplasmic reticulum Ca2+ release declines in muscle fibers from aging mice. Biophys J 2008;94:3178–88.

[53] Wang ZM, Messi ML, Delbono O. L-Type Ca(2+) channel charge movement and intracellular Ca(2+) in skeletal muscle fibers from aging mice. Biophys J 2000;78:1947–54.

[54] Renganathan M, Messi ML, Delbono O. Dihydropyridine receptor-ryanodine receptor uncoupling in aged skeletal muscle. J Membr Biol 1997;157:247–53.

[55] Renganathan M, Messi ML, Delbono O. Overexpression of IGF-1 exclusively in skeletal muscle prevents age-related decline in the number of dihydropyridine receptors. J Biol Chem 1998;273:28845–51.

[56] Boncompagni S, D'Amelio L, Fulle S, Fano G, Protasi F. Progressive disorganization of the excitation-contraction coupling apparatus in aging human skeletal muscle as revealed by electron microscopy: a possible role in the decline of muscle performance. J Gerontol A Biol Sci Med Sci 2006;61:995–1008.

[57] Damiani E, Larsson L, Margreth A. Age-related abnormalities in regulation of the ryanodine receptor in rat fast-twitch muscle. Cell Calcium 1996;19:15–27.

[58] Ryan M, Butler-Browne G, Erzen I, Mouly V, Thornell LE, Wernig A, Ohlendieck K. Persistent expression of the alpha1S-dihydropyridine receptor in aged human skeletal muscle: implications for the excitation-contraction uncoupling hypothesis of sarcopenia. Int J Mol Med 2003;11:425–34.

[59] Russ DW, Grandy JS, Toma K, Ward CW. Ageing, but not yet senescent, rats exhibit reduced muscle quality and sarcoplasmic reticulum function. Acta Physiol 2011;201:391–403.

[60] Ward CW, Reiken S, Marks AR, Marty I, Vassort G, Lacampagne A. Defects in ryanodine receptor calcium release in skeletal muscle from post-myocardial infarct rats. FASEB J 2003;17:1517–9.

[61] Yamada T, Ivarsson N, Hernandez A, Fahlstrom A, Cheng AJ, Zhang SJ, Bruton JD, Ulfhake B, Westerblad H. Impaired mitochondrial respiration and decreased fatigue resistance followed by severe muscle weakness in skeletal muscle of mitochondrial DNA mutator mice. J Physiol 2012;590:6187–97.

[62] Lamboley CR, Wyckelsma VL, Dutka TL, Mckenna MJ, Murphy RM, Lamb GD. Contractile properties and sarcoplasmic reticulum calcium content in type I and type II skeletal muscle fibres in active aged humans. J Physiol 2015;593:2499–514.

[63] Romero-Suarez S, Shen J, Brotto L, Hall T, Mo C, Valdivia HH, Andresen J, Wacker M, Nosek TM, Qu CK, Brotto M. Muscle-specific inositide phosphatase (MIP/MTMR14) is reduced with age and its loss accelerates skeletal muscle aging process by altering calcium homeostasis. Aging (Albany NY) 2010;2:504–13.

[64] Andersson DC, Betzenhauser MJ, Reiken S, Meli AC, Umanskaya A, Xie W, Shiomi T, Zalk R, Lacampagne A, Marks AR. Ryanodine receptor oxidation causes intracellular calcium leak and muscle weakness in aging. Cell Metab 2011;14:196–207.

[65] Straight CR, Ades PA, Toth MJ, Miller MS. Age-related reduction in single muscle fiber calcium sensitivity is associated with decreased muscle power in men and women. Exp Gerontol 2018;102:84–92.

[66] Hvid LG, Ortenblad N, Aagaard P, Kjaer M, Suetta C. Effects of ageing on single muscle fibre contractile function following short-term immobilisation. J Physiol 2011;589:4745–57.

[67] Hvid LG, Suetta C, Aagaard P, Kjaer M, Frandsen U, Ortenblad N. Four days of muscle disuse impairs single fiber contractile function in young and old healthy men. Exp Gerontol 2013;48:154–61.

[68] Powers SK, Jackson MJ. Exercise-induced oxidative stress: cellular mechanisms and impact on muscle force production. Physiol Rev 2008;88:1243–76.

[69] Reid MB, Moylan JS. Beyond atrophy: redox mechanisms of muscle dysfunction in chronic inflammatory disease. J Physiol 2011;589:2171–9.

[70] Prochniewicz E, Thompson LV, Thomas DD. Age-related decline in actomyosin structure and function. Exp Gerontol 2007;42:931–8.

[71] Mollica JP, Dutka TL, Merry TL, Lamboley CR, Mcconell GK, Mckenna MJ, Murphy RM, Lamb GD. S-glutathionylation of troponin I (fast) increases contractile apparatus Ca2+ sensitivity in fast-twitch muscle fibres of rats and humans. J Physiol 2012;590:1443–63.

[72] Murphy RM, Dutka TL, Lamb GD. Hydroxyl radical and glutathione interactions alter calcium sensitivity and maximum force of the contractile apparatus in rat skeletal muscle fibres. J Physiol 2008;586:2203–16.
[73] Geeves MA, Fedorov R, Manstein DJ. Molecular mechanism of actomyosin-based motility. Cell Mol Life Sci 2005;62:1462–77.
[74] Thompson LV, Durand D, Fugere NA, Ferrington DA. Myosin and actin expression and oxidation in aging muscle. J Appl Physiol 2006;101:1581–7.
[75] Balagopal P, Rooyackers OE, Adey DB, Ades PA, Nair KS. Effects of aging on in vivo synthesis of skeletal muscle myosin heavy-chain and sarcoplasmic protein in humans. Am J Physiol 1997;273:E790–800.
[76] Welle S, Thornton C, Jozefowicz R, Statt M. Myofibrillar protein synthesis in young and old men. Am J Physiol 1993;264:E693–8.
[77] Balagopal P, Schimke JC, Ades P, Adey D, Nair KS. Age effect on transcript levels and synthesis rate of muscle MHC and response to resistance exercise. Am J Physiol Endocrinol Metab 2001;280:E203–8.
[78] Moran AL, Warren GL, Lowe DA. Soleus and EDL muscle contractility across the lifespan of female C57BL/6 mice. Exp Gerontol 2005;40:966–75.
[79] Maita T, Yajima E, Nagata S, Miyanishi T, Nakayama S, Matsuda G. The primary structure of skeletal muscle myosin heavy chain: IV. Sequence of the rod, and the complete 1,938-residue sequence of the heavy chain. J Biochem 1991;110:75–87.
[80] Bobkova EA, Bobkov AA, Levitsky DI, Reisler E. Effects of SH1 and SH2 modifications on myosin: similarities and differences. Biophys J 1999;76:1001–7.
[81] Crowder MS, Cooke R. The effect of myosin sulphydryl modification on the mechanics of fibre contraction. J Muscle Res Cell Motil 1984;5:131–46.
[82] Perkins WJ, Han YS, Sieck GC. Skeletal muscle force and actomyosin ATPase activity reduced by nitric oxide donor. J Appl Physiol 1997;83:1326–32.
[83] Lowe DA, Warren GL, Snow LM, Thompson LV, Thomas DD. Muscle activity and aging affect myosin structural distribution and force generation in rat fibers. J Appl Physiol (1985) 2004;96:498–506.
[84] Zhong S, Lowe DA, Thompson LV. Effects of hindlimb unweighting and aging on rat semimembranosus muscle and myosin. J Appl Physiol 2006;101:873–80.
[85] Prochniewicz E, Thomas DD, Thompson LV. Age-related decline in actomyosin function. J Gerontol A Biol Sci Med Sci 2005;60:425–31.
[86] Yu F, Hedstrom M, Cristea A, Dalen N, Larsson L. Effects of ageing and gender on contractile properties in human skeletal muscle and single fibres. Acta Physiol (Oxf) 2007;190:229–41.
[87] Ochala J, Lambertz D, Pousson M, Goubel F, Hoecke JV. Changes in mechanical properties of human plantar flexor muscles in ageing. Exp Gerontol 2004;39:349–58.
[88] Miller MS, Callahan DM, Toth MJ. Skeletal muscle myofilament adaptations to aging, disease, and disuse and their effects on whole muscle performance in older adult humans. Front Physiol 2014;5:369.
[89] Mijnarends DM, Koster A, Schols JM, Meijers JM, Halfens RJ, Gudnason V, Eiriksdottir G, Siggeirsdottir K, Sigurdsson S, Jonsson PV, Meirelles O, Harris T. Physical activity and incidence of sarcopenia: the population-based AGES-Reykjavik Study. Age Ageing 2016;45:614–20.
[90] Kern DS, Semmler JG, Enoka RM. Long-term activity in upper- and lower-limb muscles of humans. J Appl Physiol 2001;91:2224–32.
[91] Larsson L, Din SJ, B. & Karlsson, J. Histochemical and biochemical changes in human skeletal muscle with age in sedentary males, age 22–65 years. Acta Physiol Scand 1978;103:31–9.
[92] Lexell J, Taylor CC, Sjöström M. What is the cause of the ageing atrophy? Total number, size and proportion of different fiber types studied in whole vastus lateralis muscle from 15- to 83-year-old men. J Neurol Sci 1988;84:275–94.
[93] Poggi P, Marchetti C, Scelsi R. Automatic morphometric analysis of skeletal muscle fibers in the aging man. Anat Rec 1987;217:30–4.
[94] Verdijk LB, Snijders T, Beelen M, Savelberg HH, Meijer K, Kuipers H, Van Loon LJ. Characteristics of muscle fiber type are predictive of skeletal muscle mass and strength in elderly men. J Am Geriatr Soc 2010;58:2069–75.

[95] ACSM. American College of Sports Medicine position stand. Progression models in resistance training for healthy adults. Med Sci Sports Exerc 2009;41:687–708.

[96] Borina E, Pellegrino MA, D'Antona G, Bottinelli R. Myosin and actin content of human skeletal muscle fibers following 35 days bed rest. Scand J Med Sci Sports 2010;20:65–73.

[97] Brocca L, Longa E, Cannavino J, Seynnes O, de Vito G, Mcphee J, Narici M, Pellegrino MA, Bottinelli R. Human skeletal muscle fibre contractile properties and proteomic profile: adaptations to 3 weeks of unilateral lower limb suspension and active recovery. J Physiol 2015;593:5361–85.

[98] Dutka TL, Mollica JP, Lamb GD. Differential effects of peroxynitrite on contractile protein properties in fast- and slow-twitch skeletal muscle fibers of rat. J Appl Physiol 2011;110:705–16.

[99] Andrade FH, Reid MB, Allen DG, Westerblad H. Effect of hydrogen peroxide and dithiothreitol on contractile function of single skeletal muscle fibres from the mouse. J Physiol 1998;509:565–75.

[100] Lamb GD, Posterino GS. Effects of oxidation and reduction on contractile function in skeletal muscle fibres of the rat. J Physiol 2003;546:149–63.

[101] Plant DR, Lynch GS, Williams DA. Hydrogen peroxide modulates Ca^{2+}-activation of single permeabilized fibres from fast- and slow-twitch skeletal muscles of rats. J Muscle Res Cell Motil 2000;21:747–52.

[102] Prochniewicz E, Lowe DA, Spakowicz DJ, Higgins L, O'Conor K, Thompson LV, Ferrington DA, Thomas DD. Functional, structural, and chemical changes in myosin associated with hydrogen peroxide treatment of skeletal muscle fibers. Am J Physiol 2008;294:C613–26.

[103] Reid MB, Durham WJ. Generation of reactive oxygen and nitrogen species in contracting skeletal muscle: potential impact on aging. Ann N Y Acad Sci 2002;959:108–16.

[104] Jackson MJ. Skeletal muscle aging: role of reactive oxygen species. Crit Care Med 2009;37:S368–71.

[105] Jackson MJ. Redox regulation of muscle adaptations to contractile activity and aging. J Appl Physiol (1985) 2015;119:163–71.

[106] Reid MB. Redox modulation of skeletal muscle contraction: what we know and what we don't. J Appl Physiol 2001;90:724–31.

[107] Westerblad H, Allen DG. Emerging roles of ROS/RNS in muscle function and fatigue. Antioxid Redox Signal 2011;15:2487–99.

[108] Murphy MP. How mitochondria produce reactive oxygen species. Biochem J 2009;417:1–13.

[109] Boveris A, Chance B. The mitochondrial generation of hydrogen peroxide. General properties and effect of hyperbaric oxygen. Biochem J 1973;134:707–16.

[110] Loschen G, Azzi A, Richter C, Floh L. Superoxide radicals as precursors of mitochondrial hydrogen peroxide. FEBS Lett 1974;42:68–72.

[111] Brand MD. The sites and topology of mitochondrial superoxide production. Exp Gerontol 2010;45:466–72.

[112] Tahara EB, Navarete FD, Kowaltowski AJ. Tissue-, substrate-, and site-specific characteristics of mitochondrial reactive oxygen species generation. Free Radic Biol Med 2009;46:1283–97.

[113] Fielding RA, Meydani M. Exercise, free radical generation, and aging. Aging (Milano) 1997;9:12–8.

[114] Muller FL, Song W, Jang YC, Liu Y, Sabia M, Richardson A, Remmen VAN, H. Denervation-induced skeletal muscle atrophy is associated with increased mitochondrial ROS production. Am J Physiol Regul Integr Comp Physiol 2007;293:R1159–68.

[115] Pesce V, Cormio A, Fracasso F, Vecchiet J, Felzani G, Lezza AM, Cantatore P, Gadaleta MN. Age-related mitochondrial genotypic and phenotypic alterations in human skeletal muscle. Free Radic Biol Med 2001;30:1223–33.

[116] Delbono O. Neural control of aging skeletal muscle. Aging Cell 2003;2:21–9.

[117] Holloszy JO, Chen M, Cartee GD, Young JC. Skeletal muscle atrophy in old rats: differential changes in the three fiber types. Mech Ageing Dev 1991;60:199–213.

[118] Pal R, Basu Thakur P, Li S, Minard C, Rodney GG. Real-time imaging of NADPH oxidase activity in living cells using a novel fluorescent protein reporter. PLoS One 2013;8, e63989.

[119] Nethery D, Stofan D, Callahan L, Dimarco A, Supinski G. Formation of reactive oxygen species by the contracting diaphragm is PLA(2) dependent. J Appl Physiol (1985) 1999;87:792–800.

[120] Gomez-Cabrera MC, Close GL, Kayani A, Mcardle A, VI A, J. & Jackson, M. J. Effect of xanthine oxidase-generated extracellular superoxide on skeletal muscle force generation. Am J Physiol Regul Integr Comp Physiol 2010;298:R2–8.

[121] Stuehr D, Pou S, Rosen GM. Oxygen reduction by nitric-oxide synthases. J Biol Chem 2001;276:14533–6.
[122] Sakellariou GK, Vasilaki A, Palomero J, Kayani A, Zibrik L, McArdle A, Jackson MJ. Studies of mitochondrial and nonmitochondrial sources implicate nicotinamide adenine dinucleotide phosphate oxidase(s) in the increased skeletal muscle superoxide generation that occurs during contractile activity. Antioxid Redox Signal 2013;18:603–21.
[123] Dworakowski R, Anilkumar N, Zhang M, Shah AM. Redox signalling involving NADPH oxidase-derived reactive oxygen species. Biochem Soc Trans 2006;34:960–4.
[124] Ward CW, Prosser BL, Lederer WJ. Mechanical stretch-induced activation of ROS/RNS signaling in striated muscle. Antioxid Redox Signal 2014;20:929–36.
[125] Javeshghani D, Magder SA, Barreiro E, Quinn MT, Hussain SN. Molecular characterization of a superoxide-generating NAD(P)H oxidase in the ventilatory muscles. Am J Respir Crit Care Med 2002;165:412–8.
[126] Xia R, Webb JA, Gnall LL, Cutler K, Abramson JJ. Skeletal muscle sarcoplasmic reticulum contains a NADH-dependent oxidase that generates superoxide. Am J Physiol Cell Physiol 2003;285:C215–21.
[127] Espinosa A, Leiva A, Pena M, Muller M, Debandi A, Hidalgo C, Carrasco MA, Jaimovich E. Myotube depolarization generates reactive oxygen species through NAD(P)H oxidase; ROS-elicited Ca2+ stimulates Erk, Creb, early genes. J Cell Physiol 2006;209:379–88.
[128] Hidalgo C, Sanchez G, Barrientos G, Aracena-Parks P. A transverse tubule NADPH oxidase activity stimulates calcium release from isolated triads via ryanodine receptor type 1 S -glutathionylation. J Biol Chem 2006;281:26473–82.
[129] Sullivan-Gunn MJ, Lewandowski PA. Elevated hydrogen peroxide and decreased catalase and glutathione peroxidase protection are associated with aging sarcopenia. BMC Geriatr 2013;13:104.
[130] Barrientos G, Llanos P, Hidalgo J, Bolanos P, Caputo C, Riquelme A, Sánchez G, Quest AF, Hidalgo C. Cholesterol removal from adult skeletal muscle impairs excitation-contraction coupling and aging reduces caveolin-3 and alters the expression of other triadic proteins. Front Physiol 2015;6:105.
[131] Hord JM, Botchlett R, Lawler JM. Age-related alterations in the sarcolemmal environment are attenuated by lifelong caloric restriction and voluntary exercise. Exp Gerontol 2016;83:148–57.
[132] Aranda R, Dom Nech E, Rus AD, Real JT, Sastre J, Vi AJ, Pallard FV. Age-related increase in xanthine oxidase activity in human plasma and rat tissues. Free Radic Res 2007;41:1195–200.
[133] Eskurza I, Kahn ZD, Seals DR. Xanthine oxidase does not contribute to impaired peripheral conduit artery endothelium-dependent dilatation with ageing. J Physiol 2006;571:661–8.
[134] Ryan MJ, Jackson JR, Hao Y, Leonard SS, Alway SE. Inhibition of xanthine oxidase reduces oxidative stress and improves skeletal muscle function in response to electrically stimulated isometric contractions in aged mice. Free Radic Biol Med 2011;51:38–52.
[135] Brenman JE, Chao DS, Xia H, Aldape K, Bredt DS. Nitric oxide synthase complexed with dystrophin and absent from skeletal muscle sarcolemma in Duchenne muscular dystrophy. Cell 1995;82:743–52.
[136] Buchwalow IB, Minin EA, Samoilova VE, Boecker W, Wellner M, Schmitz W, Neumann J, Punkt K. Compartmentalization of NO signaling cascade in skeletal muscles. Biochem Biophys Res Commun 2005;330:615–21.
[137] Jian Z, Han H, Zhang T, Puglisi J, Izu LT, Shaw JA, Onofiok E, Erickson JR, Chen YJ, Horvath B, Shimkunas R, Xiao W, Li Y, Pan T, Chan J, Banyasz T, Tardiff JC, Chiamvimonvat N, Bers DM, Lam KS, Chen-Izu Y. Mechanochemotransduction during cardiomyocyte contraction is mediated by localized nitric oxide signaling. Sci Signal 2014;7, ra27.
[138] Salanova M, Schiffl G, Rittweger J, Felsenberg D, Blottner D. Ryanodine receptor type-1 (RyR1) expression and protein S-nitrosylation pattern in human soleus myofibres following bed rest and exercise countermeasure. Histochem Cell Biol 2008;130:105–18.
[139] Pye D, Palomero J, Kabayo T, Jackson MJ. Real-time measurement of nitric oxide in single mature mouse skeletal muscle fibres during contractions. J Physiol 2007;581:309–18.
[140] Bredt DS, Snyder SH. Isolation of nitric oxide synthetase, a calmodulin-requiring enzyme. Proc Natl Acad Sci U S A 1990;87:682–5.
[141] Lancaster Jr JR. Simulation of the diffusion and reaction of endogenously produced nitric oxide. Proc Natl Acad Sci U S A 1994;91:8137–41.

[142] Richmonds CR, Boonyapisit K, Kusner LL, Kaminski HJ. Nitric oxide synthase in aging rat skeletal muscle. Mech Ageing Dev 1999;109:177–89.
[143] Song W, Kwak HB, Kim JH, Lawler JM. Exercise training modulates the nitric oxide synthase profile in skeletal muscle from old rats. J Gerontol A Biol Sci Med Sci 2009;64:540–9.
[144] Capanni C, Squarzoni S, Petrini S, Villanova M, Muscari C, Maraldi NM, Guarnieri C, Caldarera CM. Increase of neuronal nitric oxide synthase in rat skeletal muscle during ageing. Biochem Biophys Res Commun 1998;245:216–9.
[145] Suzuki N, Motohashi N, Uezumi A, Fukada S, Yoshimura T, Itoyama Y, Aoki M, Miyagoe-Suzuki Y, Takeda S. NO production results in suspension-induced muscle atrophy through dislocation of neuronal NOS. J Clin Invest 2007;117:2468–76.
[146] Alvarez MN, Piacenza L, Irigoin F, Peluffo G, Radi R. Macrophage-derived peroxynitrite diffusion and toxicity to Trypanosoma cruzi. Arch Biochem Biophys 2004;432:222–32.
[147] Szabó C, Ischiropoulos H, Radi R. Peroxynitrite: biochemistry, pathophysiology and development of therapeutics. Nat Rev Drug Discov 2007;6:662–80.
[148] Beckman JS, Koppenol WH. Nitric oxide, superoxide, and peroxynitrite: the good, the bad, and ugly. Am J Physiol 1996;271:C1424–37.
[149] Murakami H, Guillet C, Tardif N, Salles J, Migne C, Boirie Y, Walrand S. Cumulative 3-nitrotyrosine in specific muscle proteins is associated with muscle loss during aging. Exp Gerontol 2012;47:129–35.
[150] Pietrangelo L, D'Incecco A, Ainbinder A, Michelucci A, Kern H, Dirksen RT, Boncompagni S, Protasi F. Age-dependent uncoupling of mitochondria from Ca^{2+} release units in skeletal muscle. Oncotarget 2015;6:35358–71.
[151] Siu PM, Pistilli EE, Alway SE. Age-dependent increase in oxidative stress in gastrocnemius muscle with unloading. J Appl Physiol (1985) 2008;105:1695–705.
[152] Nuss JE, Amaning JK, Bailey CE, Deford JH, Dimayuga VL, Rabek JP, Papaconstantinou J. Oxidative modification and aggregation of creatine kinase from aged mouse skeletal muscle. Aging (Albany NY) 2009;1:557–72.
[153] Schöneich C, Viner RI, Ferrington DA, Bigelow DJ. Age-related chemical modification of the skeletal muscle sarcoplasmic reticulum Ca-ATPase of the rat. Mech Ageing Dev 1999;107:221–31.
[154] Fulle S, Protasi F, Di-Tano G, Pietrangelo T, Beltramin A, Boncompagni S, Vecchiet L, Fano G. The contribution of reactive oxygen species to sarcopenia and muscle ageing. Exp Gerontol 2004;39:17–24.
[155] Ji LL, Dillon D, Wu E. Alteration of antioxidant enzymes with aging in rat skeletal muscle and liver. Am J Physiol 1990;258:R918–23.
[156] Ji LL, Leeuwenburgh C, Leichtweis S, Gore M, Fiebig R, Hollander J, Bejma J. Oxidative stress and aging. Role of exercise and its influences on antioxidant systems. Ann N Y Acad Sci 1998;854:102–17.
[157] Leeuwenburgh C, Fiebig R, Chandwaney R, Ji LL. Aging and exercise training in skeletal muscle: responses of glutathione and antioxidant enzyme systems. Am J Physiol 1994;267:R439–45.
[158] Oh-Ishi S, Kizaki T, Yamashita H, Nagata N, Suzuki K, Taniguchi N, Ohno H. Alterations of superoxide dismutase iso-enzyme activity, content, and mRNA expression with aging in rat skeletal muscle. Mech Ageing Dev 1995;84:65–76.
[159] Hollander J, Fiebig R, Gore M, Bejma J, Ookawara T, Ohno H, Ji LL. Superoxide dismutase gene expression in skeletal muscle: fiber-specific adaptation to endurance training. Am J Physiol 1999;277:R856–62.
[160] Ji LL. Exercise at old age: does it increase or alleviate oxidative stress? Ann N Y Acad Sci 2001;928:236–47.
[161] Meister A, Anderson ME. Glutathione. Annu Rev Biochem 1983;52:711–60.
[162] Lawler JM, Cline CC, Hu Z, Coast JR. Effect of oxidant challenge on contractile function of the aging rat diaphragm. Am J Physiol 1997;272:E201–7.
[163] Richmonds CR, Kaminski HJ. Nitric oxide myotoxicity is age related. Mech Ageing Dev 2000;113:183–91.
[164] Zerba E, Komorowski TE, Faulkner JA. Free radical injury to skeletal muscles of young, adult, and old mice. Am J Physiol 1990;258:C429–35.

[165] Ferreira LF, Reid MB. Muscle-derived ROS and thiol regulation in muscle fatigue. J Appl Physiol 2008;104:853–60.
[166] Andrade FH, Reid MB, Allen DG, Westerblad H. Effect of nitric oxide on single skeletal muscle fibres from the mouse. J Physiol 1998;509:577–86.
[167] Posterino GS, Cellini MA, Lamb GD. Effects of oxidation and cytosolic redox conditions on excitation-contraction coupling in rat skeletal muscle. J Physiol 2003;547:807–23.
[168] Hunter GR, Mccarthy JP, Bamman MM. Effects of resistance training on older adults. Sports Med 2004;34:329–48.
[169] Roth SM, Ferrell RF, Hurley BF. Strength training for the prevention and treatment of sarcopenia. J Nutr Health Aging 2000;4:143–55.
[170] Trappe S, Godard M, Gallagher P, Carroll C, Rowden G, Porter D. Resistance training improves single muscle fiber contractile function in older women. Am J Physiol Cell Physiol 2001;281:C398–406.
[171] Trappe S, Williamson D, Godard M, Porter D, Rowden G, Costill D. Effect of resistance training on single muscle fiber contractile function in older men. J Appl Physiol (1985) 2000;89:143–52.
[172] Bejma J, Ji LL. Aging and acute exercise enhance free radical generation in rat skeletal muscle. J Appl Physiol 1999;87:465–70.
[173] Naito H, Powers SK, Demirel HA, Aoki J. Exercise training increases heat shock protein in skeletal muscles of old rats. Med Sci Sports Exerc 2001;33:729–34.
[174] Powers SK, Ji LL, Leeuwenburgh C. Exercise training-induced alterations in skeletal muscle antioxidant capacity: a brief review. Med Sci Sports Exerc 1999;31:987–97.
[175] Jackson MJ, McArdle A. Age-related changes in skeletal muscle reactive oxygen species generation and adaptive responses to reactive oxygen species. J Physiol 2011;589:2139–45.
[176] Ji LL, Wu E, Thomas DP. Effect of exercise training on antioxidant and metabolic functions in senescent rat skeletal muscle. Gerontology 1991;37:317–25.
[177] Hammeren J, Powers S, Lawler J, Criswell D, Martin D, Lowenthal D, Pollock M. Exercise training-induced alterations in skeletal muscle oxidative and antioxidant enzyme activity in senescent rats. Int J Sports Med 1992;13:412–6.
[178] Corpeno Kalamgi R, Salah H, Gastaldello S, Martinez-Redondo V, Ruas JL, Fury W, Bai Y, Gromada J, Sartori R, Guttridge DC, Sandri M, Larsson L. Mechano-signalling pathways in an experimental intensive critical illness myopathy model. J Physiol 2016;594:4371–88.
[179] Friedrich O, Diermeier S, Larsson L. Weak by the machines: muscle motor protein dysfunction – a side effect of intensive care unit treatment. Acta Physiol (Oxf) 2018;222, e12885.
[180] Ochala J, Gustafson AM, Diez ML, Renaud G, Li M, Aare S, Qaisar R, Banduseela VC, Hedstrom Y, Tang X, Dworkin B, Ford GC, Nair KS, Perera S, Gautel M, Larsson L. Preferential skeletal muscle myosin loss in response to mechanical silencing in a novel rat intensive care unit model: underlying mechanisms. J Physiol 2011;589:2007–26.
[181] Yamada T, Ashida Y, Tatebayashi D, Himori K. Myofibrillar function differs markedly between denervated and dexamethasone-treated rat skeletal muscles: role of mechanical load. PLoS One 2019;14, e0223551.
[182] Hasten DL, Pak-Loduca J, Obert KA, Yarasheski KE. Resistance exercise acutely increases MHC and mixed muscle protein synthesis rates in 78-84 and 23-32 yr olds. Am J Physiol Endocrinol Metab 2000;278:E620–6.
[183] Parente V, D'Antona G, Adami R, Miotti D, Capodaglio P, de Vito G, Bottinelli R. Long-term resistance training improves force and unloaded shortening velocity of single muscle fibres of elderly women. Eur J Appl Physiol 2008;104:885–93.
[184] Yarasheski KE. Exercise, aging, and muscle protein metabolism. J Gerontol A Biol Sci Med Sci 2003;58:M918–22.
[185] Dreyer HC, Drummond MJ, Pennings B, Fujita S, Glynn EL, Chinkes DL, Dhanani S, Volpi E, Rasmussen BB. Leucine-enriched essential amino acid and carbohydrate ingestion following resistance exercise enhances mTOR signaling and protein synthesis in human muscle. Am J Physiol Endocrinol Metab 2008;294:E392–400.

[186] Tipton KD, Ferrando AA, Phillips SM, Doyle Jr D, Wolfe RR. Postexercise net protein synthesis in human muscle from orally administered amino acids. Am J Physiol 1999;276:E628–34.

[187] Esmarck B, Andersen JL, Olsen S, Richter EA, Mizuno M, Kjaer M. Timing of postexercise protein intake is important for muscle hypertrophy with resistance training in elderly humans. J Physiol 2001;535:301–11.

[188] Godard MP, Williamson DL, Trappe SW. Oral amino-acid provision does not affect muscle strength or size gains in older men. Med Sci Sports Exerc 2002;34:1126–31.

[189] Welle S, Thornton CA. High-protein meals do not enhance myofibrillar synthesis after resistance exercise in 62- to 75-yr-old men and women. Am J Physiol 1998;274:E677–83.

[190] Smuder AJ, Kavazis AN, Hudson MB, Nelson WB, Powers SK. Oxidation enhances myofibrillar protein degradation via calpain and caspase-3. Free Radic Biol Med 2010;49:1152–60.

[191] Grune T, Merker K, Sandig G, Davies KJ. Selective degradation of oxidatively modified protein substrates by the proteasome. Biochem Biophys Res Commun 2003;305:709–18.

[192] Powers SK, Morton AB, Ahn B, Smuder AJ. Redox control of skeletal muscle atrophy. Free Radic Biol Med 2016;98:208–17.

Index

Note: Page numbers followed by *f* indicate figures and *t* indicate tables.

A

Acetylcholine (ACh), 61–66, 65*f*
Acetylcholinesterase (AChE), 68
Activities of daily living (ADL), 254, 282
Adenosine monophosphate-activated protein kinase (AMPK), 162–163, 211–212, 213*f*
 pathway, exercise mimetics targeting, 163
Adipocytes and myofibers, interactions between, 145–147, 148–150*f*
ADL. *See* Activities of daily living (ADL)
Age-related functional adaptations of NMJ, 66–68, 67*t*, 69*t*
Age-related loss of muscle quality, interventions to counteract, 312–313
Age-related structural adaptations of NMJ, 61–66, 62–63*f*, 65*f*, 67*t*
Aging
 and alteration in skeletal muscle, 208*f*
 mitochondrial dysfunction in, 3–11, 304–306
  altered dynamics, 5–7
  DNA damage, 5
  PGC-1a regulation, 17–18
  reactive oxygen species- induced damage, 3–4
 and mitophagy
  exercise modalities, 218–220
  practical recommendations, 218–220
 muscle stem cells with
  extrinsic changes, 118–120
  intrinsic changes, 116–118
 satellite cell function in, 116–120
 UPS and neural dysfunction in, 26–27
 vascular. *See* Vascular aging
 See also Older adults
Agrin, 73–74
AIF. *See* Apoptosis-inducing factor (AIF)
ALS. *See* Amyotrophic lateral sclerosis (ALS)
AMPK. *See* Adenosine monophosphate-activated protein kinase (AMPK)
Amyotrophic lateral sclerosis (ALS), 6
Anabolic hormones effects, on skeletal muscle, 163–165
Animal-based protein sources, 86–87
Apoptosis and autophagy, linking, 22–23
 BIM and Bcl-2, 23
 PGC-1a, 23
Apoptosis-inducing factor (AIF), 6–7
Asian Working Group for Sarcopenia (AWGS), 159, 271
Atrogin-1. *See* Atrophy gene-1 (atrogin-1)
Atrophy gene-1 (atrogin-1), 187–188
Autophagosome, 209–211
Autophagy
 and apoptosis, linking, 22–23
  BIM and Bcl-2, 23
  PGC-1a, 23
 chaperone-mediated, 209, 210*f*
 macroautophagy, 209, 210*f*
 microautophagy, 209, 210*f*
 pathway in skeletal muscle, roles of, 165
 in skeletal muscle, 209–212, 210*f*, 213*f*
Autophagy-dependent signaling, 188–190, 189*f*
Autophagy signaling defect, in sarcopenic muscle, 191*f*
 autophagy-dependent signaling, 188–190, 189*f*
 factors modulating, 193–197
  cachexia, 196–197
  denervation, 193–195
  unloading, 195–196
 molecules modulating, 192–193, 194*f*
 therapeutic strategies attenuating, 197–200
  calorie restriction, 198–199
  exercise, 197–198
  hormonal treatment, 200
  supplemental approach, 199–200
AWGS. *See* Asian Working Group for Sarcopenia (AWGS)

B

Baroreflex, 257–258
BCAA. *See* Branched-chain amino acids (BCAA)
Bcl-2, in autophagy and apoptotic pathways, 23
BDNF. *See* Brain-derived neurotrophic factor (BDNF)
BIM, in autophagy and apoptotic pathways, 23
Blood volume (BV), 258
Blow-out time (BOT), 254

Index

BOT. *See* Blow-out time (BOT)
Brain-derived neurotrophic factor (BDNF), 162–163
Branched-chain amino acids (BCAA), 87
BV. *See* Blood volume (BV)

C

CA. *See* Celiac artery (CA)
Cachexia, 196–197, 268–270
  cancer, 274–278, 276t
  condition of, 269–270, 270f
  definition of, 267–269
Calcium-induced dysregulation of mitochondria in sarcopenia, 8–11, 9f
Caloric restriction, 28–31, 30t
  for autophagy signaling defect, 198–199
Cancer cachexia, dysphagia and, 274–278, 276t
Carbonyl cyanide m-chlorophenylhydrazone (CCCP), 215
CBF. *See* Cerebral blood flow (CBF)
CCCP. *See* Carbonyl cyanide m-chlorophenylhydrazone (CCCP)
Celiac artery (CA), 255
Cell death signaling, 11–16
Central arteries, 257
Cerebral blood flow (CBF), 253
Cerebral vessels, 252–254
Chaperone-mediated autophagy (CMA), 209, 210f
Chemoradiotherapy (CRT), 277
CHF. *See* Chronic heart failure (CHF)
Chronic heart failure (CHF) dysphagia and, 281–283
Chronic obstructive pulmonary disease (COPD), 196–197
  dysphagia and, 278–281
CMA. *See* Chaperone-mediated autophagy (CMA)
COPD. *See* Chronic obstructive pulmonary disease (COPD)
C-reactive protein, 238–239
CRT. *See* Chemoradiotherapy (CRT)

CuZnSOD. *See* CuZn-superoxide dismutase (CuZnSOD)
CuZn-superoxide dismutase (CuZnSOD), 4

D

Damage-associated molecular patterns (DAMPs), 142, 143f
DAMPs. *See* Damage-associated molecular patterns (DAMPs)
Decline in Muscle quality, 296–300, 300f
Decorin, 174
Delayed onset muscle soreness (DOMS), 144
Denervation, 193–195
Denervation/reinnervation cycling process, 72
DIAAS. *See* Digestible Indispensable Amino Acid Score (DIAAS)
Dietary protein quality, 82–89
  animal-based protein sources, 86–87
  high-quality protein sources, 82–84
  leucine, 87–89, 88f
  plant-based protein sources, 84–86
Dietary protein quantity, 89–92
  protein distribution across the day, 91–92
  protein intake above RDA, 90–91
Digestible Indispensable Amino Acid Score (DIAAS), 83–85, 83t
DMD. *See* Duchenne muscular dystrophy (DMD)
DOMS. *See* Delayed onset muscle soreness (DOMS)
Duchenne muscular dystrophy (DMD), 109
Dysphagia, 268, 274–283
  and cancer cachexia, 274–278, 276t
  and chronic heart failure, 281–283
  and chronic obstructive pulmonary disease, 278–281
  definition of, 274–283

E

EDL. *See* Extensor digitorum longus (EDL)
Endplate potential (EPP), 63–64
Enobosarm (aka ostarine, MK-2866), 164
EPP. *See* Endplate potential (EPP)
ER. *See* Estrogen receptors (ER)
ESPEN-SIG. *See* European Society for Clinical Nutrition and Metabolism Special Interest Groups (ESPEN-SIG)
Estrogen receptors (ER), 125–126
European Society for Clinical Nutrition and Metabolism Special Interest Groups (ESPEN-SIG), 96
European Working Group on Sarcopenia in Older People (EWGSOP), 59–60, 96, 159–161, 271, 295–296
EWGSOP. *See* European Working Group on Sarcopenia in Older People (EWGSOP)
EWGSOP2, 271, 295–296
Exercise
  for autophagy signaling defect, 197–198
  gene set analysis of, 160–161, 160f
  modalities, for mitophagy in aging people, 218–220, 221f
  training, 208–209
Exercise-induced molecular signaling, in skeletal muscle, 161–162
Extensor digitorum longus (EDL), 122–124
Ex vivo muscle stimulation technique, 61f, 68

F

FAO. *See* Food and Agricultural Organization (FAO)
FAPs. *See* Fibroadipogenic progenitors (FAPs)
FGF21, 176–177
Fibroadipogenic progenitors (FAPs), 115–116, 119–120

Index

Fibronectin type III domain-containing protein 5 (FNDC5), 162–163
FNDC5. *See* Fibronectin type III domain-containing protein 5 (FNDC5)
Food and Agricultural Organization (FAO), 82–83
Forkhead box class O proteins (FOXO), 24, 26, 211–212, 213*f*
FOXO. *See* Forkhead box class O proteins (FOXO)

G

Gene set analysis of exercise, 160–161, 160*f*
Growth differentiation factor 8 (aka myostatin), 173–174
Growth hormones, and sarcopenic obesity, 240

H

High-quality protein sources, 82–84
Hormonal treatment, for autophagy signaling defect, 200

I

IADL. *See* Instrumental activities of daily living (IADL)
ICA. *See* Internal carotid artery (ICA)
ICCP. *See* Intergovernmental Panel on Climate Change (ICCP)
ICFSR. *See* International Clinical Practice Guidelines for Sarcopenia (ICFSR)
IGF-1. *See* Insulin-like growth factor-1 (IGF-1)
IMA. *See* Inferior mesenteric artery (IMA)
Inferior mesenteric artery (IMA), 255
Inflammaging, 73, 151–152
Inflammation
　mediators of, 144–145
　and sarcopenic obesity, 238–239
Instrumental activities of daily living (IADL), 254
Insulin-like growth factor-1 (IGF-1), 74, 175–176

Insulin resistance, 238
Intergovernmental Panel on Climate Change (ICCP), 256
Internal carotid artery (ICA), 250–251
International Clinical Practice Guidelines for Sarcopenia (ICFSR), 271
International Working Group on Sarcopenia (IWGS), 96
Intrinsic contractile dysfunction, in skeletal muscle fibers, 306–307
　reactive oxygen/nitrogen species, role of, 307–312, 308*f*
Irisin, 174–177
IWGS. *See* International Working Group on Sarcopenia (IWGS)

L

Leucine, 87–89
　impact on mTOR signaling pathway, 88*f*
　impact on muscle mass maintenance in older adults, 95–96
Leukemia inhibitory factor (LIF), 174
Leukotrienes (LT), 147–151
LIF. *See* Leukemia inhibitory factor (LIF)
Lipid accumulation, 235–237, 236*f*
Lipid mediators (LM)
　proresolving, 147–151, 152*f*
Lipopolysaccharide (LPS), 147–151
LM. *See* Lipid mediators (LM)
Loss of motor function, in sarcopenia, 16–17
　motor neurons, 16
　neural dysfunction, 16–17
Loss of vascular functions, and sarcopenia, 251–257
LPS. *See* Lipopolysaccharide (LPS)
LT. *See* Leukotrienes (LT)

M

Macroautophagy, 209, 210*f*
MAFbx/Atrogin-1. *See* Muscle atrophy F-box (MAFbx/Atrogin-1)

MCI. *See* Mild cognitive impairment (MCI)
MCU. *See* Mitochondrial calcium uniporter (MCU)
Mdm2, 218
Mechanistic/mammalian target of rapamycin complex 1 (MTORC1), 24, 211–212, 213*f*
MEPP. *See* Mini-endplate potentials (MEPP)
Metabolites, as myokines, 177–179
Microautophagy, 209, 210*f*
MicroRNAs (miRNAs), 113
　as myokines, 177–179
Mild cognitive impairment (MCI), 253
Mini-endplate potentials (MEPP), 68
MiR-489, 113
miRNAs. *See* MicroRNAs (miRNAs)
Mitochondrial biogenesis, 2
Mitochondrial calcium uniporter (MCU), 8–11, 9*f*
Mitochondrial DNA (mtDNA), 6–7
　damage, aging and, 5
Mitochondrial dysfunction, sarcopenia and, 2–3
　in aging, potential sources of, 3–11, 304–306
　altered dynamics, 5–7
　calcium-induced dysregulation, 8–11, 9*f*
　DNA damage, 5
　reactive oxygen species-induced damage, 3–4
　reduced activity, 7–8
　autophagy and apoptosis, linking, 22–23
　BIM and Bcl-2, 23
　PGC-1a, 23
　caloric restriction, 28–31, 30*t*
　cell death signaling, 11–16
　fiber type-specific loss, regulation of, 15–16
　mitochondrial-induced nuclear apoptosis, 11–14, 13–14*f*
　mitochondrial permeability transition pore, 14–15

325

Index

Mitochondrial dysfunction, sarcopenia and *(Continued)*
  loss of motor function and mobility, 16–17
    motor neurons, 16
    neural dysfunction, 16–17
  mitophagy, 18–22, 20–21*f*
  muscle wasting, 23–24
  PGC-1a regulation, 17
    in aged muscles, 17–18
    in motor neurons, 18
  sarcopenic obesity, 237–238
  UPS
    disruption in muscle and neural cells, 28
    mitophagy regulation, 27
    and neural dysfunction in aging, 26–27
    regulation, 24–26, 25*f*
Mitochondrial-induced nuclear apoptosis, 11–14, 13–14*f*
Mitochondrial permeability transition pore (mPTP), 6–8, 12–15, 13–14*f*
Mitophagy
  insufficient, in aging muscles, 21–22
  regulation and UPS, 27
  removal of dysfunctional mitochondria by, 18–21, 20–21*f*
  in skeletal muscle, 213*f*, 217*f*
    exercise modalities, 218–220, 221*f*
    Mul1, 216–218
    Mul2, 216–218
    practical recommendations, 218–220
MK-0773, 164*f*
Motor neurons, 16
  PGC-1a regulation of mitochondria in, 18
MPB. *See* Muscle protein breakdown (MPB)
MPS. *See* Muscle protein synthesis (MPS)
mPTP. *See* Mitochondrial permeability transition pore (mPTP)

MRFs. *See* Myogenic regulatory factors (MRFs)
mtDNA. *See* Mitochondrial DNA (mtDNA)
MTORC1. *See* Mechanistic/mammalian target of rapamycin complex 1 (MTORC1)
Mul1, 216–218
Mul2, 216–218
MuRF1. *See* Muscle RING Finger 1 (MuRF1)
Muscle adaptation, satellite cells and, 120–126
Muscle atrophy
  sarcopenic obesity and, 239, 240*t*
  satellite cells in, 122–126, 123*f*
Muscle atrophy F-box (MAFbx/Atrogin-1), 24–26, 25*f*
Muscle hypertrophy, satellite cells in, 120–122, 123*f*
Muscle mass
  dietary approaches to preserving and gaining, 96–98, 97*f*
  maintenance in older adults, impact of leucine on, 95–96
  regulation, 172*f*
Muscle protein breakdown (MPB), 82, 99–100
Muscle protein synthesis (MPS), 82, 84–87, 89, 91–93, 95–96, 99–100
Muscle RING Finger 1 (MuRF1), 24–27, 25*f*, 187–188
Muscle stem cells, 111–114
  with aging
    extrinsic changes in, 118–120
    intrinsic changes in, 116–118
Muscle wasting, 23–24
  and weakness, quantifications of
    in aged animals, 297*t*
    in aged human beings, 296*t*
    in inactivated animals, 299*t*
    in inactivated human beings, 298*t*
Myf5, 113
Myofiber atrophy, 71
Myofibers and adipocytes, interactions between, 145–147, 148–150*f*

Myogenesis, role of myokines in, 173–175
Myogenic regulatory factors (MRFs), 113–114
Myokines
  with biomarkers, for sarcopenia, 173*t*
  induced by exercise, systemic functions of, 162–163
  MicroRNAs and metabolites as, 177–179
  role in myogenesis, 173–175
  role in protein anabolism and catabolism, 175–177
Myonuclear domain hypothesis, 121–122
Myositis, 142
Myostatin, 145, 147*f*
Myostatin-induced muscle atrophy, 176

N

National Health and Nutrition Examination Survey, 84
NCAM. *See* Neural cell adhesion molecule (NCAM)
Neural cell adhesion molecule (NCAM), 64
Neural dysfunction in sarcopenia, mitochondrial regulation of, 16–17
Neuromuscular junction (NMJ)
  age-related functional adaptations of, 66–68, 67*t*, 69*t*
  age-related structural adaptations of, 61–66, 62–63*f*, 65*f*
  aging effects, preventing and managing, 69–70
  role in sarcopenia, 70–75
NIS. *See* Nutritional impact symptoms (NIS)
NMJ. *See* Neuromuscular junction (NMJ)
Nonsteroid anti-inflammatory drugs (NSAID), 147–151
NSAID. *See* Nonsteroid anti-inflammatory drugs (NSAID)
Nutritional impact symptoms (NIS), 275–276

Index

O

Obese sarcopenia, 145–147
Obesity
  diagnostic criteria for, 232
  sarcopenic
    diagnostic criteria for, 233–234, 234t
    growth hormones and, 240
    intervention strategies in, 240–241
    metabolism, 235–239
    muscle atrophy, 239, 240t
    pathogenesis of, 234–240, 235f
OBF. See Ocular blood flow (OBF)
Ocular blood flow (OBF), 250–251, 254
Ocular vessels, 270–271
Older adults
  dietary considerations for, 92–96
  protein intake, 93–95
  dietary protein and amino acid interventions in, 97–98
  impact of leucine on muscle mass maintenance in, 95–96
  See also Aging
OMM. See Outer mitochondrial membrane (OMM)
Outer mitochondrial membrane (OMM), 8–10, 19, 27–28

P

PAD. See Peripheral arterial disease (PAD)
Parkin pathway, in sarcopenia, 214–216, 217f
Pax7, 113–114
PDCAAS. See Protein Digestibility Corrected Amino Acid Score (PDCAAS)
PDGFRa. See Platelet-derived growth factor receptor alpha (PDGFRa)
Peripheral arterial disease (PAD), 251–252
Peripheral blood flow during exercise, role of, 250–251
Peroxisome proliferator-activated receptor a coactivator 1a (PGC-1a), 74
  in autophagy and apoptotic pathways, 23
  regulation of mitochondria, 17
  in aged muscles, 17–18
  motor neurons, 18
PG. See Prostaglandins (PG)
PINK1. See PTEN-induced putative kinase protein 1 (PINK1)
Plant-based protein sources, 84–86
Platelet-derived growth factor receptor alpha (PDGFRa), 115–116
PMNs. See Polymorphonuclear leukocytes (PMNs)
Polymorphonuclear leukocytes (PMNs), 147–151
Population Reference Intake (PRI), 89–91
PPARβ/δ pathway, exercise mimetics targeting, 163
Precocious sarcopenia, 73–74
PRI. See Population Reference Intake (PRI)
Prostaglandins (PG), 147–151
Protein anabolism, role of myokines in, 175–177
Protein catabolism, role of myokines in, 175–177
Protein Digestibility Corrected Amino Acid Score (PDCAAS), 82–85, 83t
Protein distribution across the day, 91–92
Protein intake
  considerations, for older adults, 93–95
  above RDA, 90–91
PTEN-induced putative kinase protein 1 (PINK1), 214–215, 217f
Pulsed Doppler ultrasonography, 251

R

RDA. See Recommended Dietary Allowance (RDA)
Reactive nitrogen species (RNS)
  intrinsic contractile dysfunction in skeletal muscle fibers, 307–312, 308f
Reactive oxygen species (ROS), 208, 218
  intrinsic contractile dysfunction in skeletal muscle fibers, 307–312, 308f
Reactive oxygen species-induced damage, 3–4
Recommended Dietary Allowance (RDA), 89–90, 93–94
  protein intake above, 90–91
Resistance-based exercise training, 127
RNS. See Reactive nitrogen species (RNS)
ROS. See Reactive oxygen species (ROS)

S

SA. See Synergistic ablation (SA)
Sacroplasmic retirulum, in skeletal muscle fibers
  decreased Ca^{2+} release from, 302–303
Sarcoendoplasmic reticulum ATPases (SERCA), 8, 9f, 11
Sarcopenia, 270–274
  condition of, 271–274, 272f
  definition of, 270–271
  diagnostic criteria for, 233
  See also individual entries
Sarcopenia, and mitochondrial dysfunction, 2–3
  in aging, potential sources of altered dynamics, 5–7
  calcium-induced dysregulation, 8–11, 9f
  DNA damage, 5
  reactive oxygen species-induced damage, 3–4
  reduced activity, 7–8
  autophagy and apoptosis, linking, 22–23
  BIM and Bcl-2, 23
  PGC-1a, 23
  caloric restriction, 28–31, 30t
  cell death signaling, 11–16
    fiber type-specific loss, regulation of, 15–16
    mitochondrial-induced nuclear apoptosis, 11–14, 13–14f

327

Index

Sarcopenia, and mitochondrial dysfunction *(Continued)*
  mitochondrial permeability transition pore, 14–15
  loss of motor function and mobility, 16–17
  motor neurons, 16
  neural dysfunction, 16–17
  mitophagy, 18–22, 20–21*f*
  muscle wasting, 23–24
  PGC-1a regulation, 17
    in aged muscles, 17–18
    in motor neurons, 18
  UPS
    disruption in muscle and neural cells, 28
    mitophagy regulation, 27
    and neural dysfunction in aging, 26–27
    regulation, 24–26, 25*f*
Sarcopenic obesity
  diagnostic criteria for, 233–234, 234*t*
  growth hormones and, 240
  intervention strategies in, 240–241
  metabolism, 235–239
    inflammation, 238–239
    insulin resistance, 238
    lipid accumulation, 235–237, 236*f*
    mitochondrial dysfunction, 237–238
  pathogenesis of, 234–240, 235*f*
Sarcoplasmic reticulum (SR), 8
SARM. *See* Selective androgen receptor modulator (SARM)
Satellite cells
  activity during regeneration, 114–116
  and exercise to combat sarcopenia, 126–127
  function in aging, 116–120
  morphological and anatomical characteristics of, 110*f*
  and muscle adaptation, 120–126
  in muscle atrophy, 122–126, 123*f*
  in muscle hypertrophy, 120–122, 123*f*
  in muscle regeneration, 112*f*

Sciatic nerve transection (SNT) model, 125
Secreted protein acidic and rich in cysteine (SPARC), 175
Selective androgen receptor modulator (SARM), 164
SERCA. *See* Sarcoendoplasmic reticulum ATPases (SERCA)
Skeletal muscle
  anabolic hormones effects on, 163–165
  autophagy pathway, roles of, 165
  composition of, 141
  exercise-induced molecular signaling in, 161–162
  histology of, 139–141
  inflammatory response in, 141–144, 143*f*
  type I fibers, 2
  type II fibers, 2
  vessels, 252
Skeletal muscle fibers
  age-related alterations in intracellular activation-contraction pathway in, 301–302, 301*f*
  decreased ability of cross-bridges to generate force in, 304–306, 305*f*
  decreased Ca^{2+} release from sarcoplasmic reticulum in, 302–303
  increased susceptibility of regulatory proteins to oxidative modification in, 311–312
  intrinsic contractile dysfunction in, 306–307
  reactive oxygen/nitrogen species, role of, 307–312, 308*f*
  reduced myofibrillar Ca^{2+} sensitivity in, 303–304
Skin vessels, 256
SMA. *See* Superior mesenteric artery (SMA)
SNT. *See* Sciatic nerve transection (SNT) model
Society of Sarcopenia, 98

SPARC. *See* Secreted protein acidic and rich in cysteine (SPARC)
Specialized proresolving mediators (SPMs), 147–151, 152*f*
Splanchnic vessels, 255
SPMs. *See* Specialized proresolving mediators (SPMs)
SR. *See* Sarcoplasmic reticulum (SR)
Superior mesenteric artery (SMA), 255
Supplemental approach, for autophagy signaling defect, 199–200
Synergistic ablation (SA), 121

T

Testosterone, 164*f*
Tomatidine, 164*f*
Transcranial Doppler flowmetry, 253
Tumor necrosis factor-a, in sarcopenic obesity pathogenesis, 239

U

Ubiquitin-proteasome system (UPS), 187–188
  disruption in muscle and neural cells, 28
  mitophagy regulation and, 27
  and neural dysfunction in aging, 26–27
  regulation of sarcopenia, 24–26, 25*f*
UPS. *See* Ubiquitin-proteasome system (UPS)
Ursolic acid, 164*f*

V

Vascular aging
  baroreflex, 257–258
  blood volume, 258
  central arteries, 257
  cerebral vessels, 252–254
  counteractions, 258–259
  interrelationships, 260*f*
  loss of vascular functions, 251–257
  ocular vessels, 254–255

Index

peripheral blood flow during exercise, role of, 250–251
skeletal-muscle vessels, 252
skin vessels, 256
splanchnic vessels, 255
veins, 257
VDAC. *See* Voltage-dependent anion channel (VDAC)
Veins, 257
Voltage-dependent anion channel (VDAC), 8–10

W

WHO. *See* World Health Organization (WHO)
Windkessel model, 257
WISP1. *See* WNT1 Inducible Signaling Pathway Protein 1 (WISP1)
WNT1 Inducible Signaling Pathway Protein 1 (WISP1), 115–116, 119–120

World Health Organization on chronic obstructive pulmonary disease, 278
World Health Organization (WHO), 109

X

XIAP. *See* X-linked inhibitor of apoptosis protein (XIAP)
X-linked inhibitor of apoptosis protein (XIAP), 28